Handbook of Critical Care

Handbook of Critical Care

THIRD EDITION

EDITED BY

James L. Berk, M.D.

Professor of Surgery, Case Western Reserve University School of Medicine; Attending Physician, Department of Surgery, University Hospitals, Cleveland, Ohio

James E. Sampliner, M.D.

Assistant Clinical Professor of Surgery, Case Western Reserve University School of Medicine; Director, Department of Critical Care, Meridia Hillcrest Hospital; Attending Surgeon, Mount Sinai Medical Center, Cleveland, Ohio

Foreword by

Francis D. Moore, M.D.
Moseley Professor of Surgery Emeritus, Harvard Medical School; Surgeon-in-Chief Emeritus, Peter Bent Brigham Hospital, Boston

Little, Brown and Company
Boston/Toronto/London

This book is dedicated to Richard E. Wilson, M.D., Professor of Surgery, Harvard Medical School and Chief, Surgical Oncology, Brigham and Women's Hospital, Dana-Farber Cancer Institute, whose untimely death occurred this year. Dr. Wilson's many contributions to medicine, especially to transplantation and oncology, will benefit critically ill patients for years to come. We are fortunate that one of Dr. Wilson's last contributions was to this book.

Contributing Authors

Hans-Peter Albrecht, M.D.
Institute for Physiology and Cardiology, University of Erlangen-Nürnberg, Nürnberg, West Germany

Klaus Appelbaum, M.D.
Institute for Physiology and Cardiology, University of Erlangen-Nürnberg, Nürnberg, West Germany

Stephen M. Ayres, M.D.
Dean, School of Medicine, Virginia Commonwealth University, Medical College of Virginia, Richmond, Virginia

Daniel W. Benson, M.D.
Clinical and Research Fellow, Department of Surgery, University of Cincinnati College of Medicine, Cincinnati, Ohio

James L. Berk, M.D.
Professor of Surgery, Case Western Reserve University School of Medicine; Attending Physician, Department of Surgery, University Hospitals, Cleveland, Ohio

R. Morton Bolman, III, M.D.
Professor of Surgery, University of Minnesota Medical School—Minneapolis; Professor and Chief, Division of Cardiovascular and Thoracic Surgery, University of Minnesota Hospital and Clinic, Minneapolis, Minnesota

Christopher W. Bryan-Brown, M.D.
Professor of Anesthesiology, Albert Einstein College of Medicine of Yeshiva University, Bronx, New York; Vice Chairman of Clinical Affairs, Department of Anesthesiology/Critical Care Medicine, Montefiore Medical Center, Bronx, New York

Frank B. Cerra, M.D.
Professor of Surgery, University of Minnesota Medical School—Minneapolis; Director of Critical Care and Clinical Nutrition, St. Paul-Ramsey Hospital, Minneapolis, Minnesota

William Chamberlin, M.D.
Associate Professor of Clinical Medicine, University of Chicago Pritzker School of Medicine; Director of Critical Care, Michael Reese Hospital and Medical Center, Chicago, Illinois

Kanu Chatterjee, M.B.
Professor of Medicine, University of California, San Francisco, School of Medicine; Chief, Coronary Care Unit and Associate Chief, Cardiovascular Division of the Department of Medicine, Herbert C. Moffitt Hospital, San Francisco, California

Bart Chernow, M.D., F.A.C.P.
Associate Professor of Anesthesia (Critical Care), Harvard Medical School; Associate Director, Respiratory-Surgical I.C.U., Department of Anesthesia, Massachusetts General Hospital, Boston, Massachusetts

Joseph M. Civetta, M.D.
Professor of Surgery, Anesthesiology, Medicine, and Pathology, University of Miami School of Medicine; Director, Surgical Intensive Care Unit, Jackson Memorial Medical Center, Miami, Florida

Lawrence H. Cohn, M.D.
Professor of Surgery, Harvard Medical School; Chief of Cardiac Surgery, Brigham and Women's Hospital, Boston, Massachusetts

John R. Corsetti, M.D.
Resident Physician, University of Pennsylvania Hospital, Philadelphia

William T. Couldwell, M.D.
Resident Supervisor and Clinical Instructor, University of Southern California Medical School, Los Angeles, California

Hillary F. Don, M.D.
Associate Professor of Anesthesia, University of California, San Francisco, School of Medicine, Staff Anesthetist, Veterans Administration Medical Center, San Francisco, California

Mitchell P. Fink, M.D.
Chairman, Division of General Surgery, University of Massachusetts Medical School; Director, Surgical Intensive Care Units, University of Massachusetts Medical Center, Worcester, Massachusetts

Josef E. Fischer, M.D.
Professor and Chairman, Department of Surgery, University of Cincinnati College of Medicine; Surgeon-in-Chief, Department of Surgery, University of Cincinnati Hospitals, Cincinnati, Ohio

Klaus Frank, M.D.
Institute for Physiology and Cardiology, University of Erlangen-Nürnberg, Nürnberg, West Germany

Robert J. Freeark, M.D.
Professor and Chairman, Department of Surgery, Loyola University of Chicago Stritch School of Medicine; Surgeon-in-Chief, Loyola University Hospital, Maywood, Illinois

Lorenz Frey, M.D.
Institute for Anesthesiology, Ludwig-Maximilians University; Anesthesiologist, Grobhadern Clinic, Munich, West Germany

Richard Gorlin, M.D.
Professor and Chairman, Department of Medicine, Mount Sinai School of Medicine of the City University of New York; Physician-in-Chief, Mount Sinai Hospital, New York

Manfred Kessler, M.D.
Professor of Physiology and Chairman, Institute for Physiology and Cardiology, University of Erlangen-Nürnberg, Nürnberg, West Germany

John M. Kinney, M.D.
Visiting Professor, The Rockefeller University; Senior Attending Physician in Medicine and Surgery, St. Luke's-Roosevelt Hospital Center, New York

Harry B. Kram, M.D.
Assistant Professor of Surgery and Attending Surgeon, Drew-Martin Luther King Jr. Medical Center; Los Angeles, California

Franz-Peter Lenhart, M.D.
Institute for Anesthesiology, Ludwig-Maximilians University; Anesthesiologist, Grobhadern Clinic, Munich, West Germany

George I. Litman, M.D.
Professor of Medicine, Northeastern Ohio Universities College of Medicine, Rootstown, Ohio; Chief, Division of Cardiology, Department of Internal Medicine, Akron General Medical Center, Akron, Ohio

Dwight L. Makoff, M.D.
Clinical Professor of Medicine, UCLA School of Medicine; Attending Physician, Cedars-Sinai Medical Center, Los Angeles, California

William J. Mandel, M.D.
Associate Professor of Medicine, UCLA School of Medicine, Los Angeles, California

Arthur J. Matas, M.D.
Associate Professor of Surgery, University of Minnesota Medical School—Minneapolis; Attending Surgeon and Director, Clinical Renal Transplantation, University of Minnesota Hospital and Clinic, Minneapolis, Minnesota

W. Scott McDougal, M.D.
Professor and Chairman, Department of Urology, Vanderbilt University School of Medicine, Nashville, Tennessee

Konrad Messmer
Professor and Chairman, Department of Experimental Surgery, University of Heidelberg Medical School, Heidelberg, West Germany

Michael Metzler, M.D.
Associate Professor, Department of Surgery, University of Missouri—Columbia School of Medicine; Medical Director, Surgical Intensive Care Unit, University of Missouri—Columbia Hospital and Clinics, Columbia, Missouri

Robert C. Morris, M.D.
Assistant Professor of Surgery, Loyola University of Chicago Stritch School of Medicine; Attending Surgeon, Foster G. McGaw Hospital, Maywood, Illinois

Howard S. Nearman, M.D.
Associate Professor of Anesthesiology and Surgery, Case Western Reserve University School of Medicine; Chief, Surgical Intensive Care Unit, University Hospitals of Cleveland, Cleveland, Ohio

William D. Payne, M.D.
Associate Professor of Surgery, University of Minnesota Medical School—Minneapolis; Attending Surgeon and Director, Liver Transplant Program, University of Minnesota Hospital and Clinic, Minneapolis, Minnesota

Pamela S. Peigh, M.D.
Instructor in Surgery, Harvard Medical School; Instructor, Cardiothoracic Surgery, Division of Cardiac Surgery, Brigham and Women's Hospital, Boston, Massachusetts

Klaus Peter, M.D.
Ludwig-Maximilians University; Director, Institute for Anesthesiology, Grobhadern Clinic, Munich, West Germany

Howard C. Pitluk, M.D.
Clinical Instructor of Surgery, Case Western Reserve University School of Medicine; Attending Surgeon, Mount Sinai Medical Center and Meridia Hillcrest Hospital, Cleveland, Ohio

Charles L. Rice, M.D.
Professor and Vice Chairman, Department of Surgery, University of Washington School of Medicine; Surgeon-in-Chief, Harborview Medical Center, Seattle, Washington

Robert A. Salata, M.D.
Assistant Professor of Medicine, Case Western Reserve University School of Medicine; Attending Physician and Consultant, Divisions of Infectious Diseases and Geographic Medicine, University Hospitals and Veterans Administration Medical Center, Cleveland, Ohio

James E. Sampliner, M.D.
Assistant Clinical Professor of Surgery, Case Western Reserve University
School of Medicine; Director, Department of Critical Care, Meridia
Hillcrest Hospital; Attending Surgeon, Mount Sinai Medical Center,
Cleveland, Ohio

Richard E. Sampliner, M.D.
Associate Professor of Medicine, University of Arizona College of
Medicine; Chief of Gastroenterology, University Medical Center and
Veterans Administration Medical Center, Tucson, Arizona

Warren Sherman, M.D.
Assistant Professor of Medicine, Mount Sinai School of Medicine of the
City University of New York; Assistant Attending Cardiologist and
Director, Coronary Care Units, Mount Sinai Hospital, New York,
New York

William C. Shoemaker
Professor of Surgery, UCLA School of Medicine; Vice Chairman, Drew-
Martin Luther King Jr. Medical Center, Los Angeles, California

Günther Siebenhaar
Institute for Physiology and Cardiology, University of Erlangen-
Nürnberg, Nürnberg, West Germany

John H. Siegel, M.D.
Professor of Surgery, University of Maryland School of Medicine and
Johns Hopkins University School of Medicine; Deputy Director,
Maryland Institute for Emergency Medical Services Systems, University
of Maryland Medical System, Baltimore, Maryland

Donald Silver, M.D.
Professor of Surgery, University of Missouri—Columbia School of
Medicine; Professor and Chairman, Department of Surgery, University of
Missouri—Columbia Hospital and Clinics, Columbia, Missouri

Robert L. Smith, R.R.T., R.P.F.T.
Chief Pulmonary Function Technologist, Metro Health Medical Center,
Cleveland, Ohio

Gregory G. Stanford, M.D.
Assistant Professor of Surgery, University of Texas, Southwestern
Medical School; Assistant Professor, Department of Surgery, Parkland
Memorial Hospital, Dallas, Texas

Paul M. Starker, M.D.
Assistant Professor of Surgery, Columbia University College of
Physicians and Surgeons, New York; Attending Surgeon, Overlook
Hospital, Summit, New Jersey

Joan C. Stoklosa, B.S.
Director, Cardiopulmonary Research Laboratory, Maryland Institute for
Emergency Medical Services Systems, University of Maryland School of
Medicine, Baltimore, Maryland

David E. R. Sutherland, M.D.
Professor of Surgery, University of Minnesota Medical School,
Minneapolis, Minnesota

Michael D. Tyne, M.B.A.
President and Chief Executive Officer, Karlsberger Companies,
Columbus, Ohio

Albert Joseph Varon, M.D.
Associate Professor of Clinical Anesthesiology, University of Miami
School of Medicine; Attending Anesthesiologist and Associate Director,
Surgical Intensive Care Unit, Jackson Memorial Medical Center, Miami,
Florida

Martin H. Weiss, M.D.
Professor and Chairman, Department of Neurosurgery, University of
Southern California School of Medicine, Los Angeles, California

Charles Weissman, M.D.
Associate Professor of Anesthesiology and Medicine, Columbia
University College of Physicians and Surgeons; Associate Attending
Anesthesiologist and Physician, Presbyterian Hospital, New York

Richard E. Wilson, M.D.
Professor of Surgery, Harvard Medical School; Chief, Surgical Oncology,
Brigham and Women's Hospital, Boston, Massachusetts

Lucile E. Wrenshall, M.D.
Resident, Department of Surgery, University of Minnesota Hospital and
Clinic, Minneapolis, Minnesota

Josef Zündorf
Institute of Physiology and Cardiology, University of Erlangen-Nürnberg,
Nürnberg, West Germany

Foreword

In considering the acute abdomen, it has been said that the term *acute* refers not so much to the speed of the pathologic process or its urgency, but rather to the acuteness of judgment that the surgeon must bring to bear if the patient is to be managed correctly. The same statement can be made about critical care medicine. The patient may even seem to be past the most critical stage of illness, and there may be no immediate crisis; yet each small segment of treatment that the physician or surgeon carries out is of critical importance to the patient's recovery.

These two statements have a common thread. The pathologic causes of the acute abdomen are numerous and diverse, stemming from many unrelated sources; the illnesses encountered in critical care medicine are equally numerous and varied and include diseases of the heart, lungs, circulation, brain, and viscera.

Two developments of the past 25 years in the medical and surgical care of critically ill patients have rendered a new and distinct field of hospital administration and departmental organization. The first is the improvement in the overall management of life-endangering illness through more intelligent use of blood transfusion, antibiotics, hemodialysis, and the host of techniques of metabolic care that are called into play daily for the dangerously ill person. The second development, which occurred rapidly after the advent of open heart surgery around 1960, is the improvement in, and simplification of, cardiac and respiratory assistance devices and drugs.

Most critical care units in this country today are not tied together by the disease entity involved or even by the host of details in metabolic management. Rather they are connected by the availability of cardiac and respiratory assistance, together with a team of physicians and therapists expert in the minute-by-minute management of the critically ill patient, for days or weeks at a time. The common thread is not diagnosis, or even pathology, but rather the knowledge, skills, and equipment used in care.

Many physicians of my generation remember seeing whole wards filled with poliomyelitis patients being carried through respiratory failure by the iron lung (the Drinker respirator). Manipulation of the patient within the respiratory chamber was virtually impossible because the cyclic alteration in ambient pressure was thereby lost. Yet the lives of thousands of young people were saved by this device.

For today's generation of students and residents, direct endotracheal respiratory care devices and pacemakers are so widespread in their application and so relatively simple to use that they are a "given" for the critically ill. Although they are easily moved about, are relatively inexpensive, and can produce a whole variety of maintenance patterns in the lungs and heart, the present-day devices also have negative aspects. They can still be the source of sepsis if poorly sterilized and can produce pneumothorax, atelactasis, or lethal arrhythmia if one small dial is turned to the wrong setting.

When properly used, these developments in treatment have made it possible for many young people, with their lives still ahead of them, to survive illnesses to which they formerly would have succumbed. Many patients are kept alive in such units over prolonged periods, although the mortality for certain groups may be very high (for example, patients with a combination of burns and renal failure or a combination of pulmonary insufficiency and gram-negative bacteremia). Every era has its unsolved high-mortality problems such as the latter, or new infections such as AIDS. Yet it is rare for patients with a truly hopeless long-term outlook (such as advanced cancer or late stroke) to be maintained in critical care units. It is a common public misapprehension that modern critical care methods merely prolong the misery of terminal illness or "keep people alive" who should be allowed to die. Quite the contrary, the majority of patients in critical care units today have their lives ahead of them and can recover if given the chance by expert care.

The editors, Drs. Berk and Sampliner, have put together a book that is a practical, handy reference for students and practitioners and is equally useful to nurses, respiratory therapists, and physician's assistants involved in critical care medicine.

Much of *Handbook of Critical Care* focuses on pattern recognition rather than on conventional pathologic diagnosis. The pathophysiologic patterns of respiratory alkalosis with unconsciousness, paradoxical aciduria with gastric juice loss and hypovolemia, and pulmonary ateriovenous admixture are examples of the patterns that the critical care therapist comes to recognize and learns to treat.

The intensive care therapist must always keep a sharp eye on the basic diagnosis and to the pathologic problem at hand. The therapist is cautioned to avoid the error of wasting the scarce resources of society on the very feeble elderly or the hopelessly ill patient with terminal cancer. The therapist often holds the key to long-range survival and success.

It is a pleasure to make even this small contribution to such a book. We can cheer the reader on with the thought that while modern medicine often seems to be a matter of gadgets and superspecialization—high technology—the care of the critically ill patient truly restores the physician's primary role: To look after the welfare of the *whole* patient. In critical care no physiologic system or body organ function can be spared from consideration, and through it all the intensive care provider must keep in mind the emotional adjustment of the patient, the drive to recover, the need for a frequent word of encouragement, and an abiding concern for, and understanding of, the anxiety felt by the patient's family.

Francis D. Moore, M.D.

Preface

This book is intended to be a practical guide for physicians as well as for medical students, nurses, and allied health personnel involved in the care of critically ill patients. The need for such a guide was recognized by the house officers and students at Case Western Reserve University School of Medicine.

Because an understanding of underlying theory and basic science is essential for the successful application of the various techniques and modes of therapy described, basic concepts have been included and correlated with the practical portions.

This book does not pretend to include everything that may be considered part of the large and rapidly expanding field of critical care medicine. It is intended that the text, references, and selected readings will serve as a basic source of practical information for use in the intensive care setting, as well as a foundation on which students and physicians can build.

To keep pace with the advances in critical care medicine, this edition of *Handbook of Critical Care* has been completely revised. All chapters have been thoroughly updated. Seven new chapters have been added, including discussions of ethical issues, in-situ monitoring of organs, the management of acute coronary occlusions, the surgical management of acute heart failure, the sepsis syndrome, the management of the immunodeficient patient, perioperative care of the transplant patient, and endocrine dysfunction and emergencies in critical illness.

We thank Susan Pioli, Senior Editor, Medical Division, Little, Brown and Company, and Beverly Taylor for their help in preparation of the manuscript.

J.L.B.
J.E.S.

Contents

Handbook of Critical Care

Notice

The indications and dosages of all drugs in this book have been recommended in the medical literature and conform to the practices of the general medical community. The medications described do not necessarily have specific approval by the Food and Drug Administration for use in the diseases and dosages for which they are recommended. The package insert for each drug should be consulted for use and dosage as approved by the FDA. Because standards for usage change, it is advisable to keep abreast of revised recommendations, particularly those concerning new drugs.

Ethical Issues in Critically Ill Patients: From Hippocrates and Aristotle to the Supreme Court of New Jersey

Stephen M. Ayres

The practice of medicine is first of all a search for truth—a search for the true nature of an individual's physical and mental status. It is generally believed that medicine is both an art and a science. Physicians use the scientific method when they make observations and frame hypotheses about individual patients; they use their art when exact answers are not obvious and actions based on intuition must be rapidly taken. But at these moments, just what is the "art" of the physician? The realm of philosophy, explained Bertrand Russell [27], falls somewhere between the definite knowledge of science and "groundless credulity"; it is the "art of rational conjecture." In words surprisingly close to those commonly used to describe the way physicians practice medicine, Russell suggested that

philosophy tells us how to proceed when we want to find out what may be true, or is *most likely* to be true, where it is impossible to know with certainty what is true. The art of rational conjecture is very useful in two different ways. First: often the most difficult step in the discovery of what *is* true is thinking of a hypothesis which *may* be true; when once the hypothesis has been thought of, it can be tested, but it may require a man of genius to think of it. Second: we often have to act in spite of uncertainty, because delay would be dangerous or fatal; in such a case, it is useful to possess an art by which we can judge what is probable.

Both deductive and inductive logic have been used by truth seekers. *Deductive logic,* the bedrock of theology, begins with general principles and from them develops specific inferences: for example, death occurs when the heart ceases to function, so anyone with evidence of heart function is not dead. *Inductive logic,* a major tool of science, begins with observations, from which are derived general principles. Plum and Posner [24] evaluated the outcomes of 877 patients obtained from 10 published reports and demonstrated that not a single individual with established criteria for brain death survived. Inductive reasoning thus established a new general principle for defining death that could then be deductively tested by further

clinical observation. This interplay of theory and action characterizes recorded history. Although theory frequently has governed action, observations of actual situations have more regularly led to the creation of new
theories. The physician has always stood at this intersection of philosophy
and science, of faith and reason, of the known and unknown. Hippocrates
understood this well when he bravely proclaimed that "clear knowledge
about nature can be obtained from medicine and from no other source."

Medical decision making is a complex mixture of deductive and inductive logic. Physicians carry with them an expanding data base of clinical
diagnoses and other facts. With a diagnosis such as coma, the physician
deduces a good deal about the patient's present and future situations. As
facts are collected—the beginning of spontaneous motion or evidence of
narcotic drug ingestion, for example—a new diagnosis may well be induced from the available observations. A recent case provides an example
of such clinical reasoning. An elderly patient with severe emphysema,
atrial fibrillation, and markedly abnormal blood gases was admitted to a
university teaching service. The intern conjured up a clinical picture of
"end-stage" pulmonary disease and deduced that the patient's life would
be short. He asked the patient whether he desired resuscitative measures
if he suddenly collapsed, and was answered with an emphatic Yes! The
patient gradually improved and was discharged several weeks later in a
relatively comfortable and stable condition. The intern realized that had
the patient requested that resuscitative efforts not be undertaken, he might
have died from untreated ventricular fibrillation. Presumably (and hope-
fully), these observations would lead to immediate reevaluation of the idea
of end-stage pulmonary disease. Physicians always are temporarily relying
on deductive reasoning and quickly reexamining those preliminary decisions by induction when additional observations are made.

The search for goodness, or the good act, is a recurrent philosophic
theme. Physicians generally believe that they are doing the "right thing for
my patient" when they attempt to cure illness and prevent death. Implicit
in this idea of doing good for the patient is that the physician has the
knowledge and power to improve the patient's status and is obligated to
bring the patient to this new level of betterment whether or not the patient
and the family desire it. Physicians frequently base this imperative to do
good on the Hippocratic tradition, which provides a surprisingly complete
foundation upon which to construct an ethic of critical care. "I will define
what I conceive medicine to be," stated the writers of the Hippocratic cor-
pus. "In general terms it is to do away with the sufferings of the sick, to
lessen the violence of their diseases, and to refuse to treat those who are
overmastered by their diseases, realizing that in such cases medicine is
powerless" [14]. Generations of medical students were taught the incomplete Latin formulation, *primum non nocere* ("above all, do no harm") and
used it as justification for inaction in the face of serious illness or injury.
Actually, the complete quotation from *Epidemics* is a much better summary of Hippocratic thought: "Declare the past, diagnose the present, fore-
tell the future; practice these acts. As to disease, make a habit of two things:
to help or at least to do no harm" [15]. About as good an example of common sense as ever has come down through the ages!

The critical care physician faced with the question of action or inaction is engaging in moral reasoning. The usual guide to action is called clinical experience, and the physician, using inductive logic, proceeds to follow the conventional course of action even if the outcome of that treatment cannot be predicted with reasonable certainty. Making moral choices is the essence of medical practice, but moral reasoning frequently involves making a choice between two apparently "good" options. A workable moral compass usually guides the physician toward the right action but may not be precise enough for decisions involving the use of complex technology in seriously ill patients. Like a ship approaching shoal waters, the compass may not be sufficiently reliable, and the mariner must pay attention to whatever beacons or markers are available. A group of *moral principles* serve as beacons guiding the physician toward the "best" decision.

Long-standing cultural rules, or "commandments," defining what is right and wrong constitute what is called a system or morality. Rules of behavior, the beacons of light in our metaphor, aid individuals in living a good life. Important moral principles are life, liberty, the pursuit of happiness, freedom, equality, beneficence, and utility. These traditional moral rules sometimes conflict with each other, so the correct relationship of a group of moral principles to a given situation requires some interpretation. For physicians, the Judaic and Christian presumption for life (thou shalt not kill) is a transcendent moral principle, but even that principle must be modified in certain clinical situations. And it is certainly ignored in the name of survival as societies debate the power of a first-strike nuclear attack. Even the principle of life seems to be a relative one. Physicians and others sometimes dismiss philosophers and their thoughts as irrelevant to the practical matters at hand. Yet, physicians have been some of the very best philosophers throughout the ages and, as it turned out, actually developed a pragmatic philosophy gradually adopted by armchair philosophers.

THE HISTORICAL BEDROCK

Athenian culture, the bedrock upon which classic European philosophy was developed, was based on a sharp distinction between theory and practice. In general, slaves performed the essentials of everyday life, while free men were free to reflect and philosophize. Plato (c. 427–347 B.C.), the great Idealist, believed that the ethical life was the life of reason. The cardinal virtues of wisdom, courage, temperance, and justice were immutable and timeless principles that should guide human behavior. The famed physician Hippocrates lived some 90 years (c. 460–c. 370 B.C.), a period that almost spanned the serial careers of Socrates and his pupil Plato. Although many works attributed to Hippocrates probably were written by his followers, almost all historians attribute to him *Epidemics*, Books I and III. In these works, Hippocrates provided an extensive and detailed series of clinical descriptions as he translated theory into action. A practical physician-philosopher, Hippocrates held that "clear knowledge about nature can be obtained from medicine and from no other source." [16].

Aristotle (384–322 B.C.) adopted a much more practical approach to morality than did Plato, perhaps because he was the son of a physician and observed at close hand the moral dilemmas constantly facing his father. Aristotle began his *Nicomachean Ethics* [2] with the sentence, "Every art and every inquiry, and similarly every action and pursuit, is thought to aim at some good; and for this reason the good has been rightly declared to be that at which all things aim." He went on to criticize Plato insisting on a single ideal and eternal "good" and to point out that the idea of good had to mean different things to different people. Plato's argument, Aristotle held, "seems to clash with the procedures of the sciences; for all of these, though they aim at some good and seek to supply the deficiency of it, leave on one side the knowledge of the [ideal] good." It is difficult, he continued, to know "how the man who has viewed the idea itself [of eternal good] will be a better doctor or general thereby. For a doctor seems not even to study health in this way, but the health of man, or perhaps rather the health of a particular man; it is individuals that he is healing." The Good has not universal Form regardless of subject matter or situation: sound moral judgment respects the detailed circumstances of specific kinds of cases.

Aristotle held that whereas intellectual virtue is rooted in teaching, "moral virtue comes about as a result of habit, whence also its name *ethike* is one that is formed by a slight variation from the word *ethos* [habit]." Thus, the more experienced an intensivist, the better his ethical judgment. Aristotle provided a method for determining moral virtue, that of the mean: "There are three kinds of disposition, then, two of them vices, involving excess and deficiency respectively, and one a virtue, viz. the mean." Pick the middle course, says the philosopher, and you shall be virtuous. For the critical care physician, the doctrine of the mean resembles closely the idea of "customary care."

Are philosophers useful to intensivists attempting to make life-or-death decisions? Not unless their philosophy is relevant to current problems. Stephen Toulmin, in his essay "The Recovery of Practical Philosophy," demonstrated that modern philosophers beginning with René Descartes and the Cambridge Platonists "turned ethics into abstract theory, ignoring the concrete problems of moral practice." They "assumed that God and Freedom, Mind and Matter, Good and Justice, are governed by timeless, universal 'principles' and regarded writers who focused on particular cases, or types of cases limited by specific conditions, as either unphilosophical or dishonest" [30]. John Dewey eloquently expressed the need for a *Reconstruction in Philosophy* in a 1948 introduction to his 1920 book, arguing that

the distinctive office, problems and subject matter of philosophy grow out of stresses and strains in the community life in which a given form of philosophy arises, and that, accordingly, its specific problems vary with the changes in human life that are always going on and that at times constitute a crisis and a turning point in human history [10].

Dewey concluded that

while the evils resulting at present from the entrance of "science" into our common ways of living are undeniable they are due to the fact that no systematic efforts have as yet been made to subject the "morals" underlying old institutional customs to scientific inquiry and criticism. Hence, then, lies the reconstructive work to be done by philosophy. It must be undertaken to do for the development of inquiry into human affairs and hence into morals what the philosophers of the last few centuries did for promotion of scientific inquiry in physical and physiological conditions and aspects of life [10].

Toulmin has chided those philosophers who fear to engage in applied philosophy for fear that such a useful activity might "prostitute their talents and distract them from their proper concern with quantification theory, illocutionary force, possible worlds or the nature of Erlebnis." His paper "How Medicine Saved the Life of Ethics" [31] demonstrates that the philosophic action today is at the bedside. Physicians have always known that but have sometimes hesitated to explicitly reveal the ethical basis for everyday decision making.

PHILOSOPHER-PHYSICIANS
Physicians from Hippocrates on have had to develop their own approaches to moral reasoning because of the inability of classic philosophy to deal with a rapid changing world. Toulmin's "How Medicine Saved the Life of Ethics" is rather close to Hippocrates' assertion "that clear knowledge about nature can be obtained from medicine and from no other source." While modern philosophers were turning their backs on practical ethics, a Scottish physician, John Gregory, set the stage for modern medical ethics, much as Hippocrates had done in classical times.

Gregory (1724–1773) was professor of medicine at Edinburgh University. His medical writings have generally been forgotten, but his *Lectures on the Duties and Qualifications of a Physician* [12], published in 1788, was in the Hippocratic tradition and remains as useful today as it was 200 years ago. His attempt to understand the nature of medical practice is evidenced by the subtitle *On the Method of Prosecuting Enquiries in Philosophy* that appeared in an earlier version of his tract. The *Observations* are quoted in some detail here because the original text is not widely available.

I come now to mention the moral qualities peculiarly required in the character of a physician. The chief of these is humanity; that sensibility of heart which makes us feel that for the distresses of our fellow creatures, and which of consequence incites us in the most powerful manner to relieve them. Sympathy produces an anxious attention to a thousand little circumstances that may tend to relieve the patient; an attention which money can never purchase: hence the inexpressible comfort of having a friend for a physician. Sympathy naturally engages the affection and confidence of a patient, which in many cases is of the utmost consequence to his recovery. If the physician possesses gentleness of manners, and a compassionate heart, and what Shakespeare so emphatically calls "the milk of human kindness," the patient feels his approach like that of a guardian angel ministering to his relief; while every visit of a physician who is unfeeling, and rough in his manners, makes his heart sink within him, as at the preference of one, who comes to pronounce his doom. Men of the most compassionate tempers, by being daily conversant with scenes of distress, acquire in process of time that composure and firmness of mind so necessary in the practice of physic. They can feel whatever is amiable in pity, without suffering it to enervate or unman them. Such physicians as are callous to sentiments of humanity, treat this sympathy with ridicule, and represent it either as hypocrisy, or as the indication of a feeble mind. That sympathy is often affected, I am afraid, is true; but this affectation may be easily seen through. Real sympathy is never ostentatious; on the contrary, it rather strives to conceal itself. But, what most effectually detects this hypocrisy, is a physician's different manner of behaving to people in high and people in low life; to those who reward him handsomely, and those who have not the means to do it. A generous and elevated mind is even more shy in expressing sympathy with those of high rank; being jealous of the unworthy construction so usually annexed to it. The insinuation that a compassionate and feeling heart is commonly accompanied with a weak understanding and a feeble mind is malignant and false. Experience demonstrates that a gentle and human temper, far from being inconsistent with vigour of mind, is its usual attendant; and that rough and blustering manners generally accompany a weak understanding and a mean soul, and are indeed frequently affected by men void of magnanimity and personal courage, in order to conceal their natural defects.

There is a species of good-humour different from the sympathy I have been speaking of, which is likewise amiable in a physician. It conflicts in a certain gentleness and flexibility, which makes him suffer with patients, and even apparent disappointments, the many contradictions and disappointments he is subjected to in his practice. If he is rigid and too minute in his directions about regimen, he may be assured they will not be strictly followed; and if he is severe in his manners, the deviations from his rules will as certainly be concealed from him. The consequence is that he is kept in ignorance of the true state of his patient; he ascribes to the consequences of the disease, what is merely owing to irregularities in diet, and attributes effects to medicines which were perhaps never taken. The errors which in this way he may be led into, are sufficiently obvious, and might easily be prevented by a prudent relaxation of rules that could not well be obeyed. The government of a physician over his patient should undoubtedly be absolute but an absolute government very few patients will submit to. A prudent physician should therefore prescribe such laws, as, though, not the best, are yet the best that will be observed; of different evils he should choose the least, and, at no rate, lose the confidence of his patient, so as to be deceived by him as to his true situation. This indulgence, however, which I am pleading for, must be managed with judgement and discretion; as it is very necessary that a physician should support a proper dignity and authority with his patients, for their sakes as well as his own. . . .

I may reckon among the moral duties incumbent on a physician that candor, which makes him open to conviction, and ready to acknowledge and rectify his mistakes. An obstinate adherence to an unsuccessful method of treating a disease must be owing to a high degree of self-conceit, and a belief of the infallibility of a system. This error is the more difficult to cure, as it generally proceeds from ignorance. True knowledge and clear discernment may lead one into the extreme of diffidence and humility, but are inconsistent with self-conceit. It sometimes happens too that this obstinancy proceeds from a defect in the heart. Such physicians see that they are wrong, but are too proud to acknowledge their error, especially if it is pointed out to them by one of their profession. To this species of pride, a pride compatible with true dignity and elevation of mind, have the lives of thousands been sacrificed.

Beauchamp and McCullough [5], in a small volume ideal for use in a short course in medical ethics, developed an approach to moral reasoning in medicine surprisingly similar to the principles emphasized by Gregory. They emphasize the principles of beneficence (goodness) and autonomy (freedom of choice) as key anchors in clinical decision making. Beneficence is the "sympathy" and autonomy the "indulgence" described by Gregory. But which of the two should be given precedence?

We defend the view that neither respect for autonomy nor any one moral principle has sufficient weight to trump all conflicting moral claims. The metaphor of weights moving up and down on a balance scale has often been criticized as out of place and as potentially misleading in its apparent simplicity, and this is a caution we all should heed. However, philosophers have yet to provide a more adequate way of formulating the problem of conflicting principles, and our analysis in subsequent chapters presupposes that a pluralism of (a priori) equally weighted moral principles is a fundamental feature of the moral life generally and of the moral life in medicine in particular [5].

This concept of moral balance is close to Gregory's prescription that "of different evils he should choose the least."

THE APPARENT CONFLICT OF BENEFICENCE WITH AUTONOMY

The philosopher's idea of good was given explicit form by physicians such as Hippocrates and Gregory, as well as by countless practitioners of the healing arts both before and after them. In fact, medicine and nursing are almost alone among professions in claiming to be rooted in the principle of doing good, although practitioners of law and business, for example, might claim that they, too, believe goodness to be important. Immanuel Kant (1724–1804) began his treatise on the metaphysics of morals [21] by opining that "nothing can possibly be conceived in the world, or even out of it, which can be called good without qualification except a Good Will." More recently, M. O. Kepler, in his *Medical Stewardship*, began by stating that "love for one's neighbor is absolutely fundamental to the thesis of medical ethics I wish to develop. This type of love is known as C-love or *caritas* (from the Latin) from which comes our English word 'charity,' and agape or philia from the Greek" [22].

Erik Erikson [11] took the Golden Rule as his "baseline . . . for wise and proper conduct" and pointed out that even though systematic ethicists may believe the concept too simple, the rule has "marked a mysterious meeting ground between ancient peoples separated by oceans and eras and is a theme hidden in the most memorable sayings of many thinkers." The Talmudic version of the Golden Rule, "What is hateful to yourself, do not to your fellow man," is similar to the Christian "Love thy neighbor as thyself." The Golden Rule expresses poetically the principle of beneficence but, sadly, neglects the possibility that an individual may have a different view of what is good from that of a physician. The latter might gladly submit to a coronary artery bypass operation, whereas an individual patient might not.

The idea of human rights is a relatively recent development in social evolution. When physicians and priests were one and the same, the principle of beneficence was taken for granted. Patients were expected to do what they were told, and "doctor's orders" became an everyday expression. The French philosopher Jean-Jacques Rousseau (1712–1778) spoke of human rights in his *Social Contract* [26]. In the first line of this seemingly radical work, he proclaimed that "man is born free, and he is everywhere in chains"—a statement that provided fuel for the French Revolution and inspired Patrick Henry, Thomas Jefferson, and other Americans as they planned their new democracy. The ethical principle of autonomy echoes Rousseau and the Bill of Rights in that it emphasizes the patient's primacy in making moral judgments about himself. The courts have generally held that constitutional rights permit an individual to determine what happens to himself and to his property; many of these rights have been codified in patients' bills of rights.

Rousseau pointed out that a social contract is necessary because of the inherent inequality among human beings. Some are wise, others dull; some are strong, others weak. This inequality is particularly striking in the patient-physician relationship. Whereas physicians have wide knowledge and experience, patients may understand their own needs and values but have little information about their clinical states. Only detailed conversations with patients and their families can bridge this gap in such a way that patients can make truly autonomous judgments about their own care.

A common abuse of the concept of autonomy is the refusal to tell patients the truth about their illness in an effort to protect them. Again, Dr. Gregory made important comments about the ethics of truth telling.

To a man of compassionate and feeling heart, this [truth-telling] is one of the most disagreeable duties in the profession; but it is indispensable. The manner of doing it, requires equal prudence and humanity. What should reconcile him the more easily to this painful office, is the reflection that, if the patient should recover, it will prove a joyful disappointment to his friends; and if he die, it makes the shock more gentle [12].

Physicians frequently appear to ignore the required balance between the principles of beneficence and autonomy. A good example would be a physician who recommends radical mastectomy for breast cancer and provides no options, believing he knows best. When the patient asks for a second opinion, the physician refuses, saying, "I cannot take care of you unless I can make all important decisions." Here is presumed beneficence gone amuck. Then, when the patient refuses all surgery, the physician says, kindly, "It's your life, and you are free to do anything you like." The physician is now acting as if the patient is completely autonomous.

Aside from the physician's obvious arrogance and insensitivity, the key question raised by this example must be, Is the patient completely autonomous when she refuses all treatment and leaves? She has just been told she has cancer and must have what she believes to be a destructive surgical procedure. Fear of disfigurement and death then produce uncontrollable anxiety that causes the patient to escape from the situation. Beneficence demands that the physician seek out the patient and her family and make certain that repeated efforts are made to present the true gravity of the situation. Beneficence does not mean the quick delivery of a series of commands; rather, it implies shared responsibility, patient education and understanding, and gentle persuasion where necessary. *Indeed, correctly interpreting the proper balance between these two moral principles in a given situation could be considered one of the key responsibilities of the practice of medicine.*

PATIENT AUTONOMY IN THE CRITICAL CARE SETTING

When patients become seriously ill, they may lose much of their ability to properly consider complex facts and make the kinds of decisions about their own care that they can readily make when they are in good health. In this setting, the physician *must* lean toward the beneficence model and make decisions that are believed to be in the patient's best interest. This paternalistic approach has been roundly attacked by critics of the medical profession, but it is essential in caring for the critically ill. Who would suggest, for example, that the surgeon's "paternalistic" acts of cutting, removing, and suturing of tissues during an operative procedure really violates the principle of autonomy?

Two physicians, David Jackson and Stuart Youngner [18], examined decision making in the medical intensive care unit at Case Western Reserve University Hospital in Cleveland. They discussed six patients who exhibited factors that might interfere with the ability to make autonomous decisions: ambivalence about treatment, fear of treatment because of lack of information, depression, a plea for death with dignity, and conflict with the family's perception of the patient's best interest.

Jackson and Youngner squarely faced the issue of whether ethicists or physicians should evaluate patient autonomy. Capron and Kass [9] had rather bluntly asserted that "physicians qua physicians are not expert on these philosophic questions, nor are they experts on the question of which physiologic functions decisively identify the 'living human organism'." Echoing Hippocrates, Jackson and Youngner pointed out that making difficult decisions about patient care is basic to medical practice and that terms used by ethicists and lawyers, such as "irreversible," "hopeless," and "terminal," are too vague to be useful in the clinical setting. Physicians "must be alert not to let the possibility of abuse keep them from the appropriate exercise of professional judgement. Capron and Kass are wrong; physicians qua physicians should be expert on certain philosophic questions. Physicians who are uncomfortable or inexperienced in dealing with the complex psychosocial issues facing critically ill patients may *ignore an important aspect of their professional responsibility by taking a patient's or family's statement at face value without further exploration or clarification.*" (Italics added.)

THE BURDEN-BENEFIT RELATIONSHIP IN THE CRITICALLY ILL

The balance between the risks or burdens of continued treatment relative to any anticipated benefits must be carefully considered at the same time as the relationships between beneficence and autonomy are pondered. Sometimes life itself, or the treatment proposed to sustain life, is so burdensome that the patient can claim the right to decide that the dying process be allowed to proceed. Aggressive treatment for severely burned patients was considered burdensome by one group of physicians who attempted to discover whether patients wished such painful treatment even if the chances of survival were almost nonexistent [17]. Observing that burned patients were quite lucid during the early hours of hospitalization, they carefully talked with their patients during these moments about the benefits and burdens of aggressive treatment. They opened these conversations with statements such as "You are seriously ill" or "Your life is in immediate danger." In answer to the question, "Will I die?" the authors replied, "We cannot predict the future. We can only say that, to our knowledge, no one in the past of your age and with your size of burn has ever survived this injury, either with or without maximal treatment." Twenty-four of 108 adults were determined to have an injury without precedent of survival. Twenty-one of these chose nonaggressive or ordinary care, and three requested, and received, maximal care. The authors believed the patients to be sufficiently autonomous to determine their own course of treatment, but it could also be argued that the psychologic factors associated with sudden injury required the physician to emphasize beneficence rather than autonomy.

In its "Declaration on Euthanasia," the Vatican described the problem as "due proportion in the use of remedies":

In the past, moralists replied that one is never obliged to use "extraordinary" means. This reply which as a principle still holds good, is perhaps less clear today, by reason of the imprecision of the term and the rapid progress made in the treatment of sickness. . . .

It is permitted with the patient's consent, to interrupt these means, where the results fall short of expectations. But for such a decision to be made, account will have to be taken of the reasonable wishes of the patient and the patient's family, as also of the advice of the doctors who are specially competent in the matter. The latter may in particular judge that the investment in instruments and personnel is disproportionate to the results foreseen; they may also judge that the techniques applied impose on the patient strain or suffering out of proportion with the benefits which he or she may gain from such techniques [25].

Artificial feeding, a technique that many would consider to be part of the basic humane care required for all patients, may also become burdensome in certain situations in which any benefits from such intervention are minimal. Two recent judicial decisions demonstrate how the courts have dealt with issues of benefit and burden. Elizabeth Bouvia, a 28-year-old quadriplegic woman with severe arthritic pain, had refused to take food and fluids and asked a court to be allowed to starve to death. A 1983 court decision refused her request, but in April 1986, the court of appeals agreed with Ms. Bouvia and told physicians to remove her nasogastric tube. The court ruled that removal of the tube was not a form of suicide and that the right to refuse treatment was virtually absolute. A similar decision was made by the Supreme Judicial Court of Massachusetts in the case of Paul E. Brophy, Sr. Brophy had frequently expressed the opinion that he would never wish to be maintained on life support devices, and the court upheld his wife's request to have a surgically placed feeding tube removed [28].

Withholding of nutrition and liquid seems to strike at the foundation of the beneficence principle and has been the subject of heated ethical discussion. Ethicists worry about precedent-setting positions that appear to place the unwary on a "slippery slope" toward the abyss of unethical activity. Steinbrook and Lo [28], reviewing the issue in February 1988 in a paper titled "Artificial Feeding—Solid Ground, Not a Slippery Slope," concluded that there was an emerging consensus that when the patient's wishes are known, artificial feeding may be considered to be one of the treatments that may be withheld. Three letters questioning the authors' position were published several months later. Studebaker [29] emphasized the importance of distinguishing between an individual's "right to die" and a "socially enforced 'duty to die'."

LIMITING TREATMENT IN THE CRITICALLY ILL: THE "DO NOT RESUSCITATE" ORDER

One technique for limiting care to patients when the burden of continued life appears to markedly exceed the benefits of additional treatment is the "do not resuscitate" (DNR) order. Withholding resuscitative efforts in patients who are dying clearly is justified, but the ease with which a DNR order can be written can make abuse relatively simple. Veatch [32] summarized the problem by pointing out that "patients have for some years been horrified at the thought of being trapped in terminal illness treatment without their approval. It is even worse to leave them contemplating having a nonresuscitation decision made for them without their approval." An obvious problem with DNR orders is the nonspecificity of resuscitative activities. Cardiopulmonary resuscitation includes provision of an adequate airway, electrical defibrillation, and closed cardiac massage. Electrical defibrillation is uniformly successful when correctible causes, such as acidosis or ischemia, are present. Endotracheal intubation is quite successful if the airway is occluded by food or with excessive secretions. Closed-chest massage has a variable success rate but is probably less effective than are defibrillation or intubation. Rational DNR orders should specify which of these three interventions should be withheld.

Youngner et al [33] attempted to identify the characteristics of DNR patients by studying 506 critically ill patients in a medical intensive care unit. The APACHE physiologic score was used to evaluate severity of illness. Seventy-one DNR patients had an APACHE score averaging 26.5, whereas a seriously ill subgroup of 166 patients without DNR orders had a score of 22.6. The physiologic score was 13.7 for the entire non-DNR group. DNR patients were older than non-DNR patients and frequently had serious or incapacitating chronic illness. The most common diagnoses in these DNR patients were cardiac failure, sepsis, ventilatory failure, hypovolemia, failure of oxygenation, intracranial hemorrhage, and metabolic encephalopathy.

This study identified a group of issues associated with DNR orders. As might be expected, the DNR group consumed more resources than did other patients before the DNR designation was assigned. Resource consumption fell after DNR designation was made but was still comparable to other critically ill patients. For some reason, the decision to withhold resuscitative measures was not accompanied by a reduction in other therapeutic modalities: 93 percent of patients remained on ventilators; 76 percent continued to receive vasopressors; antiarrhythmic drugs were continued in 87 percent, even though defibrillation was proscribed; 76 percent continued to receive intravenous antibiotics; and Swan-Ganz catheters were continued in 91 percent.

In editorial discussion, Veatch [32] pointed out that only 39 percent of patients were considered to have less than a 10 percent chance of surviving hospitalization, so DNR orders were commonly written for individuals where death was not inevitable. Equally bothersome was the way the DNR decision was made. According to Veatch, "In only 15% of cases were the wishes of the patient listed as a justification for not resuscitating. When Youngner et al say that the decisions tended to be made by the resident physician in conjunction with the medical intensive care unit attending physician, are they telling us that these decisions were sometimes made without the involvement and active instruction of the patient or patient's surrogate?. . . . [E]ven more provocative is the finding that four patients were not resuscitated even though there was no recorded nonresuscitation decision."

The decision to withhold any form of treatment, including resuscitation efforts, is obviously an important ethical matter. Issues of autonomy and burden must be carefully evaluated. Patients or their surrogates, as well as other members of the health care team, must participate in the decision, and some evidence of consensus must be recorded in the hospital chart. The Presbyterian–University of Pittsburgh Hospital has provided an unusually complete set of guidelines for foregoing life-sustaining treatment [7]. Drawing heavily on recommendations from the President's Commission [25], the authors provide important guidance for the documentation of decisions and the entry of orders. They emphasize that whenever a decision to withhold life-supporting techniques is made, a specific order must be written. The order must be accompanied by a detailed entry in the progress notes describing the patient's condition and the details of the details of the decision. The guidelines suggest three categories of acceptable orders: (1) "all but cardiac resuscitation," (2) "limited therapy," and (3) "comfort measures only."

ETHICAL AND LEGAL BASES FOR LIMITING OR TERMINATING TREATMENT IN THE COMATOSE PATIENT

An understanding of the balance between the principles of beneficence and autonomy, and the judgment of the benefit-burden proportion, provide caregivers with a method of making moral judgments in the unit. Those who enter the medical, nursing and other related health care professions pledge to themselves and to others that they will do all in their power to preserve and support human life. Even though caregivers must always maintain a presumption in favor of life and seek to prevent death at all cost where possible, there clearly is a group of situations in which continued life support is useless and not indicated. In these situations, life is at an end even though mechanical support permits blood to course through an otherwise lifeless person. Failure to understand that death, as much as any other human health problem, must be properly identified can produce devastating consequences for patients, families, hospital staff, and the public at large.

William Harvey discovered the circulation of the blood in the latter half of the sixteenth century and also decided that the heart was the seat of human life.

Since death is a corruption which takes place through deficiency of heat, and since all living things are warm, all dying things cold, there must be a particular seat and fountain, a kind of home and hearth, where the cherisher of nature, the original of the native fire, is stored and preserved; from which heat and life are dispensed to all parts as from a fountain head; from which sustenance may be derived; and upon which concoction and nutrition, and all vegetative energy may depend. Now, that the heart is this place, that the heart is the principle of life, and that all passes in the manner just mentioned, I trust no one will deny [13].

At almost the same time in history, Sir Francis Bacon chided the Roman philosopher Seneca and his Stoic philosophy for a complicated approach to death: "Just as I choose a ship to sail in or a house to live in, so I choose a death for my passage from life. . . . Nowhere should we indulge the soul more than in dying. . . . A man's life should satisfy other people as well, his death only himself, and whatever sort he likes best." Bacon went on to add that "it is as natural to die as to be born; and to a little infant, perhaps, the one is as painful as the other" [4]. He was echoing the moving and significant words of the author of Ecclesiastes: "For every thing there is a season, and a time to every purpose under the heaven: A time to be born, and a time to die; a time to plant, and time to pluck up that which is planted [Eccles. 3:1–2].

Definitions of death changed little over the subsequent 400 years and tended to follow William Harvey's conclusions as embodied in English common law: death is "the cessation of life," indicated primarily by "a total stoppage of the circulation of the blood" [8]. The development of mechanical ventilation, ventricular assist devices, cardiopulmonary resuscitation, and other life-sustaining techniques challenged Harvey's views. Intensive care units became filled with ventilator-dependent patients who had little hope for survival. Physicians and hospitals, acting in a spirit of beneficence, made private decisions that caused little attention until the practice of organ transplantation became widespread and the need for organs substantial. In a sense, it is unfortunate that the need for organs appeared to drive the decisions over the moment of death, as an individual came to be poised against a societal good.

"A Definition of Irreversible Coma" was published in 1968 by an ad hoc committee of the Harvard Medical School [6]. Fifteen years later, the President's Commission (see below) suggested that "using this term as synonymous with death unfortunately served to perpetuate a confusion in the medical field between the state of being permanently unconscious, as are patients in a persistent vegetative state, and that of being dead."

An attorney and a physician, Alexander Capron and Leon Kass, attempted to clarify the idea of brain death by suggesting a model statute that was published in the Law Review of the University of Pennsylvania:

A person will be considered dead if in the announced opinion of a physician, based on ordinary standards of medical practice, he has experienced an irreversible cessation of spontaneous respiratory and circulatory functions. In the event that artificial means of support preclude a determination that these functions have ceased, a person will be considered dead if in the announced opinion of a physician, based on ordinary standards of medical practice, he has experienced an irreversible cessation of spontaneous brain functions [9].

The Richmond brain case, argued in 1972, was a landmark legal precedent supporting the concept of brain death. In 1968, Thomas Tucker was pronounced dead at the Medical College of Virginia following a massive head injury. His heart was later used for one of the first heart transplants performed in the United States. His family members had not been identified, and physicians had made him an involuntary donor under the Virginia Unclaimed Bodies Act. The donor's brother subsequently stepped forward and brought suit for wrongful death against the hospital and physicians. When the case came to trial in 1972, Judge Christian Compton of the Richmond Law and Equity Court allowed the issue of brain death to be considered by the jury. A group of physicians and a medical ethicist, Joseph Fletcher, argued that life cannot exist without the brain. A seven-member jury agreed that the existing definition of death was inadequate and that the donor had died when his brain ceased to function.

Not everyone is comfortable with the brain death concept, although it is by now widely accepted in legal circles throughout the world. One philosopher, Hans Jonas [20], has viewed it as an operational tour de force rather than a reasoned definition of death itself. "We then have an 'organism' as a whole minus the brain, maintained in some partial state of life so long as the respirator and other artifices are at work. And here the question is not: has the patient died? but: how should he—still a patient—be dealt with. Now this question must be settled, surely not by a definition of death, but by a definition of man and of what life is human." The decision to terminate life support systems should not be made because the patient is brain dead, but because "it is humanly not justified—let alone, demanded—to artificially prolong the life of a brainless body. . . . On that philosophic ground, which few will contest, the physician can, indeed should, turn off the respirator and let the 'definition of death' take care of itself by what then inevitably happens." Jonas apparently agreed with the pragmatic medical decision to terminate life support but was uneasy about the theoretic underpinnings of the moral judgment.

The brain death concept became generally accepted until the Karen Quinlan tragedy began to underscore problems with its general applicability. In 1972, Jennett and Plum [19] described a group of patients who survived for prolonged periods after severe brain trauma with coma. They called this syndrome the persistent or chronic vegetative state; the public has come to know it as the Karen Quinlan syndrome. The contrast between brain death and the persistent vegetative state is perhaps best described by Korein's term *cerebral death* [23]. Cerebral death differs from brain death since in the former the midbrain, pons brainstem, and cerebellum are capable of maintaining some function.

The Supreme Court of New Jersey in 1976 ordered that Karen Quinlan be disconnected from mechanical ventilation, basing its judgment on the right of the guardian of an incompetent patient, in consultation with a hospital "ethics committee," to make informed decisions. The court held that "we consider that a practice of applying to a court to confirm such decisions would generally be inappropriate, not only because that would be a gratuitous encroachment upon the medical profession's field of competence, but because it would be impossibly cumbersome." Although two other courts followed the view of the New Jersey court, the Supreme Judicial Court of Massachusetts in the Sakiewicz decision rejected it, stating that it took "a dim view of any attempt to shift the ultimate decision-making responsibility away from the duly established courts of proper jurisdiction to any committee, panel or group, ad hoc or permanent." The resolution of this judicial conflict and the development of an emerging consensus is detailed in a later section.

On March 21, 1983, the President's Commission for the Study of Ethical Problems in Medicine and Biomedical and Behavioral Research [25] sent a most significant document to the President of the United States, the president of the Senate and the Speaker of the House of Representatives:

[We are] pleased to transmit our report on *Deciding to Forego Life-Sustaining Treatment.* This subject was not part of our original legislative mandate but was added as a natural outgrowth of our studies on informed consent, the "definition" of death, and access to health care and because it seemed to us to involve some of the most important and troubling ethical and legal questions in modern medicine.

The letter went on:

We have concluded that the cases that involve true ethical difficulties are many fewer than commonly believed and that the perception of difficulty occurs primarily because of misunderstandings about the dictates of law and ethics. Neither criminal nor civil law precludes health practitioners or their patients and relatives from reaching ethically and medically appropriate decisions about when to engage in or to forego efforts to sustain the lives of dying patients.

The President's Commission presented over 500 tightly reasoned pages to the United States government. The report generally supported the Quinlan rather than the Sakiewicz decision and provided an ethical basis for decision making in the critical care unit. It should be available to all involved in critical care.

The report emphasized that "primary responsibility for ensuring that morally justified processes of decision making are followed lies with physicians." Institutions have similar responsibilities and should develop policies regarding these important decisions. There is, however, "no substitute for the dedication, compassion, and professional judgement of physicians." Further,

The voluntary choice of a competent and informed patient should determine whether or not life-sustaining therapy will be undertaken. . . . Health care institutions and professionals should try to enhance patients' abilities to make decisions on their own behalf and to promote understanding of the available treatment options. . . . Health care professionals serve patients best by maintaining a presumption in favor of sustaining life, while recognizing that competent patients are entitled to choose to forego any treatments, including those that sustain life.

The report went on to emphasize that health care professionals do not have to take actions that violate their own professional judgment of conscience, but they may not abandon patients. Institutions may limit the availability of certain scarce resources in order to make them available where they will be most useful.

There is a more difficult problem with patients who are *incompetent* to make appropriate decisions. A surrogate—usually a family member—should be named to make decisions for an incompetent patient:

The decisions of surrogates should, when possible, attempt to replicate the ones that the patient would make if capable of doing so. When lack of evidence about the patient's wishes precludes this, decisions by surrogates should seek to protect the patient's best interests. Because such decisions are not instances of self-choice by the patient, the range of acceptable decisions by surrogates is sometimes not as broad as it would be for patients making decisions themselves.

Families, health care institutions and professionals should work together to make decisions for incompetent patients. The medical staff, administrators, and trustees should develop arrangements for consultation and review, including the formation of "ethics committees."

Legislatures and courts should develop methods for allowing individuals to designate in advance others who may make health care decisions on their behalf:

Durable powers of attorney are preferable to "living wills" since they are more generally applicable and provide a better vehicle for patients to exercise self-determination, though experience with both is limited.

Recourse to courts should be reserved for the occasions when adjudication is clearly required by state law or when concerned patients have disagreements that they cannot resolve over matters of substantial import. Courts and legislatures should be cautious about requiring judicial review of routine health care decisions for patients with inadequate decision making capacity.

JUDICIAL SUPPORT FOR TREATMENT DECISIONS
IN CRITICAL CARE

The pioneering decision of the New Jersey Supreme Court did not immediately gain judicial acceptance. The Sakiewicz court supported the concept of "substituted judgment" where a surrogate acts for the incompetent patient but insisted on judicial review rather than the review by ethics committees recommended in the Quinlan decision. The New York Court of Appeals decision in the Storar case rejected the substituted judgment concept that underlay both the Quinlan and the Sakiewicz decisions. Various public officials, including trial judges and prosecutors, equated termination of life support with euthanasia, and prosecution of physicians was threatened. Physicians were actually charged with murder in the Barber case in California for withdrawing a feeding tube at the relatives' request. The court subsequently dismissed the charges, stating that "medical procedures to provide nutrition and hydration are more similar to other medical procedures than to typical human ways of providing nutrition and hydration. Their benefits and burdens ought to be evaluated in the same manner as any other medical procedure."

Christopher J. Armstrong, associate justice of the Massachusetts Court of Appeals and a member of the National Institutes of Health Consensus Panel on Critical Care, has written and spoken about the "emerging consensus" of judicial decisions:

On matters so fraught with emotion as the withholding or withdrawing of life-sustaining treatment, there can never be perfect agreement. Although some serious problems remain, the recent court decisions from across the country seem to be falling into some definite patterns that, to me, presage substantial agreement among courts on several principles of importance to physicians and hospitals. If this reading is correct, these principles can be relied on to govern future court decisions. These principles will derive stability from the fact that they are in harmony with the traditional and accepted roles of physicians, patients, and families in determining courses of medical treatment [3].

Justice Armstrong went on to list seven "largely settled" principles:

1. A competent adult has a legal right to refuse medical treatment, a right that may be qualified in particular cases of four countervailing state interests. . . . The general state interest in the preservation of life—most weighty where the patient, properly treated, can return to reasonable health without great suffering, a decision to avoid treatment would be aberrational—carries far less weight where the patient is approaching the end of a normal life span, where the afflictions are incapacitating, and where the best that medicine can offer is an extension of suffering.
2. An incompetent patient has the same right as a competent patient to avoid treatment, and the right may be exercised in his behalf by an appropriate surrogate.
3. The family of an incompetent patient is presumptively an appropriate surrogate to act in his behalf.
4. Court proceedings are generally unnecessary to secure approval of a decision to withhold or withdraw life-sustaining medical treatment except in cases of dispute or where the incompetent patients lacks an appropriate surrogate to act in his behalf.

5. The entry of a no-code (or DNR) order on a patient's chart does not require prior judicial approval.
6. A decision to terminate medical treatment is subject to the same legal standards as a decision not to begin the treatment.
7. Rules concerning withdrawal of treatment apply equally to withdrawal of nutrition and hydration by artificial means.

TOWARD A CAREGIVER'S ETHIC

The primary ethic of critical care must be the preservation of life by competent and compassionate care. When the best care shows no hope of restoring meaningful life, physicians and nurses must be equally competent in determining levels of care appropriate to a patient's needs and abilities. From Hippocrates, Aristotle, Gregory, Dewey, Toulmin, Armstrong, and others comes a synthesis of pragmatic ethics rooted in traditional medical practice and common sense.

The first book of *Epidemics,* written by Hippocrates in the fifth century B.C., provides a strikingly modern approach to the care of the critically ill. W. H. S. Jones, an important translator of the Greek physician's works [15], reminds us that Hippocrates was writing at a time when explanations of disease moved from the idea of divine retribution to a philosophic interpretation. Hippocrates attempted to rescue medicine from the philosophers and present a scientific approach to human illness. The famous injunction to the caregiver, "To help, or at least to do no harm," appears in the section of *Epidemics I* dealing with the critically ill patient. The physician must carefully observe "all dangerous cases" and be alert for "signs" that "denote absence of crisis, pain, prolonged illness, death or a return of the same symptoms." Other signs are important, and the passage of "copious urine" was regarded as a particularly favorable sign for recovery. If death appears inevitable, the physician must provide comfort but not harm the patient by useless and burdensome treatment. This common-sense, or middle, course taken by Hippocrates and Aristotle and passed down through Gregory to the caregiver of today contains an important message: avoid the extremes of either total life support as long as possible or the premature termination of treatment when months of worthwhile life may still be possible.

Physicians, nurses, and other caregivers must be virtuous individuals who accept their professional responsibilities and who understand the application of moral principles and moral reasoning to clinical decision making. The recently published "It's Over, Debbie" [1] is a withering example of incredibly inept presumed moral reasoning. It represents the "slippery slope" so feared by those who doubt the force of human reason. Late one night, a gynecology resident "rotating through a large, private hospital" was called to see a 20-year-old woman named Debbie who was seriously ill with ovarian cancer. He began his brief note by describing how much he disliked nighttime phone calls. "I had come to detest telephone calls, because invariably I would be up for several hours and would not feel good the next day." Arriving on the floor, he quickly reviewed Debbie's chart while walking to her room. He observed, but apparently did not examine, her, and he rapidly interpreted her acute distress and pleading for relief as an autonomous decision for euthanasia. Without consulting the patient's own physician or other professionals, and apparently without discussion with an unidentified older woman who was at the bedside, he filled a syringe with morphine and abruptly ended her life.

It is obvious from the brief report that this resident physician did not fully understand the patient's clinical situation. He interpreted her unrelenting vomiting and physical inanition as representing terminal disease but made no attempt to consider how much of her debility was related to the recent chemotherapy she had received. He was apparently unwilling to spend more than a few minutes at her bedside and made no effort to consider any treatment short of euthanasia. He did not even bother to telephone the patient's own physician and, with the arrogance of ignorance, decided that the rapid termination of her life was the correct means of relieving the patient's suffering. And he published his experience so that others could admire his tough-minded approach to moral decision making.

This rather obvious example of fuzzy-headed moral reasoning seems an affront to the art of decision making. "A correct choice of therapeutic procedure in medicine," reflected Toulmin, "is the *right* treatment to pursue, not just as a matter of medical technique but for ethical reasons also" [30].

Observe, reflect, question, hypothesize, and observe again. Truth for the caregiver is achievement of a desirable outcome. The *end* is everything, as long as the means do not lead to associated undesirable consequences. Beware of absolutes that close minds and inhibit creative problem-solving. Treat each person individually while drawing on the accumulated wisdom of medicine to suggest plans of action. Strive for the greatest good possible, or at least the lesser of two evils.

Be neither complacent nor smugly overconfident that the truth is at hand. Make common cause with patients, families, and professional colleagues from all disciplines in an unabashed effort to make decisions that will lead to the very best possible conclusion. The means and ends of each clinical situation must be shared with others, so that the ethical method can be better understood. Communicate by word and in writing and, if the insight so gained is sufficiently generalizable, publish! Above all, vigorously but humbly seek the very best solution for the problem at hand!

REFERENCES

1. Anonymous. It's over, Debbie. J.A.M.A. 259:272, 1988.
2. Aristotle. Nicomachean Ethics. In *Man and Man.* New York: Random House, 1947.
3. Armstrong, C. J. Judicial Involvement in Treatment Decisions: The Emerging Consensus. In J. M. Civetta, R. W. Taylor, and R. R. Kirby, *Critical Care.* Philadelphia: Lippincott, 1988.
4. Bacon, F. Of Death, 1625. In C. W. Eliot, (ed.), *The Harvard Classics,* vol. 3. New York, 1909. P. 9.
5. Beauchamp, T. L., and McCullough, L. B. *Medical Ethics: The Moral Responsibilities of Physicians.* Englewood Cliffs, NJ: Prentice-Hall, 1984.
6. Beecher, H. K., Adams, R. D., Burger, A. D. et al. A definition of irreversible coma: Report of the ad hoc committee of the Harvard Medical School to examine the definition of brain death. *J.A.M.A.* 205:337, 1968.
7. Benesch, K., Abramson N. S., Grenvik A., et al. Medicolegal Aspects of Critical Care. Rockville, MD: Aspen Publications, 1986. Appendix A.

8. *Black's Law Dictionary 488* (4th ed., 1968). In the 5th edition (1979), an entry under "brain death" is found on p. 170.
9. Capron, A. M., and Kass, L. R. A statutory definition of the standards for determining human death: An appraisal and a proposal. University of Pennsylvania Law Review 121:87, 1972.
10. Dewey, J. *Reconstruction in Philosophy.* Boston: Beacon Press, 1948.
11. Erikson, E. The Golden Rule and the Cycle of Life. In R. J. Bulger (ed.). *In Search of the Modern Hippocrates.* Iowa City: Univ. of Iowa Press, 1987. Pp. 65–79.
12. Gregory, J. *Lectures on the Duties and Qualifications of a Physician.* London and Edinburgh: A. Strahan and T. Cadell, and W. Creech, 1788.
13. Harvey, W. Circulation of the Blood, 1628. In C. W. Eliot (ed.), *The Harvard Classics,* vol. 38, New York, 1909. P. 129.
14. Hippocrates. The Art. In W. H. S. Jones (transl.), *Hippocrates,* vol. II. London: Loeb Classical Library, William Heinemann, 1928. P. 193.
15. Hippocrates. Epidemics I. In W. H. S. Jones (transl.), *Hippocrates,* vol. I. London: Loeb Classical Library, William Heinemann, 1928. P. 165.
16. Hippocrates. Ancient Medicine. In W. H. S. Jones (transl.), *Hippocrates,* vol. I. London: Loeb Classical Library, William Heinemann, 1928. P. 53.
17. Imbus, S. H., and Zawacki, B. E. Autonomy for burned patients when survival is unprecedented. *N. Engl. J. Med.* 297:308, 1977.
18. Jackson, D. L., and Youngner, S. Patient autonomy and "death with dignity." *N. Engl. J. Med.* 301:404, 1979.
19. Jennett, W. B., and Plum, F. The persistent vegetative state: A syndrome in search of a new name. *Lancet* 1:560, 1971.
20. Jonas, H. Against the Stream: Comments on the Definition and Redefinition of Death. Philosophic Essays: From Ancient Creed to Technological Man. Englewood Cliffs, NJ: Prentice-Hall, 1974.
21. Kant, I. *Fundamental Principles of the Metaphysics of Morals,* transl. by T. K. Abbott. Buffalo: Prometheus Books, 1987.
22. Kepler, M. O. Medical Stewardship: Fullfilling the Hippocratic Legacy. Westport, CT: Greenwood Press, 1981.
23. Korein, J. The problem of brain death: Development and history. *Ann. NY Acad. Sci.* 315:19, 1978.
24. Plum, F., and Posner, J. B. *The Diagnosis of Stupor and Coma* (3rd ed.). Philadelphia: F. A. Davis, 1982.
25. President's Commission for the Study of Ethical Problems in Medicine and Biomedical and Behavioral Research. Deciding to Forego Life-Sustaining Treatment. Washington, D.C.: U.S. Gov. Printing Office, 1983.
26. Rousseau, J.-J. The Social Contract. In *Man and the State.* New York: Random House, 1947.
27. Russell, B. *The Art of Philosophizing.* Totowa, NJ: Helix Books, 1974.
28. Steinbrook, R., and Lo, B. Artificial feeding—Solid ground, not a slippery slope. *N. Engl. J. Med.* 318:286, 1988.
29. Studebaker, M. E. Letter. *N. Engl. J. Med.* 319:306, 1988.
30. Toulmin, S. The recovery of practical philosophy. *American Scholar* 57:337, 1988.
31. Toulmin, S. How medicine saved the life of ethics. *Perspect. Biol. Med.* 25:736, 1982.
32. Veatch, R. M. Deciding against resuscitation: Encouraging signs and potential dangers. *J.A.M.A.* 253:77, 1985.
33. Youngner, S., Lewandowski, W. McKlish, D. K. et al. Do not resuscitate orders: Incidence and implications in a medical intensive care unit. *J.A.M.A.* 253:54, 1985.

Design of the Intensive Care Unit

John M. Kinney
Michael D. Tyne

The ICU has correctly been referred to as the "hospital's hospital." It is here that some of the highest standards of medical, nursing, and institutional support are required. It can be efficiently run, uncrowded, and well-organized, or it can be crowded with instrumentation, disorganized, and filled with a harassed and frantic staff. The ICU presents an image to relatives and visitors that then is applied to the hospital as a whole, whether deserved or not. Unfortunately, a serious and common error is to see the design of the ICU as a problem that should be turned over entirely to architects, engineers, and hospital administrators. At the outset of any design process, it is imperative that the professional staff make every effort to educate the architects and administrators about the clinical problems they will face in the management of their life-threatened patients. It is of equal importance for the professional staff to learn from highly experienced architects how best to develop an intensive care area that will serve both patient and staff in the most efficient and sensitive way [21].

The optimum design of an ICU for a given hospital will reflect a skillful blend of broad design principles and of local circumstances, such as available space, funds, professional staff, and demands for care. In addition, the planning for a new unit should not be limited by architectural features and ICU requirements established in the past. Both medical professionals and architects should take the time to arrive at reasonable predictions about the advances in intensive care that are likely to take place in the next 10 years, and these advances should be given serious consideration during the planning stage. The medical members of the planning team play a crucial role in educating the architect regarding the impact on design of changes in patient management and instrumentation. In the same way, the architect must educate the professional staff concerning current building materials and procedures that could enhance the plans for a facility that will be used for well over a decade.

The history of intensive care units can be traced back to the early 1930s, when specialized units were established for neurosurgical care, and to the

1940s, when military hospitals designated special "shock wards" for the most severe combat casualties. The postwar period saw the development of discrete postanesthesia recovery rooms, and the poliomyelitis epidemics of the 1950s forced the grouping together of patients requiring mechanical ventilation. By the 1960s, a new kind of unit was introduced for coronary monitoring and for the postoperative care of open heart surgical patients. By the 1970s, intensive care units had been developed, along with special expertise and equipment for the care of multiple trauma and major burn cases [18,27,28]. Today's hospital is expected to be capable of providing intensive care for many, if not all, of these various medical conditions. It follows that particular ideas regarding intensive care and design features will vary among medical professionals, depending on their discipline and their training and experience. This is most obvious when considering the differences in requirements for a general surgical ICU that will be treating cases of major trauma and severe sepsis and for a medical ICU emphasizing the care of cardiology patients and continuous surveillance. Therefore, it is important that the proper medical specialists be invited to take part in the planning of an ICU that will be treating their patients.

The planning team will have to take into account a variety of projected needs. They will have to consider the needs of the community, of the institution, of the medical staff, and of the individual ICU patients. The hospital administration will have to forecast the medical needs of the community by analyzing demographic data and utilization trends to determine the appropriate number of ICU beds. Conflicting demands within the institution will stress the advantages or disadvantages of one location versus another. But in the last analysis, both available space and the convenience of the disciplines most closely related to the patient will have to determine location.

Should the new unit be as autonomous as possible, or should it depend upon general hospital functions and services whenever possible? This is a complex question whose answer will depend on cost, space availability, maximum administrative efficiency, and the quality control of satellite services. All of these issues need to be addressed before plans for a unit are finalized: otherwise, various important options will be foreclosed by both location and design [25].

The unit must be staff-oriented in ways that too frequently are ignored, particularly in relation to the needs of the nursing staff. The extra effort demanded of the intensive care nurse as the result of careless or inadequate ICU design can make an insidious contribution to high turnover rate and to the costly training of new nursing personnel. A pleasant and efficiently designed ICU can pay major dividends to the hospital when it comes to nursing recruitment. We have seen individuals who were being recruited as floor nurses gain a strongly favorable impression of an institution as a result of touring the ICU.

One of the most frequent problems encountered in many intensive care units is that of "overutilized" space. Nowhere is this problem more evident than in the nursing station, where the same area is expected to serve for patient surveillance, medicine preparation, direction of visitors, attention to monitoring screens, and the writing of nursing notes. In the same space, physicians will be discussing their patients, examining x-rays, writing notes, and using the telephones. This concentration of activities can lead to errors, stress, and short tempers. Because the ICU and the emergency room place unusual demands on staff, extra attention and thought need to be given to their efficiency and comfort.

We have too often heard that the critically ill patient is indifferent to the environment, being "too sick to know, or care." While this admittedly is true for some patients, it certainly is not so for all. The ICU environment far too often needlessly enhances fearfulness. Abrasive sights and sounds, as well as glaring lights, contribute to unnecessary stress. While it is essential for the patient to maintain reassuring contact with the staff, it is equally important to reduce stress-producing factors that are incorporated solely for the convenience of the nurse and the physician [7]. These *patient-oriented* aspects of design are discussed in more detail elsewhere in this chapter.

The good ICU will be the "hospital's hospital," providing a window into the attitudes and efficiency of the medical care throughout the institution. In addition, an excellent ICU is a superb educational and training facility for the house staff. Planning a new unit is a challenge for the planning team and those responsible for supporting services, who must project important trends in medical care for a facility that must operate smoothly for a decade or more. For those who are involved in planning such a facility, we offer the following considerations of different aspects of ICU design that we feel have been well established by both medical and architectural experience.

BED NEED

Few other inpatient units experience the fluctuations in census that an ICU does. An ICU that is always at maximum capacity may be too small or may be inappropriately utilized, whereas one with a consistently low occupancy imposes a high operational cost per bed. A careful balance must be achieved between the size of the unit and the ability to admit a patient in urgent need of a bed. Determining the precise number of critical care beds needed is difficult. A number of factors should be considered in making this determination, including admission and discharge criteria, total hospital bed capacity, and cost-effective occupancy.

The first step in determining the appropriate number of beds involves an examination of which patients belong in the ICU. Cullen, et al. [4] have noted two functions for the ICU: (1) monitoring of a patient's vital functions and their maintenance at levels as close to normal as possible; and (2) provision of definitive therapy to patients with acute but reversible life-threatening dysfunctions of vital systems. The Task Force on Guidelines for the Society of Critical Care Medicine [26] expressed a similar opinion in stating that "eligibility for ICU admission and discharge is also based on the reversibility of the clinical problem as well as the likely benefits of ICU treatment and expectation of recovery." The Task Force suggested a triage system for allocating ICU beds, with patients requiring intensive treatment having priority over those requiring intensive monitoring and the lowest priority given to those who are terminal or are critically ill with a poor prognosis for recovery. The last-named group has received a great deal of attention in recent years. Given the fact that these patients are sicker, it is not surprising that the greater proportion of cost and effort is spent on those who do not survive. As Hudson [12] has noted, "Not everyone should be in an ICU when he dies." Each institution must decide whether or not ICU beds should be allocated to this third group of patients, since this consideration will influence the total number of ICU beds. Of course, in many institutions, and particularly in small community hospitals, the level of nursing care needed for these patients can only be found in intensive care.

One approach to determining the number of intensive care beds is to use a percentage of total medical/surgical beds. A Veterans Administration standard [29] suggested 15 percent of adult medical beds or 20 percent of adult surgical beds, or approximately 17.5 percent of adult medical/surgical beds. A survey [1] of American Hospital Association member hospitals indicated that intensive care beds account for approximately 9 to 11 percent of adult medical/surgical beds for hospitals with fewer than 200 beds and 12 to 13 percent for those hospitals with 200-plus beds. The percentage appears to increase slightly with the total bed capacity of the institution. In a children's hospital, one typically finds 25 to 30 percent of all the beds devoted to critical care [19].

A more precise calculation entails use of historical utilization data and projections of future volume in conjunction with an evaluation of admission and discharge criteria. One then sets an occupancy goal to determine the number of beds needed. Average ICU occupancy is below that typically found in other units. However, regulatory agencies typically set 75 to 80 percent as the occupancy criteria. The Poisson formula uses the projected average daily census (ADC) and the desired probability of having a bed when one is needed. The formula follows:

$$\text{Beds needed} = \text{ADC} + Z\sqrt{\text{ADC}}$$

A table of various probabilities and the associated Z value follows.

P	Z
99%	2.33
95%	1.65
90%	1.28
85%	1.04

One must also take into account desired average occupancy. A higher probability of bed availability yields a lower census.

In summary, determination of bed need takes a careful evaluation of the appropriateness of admission and discharge criteria, the type of patient admitted, length of stay, desired occupancy, and availability-of-a-bed criteria. Also to be considered are whether the hospital has a step-down or intermediate care unit and the quality of nursing on the medical-surgical units as an inducement or deterrent to early ICU discharge [8,9].

ICU LOCATION

Historically, the optimal location for an ICU was considered by most to be contiguous to the surgical suite, if not an actual extension of the recovery room [13]. Today, the issue of ICU location is influenced by many variables. With ICUs now supporting many nonsurgical disciplines, including cardiology, neurology, neonatology, and others, and with ICUs growing in numbers of beds and area in proportion to the total hospital, there often is not enough space on the surgical suite floor to accommodate the ICU. The proximity of the ICU to the emergency department can enhance the ease and convenience of transferring an unstable patient who requires continuous life support. The ICU does not need to be near support services such as radiology and respiratory therapy, as long as the distance is not too great for moving bulky equipment to the unit. Figure 2-1 illustrates the various interdepartmental relationships.

A modern, well-designed hospital depends greatly upon its vertical transportation core (elevators) to expedite movement of patients, staff, and supplies, independent of visitor traffic. High-speed elevators must link departments in hospitals that are increasingly vertical on dense, urban sites. But where a horizontal relationship between major hospital departments is possible, a high priority should be given to locating ICUs in close proximity with surgery and the other departments noted above.

The historical functional relationship between the ICU and the recovery room no longer drives the decision to co-locate these two services. However, hospitals with fewer than 100 to 150 beds may still find that the ICU works well near the recovery room and that this arrangement is cost effective in terms of providing physician coverage together with sharing of staff and equipment. This is particularly true if the ICU has a high proportion of postoperative cases and an anesthesiologist is medical administrator of the recovery room and the ICU [13].

In hospitals of 150 to 300 beds, the ICU usually functions independently of the recovery room, because the required number of beds cannot be accommodated in or contiguous to recovery. ICUs in medium-sized hospitals tend to be multispecialty units. Once the number of beds exceeds the standard maximum capacity of 12 to 15, units should be split into more manageable components. Six beds is the generally accepted minimum unit size. At this scale, the importance of the interrelationship between the ICUs may supersede that between the ICU and the recovery room.

Institutions of 300 or more beds, particularly teaching hospitals or referral centers, may determine that requirements for a specific service justify intensive care specialization to support centers of excellence. Most frequently seen are units dedicated to high-risk neonatal, cardiac, pulmonary, burns, and postoperative cardiac and neurosurgical patients [6]. In the case of multiple ICUs, the trend has been toward the development of a clustering of beds with satellites of various ancillary departments, such as respiratory therapy, lab, and pharmacy, serving all units. Clustering facilitates

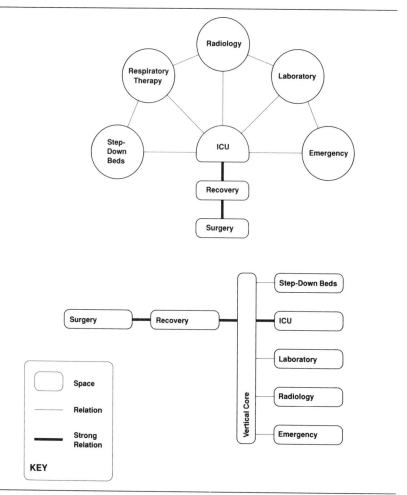

Fig. 2-1. Interdepartmental relationships.

ancillary support, permits flexible staffing, and can provide economies in
the sharing of support space and equipment. The link to anesthesiology is
usually not necessary, as units are run by their own intensivists. The requirement for proximity to major support services may be eliminated by
placing satellites of the services within the ICU suites. This point is discussed later in the chapter.

A few large hospitals have chosen to decentralize their ICUs in favor of
enhancing the integrity of a clinical service. In these instances, for example, the cardiac care unit (CCU) is adjacent to the cardiology and cardiovascular surgery nursing units and the neuro ICU is adjacent to the neurology and neurosurgery nursing units. In a few cases, research and
ambulatory care programs of the services have even been placed on the

same level as the inpatient units, for reasons of improved continuity of care, increased staffing efficiency, etc. This scheme is possible only when individual components, including the ICUs, are large enough to stand alone and operate economically. Also, the site and building conditions must be such that a scheme such as this can operate effectively.

Another factor to be considered in choosing a location for an ICU is the relationship to step-down nursing units. Step-down beds are used for patients who do not need skilled ICU care but require continued monitoring. Many ICUs suffer from overcrowding because of an inadequate number of beds or an inadequate level of staffing capable of providing intermediate care. Some hospitals are now faced with an inadequate number of step-down beds due to financial pressures to move patients out of the intensive care environment and to the general increasing acuity of the general inpatient population. These pressures have resulted in the introduction of monitoring on general acute units, as well as changing space and operational requirements on those units. Some of those requirements include upgrading of the units to provide telemetry or portable monitoring, more private rooms, larger equipment storage areas, aggressive in-service training for nursing staff, and more flexible arrangements to provide adequate staffing as acuity shifts on these units.

Some institutions are now considering consolidating the three levels of care (intensive, step-down, and acute) into two (intensive and acute), with step-down absorbed by the acute units. A major advantage of consolidation is reduction of the number of transfers of patients from unit to unit. As lengths of stay decline, it is difficult for the patient, family, and staff to adjust to the disruptions caused by multiple transfers. Transfers are also expensive and time consuming. Some institutions have evolved toward two-level care as the demand for step-down beds has forced upgrades on the acute units. Others have made a conscious investment in anticipation of future changes in the health care system.

DESIGN OF THE ICU

Once the appropriate number of beds and the optimal location for the ICU have been determined, discussions about operation and design should begin. Replacement of the ICU in new construction is ideal but often not possible. In new construction, the shape of the unit results from decisions regarding functional relationships, total area and traffic, and work flow. In renovated space, the shape of the existing wing controls the design of the unit. In either case, the design goal is to optimize the functional characteristics of the unit. Regardless, proposed designs must incorporate adequate exterior wall area to accommodate appropriate patient room dimensions and windows for each patient area. Usually, a square-shaped wing is more satisfactory than a rectangular one.

The ICU consists of three zones of activity: (1) patient bed area, (2) staff areas, and (3) unit support areas. Figure 2-2 illustrates the functional relationships among these three components. Several factors have led to an increase in the size of all three areas. Increased patient acuity and the multiplicity of equipment require a larger patient area. The staff area (locker

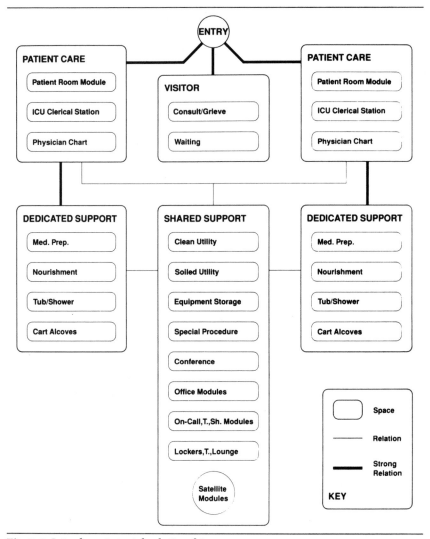

Fig. 2-2. Intradepartmental relationships.

rooms, lounges, conference rooms, on-call rooms, clerical centers) has increased because of a shift in patient management to a team approach, which often requires that staff from other departments be located in or near the ICU. Teaching hospital ICUs must accommodate fellows, residents, and medical students, plus nursing and paramedical technologist students. Demand for unit support space has intensified to accommodate the increasing amounts of supplies and equipment used in the ICU and also to provide for support department satellites.

In general, the ratio of total unit square footage per bed has increased. This ratio can range from approximately 450 to 500 square feet per bed in a community hospital up to 600 square feet per bed in a teaching hospital with a large cluster of ICU beds. Another useful ratio in estimating total unit size is 2.5 to 3 times the size of the bed space [26].

Hudson [12] has proposed that the ICU should be designed to meet four goals: (1) direct observation of the patient as part of the monitoring function, (2) the surveillance of physiologic monitoring, (3) the provision of routine and emergent therapeutic interventions, and (4) the recording of patient information. Under these general criteria, the actual design is based on the specific needs of the unit. Thus, identification of the type of patient, acuity, monitoring requirements, etc., at the beginning of the planning process is vital [17].

Patient Bed Area

The design of an ICU reflects a balance between maximum surveillance (and minimum privacy) of the open room with curtained bed areas and the minimum surveillance (and maximum privacy) of the individual room. The ideal design is sufficiently flexible to enhance surveillance when that is particularly required or to enhance privacy when that is appropriate. The first-generation ICUs generally adopted an open design, primarily because the ICU evolved as an extension of the recovery room. However, the use of private rooms with total or partial glass walls and breakaway doors is more common today [2,20,24].

The open bay design has a number of advantages: (1) better access to the patient, (2) the ability to encroach on floor space of an adjacent cubicle when there is a shortage of space for equipment for a patient, and (3) easier monitoring of two patients by a single nurse. For those units in which length of stay is short and patients are semiconscious, this design may be appropriate. As noted by Kinney, however, "No patient's bed should remain exposed simply because it is necessary for surveillance to be maintained from the nurse's station to a more distant bed" [13,14].

There has been a shift toward the enclosed private room with glass breakaway doors or sliding glass doors. This design enhances visibility and the ability to move patients with equipment in and out of the area. Although visibility remans vital to nursing practices—and, in fact, is dictated by some building codes—sophisticated monitoring devices can be used successfully to supplement visualization of the patient.

The high risk of cross-infection in an open ICU is often used as a justification for solid partitions. Studies on the relationship between ICU design and nosocomial infection have been inconclusive. One group of researchers studied an open unit and repeated the study after the unit had been converted to a closed unit with walls and sinks in each patient room [5,22]. The researchers collected microbiologic data on patients at various points of their stays, counted staff interactions with patients and the frequency of hand washing, and took air samples. They found that over one-half of the nosocomial infections in both units were caused by organisms present in the patient at the time of admission, and that although the number of staff interactions decreased in the closed unit, the decrease was not statistically significant. Of greatest interest is the finding that the frequency of hand washing was not affected by the presence of sinks in the closed unit. The study concluded that "excellent facilities alone do not result in increased frequency of hand washing after potentially contaminating activities" and that "in-service education would appear to be of greater importance than the availability of sinks for hand washing" [5,22]. It must be noted, however, that this does not imply that the availability of hand-washing sinks is irrelevant. Given the increasing acuity of the ICU patient and the resultant demands on staff, any reasonable means to improve access and adherence to hand washing should be a priority in unit design [3,18]. Given effective in-service education, the presence of sinks can facilitate hand-washing frequency.

It should be noted that a closed unit is more costly to construct than an open unit. Of no less importance is benefit of the private room to the patient in terms of greater privacy; fewer distractions from excess noise, traffic, and light; the ability to initiate patient and family education; and the ability to provide grieving and counseling space within the patient area. In addition, private-room patients suffer less anxiety related to watching other acutely ill patients and misinterpreting procedures being done on them. One of the most effective ways to reduce pain is to decrease any underlying fears.

The recommended size of the patient area has increased since the initial development of ICUs. In an open unit, each patient area should be a minimum of 150 square feet. A private room should be in the range of 170 to 225 square feet. Isolation rooms should be larger, at 250 square feet. The Task Force on Guidelines of the Society of Critical Care Medicine suggested 150 to 200 square feet for open units and 225 to 250 square feet for closed units [26]. There must be a minimum of 8 feet between beds in both adult and pediatric units that are in an open configuration [3].

Space needs in neonatal ICUs are different because of the size of the patient bed and the fact that such units typically are open. A level-III neonatal patient area should contain 100 to 120 square feet. Level-II bed areas should be approximately 80 square feet in size [8,30].

Another consideration in patient area design is the location of electrical outlets, gases, and suction. Typically, these devices are built into the head wall; the alternative is a ceiling-mounted or a freestanding power column. The essential concern is simultaneous access to the head of the patient and to adequate numbers of gas and electrical outlets. Another concern is accommodation of equipment such as monitors and infusion pumps. Every effort should be made to use vertical services for equipment placement, freeing up floor space to improve access to the patient.

Other features of the patient area should include a large clock, a calendar, and a window to the outside to maintain time and day/night orientation. Depending on the type of ICU and the philosophy of care, furnishings may include chairs, a patient wardrobe, bedside stand, lockable storage cabinets and/or drawers, and sink and charting area (waist-high) for staff. The charting area should be able to accommodate a computer terminal and appropriate wiring. A toilet is required in each isolation room, whereas a toilet in each patient area is desirable but not required. If the unit typically has a high census of infectious patients and an inadequate number of isolation rooms, a toilet in each area is an asset. When space is at a premium, use of a "Pullman" toilet may meet the need for toilet facilities.

Staff Areas

Nurses' Station

The ICU nurses' station is quite different from that on a typical medical/surgical nursing unit. The level of activity is higher, as is the acuity of the patients. The nursing station must be located such that direct visual surveillance of all patients is possible. The distance between the station and each bed should be as short as possible. The corridor around the station should be of sufficient width to accommodate the movement of staff, equipment, and supplies. The required minimum of 8 feet is often exceeded. The nursing station should contain a work area for the ward clerk, as well as an adequate writing surface for physicians, nurses, and other technical and support staff. The station should also include adequate space for storage of records, forms, and supplies, for some type of chart rack system, and for monitoring and closed-circuit television screens. A physician dictation area with telephone hookup can be located in the station or in a proximate physician workroom.

Careful analysis of the number of people and the types and volume of equipment will dictate the size of the nurses' station. The ultimate design enhances performance of the activities accomplished here by differentiating among computer work areas, stand-up charting counters, dictation cubicles, etc.

The medication preparation area often is inappropriately located within the nursing station. Studies of nurses preparing and administering drugs on a conventional unit have shown that on average, 18 percent, or one medication in six, is in error [10]. Two major causes of medication error are haste and interruption, and medication errors are more serious in the ICU because of the acuity of the patients. Thus, the medication area should be located away from the nursing station functions at a place where there is no visual surveillance of the patients and no possibility of phone interruptions. Equipment includes a counter top, a medication refrigerator, shelving, a locked narcotics cabinet, a sink with hot and cold water, and facilities for whatever unit dose system is in place.

Clean and Soiled Utility

Codes require separate processing areas for clean and soiled items. The clean utility should contain a limited inventory of clean storage (procedure trays, bandages, pads, etc.) and intravenous solutions. The room should also include a sink, a work counter, and a supply distribution/storage system. Whether the supply system operates via exchange carts or par-level restocking, wire carts are the storage system of choice, because they are easier to clean and more sanitary than are solid shelving systems. The linen cart may also be stored in this room, or it may be stored in a separate room or alcove.

A soiled utility room must be accessible to but separate from other work areas. Here are held bagged waste material and disposables, soiled reusable items awaiting transfer to central supply, and soiled linens. The room should contain a sink, hopper, and bedpan flusher. If each patient room has a toilet with bedpan flusher, the soiled utility room can be smaller.

Storage
The unit must have alcoves and storerooms for crash carts, defibrillators, stretchers, ventilators, scales, portable x-ray machine, IV poles, stretchers, and other equipment. Space requirements vary according to the size of the unit and inventory requirements. If a well-functioning equipment distribution system is in place, this area may be smaller. Given very high construction costs, it may be more cost-effective to store idle equipment in a central storage facility than in the ICU.

Nourishment Area
This area provides storage and preparation space for patient nourishments. The size and amount of equipment will depend on the hospital's dietary service. Once again, given the number of higher-priority and better uses for expensive space, it is recommended that space for this function be limited in the ICU. The area should include a small refrigerator, a counter, a sink, an ice maker, a microwave oven, and minimal storage cabinets.

Special-Procedures/Treatment Room
The trend in recent years has been to perform as much diagnostic and therapeutic work as possible in the ICU patient room, in order to keep patient transport to an absolute minimum. This has meant an ever-increasing amount of space devoted to each patient area. For such procedures as inserting indwelling arterial lines, Swan-Ganz catheters, and pacemakers, guidance is generally provided by a fluoroscopic C-arm unit. If this is done in the patient room, the patient must be on a radiographically transparent bed. The patient room must be large enough to accommodate not only staff, C-arm, and life-support equipment, but also adequate shielding to protect staff and all other patients from excessive radiation exposure.

An alternative in large ICUs is to provide a special-procedures room with C-arm, fluoroscopic, or cardiac catheterization equipment. These rooms range in size from 300 to 600 square feet. The decision as to whether or not to provide a special-procedures room depends on the distance and inconvenience of using facilities in imaging services or cardiology, as well as the frequency such a facility would be used. Both capital and operating costs are issues to contend with.

Department Satellites
Other departments will need staff and support space in the ICU, on a part-time or a full-time basis. Dietary, social service, chaplaincy, and other departments may share a consultation room, or each may require a dedicated office, depending on the scope of services provided and the number of patients served.

The need for laboratory, respiratory therapy, or pharmacy satellites depends on the proximity of these departments to ICU and the ability of the central department to respond to ICU staff and patient needs. Sometimes the desired accessibility can be enhanced by mechanical conveyance (pneumatic tube, dumbwaiter, etc.) or by expanded computer interface.

The decision to provide a satellite should take into account not only the cost of the space and equipment, but also operating costs and quality control issues. The hospital must consider the volume of service to be provided by the satellite, the scope of services to be rendered, the hours of operation and the corresponding number of skilled technicians or professionals required, duplication of expensive equipment, quality control, security, and access to professional staff for support and training.

Unit Support

Various nonclinical areas are vital components of any ICU. These areas, which should be clustered away from the busy traffic areas and can be located outside the inner clean core although adjacent to the ICU, include the following:

Conference room—with x-ray view boxes and audiovisual capability.
Staff lounge—with microwave oven, refrigerator, and comfortable furniture.
On-call rooms—with a bed and desk, access to shower and toilet, and telephone or intercom connection to the ICU.
Offices—for medical director, secretaries, head nurse, clinical nurse specialist, etc.; consider shared office for dietitian, social worker, home care coordinator, etc., depending upon size of unit.
Male and female lockers/toilets/showers—should be contiguous to staff lounge.
Family waiting—on average, 1.5 to 2 seats per bed is adequate; should be comfortable and relaxing; seating should be in small clusters, affording some privacy to family groups; areas should include house and public telephones and adjacent toilet facilities.
Grieving room—should be adjacent to family waiting, social work, or pastoral care offices; should seat four to six or more people in a comfortable environment with indirect lighting.
Housekeeping closet—in the unit; should not serve other departments or nursing units; must be large enough to store all supplies and equipment kept by housekeeping on the unit and must include a floor sink.

Figure 2-3 is a generic schematic of two 8-bed ICUs that illustrates some of the principles discussed above, such as patient visibility, separation of work areas, and optional departmental satellite locations.

Space Requirements for Nutrition

Space requirements for nutritional care are sometimes ignored in designing an ICU on the basis that the average length of stay in the unit is too short for nutritional deficits to make any difference. Further, it is assumed that whatever deficits may occur will be made up upon discharge to another part of the hospital. There is growing awareness of the fallacies in this attitude, which ignores the following points.

1. Malnutrition develops more quickly in acutely ill patients.
2. Malnutrition may have been present but unsuspected at the start of the ICU patient's acute condition.

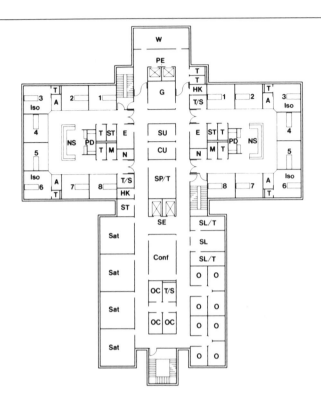

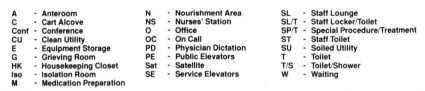

LEGEND

A	- Anteroom	N	- Nourishment Area	SL	- Staff Lounge
C	- Cart Alcove	NS	- Nurses' Station	SL/T	- Staff Locker/Toilet
Conf	- Conference	O	- Office	SP/T	- Special Procedure/Treatment
CU	- Clean Utility	OC	- On Call	ST	- Staff Toilet
E	- Equipment Storage	PD	- Physician Dictation	SU	- Soiled Utility
G	- Grieving Room	PE	- Public Elevators	T	- Toilet
HK	- Housekeeping Closet	Sat	- Satellite	T/S	- Toilet/Shower
Iso	- Isolation Room	SE	- Service Elevators	W	- Waiting
M	- Medication Preparation				

Fig. 2-3. Typical critical care floor plan.

3. The clinical appearance of early weight loss and depletion is often obscured by fluid retention.
4. It is becoming recognized that loss of function can occur with smaller degrees of nutritional deficit than previously thought.
5. Every physician must decide how to estimate the extent of nutritional deficit in any patient and how much deficit is acceptable before aggressive nutritional support is undertaken.

The ICU for cardiac monitoring must provide nutritious meals that follow certain requirements, but this task can be handled by a competent dietitian who utilizes a diet kitchen on the ICU or orders special foods from a central dietary department. But the growth of intensive care has been accompanied by advances not only in monitoring, but also in mechanical life support systems and in pharmacology. These developments over the past 20 years have been paralleled by growing availability of specialized products, both enteral and parenteral, that can be utilized in a safe and effective manner [15,16].

Nutrition support should be represented in the plans for an ICU just as the pharmacy is represented. There is a recurrent need to decide whether the unit should be autonomous, with its own solution preparation area, or should depend on the hospital-wide nutritional support service. Even in the latter case, some space will have to be allocated to nutritional functions in the unit, in order to address the need for storage of some solutions and for desk and file space for preparation and analysis of nutritional activities in the ICU and nutritional assessment of patients.

Systems

Materials Management

Modern materials management systems relieve caregivers of the mundane tasks of purchasing, receiving, storing, transporting, inventorying, and restocking, thus allowing caregivers to focus on patient care. For such a system to work, it is essential that the materials management staff share the caregiver's concern for the patient. At the same time, requirements for service must be fiscally responsible in terms of maintaining reasonable inventory levels in the hospital and in the ICU. The desire to maintain a large inventory of supplies in the ICU is detrimental in three ways: (1) large volumes of supplies require copious amounts of space, which reduces the area available for patient care (ICU space costs two to three times the cost of storage in materials management); (2) low turnover of supplies leads to outdated sterile supplies; and (3) the money invested in excess supplies reduces the hospital's cash flow and can impair the institution's financial viability.

Two materials management systems address these needs. The first, the exchange cart system, provides full rotation of the stock whenever the carts are exchanged, keeps the supplies in a preestablished location on the unit, provides a system to clean the storage racks, eliminates the need for inventorying on the unit, and allows supply restocking with minimum disruption in the ICU.

A quality alternative system is par-level stocking, which is fully managed by the materials management staff. In this system, supply levels would be inventoried daily by materials personnel. Advantages include transport of fewer supplies through the hospital (unused supplies remain on the unit rather than being returned to stores), less capital tied up in expensive exchange carts, and the ability to manage supplies in more than one location in the ICU. Disadvantages include the need for inventorying, restocking, and checking for out-of-date supplies on the units—procedures that can be disruptive to caregivers and present the potential for unwanted noise.

Both systems can respond to long-term and short-term changes in demand. Monitoring of average daily usage of each item and of day-to-day fluctuation in demand allows the setting of appropriate par levels for restocking. Should the ICU get one or more patients requiring supplies in larger-than-normal quantities (i.e, for burn care or dialysis), the ICU staff can notify materials management to temporarily increase the par level for specific items or to add items not usually on the list. In any event, feedback and communication are essential to the maintenance of an effective restocking system. It is also essential to have a backup system for quickly providing needed items. A mechanical system, such as a dumbwaiter or mechanical cart that connects materials management directly to the ICU, is ideal. A 24-hour stat delivery service or a nearby backup supply cart can be effective alternatives. Requiring the nursing supervisor to obtain supplies from the storeroom and deliver them to ICU is not a practical alternative.

Data Processing and Communications Systems
The explosive growth of computer technology has made computers a common feature of the modern ICU. However, the computer has often been introduced into an environment in which neither the design nor the standard operating procedures have allowed optimum use.

Early computers in hospitals were most useful for handling finances, billing, and inventory. Computer applications in the ICU proved much more challenging. An early application was the transmittal of laboratory reports to terminals on the ICU, where a printout was made for the patient record. The collection and storage of bedside physiologic monitoring data have proved to be more difficult to develop and effectively blend with the biochemical data from the laboratory, especially in a form suitable for a permanent medicolegal record.

It has become apparent that medical professionals think about data much more effectively when it is properly graphed than when it is presented as columns of figures. The challenge has been to understand how to organize patient data to assist and enhance clinical "pattern recognition" [23]. Improved graphic presentation of patient data will become progressively available, but the increased amounts of memory and storage capability will require space in the unit or in a remote location equipped with adequate facilities for data transmission.

A decision is required as to whether the ICU should be as autonomous as possible in data processing capabilities, or whether it should share the hospital's central facilities—including a mainframe computer that probably was not intended for tasks such as processing of data from patient monitoring. In planning for the future, it is essential to allow for extensive computerization within the ICU, for both administrative and patient care purposes. Administrative capabilities include ordering tests and therapy, receiving reports, tracking patient charges, and maintaining the patient record.

The introduction of physiologic monitoring at the bedside has increased the volume of ICU patient data available to the caregiver [10]. Computer applications for collecting, storing, and manipulating data are steadily being expanded, to reduce the "overload" of information presented as part of patient management. Data processing systems have been used, with caution, to "close the loop"—that is, to analyze patient data and activate the administration of medication or increments of a blood transfusion depending upon the patient's condition. However, the most impressive system for recognizing and interpreting all kinds of patient data at the bedside is still the experienced ICU nurse!

The patient care computer typically is a separate system that may be centralized in one location or decentralized through placement of a data processing unit at each bedside. The variety of available equipment is extensive, and each hospital must evaluate which system is best for its requirements. However, it can be generalized that the future requirements for data transmission to and from each ICU patient bedside will continue to grow. Fiberoptic cables have become the technology of choice for broadband, high-volume data transmission. At present, the premiums for installing fiberoptic cables are only 20 percent over the cost of installing traditional twisted-pair copper wiring and 10 percent over that of coaxial cables. Provision should be made for future expansion for systems not yet envisioned. This can be done by making it possible to add cabling in the future or by installing spare data lines during construction. If a central computer is not planned initially, it would be appropriate to designate a 100-to-150-square-foot room that could be used for this purpose in the future. Cabling should be run so that it can be accessed in this room. Until the time the room is actually used for the computer, it can be used as an office, for storage, or for any other functions that could be relocated easily.

An additional piece of equipment being installed in some ICUs is the gas chromatograph, which could be installed in the computer room. Sampling tubes must be run to each patient's bedside, much like fiberoptic cable. Ideally, the data output of the gas chromatograph should feed into the patient care computer.

An additional benefit of computer systems is the capability to provide administrative and patient care data to the physician's office, which allows the physician to check on the patient more frequently without telephoning the nursing station. By this means, the physician can also order tests, prescribe treatment, and complete charts more easily.

The transfer of information in the ICU should not victimize the patient. Printers and keyboards that are near the patient should be as quiet as possible; touch-sense screens on video display terminals are easy to use and facilitate staff training. Telephone and intercom systems in the new ICU should permit turning off the ringer on patient telephones and incorporate pleasant-sounding rings or loudness controls on telephones in the nursing station and other phones that can be heard by patients. The intercom system should permit contact with staff throughout the unit, including the special-procedures room, the director's office, and staff lounges.

Clinical data processing in the ICU can be expected to play an increasingly important role in patient care in the coming years. But a related aspect of data processing in the ICU has received too little attention: namely, how will the records room deal with the expanding amount of ICU data from each patient? Should the ICU have sufficient space and personnel to permit the data from each patient day to be reduced and summarized for permanent storage? Or should the ICU provide even greater storage capability, to postpone the task of data reduction for many days, or even until patient discharge?

Environmental Systems

The capabilities of the ICU's environmental systems are dictated by building codes and by the hospital's budget. The optimum system is rarely affordable. For example, it may not be practical to provide a system through which each patient room can be individually switched from positive to negative air pressure for isolation or reverse isolation. Likewise, it is expensive to provide a separate temperature control for each office and storage room on the unit. However, the temperature of each patient room should be individually adjustable. Because of the complexities of heating/ventilating/air conditioning (HVAC) systems and the potential of linking new systems to existing air handlers, heat sources, and chilled water sources, decisions about environmental systems should be deferred until a competent hospital HVAC engineer is hired for the project. Such an engineer is as important for renovation projects as for new construction, because of the incapacity of some older buildings to accommodate the mechanical components of a modern HVAC system for an ICU. Frequently, it is found that space for the associated mechanical systems is so limited in existing structures that the only alternative is to place the ICU in new construction.

Patient Environment

Rest and sleep are essential components of the recovery process, yet both are often difficult in the ICU. Rest may elude the patient due to noise; lack of privacy; annoying bright or flashing lights; and the lack of familiar identifiable events, which results in a tendency to disorient the patient and increase stress [7].

Interest in the physiology of sleep and its relationship to clinical recovery will undoubtedly increase over the coming years, and it can be anticipated that the time will come when a quantitative indication of a patient's night sleep will be included in the next day's summary of his physiologic state. Until we can quantitate the quality of sleep better, it is wise to make every effort possible in the ICU to provide a "sleep possible" environment.

Control of the following elements can substantially increase patient comfort and improve the patient's ability to rest and recover.

Temperature

In each patient room or cubicle, air flow and temperature should be controlled to match the needs of the patient. Air should not blow directly on the patient.

Lighting

The patient area should have a lighting system that provides indirect lighting for general care and reduced lighting at night time. Switchable direct lighting is needed over each patient bed for examination or procedures and should be used on a need basis. Other lights on the unit should be shielded, to prevent glare.

Windows
Windows are now required by code in all ICU patient rooms. However, their importance in the ICU often is not fully recognized. Sunlight, or at least daylight, appears to play an important emotional role in preventing sensory affective disorder (SAD), which is now recognized as a genuine clinical entity. Is it possible that the ICU depressions that have been written about in the past could have been aggravated by lack of natural light?

Windows, along with a clock and calendar, help to orient the patient to day-night cycles and the passage of time. Windows oriented to provide a view of the city or landscape allow the patient to focus on something besides illness or pain. The windows should be fitted with drapes or blinds so that direct sunlight does not fall on the patient's eyes and that the brightness of the room can be controlled to prevent excessive solar thermal gain.

Privacy
Walls, curtains, and other visual barriers should be designed so as to provide patient-to-patient visual privacy while allowing the staff to keep an eye on patients.

Noise
Intensive care units can be exceedingly noisy places. Because studies have shown that disruptive noise creates stress and can affect heart and respiration rates, it is appropriate to find ways to reduce unwanted noise in the ICU [7]. Sources of noise include monitors and alarms within the patient room/module and elsewhere in the ICU, printers, various mechanical sounds from respirators, the HVAC system, oxygen bubbling through a humidifier, and the sounds generated by opening supply packets, tearing paper from a printer, the paging/nurse intercom, moving furniture and equipment, beepers, and general talking on the unit. Such sounds are particularly disruptive when they have no relevance to the patient. The fact that the patient cannot control the noise factor may lead to frustration, thereby adding stress to an already stressful situation. Efforts should be made during the design process to incorporate low-noise equipment, shield noisy items to reduce the sound level reaching the patient, incorporate sound-absorbing materials into walls, ceiling and floors wherever possible, and keep noisy items and areas (i.e., conference rooms, lockers, printers, paging speakers, alarms, and nursing stations) as shielded from the patient room as possible [11].

Room Decor
Make the patient environment warm and comfortable from the patient's perspective through use of soft, restful colors and textures. A picture or something of visual interest provides an area for the patient to focus on in addition to the window.

BUILDING AND LIFE SAFETY CODE COMPLIANCE

Stringent building and life safety codes and standards govern both the design and the operation of all health care facilities. These rules and regulations are promulgated by many different local, state, federal, and quasi-voluntary agencies (such as Joint Commission on Accreditation of Healthcare Organizations). Not infrequently, various codes and standards appear to be in conflict. Further, codes are subject to differing interpretations by individuals even within the same agency. Finally, because codes and standards often deal with highly technical aspects of building construction, the user should rely on the design professional—i.e., architect or engineer—to accept responsibility that applicable codes are met for any new or renovated construction.

REFERENCES

1. *AHA Guide.* Chicago: American Hospital Association, 1988.
2. Berk, J. L., and Sampliner, J. E. *Handbook of Critical Care* (2nd ed.). Boston: Little, Brown, 1982.
3. Committee on Hospital Care of the American Academy of Pediatrics and the Pediatric Section of the Society of Critical Care Medicine. *Guidelines for Pediatric Intensive Care Unit.* Baltimore: Williams & Wilkins, 1983.
4. Cullen, D. J., Ferrara, L. C., Briggs, B. A., et al. Survival, hospitalization charges and follow-up results in critically ill patients. *N. Engl. J. Med.* 294:982, 1976.
5. Garner, J. S. *Isolation Techniques in Critical Care Units.* Germantown, MD: Aspen Systems Corporation, 1980.
6. Grenvik, A. Specialty Intensive Care Units. In *Hospital Special-Care Facilities.* New York: Academic, 1981.
7. Hansell, H. N. The Behavioral effects of noise on man: The patient with intensive care unit psychosis. *Heart and Lung* 13:59, 1984.
8. Haynie, W. E., and Hayet, L. Neonatal ICU Meets Present, Future Demand." *Hospitals* Feb. 16, 1980:145.
9. Health Services and Promotion Branch, Department of National Health and Welfare. *Evaluation and space programming methodology for special care units.* Montreal: The Minister of National Health and Welfare, November, 1979.
10. Hill, D. W. Monitoring Equipment and Unit Design. In J. Tinker and M. Rapin (eds.), *Care of the Critically Ill Patient.* New York: Springer-Verlag, 1983.
11. Hilton, A. The hospital racket: How noisy is your unit? *Am. J. Nurs.* 87:59, 1987.
12. Hudson, L. D. Design of the intensive care unit from a monitoring point of view. *Respir. Care* 30:549, 1985.
13. Kinney, J. M. Design of the Intensive Care Unit. In J. L. Berk and J. E. Sampliner (eds.), *Handbook of Critical Care* (2nd ed.). Boston: Little, Brown, 1982.
14. Kinney, J. M., Bendixen, H. H., and Powers, S. R. (eds.). *Manual of Surgical Intensive Care.* Philadelphia: Saunders, 1977.
15. Kinney, J. M. Nutrition in the intensive care patient. *Crit. Care Clin.* 3:1, 1987.
16. Kinney, J. M., Elwyn, D. H., and Carpentier, Y. A. The Intensive Care Patient. In J. M. Kinney, K. N. Jeejeebhoy, G. L. Hill, O. E. Own (eds.) *Nutrition and Metabolism in Patient Care.* Philadelphia: Saunders, 1988. P. 656.
17. Kruse, J. A., et al. Comparison of clinical assessment with APACHE II for predicting mortality risk in patients admitted to a medical intensive care unit. *J.A.M.A* 260:1739, 1988.

18. Laufman, H. In *Hospital Special-Care Facilities*. New York: Academic, 1981.
19. The National Association of Children's Hospitals and Related Institutions, Inc. *Study to Quantify the Uniqueness of Children's Hospitals*. Wilmington, DE, 1978.
20. Office of Medical Application of Research and National Institutes. Critical care medicine. In *J.A.M.A.* 250:798, 1983.
21. Piergeorge, A. R., Cesarano, F. L., and Casanova, D. M. Designing the Critical Care Unit: A Multidisciplinary Approach. In *Critical Care Medicine*. Baltimore: Williams & Wilkins, 1983. P. 541.
22. Preston, G. A., Larson, E. L., and Stamm, W. E. The effect of private isolation rooms on patient care practices, colonization and infection in an intensive care unit. *Am. J. Med.* 70:641, 1981.
23. Putsep, E. *Modern Hospital*. London: Lloyd-Duke, 1979. P. 321.
24. Shoemaker, W. C., Thompson, L. W., and Holbrook, P. R. *Textbook of Critical Care*. Philadelphia: Saunders, 1984.
25. Stoddart, J. C. *Design, Staffing, and Equipment Requirements for an Intensive Care Unit*. International Anesthesiology Clinics, 1981 19(2) 77–95 J. C. Stoddart, 1980.
26. Task Force on Guidelines. The Society of Critical Care Medicine. Recommendations for critical care unit design. *Crit. Care Med.* 16(8):796, 1988.
27. Why Build Special Care Units? *Hospitals* Feb. 16, 1980. P. 78.
28. Yu, P. Historical aspects of intensive coronary care. *Curr. Probl. in Cardiol.* 5(8):5, 1980.
29. Office of Construction. *Planning Criteria for VA Facilities*. Washington, D.C.: Veterans Administration, 1980.

Multiple Organ Failure

James L. Berk

The reader may wonder why the chapter on multiple organ failure (MOF) appears near the beginning of the book rather than near the end. It is true that multiple organ failure occurs late in the course of a critically ill patient and often marks the terminal phase of the illness; accordingly, it would logically appear in sequence after the chapters dealing with specific organ systems. However, even though the multiple organ failure syndrome appears to result from a systemic response of the host to uncontrolled illness, and definitive therapy to control the humoral substances thought to be responsible is not yet clinically available, much can be done to help prevent multiple organ failure. Several common factors contributing to multiple organ failure can be treated, and, in addition, failure of individual organs can be treated, which if uncorrected can contribute to failure of other organs and result in progressive multiple organ failure. Thus, meticulous attention to details early in the illness of a critically ill patient in many instances may prevent multiple organ failure late in the illness. It is my intent that by presenting this chapter early, the reader will gain an understanding of the many identifiable factors involved in the pathogenesis of multiple organ failure. Such an understanding, it is hoped, will make the ensuing chapters more closely interrelated and more meaningful.

Advances in organ system support and monitoring have permitted the prolonged survival of critically ill patients and thereby created a new syndrome called Multiple Organ Failure. This syndrome commonly follows severe trauma or major surgery and is frequently associated with uncontrolled sepsis, but it may occur with any type of serious illness, such as gastrointestinal hemorrhage, pneumonia, pancreatitis, diverticulitis, or shock from any cause.

During the 1930s and early World War II cardiovascular collapse, or shock, was the major limitation to survival. An understanding of the role of blood loss in shock and the introduction of blood-banking techniques permitted the salvage of many patients with massive blood loss. By the end of World War II, acute renal failure following trauma had become the condition that limited survival; subsequently, the use of dialysis permitted the survival of many patients with established renal failure. During the Vietnam conflict, rapid evacuation and prompt fluid replacement resulted in survival from previously fatal injuries, and acute respiratory failure, referred to as shock lung, became recognized. Thus, the successful treatment of one failing organ has permitted longer survival and the subsequent failure of other organs.

Many of the surviving patients whose organ systems are good enough will develop a hypermetabolic-hyperdynamic state with a high cardiac index, low peripheral resistance, increased oxygen consumption, and excessive protein catabolism producing severe body wasting. Multiple organ failure seems to be a response to the hyperdynamic-hypermetabolic state, and inadequate cellular perfusion relative to metabolic needs seems to be its hallmark. Survival does not appear to be predictable from the usual admission severity scores, but visceral blood flow and oxygen consumption do appear to be major determinants of survival [1, 14, 16, 21, 32].

Many humoral substances—e.g., catecholamines, thyroxin, glucagon, insulin, corticosteroids, growth hormone, histamine, myocardial depressant factor, lysosomal enzymes, prostaglandins, complement, kinins, endotoxin, proteases, serotonin, free-oxygen radicals, fibronectin, interleukins, cachectin, and neuropeptides—are released or activated by perfusion deficits, hypoxia, invading microorganisms, and injured or dead tissue and are responsible for the metabolic, circulatory, and immunologic changes observed in critically ill patients. Some of the effects of these substances are compensatory early in the course of the illness, but if the illness continues unabated, it appears that these mediator substances contribute to the development of multiple organ failure [3, 4, 6, 8, 13, 15, 17, 19, 37].

Control of the mediator substances ultimately will be the treatment of choice for multiple organ failure, but, unfortunately, this modality is still largely investigational. Corticosteroids—long a controversial drug in critically ill patients—in pharmacologic doses have not improved survival in patients with multiple organ failure [33]. Thus, the best treatment of multiple organ failure is prevention. One must promptly identify the known factors that can contribute to organ failure, including both those common to all organs and those specific for individual organs. Correct the primary initiating illness as soon as possible: treat perfusion deficits, eliminate infectious foci, debride necrotic tissue, and stabilize fractures. Provide adequate oxygenation and ventilation, along with sufficient nutrition to prevent malnutrition. Monitor individual organ function to detect problems before overt organ failure occurs and be aware of the possible deleterious effects of therapy. Failure of an organ that has not been or can no longer be corrected may affect other organs and set up a vicious cycle of failing organs—a physiologic domino effect. Finally, a stage is reached at which the treatment of one failing organ results in the failure of other organs, making survival unlikely. The greater the number of failing organs, the less likely is survival [8, 36].

Trauma may affect organ function directly (e.g., a myocardial contusion) or indirectly, due to circulatory and respiratory failure. Prompt resuscitation with establishment of an airway, adequate oxygenation and ventilation, and appropriate fluid replacement, followed by required surgery—which may include hemostasis, debridement of devitalized tissues, repair of damaged viscera, or stabilization of fractures—may prevent multiple organ failure much later in the course of illness.

Following major surgery, trauma, and other critical illnesses, there is an increased energy requirement and a negative nitrogen balance related to stress. Both are greatly increased by the hypermetabolic state. Caloric requirements may approach 40 to 70 cal/kg/day, or 5000 cal/day, in the hypermetabolic state. Three liters of 5% dextrose in water will supply 600 calories. Protein losses may approach 250 gm/day, with additional losses of 10 to 50 gm/day in patients with burns, draining fistulas, pancreatitis, peritonitis, or intestinal obstruction. Severe malnutrition can develop in a few days, with patients losing more than 3 lb of muscle and other organ tissue per day. Studies in surgical patients have shown that an acute loss of 30 percent of body weight in 30 days is uniformly fatal.

Malnutrition is a common and major contributing factor to multiple organ failure. In addition to starvation, the metabolic changes of the hypermetabolic state of critical illness must be understood and treated. In the hypermetabolic state the resting energy expenditure increases. Differing from starvation, in which the carbon source for oxidation is glucose in the early stages and mostly fatty acids and ketones later, in the hypermetabolic state there is mixed substrate oxidation. The fraction of total energy expenditure derived from glucose is significantly reduced, and the fraction derived from the direct oxidation of amino acids is significantly increased. The remainder of the energy expenditure is derived from the direct oxidation of fats, probably the medium- and long-chain variety. As organ failure progresses, still more is derived from amino acids. Paradoxically, despite the severely increased catabolism of protein stores, total body protein synthesis is decreased, resulting in marked and rapid protein depletion, primarily of skeletal muscles and abdominal viscera. Additional nutrition over and above that required to prevent starvation is needed to prevent substrate-limited metabolism and loss of organ structure and function. Glucose has a protein-sparing effect but caloric intake in excess of 50 kcal/kg does not continue to have an appreciable additive effect on the severe protein catabolism and may produce untoward effects, including the fatty liver syndrome, hyperglycemia with hyperosmolar complications, and increased resting energy expenditure and CO_2 production—the latter resulting in increased ventilation and the potential for respiratory failure. To prevent these problems in patients with the hypermetabolic state, the glucose load generally should not exceed 5 mg/kg/min, the nonprotein caloric load should not exceed 35 to 40 cal/kg/day, and the caloric/nitrogen ratio should be no more than 100 nonprotein calories per gram of administered nitrogen. Because there is variability, however, measurement of the resting energy expenditure may be helpful.

Intravenous emulsions of long-chain fatty acid triglycerides, when substituted for glucose calories, can control many of the problems associated with excess glucose administration. They also have been shown to have a protein-sparing effect at least equivalent to that of glucose and to assist in maintaining organ structure and function. Doses greater than 2 to 3 gm/kg/day may induce fatty liver. Current recommendations are that fatty emulsions supply 30 to 40 percent of the nonprotein calories and that their clearance be monitored.

Studies have shown that the administration of large amounts of amino acids modified to include branched-chain amino acids and to reduce amino acids that are potentially hepatotoxic and that promote gluconeogenesis (already markedly increased) can increase total body protein synthesis, so that nitrogen balance can be achieved in many instances. The current recommendation is to begin at 2 gm/kg/day and to adjust the dose until nitrogen equilibrium is established.

Thus, it is clear that the correct amounts and mix of glucose, fat, and amino acids supplied for alimentation are important in preventing MOF and, conversely, that incorrect amounts and mix can contribute to organ failure [5, 7, 8, 9, 11, 35].

Critically ill patients with alimentary tract dysfunction should receive early total parenteral nutrition (TPN), to supply the increased energy required for fuel and the proteins needed to make essential enzymes and to maintain cellular structure. If the patient cannot be expected with reasonable certainty to take and absorb adequate oral nutrition within 5 to 7 days, parenteral hyperalimentation should be begun as soon as the patient is hemodynamically stable. Withholding TPN because of its possible risks and because it is anticipated that the patient will be able to take nutrition orally "in a few days" frequently results in malnutrition due to unforseen problems and delays.

Enteral feeding is an underused modality of supplying nutrition for critically ill patients. With the feeding tube placed distal to the pylorus at surgery, under fluoroscopy, or by endoscopy, aspiration has been rare and effective absorption has been achieved in the presence of mild ileus. In addition to avoiding the complications of parenteral nutrition, enteral feeding may have benefits over the intravenous route such as prevention of stress ulcers and hepatic dysfunction, and, in this regard, it may alter the progression of multiple organ failure [12, 27].

Remember! Malnutrition is a major factor contributing to MOF and can be prevented.

Injured, postoperative, and critically ill patients may develop an altered immune response and decreased resistance to infection [6, 13, 22, 28, 29]. This state of acquired immunodeficiency can be an important factor in the development of sepsis from contamination or in the inability of the patient to combat an established infectious process. The degree of suppression is related to the magnitude of the stress. Additional factors that contribute to the decreased immune response are anesthesia, shock, blood loss, sepsis, malnutrition, liver disease, and drugs (e.g., corticosteroids and Imuran). Depressed neutrophil antibacterial activity and depressed lymphocyte function have been demonstrated in patients following trauma and elective surgery. A deficiency of opsonins (serum proteins that interact with organisms to increase cellular recognition and removal by phagocytosis) has been demonstrated in patients following trauma. Systemic reticuloendo-thelial (RE) system depression occurs after trauma and in a variety of shock states. Failure of the hepatic RE system may permit bacteria from the gastrointestinal tract to enter the pulmonary circulation and contribute to a continuing septic state [34].

With contamination, bacteremia is more likely to occur and, in turn, may cause further impairment of the RE system. In addition, many seriously ill patients do not exhibit a skin reaction when antigens are injected into the skin. This anergy or depression of the delayed hypersensitivity response has been correlated with depressed neutrophil function and is associated with an increased incidence of infection, septicemia, and death related to the infection. Erosion of the body cell mass has been correlated with the anergic state. Adequate nutrition and aggressive surgical drainage of the infection will restore the delayed hypersensitivity response, improve abnormal cellular and serum components of host defense, and increase survival. Late nutrition after the development of septic complications may not correct contracture of body cell mas and the anergic state. Thus, stress, trauma, drugs, inadequate nutrition, and infection itself can alter the host immune response and defense against infection, which, when established, can result directly in multiple organ failure.

Adult Respiratory Distress Syndrome (ARDS) is the name most often given to acute respiratory failure occurring in critically ill patients. Many other names, depending on the clinical setting, have also been given to this syndrome (Table 3-1).

In most critically ill patients who develop multiple organ failure, the lung is usually the first organ to fail, and other organs follow in a characteristic sequential pattern. This pattern, together with the associated finding of impaired peripheral oxygen utilization in patients with ARDS, adds support to the concept that systemic factors play a major role in the pathogenesis of ARDS and multiple organ failure [20]. In addition, the lung appears to be a key organ in the development of multiple organ failure [2]. The failing lung may be a source of inflammatory mediators that can damage downstream organs, or failure of the lung's metabolic clearance activity may permit still more toxic substances to reach distal organs. As pulmonary failure progresses, particularly in situations in which the complement system is strongly activated, hypoxia appears to contribute to multiple organ failure. The majority of patients dying with ARDS die of multiple organ failure and hemodynamic instability, rather than impaired gas exchange [2, 17, 18, 25, 26, 38].

Even though ARDS appears to be a systemic response to uncontrolled illness and definitive treatment is not yet available, it should not be concluded that little can be done other than respiratory support and control of the basic illness. The old concept that ARDS can be diagnosed by a chest x-ray and that it is progressive, usually resulting in death regardless of the treatment, has long been put to rest. Acute respiratory failure can be diagnosed, but there is no way to make a definitive diagnosis of ARDS except by exclusion and in retrospect. X-ray patterns are suggestive but not diagnostic.

Table 3-1. Synonyms for acute respiratory failure in the critically ill patient

Shock lung
Posttraumatic pulmonary insufficiency
Respiratory distress syndrome (RDS)
Acute respiratory distress syndrome (ARDS)
Adult respiratory distress syndrome (ARDS)
Acute respiratory failure
Congestive atelectasis
Da Nang lung
Hemorrhagic atelectasis
Pump lung
Posttransfusion lung
Progressive pulmonary consolidation
Respiratory lung
Stiff lung syndrome
Traumatic lung
Transplant lung
White lung syndrome
Adult hyaline membrane disease
Pulmonary hyaline membrane disease
Noncardiac pulmonary edema
Wet lung of trauma
Respiratory insufficiency syndrome
Progressive respiratory distress
Progressive pulmonary consolidation
Hemorrhagic lung syndrome
Bronchopulmonary dysplasia

   As is the case with other failing organs, the best treatment for acute respiratory failure is prevention and in this respect a great deal can be done. Acute respiratory failure occurs frequently if the PaO_2 is evaluated in relation to the fraction inspired oxygen. When respiratory failure is diagnosed, ventilation and oxygenation should be supported by whatever means are required. The underlying illness should be corrected as soon as possible. Treat shock and ensure adequate total body perfusion including that required for the hypermetabolic-hyperdynamic state. In critically ill patients with unexplained tachypnea and respiratory alkalosis and an inappropriately low PaO_2, suspect infection. Often the pulse, temperature, and white blood count are increased, but not always. The source of sepsis may not be obvious and must be actively sought not only by careful physical examination but by x-ray, ultrasound, scans, CT and MRI. Adequate treatment of the infection including drainage of an abscess can reverse progressive respiratory failure and prevent multiple organ failure. Conversely, survival is not likely, regardless of all other medical care, if the

Table 3-2. Causes of acute respiratory failure in the critically ill patient

1. Fluid overload
2. Left heart failure
3. Trauma: fractured ribs, flail chest, pneumohemothorax, contusion of lung and heart
4. Sepsis
5. Shock
6. Atelectasis
7. Inadequate tracheobronchial toilet
8. Thromboembolism
9. Fat embolism
10. Aspiration pneumonia
11. Bacterial pneumonia
12. Viral pneumonia
13. Abdominal distention
14. Multiple blood transfusions—particulate matter
15. Oxygen toxicity
16. Ventilator injury
17. Cardiopulmonary bypass
18. Humoral substances
19. Transfusion reactions
20. Head injuries
21. Burns
22. Drug abuse—heroin pulmonary edema
23. Anaphylaxis
24. Metabolic—hypophosphatemia
25. Preexisting lung disease

abscess is not adequately drained. Supply required nutrition early to prevent malnutrition. In addition, many other factors, sometimes neglected, are additive and can contribute to respiratory failure, many of which can be prevented or treated (Table 3-2). Early attention to details can prevent progressive pulmonary insufficiency several days later.

Because the low PaO_2 in patients with incipient ARDS results in part from interstitial edema due to increased capillary permeability, it is easy to understand why these patients are particularly vulnerable to a fluid overload or left heart failure, which together, in my experience, contribute to acute respiratory failure in a high percentage of critically ill surgical patients admitted to the ICU. Avoid overhydration following resuscitation from all types of shock. If high-output renal failure is not present, hourly urine outputs greater than 50 ml/hr suggest overhydration and set the stage for pulmonary failure several days later. Overhydration is not uncommon in small, critically ill patients in an antidiuretic state who are receiving intravenous fluids for prolonged periods. A patient may require no more than 1000 to 1200 ml/day maintenance yet may receive 2000 to 3000 ml/day or much more for several days. Patients who are particularly susceptible to pulmonary failure from overhydration are the elderly and those with congestive heart failure, chronic pulmonary disease, advanced sepsis, and lung trauma. Accurate intake and output measurements and daily weights are essential to prevent fluid loading. Overhydration can develop insidiously. Remember that a patient can become overhydrated and develop pulmonary insufficiency without an elevated central venous pressure or pulmonary capillary wedge pressure. Once detected, over-hydration should be treated vigorously by fluid restriction and the administration of diuretics as necessary.

In critically ill patients, deep breathing, coughing, turning, and early ambulation are essential to prevent mucous plugs, which can lead to ventilation-perfusion inequalities, alveolar collapse, and pneumonia. Patients on a ventilator can sit in a chair and even walk. Chest physical therapy and postural drainage will help avoid mucous plugs. Oversedation permits patients to lie flat on their backs for long periods without moving or coughing, setting the stage for atelectasis and pneumonia and progressive pulmonary problems. Adequate humidity must be provided to prevent inspissated secretions and injury to the respiratory ciliary action. Tracheobronchial aspiration should be used as necessary in patients who retain secretions.

Paralytic ileus is extremely common in critically ill patients. Abdominal distention causes elevation of the diaphragm, basilar atelectasis with shunting, and a decreased vital capacity. Nasogastric suction should be begun early. Premature oral feeding may result in additional abdominal distention and further compromise of pulmonary function. Aspiration pneumonia is not infrequent and often goes unrecognized as a cause of respiratory failure, particularly in obtunded, debilitated patients and in patients receiving gastric tube feedings.

Prolonged use of concentrations of oxygen above 50% may cause pulmonary damage (oxygen toxicity) and should be avoided. However, it is better to use 100% oxygen until the blood gas measurements are reported than to permit 1 minute of hypoxia. A PaO_2 greater than 80 torr is usually unnecessary. Positive end expiratory pressure (PEEP) should be considered early; but remember that although PEEP may result in an increased PaO_2, the cardiac output may be decreased, so that the oxygen transport may actually be decreased. Measurements of the cardiac output, blood gases, and hemoglobin concentration and correction of any abnormalities are essential to ensure adequate oxygen transport and tissue oxygenation.

In critically ill patients, particularly those with congestive heart failure, prolonged immobilization, or a malignancy, a high index of suspicion should be maintained for pulmonary emboli, another cause of respiratory failure. Not infrequently, the fall in the PaO_2 is transient. Remember that a friction rub, hemoptysis and a classical wedge-shaped shadow on the x-ray appear late and are signs of pulmonary infarction, not pulmonary embolism. If treatment is withheld until infarction is obvious, the patient may die of a subsequent embolus. The diagnosis should be suspected early in the appropriate clinical setting. Remember that the chest x-ray and electrocardiogram may not be abnormal. A lung scan may be diagnostic if there are no other abnormalities on the chest x-ray, but a pulmonary angiogram is definitive.

Embolization of particulate matter from multiple blood transfusions has been implicated in pulmonary insufficiency. If blood loss is excessive and transfusions exceed 4 units, blood filters should be used. Dacron-wool and polyester mesh of 25 to 40 microns appear to be effective and should be changed after every 3 units of blood.

Trauma can directly or indirectly result in respiratory failure. Fractured ribs and a flail chest may be obvious, but pulmonary or myocardial contusions may not be. A pneumothorax or hemothorax secondary to the fractured ribs may appear sometime after admission. A subclavian venopuncture, particularly when followed by positive-pressure anesthesia, use of a ventilator, or PEEP, may result in an unrecognized pneumothorax. Prompt, adequate debridement of all devitalized tissue can prevent a nidus for infection and subsequent respiratory failure. Consider fat emboli in patients with long bone fractures following major trauma. Early fixation of fractures permits early mobilization, with the attendant beneficial effects on cardiac, pulmonary, and gastrointestinal function and on nitrogen balance.

The use of vasoactive drugs can lead to ventilation-perfusion inequalities caused by a redistribution of the pulmonary microcirculatory blood flow and can contribute to pulmonary insufficiency. These drugs should be used only when necessary and with appropriate monitoring of blood gases.

With the routine use of automated multichannel blood chemical analyses, hypophosphatemia became recognized as a cause of acute respiratory failure as well as of MOF. The common clinical setting for hypophosphatemia is in the nutritionally depleted, critically ill patient receiving hyperalimentation (the phosphorus moves with glucose into the cells) and antacids (which bind phosphorus), who is being dialyzed (with a phosphate-poor bath). Alcoholic patients are particularly susceptible. Again, prevention through administration of additional phosphate in the hyperalimentation fluid when necessary is important. Once hypophosphatemia becomes established, intravenous phosphate may be lifesaving.

In summary, acute respiratory failure in critically ill patients may result from one or more specific causes, frequently unrecognized—all of which can contribute to acute pulmonary failure. Attention to details can often prevent respiratory failure, but if it should occur, early detection and correction of the contributory problems together with required pulmonary support can frequently prevent progressive respiratory failure—a key factor contributing to multiple organ failure. Routine ordering of deep breathing and coughing and administration of mucolytic agents and incentive-type spirometers will not by themselves prevent acute respiratory failure. Close patient observation and attention to details will in many instances prevent respiratory failure and subsequent MOF.

Cardiac failure is not only a major cause of acute respiratory failure due to pulmonary edema (backward failure), but also a major cause of MOF due to decreased organ perfusion (forward failure). Backward failure usually, but not always, precedes forward failure. Cardiac failure frequently occurs insidiously in critically ill patients, particularly those with preexisting heart disease, as a result of the increased circulatory requirements imposed by the hypermetabolic-hyperdynamic state associated with stress, trauma, and sepsis or the reduced coronary perfusion associated with low-flow states. In the hyperdynamic state the increased oxygen demand must be met by an increased cardiac output. If the cardiac output cannot increase sufficiently to meet the increased oxygen demand, survival becomes unlikely. An increased cardiac output associated with a decreased ejection fraction is evidence of beginning heart failure [30, 31]. Hypovolemic, septic, and cardiogenic (sometimes from a silent myocardial infarction) shock may be present and contribute to decreased coronary perfusion even though the classical signs of shock—low blood pressure, cold, clammy, pale skin—are absent. Fluid overload, hypoxemia from respiratory failure, acidosis, and electrolyte abnormalities may also contribute to cardiac failure. Pericardial tamponade or a myocardial contusion following trauma can also result in decreased cardiac function. In addition, a decreased cardiac output, and hence decreased coronary flow, can be caused by positive pressure ventilation, PEEP, and vasopressors, particularly in a patient with a failing heart. Left heart failure should be detected and treated long before frank pulmonary edema and hypotension occur. Remember that the PaO_2 often falls before congestive heart failure can be detected clinically, that the central venous pressure may be normal in 30 to 50 percent of critically ill patients with significant left heart failure, and that even young, previously healthy, critically ill patients can develop left and/or right heart failure. A Swan-Ganz flow-directed catheter should be placed early. Critically ill patients have little tolerance for delays in diagnosis and in beginning definitive treatment. Diuretics may suffice, but depending on the hemodynamic findings, vasodilators, inotropic agents, or mechanical circulatory support may be necessary. Cardiac failure, left or right, is a major, often unrecognized, cause of multiple organ failure.

Abnormalities of hepatic function frequently occur in critically ill patients. Following trauma or surgery, a slight transient jaundice appears within 2 to 4 days as a result of mild hepatocyte dysfunction, multiple transfusions, hematoma resorption, drugs, and anesthesia. This transient jaundice has no prognostic significance. A larger increase in bilirubin, plus an increase in liver enzymes, occurs later—usually 1 to 3 weeks after injury. Severe infection is present in the vast majority of patients. The patient typically is in a hyperdynamic state and frequently has pulmonary failure. There are several other known causes of hepatic failure. Hypoperfusion resulting from traumatic and hypovolemic shock occurs early; that from cardiogenic and septic shock usually occurs later. Low-flow states may not be clinically obvious, and appropriate hemodynamic monitoring is essential for early detection. Damage to the hepatic parenchyma may occur early and abnormal function may appear later, very much like acute tubular necrosis. Hypoxia from acute respiratory failure plays an important role in the pathogenesis of liver failure. Hepatic vasoconstriction—either endogenous, related to stress, or exogenous, from vasoactive drugs—may contribute to hypoperfusion. Liver injury per se is not likely to cause liver failure unless a massive resection is accompanied by shock or sepsis. Sepsis has a direct effect on the Kupffer cells and hepatocytes, resulting in impairment of enzymatic function and bile transport. Malnutrition, a major cause of liver failure, results in failure of the liver to synthesize essential substances (e.g., decreased serum albumin and coagulation factors) and failure of energy-dependent mechanisms. Bile salt excretion into bile is energy dependent and can contribute to hepatic bile stasis. Impairment of hepatocellular sodium and potassium transport, also energy dependent, can result in increased intracellular water and cell swelling. Lastly, anesthetics such as halothane and drugs such as tetracycline, chlorpromazine, and heroin can result in liver damage. Progressive failure of synthetic, metabolic, and phagocytic functions of the liver are important factors in the progression of MOF [10, 24].

Acute renal failure due to acute tubular necrosis may follow low-flow states, including hypovolemic, cardiogenic, and septic shock. Remember that hypotension need not be present. Otherwise, acute renal failure, when part of the multiple organ failure syndrome, typically occurs later in the illness, after hepatic failure. Hypoxia resulting from acute respiratory failure, particularly if associated with decreased perfusion, is a common factor contributing to acute renal failure. In addition, advanced sepsis, such as an undrained abscess, appears to have a direct effect on the kidney in producing renal failure. Transfusion reactions, myoglobin from a crush injury, and increased bilirubin from any cause when associated with hypotension may result in renal failure. Nephrotoxic drugs (e.g., gentamicin, kanamycin, cephalosporins, methicillin, and methoxyfluorane) are also common causes of renal failure. Occlusion of the renal blood vessels may occur in disseminated intravascular coagulation, shock, and severe infections. Renal vasoconstriction from vasoactive drugs has been implicated in renal failure. Prompt fluid replacement, adequate respiratory and circulatory support, drainage of abscesses, and awareness of potentially nephrotoxic drugs may avoid renal failure in many instances. Established renal failure is treated by dialysis.

Coagulopathies are common in the critically ill patient. Massive blood transfusions greater than 10 units per 24 hours will cause a decrease in platelets and factors 5 and 8, which are not stored in bank blood. One unit of fresh blood should be given for every 4 units of bank blood. Disseminated intravascular coagulation (DIC) follows severe trauma, sepsis, shock, and incompatible blood transfusions and may cause consumption of clotting factors, resulting in bleeding; or if fibrinolytic activity is insufficient, the microcirculation may become obstructed by thromboses, which can lead to cellular necrosis and multiple organ failure. Hyperfibrinolysis follows extensive trauma, acute hypoxia, and shock and can lead to excessive bleeding. Drugs such as chloramphenicol can depress the bone marrow and lead to thrombocytopenia and bleeding disorders. Dextran, if given in amounts greater than 1.5 liters per day—or less if there are decreased platelets—may cause decreased platelet adhesiveness and an increase in thrombus lysibility. Hepatic insufficiency causes a decreased synthesis of coagulation factors 5 and 7 to 10, increased fibrinolysis, and platelet dysfunction. Renal failure causes platelet dysfunction, which can be improved by dialysis. Sepsis, particularly gram-negative septicemia, results in decreased platelets due either to chronic DIC or to a primary effect. Again, prevention is the best treatment of coagulopathies. Otherwise, early treatment of causes and replacement of factors, when possible, may help prevent excessive bleeding, which, particularly if stress ulcers are present, can lead to a perfusion deficit and MOF.

Stress bleeding and absorptive and barrier dysfunction of the stomach and proximal small bowel occur in critically ill patients, many of whom are already suffering from respiratory failure, some degree of hepatic failure, and a coagulopathy. Many have been ill for some time and are malnourished.

Recent studies have suggested that upper gastrointestinal bleeding occurs in approximately one-third of critically ill patients with septicemia. Usually, there are multiple erosions in the body and fundus of the stomach, which have been referred to as acute hemorrhagic gastritis. Less commonly, there is a single, acute, peptic-type ulcer in the antrum or duodenum. The etiology of stress bleeding is controversial. Most authorities agree that acid is necessary, but they have found little correlation between acid hypersecretion and stress ulcers, except following head injury. Back diffusion of acid due to loss of the mucosal integrity may explain the lack of correlation and may result in cellular damage. Hypoperfusion of the mucosa, as seen in various types of shock, and hypoxia appear to play important roles in the pathogenesis of stress bleeding. Vasoactive drugs may cause vasoconstriction and add to the ischemia. High metabolic demands and rapid turnover of mucosal cells at a time of a deficiency of high-energy intermediates and protein substrates (malnutrition) appear to be major causes of cellular necrosis and stress bleeding. Aspirin and corticosteroids may contribute to mucosal damage.

The factors involved in the pathogenesis of stress bleeding should be prevented or corrected early. An adequate blood volume, along with satisfactory cardiac function, ventilation, and oxygenation, should be maintained to prevent hypoperfusion and hypoxia. Coagulation abnormalities should be corrected, if possible, using platelets, fresh frozen plasma, and vitamin K. Sepsis should be prevented by early use of antibiotics, appropriate debridement of devitalized tissue, and prompt drainage of pus. Early total parenteral nutrition to prevent malnutrition in critically ill patients is essential. Installation of antacids to maintain the gastric pH greater than 3.5, or possibly greater than 6, appears to be beneficial in preventing stress bleeding. H_2 blocking drugs, such as cimetidine and ranitidine, have been used routinely in patients with stress ulcer bleeding, but recent studies have suggested that these drugs may not be effective and that their use may result in potentially serious complications. Sucralfate, a member of the sulfhydryl group, appears to prevent and heal mucosal injury, and as yet, serious complications have not been reported. If the bleeding cannot be controlled, surgery should be considered. Regardless of the treatment, if the stress is not removed—e.g., if infection is not adequately controlled—the patient most likely will not survive.

Growing evidence suggests that the persistence of sepsis and subsequent multiple organ failure in critically ill patients may result from colonization of the proximal gut with enteric organisms and impairment of the normal barrier function of the gastrointestinal tract, which together may allow the bowel to serve as a reservoir of pathogens [6, 23]. These organisms can enter the portal circulation, and with hepatic dysfunction, they can pass into the pulmonary circulation and fuel an ongoing infectious process. Oral and pharyngeal colonization can result in direct aspiration of enteric organisms and pneumonia. Raising the gastric pH by antacids or H_2 blockers and the use of systemic antibiotics can contribute to bacterial overgrowth and make a critically ill patient even more vulnerable to pneumonia. Sucralfate does not have an effect on acid secretion and may prove to be the cytoprotective agent of choice.

In critically ill patients, organ systems often fail in a sequential pattern. Respiratory failure usually occurs first, followed in order by cardiac, hepatic, renal, hemotologic, and gastrointestinal failure. This pattern results from the frequency of occurrence of causative factors, which result in the failure of specific organs, organ susceptibility to common factors (i.e., low-flow, hypoxia, malnutrition, and sepsis), preexisting organ disease, and the effect of failure of one organ on others.

Many factors contribute to pulmonary failure, so it is not surprising that this disorder occurs commonly in critically ill patients. The resultant hypoxia, if uncorrected promptly, contributes to failure of other organs.

Cardiac failure usually results from a combination of preexisting disease, low-flow states, hypoxia, and increased cardiac work due to the hypermetabolic-hyperdynamic state. It often occurs insidiously and may not be recognized, even though it contributes to respiratory failure and decreased organ perfusion, both of which contribute to multiple organ failure. As tissue hypoxia and ischemia increase, anaerobic metabolism increases and lactic acidosis occurs, which, in turn, will tend to decrease cardiac function still more.

As sepsis, malnutrition, hypoxia, or hypoperfusion continue, the liver begins to fail. Failure of protein synthesis for cell structure and essential substances leads to further MOF. Decreased plasma albumin concentration results in generalized edema, which can adversely affect the function of all organs. Decreased synthesis of clotting factors will contribute to a coagulopathy, which very likely has already begun to develop. Progressive hepatic failure will contribute to renal failure by way of the increased bile pigments and also through unknown humoral effects—the hepatorenal syndrome.

When pulmonary and cardiac failure occur simultaneously, particularly in association with continued sepsis and hepatic dysfunction, renal failure becomes likely. Of course, if the patient is receiving a nephrotoxic antibiotic, if a major transfusion reaction takes place, or if the patient has been in shock, renal failure can occur independently.

Following shock, if no other factors contributed to specific organ failure, renal and, later, hepatic failure would be most likely to occur, because these organs are more susceptible to low-flow states. The lungs, kidneys, liver, and coagulation factors, in that order, appear to be more susceptible to sepsis than the heart.

Coagulopathy usually begins after prolonged sepsis and starvation and progresses as pulmonary, hepatic, and renal failure occur. A marrow-depressant drug, such as chloramphenicol, can cause a coagulopathy at any time.

With continued sepsis, malnutrition, respiratory and/or cardiac failure, and, often, renal and hepatic failure, stress bleeding occurs. Bleeding will be worse if a coagulopathy is present or if the patient is being dialyzed and the heparin used regionally is not fully reversed—not a rare occurrence. It is likely that gastrointestinal bleeding will occur earlier if the patient has an ulcer diathesis, has received ulcerogenic drugs, and did not receive adequate prophylactic ulcer therapy. If as a result of gastrointestinal bleeding, hypoperfusion and shock occur, all organs will deteriorate even more rapidly.

As MOF progresses, a point is reached at which a vicious cycle begins, and the treatment of one failing organ makes the function of another worse. Mechanical ventilation or PEEP will improve oxygenation and ventilation but will tend to decrease further the output of a failing heart. Diuretics will decrease pulmonary edema and improve respiratory function, but frequently they will decrease the output of a failing heart further by decreasing the required elevated preload. Conversely, giving fluids to increase the preload of a failing heart to increase the cardiac output and tissue perfusion worsens pulmonary failure. In addition, inotropic agents required to increase the output of a failing heart will cause a redistribution of a pulmonary blood flow and increase the pulmonary shunt, causing still more hypoxia. Thus, when pulmonary and cardiac failure occur simultaneously, a point is reached at which the treatment of one makes the other worse, and progressive failure of both results in MOF.

Similarly, the treatment of cardiac and renal failure may not be compatible. The removal of water by dialysis may decrease the required preload of a failing heart and result in hypotension. Intravenous fluid and albumin given to reverse the not-uncommon hypotension associated with dialysis may mitigate some of the beneficial effect of dialysis. Vasopressors, also given to raise a falling blood pressure during dialysis, very likely will adversely affect the failing heart by increasing the afterload.

When cardiac, pulmonary, or renal failure is present, the volume of parenteral nutrition may be limited. When renal or hepatic failure occur, volume and protein content of parenteral nutrition may be limited. As malnutrition progresses, it will result directly in failure of all organ systems and indirectly in failure by contributing to a decreased immune response and enhancing sepsis. As sepsis continues, antibiotics that might be beneficial in controlling the infection may have to be withheld, because of toxic effects on failing kidneys, liver, or bone marrow.

In summary, the best treatment of multiple organ failure is prevention of the many factors that result in a chain of events leading to organ failure. If this is not possible, early detection of failing organs and correction of specific causative factors are mandatory to prevent MOF. Attention to details early on may prevent progressive MOF much later. Adequate perfusion, tracheobronchial toilet, ventilation, and oxygenation should be maintained, abnormalities of which may not always be obvious. Infection should be prevented by judicious use of antibiotics and by appropriate surgery when necessary. Malnutrition should be prevented. If failure of an organ is suspected, do not base therapy on assumptions: it may take several hours to learn that the therapy was not effective, during which time the patient may rapidly deteriorate further. Rather, make definitive measurements so that correct therapy can be begun promptly and maintained precisely. Critically ill patients have no tolerance for the wrong therapy or delays in the correct therapy. Failure of one organ affects the function of other organs, and in time a vicious cycle occurs as treatment of one failing organ adversely affects the function of other organs. At this point, progressive multiple organ failure results and survival becomes unlikely.

REFERENCES

1. Baue, A. E. Recovery from multiple organ failure. *Am. J. Surg.* 149:420, 1985.
2. Bell, R., Coalson, J., and Smith, J. Multiple organ system failure and infection in adult respiratory distress syndrome. *Ann. Intern. Med.* 99:293, 1983.
3. Beutler, B., and Cerami, A. Cachectin: More than a tumor necrosis factor. *N. Engl. J. Med.* 316:379, 1987.
4. Border, J. R. Hypothesis: Sepsis, multiple systems organ failure, and the macrophage. *Arch. Surg.* 123:285, 1988.
5. Bower, R. H., Muggin-Sullam, M., Vallgren, S., and Fisher, J. Branched chain amino acid enriched solutions in the septic patient: A randomized prospective trial. *Ann. Surg.* 203:13, 1986.
6. Carrico, C. J., Meakins, J. L., Marshall, J. C., Fry, D. E., and Maier, R. Z. Multiple-organ-failure syndrome. *Arch. Surg.* 121:196, 1986.
7. Cerra, F. B. Hypermetabolism, organ failure, and metabolic support. *Surgery* 101:1, 1987.
8. Cerra, F. B. The hypermetabolism organ failure complex. *World J. Surg.* 11:173, 1987.
9. Cerra, F. B. The effect of stress level, amino acid formula, and nitrogen dose on nitrogen retention in traumatic and septic stress. *Ann. Surg.* 205:282, 1987.
10. Cerra, F. B., Siegel, J. H., and Border, J. Hepatic failure of sepsis. *Surgery* 86:409, 1979.
11. Cerra, F. B., Mazuski, J., Chute, E., and Teasley, K. Branched chain metabolic support. *Ann. Surg.* 199:286, 1984.
12. Cerra, F. B., Shronts, E. P., and Konstanstinides, N. N. Enteral feeding in sepsis: A prospective randomized double-blind trial period. *Surgery* 98:632, 1985.
13. Christou, N. V., Mannick, J. A., and West, M. A. Lymphocyte-macrophage interactions in the response to surgical infections. *Arch. Surg.* 122:239, 1987.
14. Dahn, M. S., Lange, P., Lobdell, K., and Hans, B. Splanchnic and total body oxygen consumption differences in septic and injury patients. *Surgery* 101:69, 1987.
15. DeCamp, M. M., and Demling, R. H. Posttraumatic multisystem organ failure. *J.A.M.A.* 260:530, 1988.
16. Filkins, J. P. Monokines and the metabolic pathophysiology of septic shock. *Fed. Proc.* 44:300, 1985.
17. Goris, R. J. Pathophysiology of multiple organ failure with sepsis. *Med. Klin.* 82:546, 1987.
18. Goris, R. J. Prevention of ARDS and MOF by prophylactic mechanical ventilation and early fracture stabilization. *Prog. Clin. Biol. Res.* 236:163, 1987.
19. Hyers, T. M., Gee, M., and Andreadis, N. A. Cellular interactions in the multiple organ injury syndrome. *Am. Rev. Respir. Dis.* 135:952, 1987.
20. Kariman, K., and Burns, S. Regulation of tissue oxygen extraction is dis-

turbed in adult respiratory distress syndrome. *Am. Rev. Respir. Dis.* 132:109, 1985.

21. Kumon, K., Tanaka, K., and Hirata, T. Organ failure due to low cardiac output syndrome following open heart surgery. *Jpn. Circ. J.* 50:329, 1986.

22. MacLean, L. V., and Meakins, J. L. Host resistance in sepsis and trauma. *Ann. Surg.* 182:207, 1975.

23. Marshall, J.C., Christou, N.V., Horn, R., and Meakins, J. L. The microbiology of multiple organ failure. *Arch. Surg.* 123:309, 1988.

24. Matuschak, G. M., and Martin, D. J. Influence of end-stage liver failure on survival during multiple systems organ failure. *Transplant. Proc.* XIX:40, 1987.

25. Mayers, I., Stimpson, R., and Openheimer, L. Delayed resolution of high-pressure pulmonary edema or capillary leak. *Surgery* 101:450, 1987.

26. Montgomery, A., Stager, M., and Carrico, J. Causes of mortality in patients with the adult respiratory distress syndrome. *Am. Rev. Respir. Dis.* 132:485, 1985.

27. Moore, E. E., and Jones, T. N. Benefits of immediate jejunostomy feeding after major abdominal trauma—A prospective randomized study. *J. Trauma* 26:874, 1986.

28. Nishijima, M. K., and Takezawa, J. Serial changes in cellular immunity of septic patients with multiple organ-system failure. *Crit. Care Med.* 14:87, 1986.

29. Nohr, C. W., Christou, N. V., and Rode, H. In vivo and in vitro humoral immunity in surgical patients. *Ann. Surg.* 200:373, 1984.

30. Parker, M. M., Shelhamer, J. H., and Bacharach, S. L. Profound but reversible myocardial depression in patients with septic shock. *Ann. Intern. Med.* 100:483, 1984.

31. Parrillo, J. E., Burch, C., and Shelhamer, J. H. A circulating myocardial depressant substance in humans with septic shock: Septic shock patients with a reduced ejection fraction have a circulating factor that depresses in vitro myocardial cell performance. *J. Clin. Invest.* 76:1539, 1985.

32. Pearl, R. H., Clowes, G. H., Hirsch, E. F., and Loda, M. Prognosis and survival as determined by visceral amino acid clearance in severe trauma. *J. Trauma* 25:777, 1985.

33. Reines, H. D., Halushka, P. V., and Cook, J. A. Lack of effect of glucocorticoids upon plasma thromboxane in patients in a state of shock. *Surg. Gynecol. Obstet.* 160:320, 1985.

34. Saba, T. M., and Jaffe, E. Plasma fibronectin: Its synthesis by vascular endothelial cells and role in cardiopulmonary integrity following trauma as related to reticuloendothelial function. *Am. J. Med.* 68:577, 1980.

35. Saito, H., Trocki, O., and Wang, S. Metabolic and immune effects of dietary arginine supplementation after burn. *Arch. Surg.* 122:784, 1987.

36. Shen, T. F., and Zhang, S. Acute renal failure in multiple organ system failure. *Arch. Surg.* 122:1131, 1987.

37. Watters, J. M., Bessy, P. Q., and Dinarello, C. A. Both inflammatory and endocrine mediators stimulate host response to sepsis. *Arch. Surg.* 121:179, 1986.

38. Weigelt, J. A. Current concepts in the management of the adult respiratory distress syndrome. *World J. Surg.* 11:161, 1987.

General Care of the Critically Ill Patient

James E. Sampliner
Howard C. Pitluk
Richard E. Sampliner

The critically ill patient often enters the intensive care unit (ICU) after a catastrophic event. Whether coming from the emergency room or the operating room, the patient usually is disoriented, sedated, or comatose. Once fully awake, the patient is not only confronted with complex equipment, but usually is immobilized by tubes, lines, and even restraints. Confusion, fear, and pain can be overwhelming, especially if an endotracheal tube renders verbal communication impossible. The physicians and the ICU staff must begin to humanize this environment. Time must be taken to explain the illness, the equipment, and invasive procedures. An informed, cooperative patient often requires less sedation and is easier to treat. Concern, compassion, and kindness are cornerstones of the delivery of quality critical care.

The ICU can also be a stressful environment for physicians and staff. Critically ill patients requiring constant bedside attention intensify the emotional strain placed on the medical staff. The workload is often so demanding that little time is available even for short breaks. To prevent staff burnout, several measures can be taken. First, a lounge in or near the unit should be provided for relaxation. When feasible, periodic rotation of the ICU staff to step-down areas is helpful in controlling the emotional stress associated with critical illness. During slow periods on the ICU, continuing education programs can be held to augment daily teaching rounds. In these sessions staff members should be encouraged to verbalize their feelings toward patients. This format of rotation, education, and verbalization is most helpful in maintaining the proper mental attitude vital for the successful treatment of the critically ill.

APPROACH TO THE CRITICALLY ILL PATIENT

General Approach

The management of critically ill patients presents a complex, dynamic problem to the physician staff. Although no one routine format will suffice for every ICU patient, a general design for patient care can be outlined [1]. Optimal therapy requires a multidisciplinary approach. Just as the human organism is an integrated network of separate but interdependent systems, so must the care of the critically ill be viewed. To maximize efficiency and minimize confusion and conflict one physician must coordinate the efforts of all the professionals caring for a given patient.

Because of the complex nature of critical illness, there is a tendency to treat the patient as an abstraction. To avoid this, the ICU physicians and staff should make a special effort to maintain personal contact with the patient. This is vital, and in turn, patients must be able to express their feelings to those responsible for their care. When the patient is intubated, special measures, such as a writing board, need be provided. All procedures should be explained to the conscious patient and psychologic support provided.

Measures to control patient anxiety are critical. Orientation to time and place, noise restriction, maintenance of diurnal patterns, prevention of sleep deprivation, and verbal as well as physical, "hands on," contact will help ensure a successful treatment result [9]. As an adjunct, diazepam (Valium) in daily divided doses of 8 to 30 mg can be utilized.

Two other psychopathologic problems can be seen on the ICU [18]. The first is depression. Because most stays on the ICU are relatively short, an acute reactive depression is most common. With a protracted stay, a patient may well develop a major depression, complete with psychotic symptoms. Recognition of these states is important in order to obtain early psychiatric consultation. Remember, it is initially better to discuss the underlying psychologic conflicts with the patient than to mask the problem by instituting antidepressant drugs.

The second, and more common, psychiatric abnormality encountered is that of delirium. Diagnosis featuring the triad of confusion, memory deficit, and disorientation must be made promptly, so that treatment can be instituted to gain control of the agitated patient. Haloperidol (Haldol) is an effective agent to use in gaining control. An initial dose of 2 to 5 mg intramuscularly may be given. Smaller doses (1–2 mg) may then be repeated as needed for control. Restraints may be necessary until the medication takes effect.

As a final means of alleviating patient anxiety, staff discussion must be held far enough from the bedside so as not to frighten the listening patient. Time must be spent after rounds to discuss treatment and prognosis, answer any questions, and communicate with patients and their families in an open atmosphere of mutual trust and understanding.

It must be remembered that the ICU offers its facilities to patients with a chance for survival [6]. On occasion, discontinuation of life-support systems may spare a patient and the family undue emotional and financial suffering. The dilemma of whether to continue aggressive critical care or to offer only supportive care generates ethical and emotional problems for physicians, nursing staff, and patients' families. Solutions are not easy, but they must be arrived at with all involved reaching unanimity on this most difficult and painful task.

Subsequent chapters will provide specific information concerning each vital organ system involved in critical care. However, a precise general care plan is a necessity in the treatment of the critically ill patient. Each organ system must be monitored, protected, and treated as necessary. Deterioration of one organ system may contribute to or be the harbinger of other organ failure. Critical care involves the care of the whole patient. The following format will supply a proper approach to this patient.

History and Physical Examination

Obtain as complete a history as possible, either from the patient or from family members. Pay particular attention to allergies, medications, bleeding disorders, and all significant past medical problems.

A thorough physical examination is essential. Repeat exams must be carried out frequently, with special attention paid to and a careful search for any sign of change. Despite all the sophisticated monitoring devices available, there is no substitute for physically touching and examining the patient!

Baseline Studies

Simultaneously with the history and physical examination, baseline physiologic measurements (e.g., weight, vital signs) and laboratory profiles must be obtained. Do not forget the clotting profiles. All indwelling lines should be noted and dated, and all medications reviewed for route of administration as well as continued need. Prior to order writing, the physician should have a clear, succinct list of patient problems and goals of therapy, so that the orders will reflect proper care in every area.

Writing the Orders

Following are some general rules for order writing:

1. Orders should be written early each morning and periodically updated throughout the day, depending on the patient's stability.
2. Orders must be written clearly and should be reviewed with the bedside nurse, so that transcription errors can be avoided and urgent intervention not delayed.
3. Orders should be written in a systematic fashion (organ system by organ system), so that no area is neglected.

Activity

Although most will be confined to bed, critically ill patients should be encouraged to move actively in bed, to turn or be turned frequently and to engage in leg exercises.

Diet

Diets of critically ill patients vary widely with the individual situation, and specific nutritional considerations are dealt with in Chapter 21. Remember that it is vital to start some form of nutritional support early in critical illness.

Intravenous Fluids

The orders for intravenous fluids should include the type of solution to be administered, the rate, and the appropriate line to be used. With multiple infusion sites and many piggyback additives being used in most ICU patients, be careful not to fluid-overload the patient. A well-designed ICU flow sheet, on which all sources of intake and output are separately listed, assists in this task, as does the use of daily weights. It is also desirable to reevaluate fluid orders each shift, based on input, output, and electrolyte change. In patients with abnormal gastrointestinal losses (e.g., fistulae, excessive nasogastric tube suction) aliquots of fluid can be sent for electrolyte analysis to assist with proper selection of fluid replacement.

Laboratory Investigations

Laboratory tests should be ordered because of need, not just because the patient is on the ICU. Overordering of blood tests can certainly contribute to an ICU anemia. Attention should be directed to the exact details for any special procedures (e.g., use of arterial versus venous blood), the times that tests are to be done, and other specific instructions.

OSMOLALITY. Determination of serum osmolality, which is frequently helpful in the care of the critically ill patient, can be done in the laboratory using a freezing-point depression. When this is not available, the following formula may be used:

$$\text{Osmolality (mOsm/kg)} = 1.6 \,(Na) + BUN/2.8 + \text{blood glucose}/18$$

In most situations the calculated serum osmolality will be 5 to 8 mOsm/kg less than that measured by the freezing-point depression method. The calculated osmolality should not be substituted routinely for actual measurements, since in some situations there will be a substantial discrepancy between calculated and measured osmolalities (e.g., in uremia, hyperlipemia, and multiple myeloma).

Medications

Each medication, along with its proper dose, frequency, and route of administration, must be specifically indicated. Again, remember that multiple intravenous medications can represent a large volume of fluid in the volume-sensitive patient.

The possibility of drug interactions must also be kept in mind. Many hospital pharmacies have set up computerized drug surveillance programs to alert the physician to potential interactions, as well as to adverse reactions. *Drug Interactions* is an excellent book to keep on the ICU for immediate reference [8].

Diagnostic Procedures

Included in the orders for diagnostic procedures are electrocardiograms, roentgenograms, and all special procedures. Studies must be planned so that circulating radionuclides do not interfere with each other or barium does not obscure a possible computed tomography (CT) scan. Direct discussion of the procedure with the consulting radiologist or technician is most helpful in obtaining a test that will give a good result.

Instructions to the Nursing Staff
The orders for the nursing staff should include instructions pertaining to tubes, drains, dressings, intravenous lines, and patient activity. Reiteration of care instructions to the bedside nurse each morning on rounds is a useful practice. Orders concerning the notification of the physician should include detailed instructions covering changes in vital signs, urine output, or any other significant monitored parameter. Other orders should relate to the patient's comfort and basic needs (e.g., pain and sleep medications, laxatives, psychologic support).

Special Considerations
The goal of therapy in the critically ill patient is to normalize each organ system so as to prevent the onset of organ failure, or to correct as quickly as possible any existing abnormalities in these systems. As the heart, lung, kidney, etc., are target organs of multisystem organ failure, so is the gastrointestinal (GI) tract. In fact, there is increasing evidence today that the GI tract may have an active role in the pathogenesis of multiple organ system failure [5]. Thus, it is important to look closely at several gastrointestinal problems seen in critical illness.

Gastrointestinal Bleeding
In the critical care setting, prevention of gastrointestinal bleeding must be emphasized. Although the role of pH control and the precise pH end point for therapy remain controversial, the standard of care in the high-risk patient requires prophylaxis for stress bleeding. Although the frequency of clinically significant bleeding is low, patients with extensive burns, polytrauma, sepsis, renal failure, and respiratory insufficiency are at increased risk. Hourly doses of antacids to keep the pH above 4.5 and the intravenous use of H_2-receptor blockers, or both, should be effective [14].

Recent, controversial studies have suggested an increased risk of nosocomial pneumonia from pH control therapy, a problem avoided by the use of a cytoprotective agent, such as sucralfate, at a dose of 1 gm every 6 hours [7, 17].

Hematemesis, melena, or profuse rectal bleeding signals a "red alert" in the ICU. Bleeding that results in changes in vital signs requires volume stabilization and immediate investigation of the source. Esophagogastroduodenoscopy is the first diagnostic step for hematemesis and/or melena. After the stomach has been lavaged through a large-bore oral tube, upper endoscopy will most often define the site of bleeding, permitting the institution of a specific treatment plan. Large esophageal varices, (> 5 mm) bleeding ulcers, focal erosions, or "visible vessels" in ulcers can be injected with sclerosant or cauterized with multipolar electrocautery or heater probe [10, 13]. The rate of success for these local measures is very high, and they should be the first-line approach in critically ill patients, prior to surgical intervention.

When bright red blood is coming from the rectum, rectal examination to rule out any local bleeding point is the first diagnostic step. If not yet done, upper endoscopy may still be necessary to rule out a bleeding source proximal to the distal duodenum. When upper endoscopy is negative, a tagged red cell study may localize a segment of the colon as the site of bleeding. If this study is positive, two possible routes of therapy are available. Angiography with selective visceral artery catheterization not only can be diagnostic, but also can be therapeutic when local Pitressin infusion is used [2]. If Pitressin is used, peripheral arterial and central venous lines are inserted and a Foley catheter is placed. The patient is sent to the x-ray department with a constant infusion pump (e.g., Holter or IVAC) for continuous intra-arterial infusion and with a Pitressin mixture of 200 clinical units in 500 ml of 5% D/0.25% saline (0.4 units/ml). With the intra-arterial catheter in place, Pitressin is then infused at 0.2 units per minute for 20 minutes. A postinfusion angiogram is required to observe vasoconstriction of the distal branches of the perfused vessel and cessation of extravasation. (The infusion rate may be appropriately adjusted in order to meet these radiologic criteria.)

After angiography the patient is transferred to the ICU for infusion at the determined rate to control bleeding. This infusion should be continued for at least 12 hours, and then the Pitressin concentration should be slowly reduced over the next 1 to 2 days, to avoid Pitressin rebound bleeding. Once the Pitressin has been discontinued, a short perfusion time with saline should be carried out before removal of the catheter. In addition, the following should be done:

1. Monitoring of vital signs, including central venous pressure, urinary output, and daily weight.
2. Daily KUB to check catheter position.
3. Careful observation for bradycardia, water intoxication, and post-Pitressin diuresis.
4. Good catheter maintenance, including an aseptic catheter puncture site, a close check of distal pulses, and the curtailment of leg movement to prevent catheter displacement and possible arterial injury.

Following catheter removal, adequate local pressure should be provided to control bleeding from the puncture site. Strict control of additional fluid administration must be maintained in view of the added volume of intra-arterial perfusion.

The other modality employed in lower GI bleeding is colonoscopy. In an ideal examination, the patient first undergoes colonic lavage, usually with 4 liters of a polyethelene glycol–electrolyte solution. If an ileus is present, this preparation should be excluded. Not only can the colonoscope define the source of bleeding (i.e., vascular, diverticular, neoplasia), but in angiodysplastic lesions it can be used therapeutically to cauterize the source of bleeding.

Adynamic Ileus
Motility problems of the GI tract are common in the critically ill patient. As the advantages of enteral nutritional support become clear (see Chap.

21), the loss of a functional GI tract becomes more important. Unfortunately, this is the norm in the critically ill patient. The causes of ileus include laparotomy; trauma; head injury; retroperitoneal, pelvic, and spinal cord injury; metabolic abnormalities; intra-abdominal sepsis; pneumonia; and the use of anticholinergic, opiate, and psychotropic medications.

Physical examination usually reveals a distended quiet abdomen. Plain abdominal x-rays are usually confirmatory and show distended loops of small and large bowel. Treatment of adynamic ileus is supportive (nasogastric suction and intravenous fluids), as the process is self-limited. If return of bowel function is delayed beyond the usual 3-to-5-day period, a vigorous search must be made for treatable causes of bowel dysfunction. At this point, review all orders to ascertain that excessive medication is not contributing to the problem. Recheck electrolytes, making sure the patient is not hypokalemic, hypocalcemic, or hypomagnesemic. Remember that myxedema can be a hidden cause for ileus. Finally, total parenteral nutrition can in and of itself delay the return of bowel function.

Mechanical small-bowel obstruction must be ruled out. Previous abdominal surgery, missed external herniae, wound dehiscence, intra-abdominal abscess, or a smouldering pancreatitis can all be implicated in bowel dysfunction. Sigmoidoscopy, colonoscopy, contrast studies (i.e., barium enema), and CT scan may be helpful in making a diagnosis [11].

Diarrhea

Physiologically, diarrhea can be defined as a stool volume greater than 200 gm in 24 hours in an individual on a "Western diet." In an intensive care setting, large volume stool output raises certain questions. What is entering the patient's gut? Antacids and tube feedings may need to be altered. What is exiting the gut? Stools should be checked for white cells, culture and sensitivity, ova, and parasites and *Clostridium difficile* toxin. The presence of white cells indicates violation of the colonic mucosa with infection or inflammation, or both, and is an indication for flexible sigmoidoscopy. Abnormal mucosa should be biopsied for etiologic clues. The observation of yellowish plaques of pseudomembranous colitis due to *C. difficile* enables initiation of appropriate antibiotic therapy prior to the availability of the toxin results. If the stools are liquid, sodium and potassium should be determined in supernatant stool water for detection of an osmotic gap: $(Na + K) \times 2 -$ plasma osmolality = the osmotic gap. An osmotic gap greater than 160 indicates carbohydrate malabsorption or excessive intake of an osmotic agent [16]. Recently, severe hypoalbuminemia has been associated with diarrhea in critically ill patients [3]. Preliminary evidence suggests that a peptide-based enteral diet with less fat will lead to resolution of diarrhea and repletion of the serum albumin [4].

Acute Acalculous Cholecystitis

Difficult to diagnose, increasing in frequency, and potentially life-threatening, acute acalculous cholecystitis must be recognized early and treated vigorously. Symptoms and signs of this disease entity on the ICU are variable. Right-upper-quadrant pain, unexplained fever, leukocytosis, and elevated amylase, bilirubin, and/or alkaline phosphatase may help lead to a diagnosis. Ultrasonography is a useful diagnostic tool showing gallbladder dilatation, wall edema (> 3.5 mm thickness is significant) or biliary sludge. Hepatobiliary radionuclide scanning can also be helpful in demonstrating cystic duct obstruction. Many of the above findings are nonspecific in the critically ill patient, but the addition of associated risk factors such as prolonged narcotic use, NPO, and mechanical ventilation increases the likelihood of this diagnosis [15].

The pathogenesis of acute acalculous cholecystitis is multifactoral, but in general, rapid distension of the gallbladder compromises circulation to the gallbladder, leading to an acute development of necrosis. Therefore, once the diagnosis is made, prompt surgical intervention is indicated. Cholecystostomy performed under local anesthesia is the procedure of choice in the ICU patient unless extensive necrosis or perforation of the gallbladder necessitates cholecystectomy [12].

REFERENCES

1. Artz, J. S., et al. Application of a critical care monitoring program in the diagnosis and management of critically ill patients in a community hospital. *Crit. Care Med.* 2:42, 1974.
2. Baum, S., et al. Gastrointestinal hemorrhage: Angiographic diagnosis and control. *Adv. Surg.* 7:149, 1973.
3. Brinson, K. R., and Kolts, B. E. Diarrhea associated with severe hypoalbuminemia as an indicator of diarrheal incidence in critically ill patients. *Crit. Care Med.* 15:506, 1987.
4. Brinson, K. R., and Kolts, B. E. Diarrhea associated with severe hypoalbuminemia: A comparison of peptide-based chemically defined diet and standard enteral alimentation. *Crit. Care Med.* 16:130, 1988.
5. Carrico, C. J., Meakins, J. L., Marshall, J. C. et al. Multiple organ failure syndrome. *Arch. Surg.* 121:196, 1986.
6. Clinical Care Committee of the Massachusetts General Hospital. Optimum care for hopelessly ill patients. *N. Engl. J. Med.* 295:362, 1976.
7. Driks, M. R., Craven, O. E., Celli, B. R., et al. Nosocomial pneumonia in intubated patients given Sucralfate as compared with antacids or histamine Type 2 blockers. *N. Engl. J. Med.* 317:1376, 1987.
8. Hansten, P. D. *Drug Interactions* (6th ed.). Philadelphia: Lea & Febiger, 1988.
9. Kiely, W. F. Psychiatric aspects of critical care. *Crit. Care Med.* 2:139, 1974.
10. Laine, L. Multipolar electrocoagulation in the treatment of active upper gastrointestinal tract hemorrhage. *N. Engl. J. Med.* 316:1613, 1987.
11. Norwood, S. H., and Civetta, J. M. Abdominal CT scanning in critically ill surgical patients. *Crit. Care Med.* 13:350, 1986.
12. Orlando, R., Gleason, E., and Drezner, A. J. Acute acalculous cholecystitis in the critically ill patient. *Am. J. Surg.* 145:472, 1983.
13. Panes, J., Viver, J., Forne, M., et al. Controlled trial of endoscopic sclerosis in bleeding peptic ulcers. *Lancet* 2:1292, 1987.
14. Priebe, H. J., et al. Antacid versus cimetidine in preventing acute gastrointestinal bleeding. *N. Engl. J. Med.* 302:426, 1980.
15. Savino, J. A., Scalea, T. M., and DelGuercio, L. R. Factors encouraging laparotomy in acalculous cholecystitis in the critically ill patient. *Am. J. Surg.* 145:472, 1983.
16. Shiau, Y., Feldman, G. M., Resnick, M. A., et al. Stool electrolytes and osmolality measurements in the evaluation of diarrheal disorders. *Ann. Intern. Med.* 102:773, 1985.

17. Tryba, M. Risk of acute stress bleeding and nosocomial pneumonia in ventilated intensive care patients: Sucralfate versus antacids. *Am. J. Med.* Suppl.
3B:117, 1987.
18. Weiss, H. J. Psychological aspects of intensive care. In J. L. Berk and J. E.
Sampliner (eds.), *Handbook of Critical Care* (2nd ed.). Boston: Little, Brown,
1982.

SELECTED READINGS

American College of Surgeons. *Manual of Preoperative and Postoperative Care*
(3rd ed.). Philadelphia: Saunders, 1983.

Beal, J. M. (ed.) *Critical Care for the Surgical Patient.* New York: MacMillan,
1982.

Behrendt, D. M., and Austin, W. G. *Patient Care in Cardiac Surgery* (4th ed.).
Boston: Little, Brown, 1985.

Cerra, F. G. *Manual of Critical Care.* St. Louis: Mosby, 1987.

Civetta, J. M., Taylor, R. W., and Kirby, R. *Critical Care.* Philadelphia: Lippincott,
1988.

Dantzker, D. R. *Cardiopulmonary Critical Care.* New York: Grune & Stratton,
1986.

Goldberger, E. *A Primer of Water, Electrolyte and Acid-Base Syndromes* (7th
ed.). Philadelphia: Lea & Febiger, 1986.

Kinney, J. M., et al. *American College of Surgeons Manual of Surgical Intensive
Care.* Philadelphia: Saunders, 1987.

Luce, J. M., and Pierson, D. J. *Critical Care Medicine.* Philadelphia: Saunders,
1988.

Neville, W. E. *Intensive Care of the Surgical Cardiopulmonary Patient* (2nd ed.).
Chicago, London: Year Book, 1983.

Parillo, J. E. *Current Therapy for Critical Care Medicine.* New York: Decker,
1987.

Rippe, J. M. *Manual of Intensive Care Medicine* (2nd ed.). Boston: Little, Brown,
1989.

Shoemaker, W. C., et al. *Textbook of Critical Care* (2nd ed.). Philadelphia: Saunders, 1988.

Washington University Manual of Medical Therapeutics (26th ed.). Boston:
Little, Brown, 1989.

Noninvasive Diagnostic Techniques in Critical Care

George I. Litman

Noninvasive diagnostic procedures involve no incising or puncturing of the skin and therefore result in few, if any, complications. Radioisotope studies do use intravenous injection but are otherwise noninvasive, as are computed tomography, ultrasound, and magnetic resonance imaging. Each provides specific information, but they can also be complementary. With portable gamma cameras and ultrasound units, these techniques can be taken to the bedside of even the most critically ill patient. The purpose of this chapter is to introduce these noninvasive procedures and relate them to specific critical care problems.

ULTRASOUND

Ultrasound has a frequency of greater than 20,000 cycles per second (Hertz, or Hz). Medical sonography employs frequencies between 1 and 20 Hz. Ultrasound is produced by a crystal enclosed within a transducer positioned on the chest wall or abdomen. It travels through the body tissues at a speed of 1540 m/sec in the form of a beam whose shape is determined by the size of the transducer, the frequency of the crystal, and the degree of focusing. The echoes reflected from blood-tissue interfaces are detected by the transducer, amplified, and then displayed on a monitor for videotape and strip-chart recording [12, 23, 65].

ECHOCARDIOGRAPHY

M-mode echocardiography produces a one-dimensional image of cardiac structures with excellent temporal resolution. Two-dimensional real-time

I would like to thank Andrew Kurman, M.D., of the Department of Radiology at Akron General Medical Center for providing the MRI figure used in this chapter and the Cardiac Function Laboratory at Akron General for assistance in obtaining the echocardiographic figures. I would also like to thank Joel Walker of the Biomedical Communications Department at Akron General for his assistance in preparing the photos used in the chapter. Finally, I would like to thank my secretary, Nancy Hooper, for her assistance in completing the chapter.

echocardiography produces a planar image providing details of the structure and motions of the heart. Doppler echocardiography characterizes the flow of blood, and the hybrid formed by the superimposition of two-dimensional and pulsed Doppler data is termed *color-flow mapping.* When displayed in color, Doppler flow imaging is quite dramatic, but the technology is extremely complex and expensive [20, 23, 55, 62, 78].

Since ultrasound is transmitted poorly through bone and air, obtaining an adequate echocardiogram depends on finding an "acoustic window." Critically ill patients pose significant problems in this regard, because they might be restless or uncooperative, and it might not be possible to position them properly. In many patients, mechanical ventilation and positive end expiratory pressure result in hyperinflation of the lungs, precluding adequate ultrasound imaging of the heart. In patients requiring more than 10 cm of positive end expiratory pressure, images are usually poor. Even the most proficient personnel might not obtain complete information from a particular study [66].

Specific Indications

Pericardial Effusion

Echocardiography is currently the most sensitive and specific procedure for the diagnosis of pericardial effusion. Detection and serial follow-up of the presence and approximate amount of pericardial fluid are more accurate with echocardiography than with any other method [24, 25, 35].

A pericardial effusion appears as an echo-free space behind the epicardial surface of the posterior wall and in front of the pericardium. Where a small effusion exists, this echo-free space will be small, and the epicardial-pericardial separation will occur primarily during systole. As the effusion becomes larger, this separation is increased and is present during both systole and diastole. With a larger effusion, an echo-free space is also seen in front of the right ventricular wall [24, 25, 35].

When a large pericardial effusion is present, the heart may swing like a pendulum in the pericardial sac with each cardiac cycle [91]. The echocardiogram will detect the abnormal motion of all cardiac walls, including the septum, moving in the same direction with each heartbeat [48].

Several causes of false-negative and false-positive diagnoses have been identified, especially during the use of M-mode echocardiography. Among the false-positive causes are pleural effusion, dilated descending aorta, pericardial fat pad, and tumor encasing the heart. Two-dimensional (2D) echocardiography improves the sensitivity and specificity of the diagnosis of pericardial effusion [66].

False-negative studies may occur with loculated effusion and clotted blood. Therefore, a blood clot in the posterior pericardium may not be detected—clearly a disadvantage, especially in the trauma patient [39, 42].

Cardiac Tamponade

Two-dimensional echocardiography is highly specific for the detection of cardiac tamponade caused by pericardial effusion (Fig. 5-1). Although a large effusion is more likely to produce cardiac tamponade than is a small

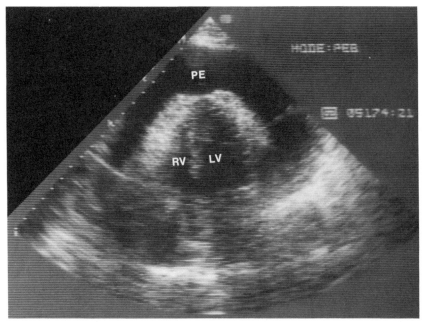

Fig. 5-1. An apical four-chamber view demonstrating a large pericardial effusion (PE). RV = right ventricle; LV = left ventricle.

one, other factors also contribute, including the speed of fluid accumulation, pericardial compliance, the size of the heart, and intravascular volume. The development of cardiac tamponade is a hemodynamic process. Echocardiographic findings of tamponade include the presence of pericardial effusion, respiratory variations in left ventricular dimensions, right ventricular diastolic compression, left atrial diastolic compression, and right atrial diastolic compression. The latter sign appears to be the most sensitive indicator of pericardial tamponade [41, 42, 56, 81].

Aortic Dissection
Acute dissection of the thoracic aorta is among the most lethal of all medical emergencies. In a review of 425 cases by Hirst et al., 21 percent of patients were dead within 24 hours, and 49 percent died within 4 days of the onset of symptoms [34]. Early diagnosis and aggressive treatment of these patients may prolong survival and allow time for potentially definitive surgery.

Echocardiography can be valuable in the diagnosis of proximal aortic dissection by demonstrating the separation of aortic layers and the presence of aortic valve regurgitation [8, 59, 94]. Nanda et al. first reported the echocardiographic findings of the demonstration of a false lumen, dilation of the aortic root, widening of both anterior and posterior walls, and preservation of normal aortic valve motion [60]. Recently, Iliceto et al., utilizing color-flow Doppler imaging, demonstrated the possibility of comprehensive evaluation of flow dynamics in aortic regurgitation. The 2D echo can frequently identify the intimal flap and the dilated aorta [36]. Pulsed Doppler may help identify the true lumen from the false lumen. Doppler flow imaging offers another, somewhat dramatic, display of the pathology in patients with aortic dissection—demonstrating blood flow passing through the true lumen with no flow recorded in the false lumen [14, 94]. An important aspect of the color Doppler technique in the evaluation of patients with aortic dissection is its ability to characterize the severity of associated aortic regurgitation [40, 69, 70].

Unlike angiography, this new imaging technique is totally noninvasive and easily repeatable, and therefore particularly useful in seriously ill patients in whom serial evaluations need to be carried out.

Despite these major advances, the diagnosis of dissecting aortic aneurysm and the definition of its origin and extent might necessitate contrast angiography.

Acute Aortic Valve Regurgitation

Acute aortic valve regurgitation may occur as a result of infective endocarditis or of acute traumatic rupture [54, 97]. Echocardiography combined with 2D and Doppler studies can assist in defining the etiology as well as the significance of the aortic valve regurgitation [69, 70, 77]. Dense, irregular echoes from one or more leaflets may represent the vegetations of endocarditis [77, 97]. These are usually seen best during diastole; but with newer 2D systems and varying views, the angle may be more important than timing. A flail leaflet prolapsing into the left ventricular outflow tract in diastole suggests valve disruption. With the new color-flow techniques, prosthetic valve dysfunction potentially can be evaluated, allowing for determination of the location and severity of regurgitant valves [40, 69].

Acute severe aortic regurgitation usually demonstrates early coaptation of the mitral leaflets in diastole, before the QRS on a simultaneously recorded electrocardiogram [92]. In contrast to chronic aortic regurgitation, exaggerated wall motion and a markedly dilated ventricle are not seen.

Mitral Valve Regurgitation

New color-flow and 2D Doppler echo studies have allowed for evaluation and quantification of mitral valve regurgitation. The etiology of severe acute mitral valve regurgitation usually is secondary to bacterial endocarditis, rupture of mitral valve leaflet, flail mitral valve, or papillary muscle or chordal rupture (Figure 5-2). These conditions are well-visualized by these newer echocardiographic techniques, allowing not only for etiologic differential, but for hemodynamic quantification as well [58, 86].

Prosthetic valve dysfunction is particularly well evaluated by the newer echocardiographic color flow method [1, 21, 64].

Acute Myocardial Infarction

Several significant complications of myocardial infarction can be readily and specifically diagnosed by echocardiography. Significant left ventricular dysfunction and regional wall motion abnormality are readily noted on

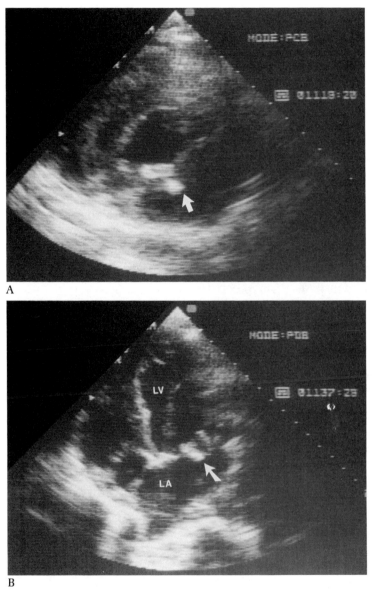

A

B

Fig. 5-2. A. Cross-sectional two-dimensional view of mitral valve in a 24-year-old female drug addict showing dense echoes of vegetations of endocarditis (arrow). B. Four-chamber view of same patient demonstrating large vegetations of endocarditis on mitral valve leaflet (arrow). RV = right ventricle; LV = left ventricle; LA = left atrium.

2D echo study. This can explain hypotension and congestive failure in patients with myocardial infarction [66].

Acute rupture of the interventricular septum may be confirmed by visualization of the septal defect and/or dilation of the right ventricle [57]. Additionally, Doppler and color-flow mapping demonstrate this intracardiac shunt [66].

Acute mitral regurgitation may result from rupture of a papillary muscle or chorda tendineae. In this setting, echocardiography may reveal the characteristic motion of a flail mitral leaflet [57]. Doppler studies aid in qualitative evaluation of mitral regurgitation [58].

A large ventricular aneurysm may produce cardiogenic shock. Echocardiography will demonstrate a dyskinetic segment of the left ventricle [44, 95]. In right ventricular infarction, echocardiography reveals a dilated right ventricle with segmental wall motion abnormalities. On occasion, ventricular rupture occurs and produces a pseudoaneurysm. Specific echocardiographic findings include demonstration of the aneurysm, along with pericardial fluid [95].

Ultrasound
The diagnostic accuracy of portable sonograms appears to warrant its continued use in the critical care environment. It is probably the most important screening method for the detection of an intraabdominal sepsis source or hydronephrosis. Harris et al. confirmed this impression in a study performed at the Massachusetts General Hospital Intensive Care Unit [32].

NUCLEAR MEDICINE
Lung Scanning
Following intravenous injection of technetium-labeled albumin particles, special gamma-counting cameras can be used to scan the distribution of the resulting radioactivity in the lungs. This technique has proved valuable in detecting the presence of pulmonary arterial emboli.

Pulmonary Embolism
Pulmonary embolism is a common, recurrent, age-related phenomenon that can occur without warning in its most lethal form. It accounts for 50,000 to 100,000 deaths each year in the United States. Pulmonary embolism must be considered in the differential diagnosis of every acute cardiorespiratory disorder.

The lungs lend themselves well to the study of regional function with radioactive tracer techniques [28, 31]. This method accurately reflects the distribution and severity of perfusion abnormalities from any cause [90]. Because of its relatively noninvasive nature, the perfusion lung scan has become the principal screening procedure for patients suspected of suffering a pulmonary embolus.

When multiple views are obtained, a normal lung scan essentially excludes any clinically detectable pulmonary embolism. When the scan is abnormal, the likelihood of embolic phenomena can be determined from the nature of the observed defects. Lung scans with a high probability of pulmonary embolism demonstrate multiple wedge-shaped or concave defects that follow a segmental vascular distribution. Low-probability scans show nonsegmental and nonvascular distributions of perfusion defects. A chest x-ray obtained in conjunction with the lung scan enhances its diagnostic specificity. A concave peripheral perfusion defect in the presence of a normal chest roentgenogram is likely to be caused by an embolus.

In a recent study, 75 percent of scans with high probability for embolus were confirmed by pulmonary angiography. With a normal scan, the angiogram was also normal [28]. In the Urokinase Pulmonary Embolism Trial, among 10 patients with a large embolus in the proximal main pulmonary artery, none of the lung scans were normal [90]. False-positive tests are encountered in a variety of pulmonary and cardiac conditions, such as neoplasms, pneumonia, atelectasis, chronic bronchitis, and chronic obstructive pulmonary disease. These can usually be identified on chest x-ray.

In combination with a normal Xenon 133 ventilation study, an abnormal lung scan is virtually diagnostic of pulmonary embolism. On the other hand, in a patient with an abnormal perfusion lung scan and a matching abnormal ventilation study, the presence of pulmonary embolism is less likely but cannot be absolutely excluded [52]. With the increased specificity attainable by combining ventilation and perfusion scans, it is possible to limit pulmonary angiography to patients who do not meet these criteria or who have coexisting pulmonary embolism and chronic obstructive pulmonary disease.

Although high-probability ventilation-perfusion scans most likely indicate pulmonary embolism, pulmonary angiography is recommended when the patient may be at high risk of bleeding from anticoagulation, when considering thrombolytic therapy, or when the need for vena caval interruption is present. With indeterminate scans or substantial clinical evidence for alternative diagnoses, angiography will be necessary [2].

Cardiac Isotope Imaging

The use of radioisotopes in clinical cardiology represents an exciting advance in nuclear medicine. These noninvasive techniques permit easy evaluation of the size and function of the cardiac chambers and allow visualization of the physiologic adequacy of blood flow to the myocardium. Maximum information is obtained when a combination of thallium 201 (^{201}T1) and technetium 99 pyrophosphate (^{99m}Tc PYP) is used in addition to dynamic ventriculography with ^{99m}Tc-labeled albumin or red cells [6].

When ^{99m}Tc is bound to human albumin and injected intravenously, ^{99m}Tc displays the dimensions of the great vessels and chambers of the heart. It is thus used to calculate the size and functional capabilities of the heart, expressed as cardiac output or systolic ejection fraction. In addition, ^{99m}Tc albumin can detect intracardiac shunts and abnormal wall motion [67], and ^{99m}Tc PYP reveals the blood flow distribution in the myocardium but is eventually concentrated in regions of acute myocardial ischemia and infarction.

The myocardial blood flow is also demonstrated by [201]T1, the agent of choice for perfusion scanning [84, 85]. After intravenous injection, [201]T1 uptake will be seen in the normally perfused left ventricular myocardium of the resting patient. Since the muscle mass of the right ventricle is much less than that of the left, visualization of the right ventricle is usually abnormal. Areas with decreased or absent flow are identified as cold spots. An area with compromised circulation only during exercise is ischemic, whereas an area with a consistent perfusion defect at rest exhibits the scar of a previous infarction. A hypertrophied area of myocardium may show greater-than-normal uptake. Therefore, the evaluation of a [201]T1 scan permits (1) determination of the size, shape, and position of the heart; (2) definition of areas of ischemia or infarct; (3) visualization of an abnormal right ventricle; and (4) measurement of the thickness of the myocardium in some cases.

The future of myocardial imaging may well lie with three-dimensional image reconstruction [43]. Ter-Pogossian and colleagues have accomplished this with a positron-emitting tracer and positron-tomographic cameras [89]. However, a positron-based technique requires the availability of a cyclotron and of expensive detection equipment—formidable requirements that place these techniques beyond the reach of the average institution.

Acute Myocardial Infarction

When employed 6 to 8 hours after the onset of symptoms, [201]T1 is most sensitive for the indication of an acute myocardial infarction [71]. When used in evaluating over 1600 patients with recent episodes of chest pain, [201]T1 scintigraphy was helpful in identifying those with infarcts [96]. However, the most common cause of focal defects in [201]T1 scanning in non-symptomatic patients at rest is scar tissue from old myocardial infarction.

If radioisotopic imaging is delayed, ^{99m}Tc PYP becomes the agent of choice, because it is selectively taken up by infarcted cardiac cells and appears as a hot spot on the scintigram, delineating the site and extent of the damaged area [9, 10, 68]. The ^{99m}Tc PYP scan becomes positive 10 to 12 hours after infarction and then becomes increasingly positive for 24 to 72 hours. Therefore, it is suggested that the ^{99m}Tc PYP scintigram be obtained within 48 hours after suspected infarction and repeated 48 hours later if the initial scan is equivocal or negative in the face of high clinical suspicion. Repeat studies are also beneficial in determining whether there was extension of infarcted areas [100, 101].

Recent developments in monoclonal antibody technology and labeling techniques have permitted production of pure and specific antimyosin antibodies. Myocardial injury and necrosis result in cell membrane disruption, leaving intracellular myosin exposed to extracellular fluids. Radiolabeled antimyosin antibodies administered intravenously under these circumstances localize at the infarction site. Compared with the ^{99m}Tc pyrophosphate technique, which is affected by radiotracer uptake in the ribs and spine, the labeled-antibody approach is probably more accurate in positively identifying the site of tissue damage.

These new noninvasive techniques are particularly advantageous when other diagnostic methods are inadequate. It is impossible to distinguish between subendocardial ischemia and infarction on the basis of electrocardiogram findings alone. Intraventricular conduction defects, such as left bundle branch block, obscure the electrocardiogram changes of an acute myocardial infarction. No history is available from patients who arrive at the hospital comatose, and serum enzyme measurements may not be positive in patients who present hours or days after the onset of symptoms. In the perioperative and postoperative periods, especially following coronary artery revascularization, patients may have chest pain and elevated serum enzymes, obscuring the diagnosis of a new infarct. With portable gamma cameras now available, these studies can be performed in the intensive care setting.

Myocardial Contusion

Today, more patients survive transport to an emergency medical facility following severe blunt chest injury and penetrating wounds of the heart as a result of improved on-the-scene resuscitative techniques. Standard evaluation begins with a thorough physical examination, with special attention paid to the structural integrity of the bony thorax, the adequacy of respiration and circulation, and the peripheral pulses [33]. Despite chest x-ray and electrocardiographic data, myocardial contusion is easily overlooked and may present formidable complications during the recovery period [49].

Regardless of etiology, ^{99m}Tc PYP will identify myocardial necrosis if some blood flow is present and a critical mass of tissue is involved [68, 101]. A scintigram should be obtained for any victim of major blunt chest trauma, even without suggestive electrocardiographic findings such as premature ventricular contractions or minor intraventricular conduction disturbances [102]. The timing of the scan is the same as that for an acute myocardial infarction. If the scan is positive, the patient must be monitored closely for arrhythmias, congestive failure, and other complications of acute infarcts.

Gated radionuclide angiography appears to have two limited but important roles in the evaluation of cardiac contusion: (1) in hemodynamically unstable patients, a portable scan may distinguish between cardiac and noncardiac etiologies for the hemodynamic instability; (2) patients with persistent electrocardiographic abnormalities should be scanned to rule out the possibility of ventricular aneurysm, a reported lethal complication of cardiac contusion. Also, the gated scan may be useful in the preoperative evaluation of cardiac function in stable patients with other evidence of cardiac injury who may require serious and urgent surgery [26].

Myocardial Function and Shunt Determinations

Radioisotopic angiography can be performed using ^{99m}Tc-labeled human albumin or red cells. These studies have been improved by computer technology that enables evaluation of ventricular wall motion, cardiac output, and systolic ejection fractions. It is now possible to determine cardiac function noninvasively in the critically ill patient [5].

In addition, radioisotopic angiography permits detection and calculation of intracardiac shunts. Shunts, such as ventricular septal defects, may be congenital or may result from myocardial infarction or blunt chest trauma.

COMPUTED TOMOGRAPHY

The operation of computed tomography (CT) scanners involves the axial rotation of an x-ray beam around the patient. Detectors opposite the x-ray source measure the attenuation of the x-rays after they have passed through the tissue. After the data are collected in multiple projections, a computer calculates the attenuation coefficient of each point of a matrix, thus producing an image of the scanned sections. The image is stored and may be recorded photographically [87, 88].

Computed tomography differs from conventional shadow radiography and tomography because the x-ray beam is thinly collimated to reduce the effect of scatter, the detector system (sodium iodide crystal or xenon gas) has a greater response capability than does a conventional photographic plate, and a computer is used that resolves the summed x-ray projection data perceived by the detector into discrete linear attenuation coefficients [98].

The field of computed tomography has seen the development of a number of refinements, including fast CT, cine CT, and gated CT. Its usefulness as a diagnostic tool has been overwhelming. It provides excellent diagnostic information across the spectrum of intracranial disease [17, 22, 46]. It fulfills a major role as a low-risk, painless, and noninvasive method of evaluating the abdominal cavity [38, 74, 75, 80]. Several studies have demonstrated the possibility of performing CT scans even in the most severely ill patients [29, 61, 74, 93].

Central Nervous System: Intracranial Lesions

Computerized tomography allows clear imaging of discrete cranial lesions—sagittal, coronal, horizontal, or oblique. The radiation dosage from a complete series of CT scans—approximately 4 rads—roughly equals that of six routine skull x-ray series.

Computerized tomography is estimated to be 90 to 98 percent accurate in the imaging of intracranial lesions and is thus one of the most effective medical detection systems available [15].

Although computerized tomography may demonstrate skull fractures, it is of much greater value with extracerebral and intraparenchymal hematomas [17]. Acute epidural and subdural hematomas are readily detectable, as are intraparenchymal hematomas. The hematoma retains a high density for 2 to 4 weeks, after which time blood is partially absorbed, giving the lesion about the same density as surrounding brain tissue [46, 63].

Granulomas and abscesses can be detected on CT scans. Although some contain calcium, most show up only after injection of intravenous contrast. Abscesses usually have thin, regular walls [63].

Nearly all tumors occupy significant space and thus cause displacement and distortion of normal structures [15, 16]. Some are calcified, others are hemorrhagic. Almost all visualize better after contrast injection. Some tumors have radiologic characteristics that permit the pathologic diagnosis from CT scanning alone [46]. A clinical "stroke" may represent an arterial or venous infarct or a hemorrhage. Arterial infarcts conform to the arterial territory involved and appear 24 hours after the stroke, leading to focal atrophy in about 6 weeks. Arterial infarcts sometimes become hemorrhagic, and thus anticoagulation therapy is absolutely contraindicated in those patients with hemorrhagic infarcts on CT scan.

Venous infarcts, which characteristically are hemorrhagic and scattered, do not follow arterial distribution. Hemorrhage due to hypertension typically occurs in the external capsule but may extend to the brain parenchyma or the ventricle.

Intracerebral and subarachnoid hemorrhage may result from arteriovenous malformation. The vessels are usually visible after intravenous contrast. CT also visualizes the thrombosed portion of a giant aneurysm. Angiography is still necessary to visualize the base of an aneurysm and its relation to adjacent vessels and vascular spasm, as well as to delineate vessel lacerations or traumatic fistulas [73, 98].

If a patient with suspected intracranial bleeding demonstrates altered mentation, papilledema, or focal neurologic findings, a CT scan should be the initial procedure. A lumbar puncture may precipitate transtentorial herniation if the bleeding is a result of a mass lesion or a ruptured aneurysm. The CT scan visualizes the bleeding and may indicate the need for emergency angiography [16, 73, 103]. In addition, the CT scan may provide important prognostic information when done within 24 hours after head injury in comatose patients [93].

Chest

CT serves as an effective method for defining vascular mediastinal masses, aortic aneurysms, and aortic dissections. With thoracic aortic aneurysm, the transverse scans display a markedly dilated ascending aorta and depict areas of calcification along its outer margin [30]. The presence of peripheral calcification favors a true aneurysm as opposed to a dissecting aneurysm. This can be seen before the infusion of contrast medium, which confirms that the mass is indeed vascular [29].

True aortic aneurysm can be distinguished from classic aortic dissection. False and true lumens may opacify differently. Unequivocal diagnosis of dissection on CT scan requires visualization of the intimal flap [30, 51].

CT scanning has been used to demonstrate tracheal esophageal fistula [47]. Additionally, Golding et al., utilizing CT scanning of the chest in intensive care patients, noted its usefulness when more morphologic information is necessary [29]. Those patients whose deterioration or failure to improve is attributed to a thoracic cause unexplained by chest x-ray are likely to gain from CT scanning. Lesions located in the mediastinum on the pleural and chest wall, as well as localized lung lesions, are well demonstrated by CT [29].

Abdominal Computed Tomography

Pancreas
Computed tomography appears to be more reliable in the demonstration of the normal and abnormal pancreas than almost any other procedure.

Abdominal CT scanning is worthwhile in the evaluation of pancreatic carcinoma and pancreatitis, especially with abscesses, pseudocysts, or phlegmon [80]. Kalmar, Mathews, and Bishop, in a study of 214 patients with pancreatitis, demonstrated the effectiveness of CT scanning in evaluating local changes in the inflamed pancreas and extrapancreatic inflammatory changes and complications [38]. Many patients with acute pancreatitis were found to have thickened perirenal fascia, ileum, and pleural effusion. Reliable signs of chronic pancreatitis, in addition to gland enlargement, include calcification, pseudocyst, atrophy, and pancreatic duct dilation [38]. The CT scan can often distinguish between pancreatic abscess and phlegmon and is an easily performed test for evaluation of changes in pancreatic pseudocyst.

Jaundice

Computed tomography has been shown to be a practical and accurate method of distinguishing between obstructive and nonobstructive jaundice. Normal intrahepatic ducts are usually not identifiable on scans. Dilated intrahepatic bile ducts appear as linear branching or circular, low-density structures that are less dense than the adjacent portal vein branches [80].

Retroperitoneal Space

The retroperitoneal space, one of the most inaccessible areas of the body to conventional radiography, is readily visualized with CT scanning. Location and identification of abscesses, hemorrhage, and mass lesions are possible and practical.

Hemorrhage is seen as a more-or-less diffuse mass. Retroperitoneal hemorrhage can occur as a result of external trauma, internal trauma to vessels cannulated for various reasons, a leaking abdominal aneurysm, bleeding diathesis, anticoagulation, or certain neoplasms [83].

A number of studies have demonstrated that CT is effective in identifying a well-defined abdominal abscess in a variety of patients [75, 76, 79]. However, Norwood and Civetta, in a recent study of critically ill surgical patients in whom abdominal CT scanning was performed, found that for septic patients, even when the scans were positive, the information did not usually influence clinical decision making [61]. The CT scan should only be employed in these critically ill patients to confirm the diagnosis of intraabdominal abscess, and thus to diminish the incidence of negative reexploration, rather than to discover a specific diagnosis in the patient with multiple system failure [61].

MAGNETIC RESONANCE IMAGING

Magnetic resonance imaging (MRI) may be the most significant advance since the development of x-radiography, in that it is an apparently safe way to look inside the body that is noninvasive. It is nonionizing; it generates intravascular and soft tissue contrast without the need for contrast medium; it is intrinsically three-dimensional, allowing images to be obtained from any plane-orientation; it can image structures without interference from bone; and it has the potential to evaluate biochemical composition and reaction and disease-related changes [11, 13, 53].

The magnetic resonance images are obtained by placing the patient within a powerful, highly uniform, static magnetic field. Magnetized protons (hydrogen nuclei) within the patient align like small magnets in this field. Radio-frequency pulses are then used to create an oscillating magnetic field perpendicular to the main field from which the nuclei absorb energy and move out of alignment with the static field in a state of excitation. As the nuclei return from excitation to the equilibrium state, a signal induced in the receiver coil of the instrument by the nuclear magnetization can then be transformed by a series of algorithms into diagnostic images. Magnetic resonance images are based on proton density and proton relaxation dynamics. Proton characteristics vary according to the tissue under examination and reflect physical and chemical properties [13, 55, 72].

Of extreme concern during MRI studies is that the patient's body contains no ferromagnetic objects, such as aneurysm clips, shrapnel, or bullets, or implanted devices, such as pacemakers or electrical leads. The strong magnetic fields could easily dislodge these objects and inactivate devices. Despite early concerns, imaging in patients with weight-bearing prostheses or prosthetic valves is now felt to be safe.

Significant danger can arise from loose ferromagnetic objects in the imaging room that can be attracted to the magnet and thus become high-speed flying projectiles.

Unfortunately, with gradient and receiver coils in place, the internal diameter of current imaging systems is frequently reduced to approximately 60 cm. This can lead to claustrophobia in predisposed patients. Some obese patients cannot be examined.

Technological advances now evolving—such as cine MRI; improved surface coils; respiratory, cardiac, and peripheral gating; and fast screening—may resolve the current problem of slow scan-acquisition time.

The strong static magnetic field, which interferes with proper functioning of the usual life support equipment, and the small bore of the magnet make it difficult to examine some critically ill patients. A recently described method of physiologic support and monitoring of critically ill patients during MRI utilizes modified ventilators, in which ferromagnetic parts are replaced with plastic, stainless steel, and aluminum compounds, and modified physiological monitoring equipment. With this method, patients can be imaged without interruption of life support systems [7].

The uses of the MRI in critically ill patients are limited because of the above-noted technological problems. But the full potential of MRI has not been reached, and continuing refinement of equipment, contrast agents, and software may be anticipated.

The Brain
MRI provides superior sensitivity to CT scanning in many neurologic conditions, including head trauma and ischemia. Because of the absence of bone artifacts, which are seen on CT, MRI is superior at the vertex, in the posterior fossa, near the walls of the middle fossa, at the base of the skull, and in the orbit.

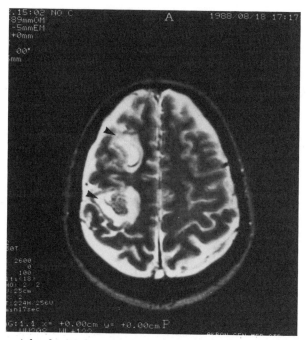

Fig. 5-3. T_2-weighted MRI demonstrating a subacute intracerebral hematoma (upper arrow) and an acute intracerebral hematoma (lower arrow). This 58-year-old male had acute venous sinus thrombosis.

Subacute hematoma is readily detected by MRI, whereas it may be much less conspicuous on CT. CT is more sensitive in acute hemorrhage, whereas MRI is more sensitive in subacute hemorrhage [11, 82] (Fig. 5-3).

In head trauma, MRI has proved useful in the detection of intracranial hemorrhage, including hemorrhagic contusions and shearing injuries. During the first 1 to 3 days after injury, however, CT is preferable not only because examination time is shorter, but also because hemorrhage at this time is more reliably demonstrated by CT.

The Aorta

MRI permits visualization of the aortic root and detects intramural hemorrhage, wall separation, and intimal flap. It permits the distinction between aortic dissection and aneurysm of the thoracic and abdominal aorta. It can accurately delineate aortic size, changes in aneurysm dimensions, and aortic aneurysm bleeding [4, 18, 27, 50].

DIGITAL SUBTRACTION ANGIOGRAPHY

Digital subtraction angiography (DSA) utilizes standard angiographic images by processing them through a high-speed digital computer. Adequate visualization of major arterial systems can be obtained with low concentrations of contrast material at fluoroscopic energy levels. Although this procedure has had some role in screening and diagnosis, its use in critical situations has seemingly been limited. A recent study evaluated a small portable video-image-processing system in the intensive care unit. The technique showed promise in evaluation of pulmonary emboli, cardiac chambers, and aortic arch [19, 37].

CONCLUSION

Noninvasive diagnostic procedures, increasingly available and safe, have demonstrated unique potential in the evaluation of the critically ill patient. The portability of excellent imaging systems has extended the utility of ultrasound and nuclear techniques. Improvements in computed tomography and the development of nuclear magnetic resonance imaging have extended the scope of noninvasive diagnosis. Future technological developments hold the promise of bringing these latest techniques to critically ill patients.

REFERENCES

1. Alan, M., Rosman, H. S., Lakier, J. B., et al. Doppler and echocardiographic features of normal and dysfunctioning bioprosthetic valves. *J. Am. Coll. Cardiol.* 10:851, 1987.
2. Alderson, P. O., and Martin, E. C. Pulmonary embolism: Diagnosis with multiple imaging modalities. *Radiology* 164:297, 1987.
3. Amparo, E. G., Higgins, C. B., Hoddick, W., et al. Magnetic resonance imaging of aortic disease. *A.J.R.* 143:1203, 1984.
4. Amparo, E. G., Higgins, C. B., Hricak, H., et al. Aortic dissection: Magnetic resonance imaging. *Radiology* 155:399, 1985.
5. Bacharach, S. L., Green, M. V., Boker, J. S., et al. A real-time system for multi-image gated cardiac studies. *J. Nucl. Med.* 18:79, 1977.
6. Beller, G. Nuclear cardiology: Current indications and clinical usefulness. *Curr. Probl. Cardiol.* 10:1, 1985.
7. Bennett, G. H., Ropper, A. H., and Johnson, K. A. Physiological support and monitoring of critically ill patients during magnetic resonance imaging. *J. Neurosurg.* 68:246, 1988.
8. Brown, O. R., Popp, R. L., and Kloster, F. E. Echocardiographic criteria for aortic root dissection. *Am. J. Cardiol.* 36:17, 1975.
9. Buja, L. M., Tofe, A. J., Kulkarni, P. V., et al. Sites and mechanisms of localization of technetium-99m phosphorus radiopharmaceuticals in acute myocardial infarcts and other tissues. *J. Clin. Invest.* 60:724, 1977.
10. Burno, F. P., Cobb, F. R., Rivas, F., and Goodrich, J. K. Evaluation of 99m technetium stannous pyrophosphate as an imaging agent in acute myocardial infarction. *Circulation* 54:71, 1976.
11. Bydder, G. M., and Steiner, R. E. NMR imaging of the brain. *Neuroradiology* 23:231, 1982.
12. Christensen, E. E., Curry, T. S., and Dowdey, J. E. *An Introduction to the Physics of Radiology.* Philadelphia: Lea & Febiger, 1978. Pp. 361–394.
13. Council on Scientific Affairs of the American Medical Association, Report of the Magnetic Resonance Imaging Panel. Magnetic resonance imaging of the cardiovascular system: Present state of the art and future potential. *J.A.M.A.* 259:253, 1988.
14. Dagli, S. V., Nanda, N. C., Roitman, D, et al. Evaluation of aortic dissection by Doppler color flow mapping. *Am. J. Cardiol.* 56:497, 1985.
15. Davis, D. O. CT in the diagnosis of supratentorial tumors. *Semin. Roentgenol.* 12:97, 1977.

16. Davis, K. R., Poletti, C. E., Roberson, G. H., Tadmor, R., and Kjellberg, R. N. Complementary role of computed tomography and other neuroradiologic procedures. *Surg. Neurol.* 8:437, 1977.

17. Davis, K. R., Taveras, J. M., Roberson, G. H., Ackerman, R. H., and Dreesball, J. N. Computed tomography in head trauma. *Semin. Roentgenol.* 12:53, 1978.

18. Dooms, G. C., and Higgins, C. B. The potential of magnetic resonance imaging for the evaluation of thoracic arterial disease. *J. Thorac. Cardiovasc. Surg.* 92:1088, 1987.

19. Duff, T. A., Turski, P. A., Sackett, J. F., et al. Evolving role of digital subtraction angiography in neurosurgical practice. *Neurosurgery* 11:430, 1982.

20. Duncan, W. J. *Color Doppler in Clinical Cardiology.* Philadelphia: Saunders, 1988.

21. Effron, M. K., and Popp, R. L. Two-dimensional echocardiographic assessment of bioprosthetic valve dysfunction and infective endocarditis. *J. Am. Coll. Cardiol.* 2:597, 1983.

22. Evens, R. G. New frontiers for radiology: Computed tomography. *A.J.R.* 126:1117, 1976.

23. Feigenbaum, H. *Echocardiography* (4th ed.). Philadelphia: Lea & Febiger, 1986.

24. Feigenbaum, H., Waldhausen, J. A., and Hyde, L. P. Ultrasound diagnosis of pericardial effusion. *J.A.M.A.* 191:107, 1965.

25. Feigenbaum, H., Zaky, A., and Waldhausen, J. A. Use of ultrasound in the diagnosis of pericardial effusion. *Ann. Intern. Med.* 65:443, 1966.

26. Fenner, J. K., Knopp, R., Lee, B., et al. The use of gated radionuclide angiography in the diagnosis of cardiac contusion. *Ann. Emerg. Med.* 13:688, 1984.

27. Geisinger, M. A., Risius, B., O'Donnell, J. A., et al. Thoracic aortic dissection: Magnetic resonance imaging. *Radiology* 155:407, 1985.

28. Gilday, D. L., Poulore, K. P., and DeLand, F. H. Accuracy of detection of pulmonary embolism by lung scanning correlated with pulmonary angiography. *A.J.R.* 115:732, 1972.

29. Golding, R. P., Knape, P., Strack van Schijndel, R. J. M., et al. Computed tomography as an adjunct to chest x-rays of intensive care patients. *Crit. Care Med.* 16:211, 1988.

30. Goodwin, J. D., Herfkens, R. J., Skioldebrand, C. B., et al. Evaluation of dissections and aneurysms of the thoracic aorta by conventional and dynamic CT scanning. *Radiology* 136:125, 1980.

31. Greenspan, R. H. Does a normal isotope perfusion scan exclude pulmonary embolism? *Invest. Radiol.* 9:44, 1974.

32. Harris, D. R., Simeone, J. F., Mueller, P. R., and Butch, R. J. Portable ultrasound examinations in intensive care units. *J. Ultrasound Med.* 4:463, 1985.

33. Hipona, F. A., and Paredes, S. The radiologic evaluation of patients with chest trauma. *Med. Clin. North Am.* 59:65, 1975.

34. Hirst, A. E., Johns, V. J., Jr., and Kime, S., Jr. Dissecting aneurysms of the aorta: A review. *Medicine* 37:217, 1958.

35. Horowitz, M. S., Schultz, C. S., Stinson, E. B., Harrison, D. C., and Popp, R. L. Sensitivity and specificity of echocardiographic diagnosis of pericardial effusion. *Circulation* 50:239, 1974.

36. Iliceto, S., Nanda, N. C., and Rizzon, P. Color Doppler evaluation of aortic dissection. *Circulation* 75:748, 1987.

37. Janssen, J. H. A., Ackermans, J., Tijdens, F., et al. Bedside digital subtraction angiography in critical medicine. *Crit. Care Med.* 12:1067, 1984.

38. Kalmar, J. A., Mathews, C. C., and Bishop, L. A. Computerized tomography in acute and chronic pancreatitis. *South. Med. J.* 77:1393, 1984.

39. Kerber, R. E., and Payvandi, M. N. Echocardiography in acute hemopericardium: Production of false negative echocardiograms of pericardial clots. *Circulation* 56 (suppl. 3):III–24, 1977.

40. Kitabatke, A., Ito, H., Inoue, M., et al. A new approach to noninvasive evaluation of aortic regurgitant fraction by two-dimensional Doppler echocardiography. *Circulation* 72:523, 1985.

41. Kronzon, I., Cohen, M. L., and Winer, H. E. Diastolic atrial compression: A sensitive echocardiographic sign of cardiac tamponade. *J. Am. Coll. Cardiol.* 2:770, 1983.

42. Kronzon, I., Cohen, M. L., and Winer, H. E. Cardiac tamponade by loculated pericardial hematoma: Limitations of M-mode echocardiography. *J. Am. Coll. Cardiol.* 1:913, 1983.

43. Kuhl, D. E., and Edwards, R. Q. Cylindrical and section radioisotope scanning of the liver and brain. *Radiology* 83:926, 1964.

44. Lebovitz, A. J., Miller, L. W., and Kennedy, H. L. Mechanical complications of acute myocardial infarction. *C.V.R. & R.* 5:948, 1984.

45. Lee, J. K. T., Ling, D., Herken, J. P., et al. Magnetic resonance imaging of abdominal aortic aneurysms. *A.J.R.* 143:1197, 1984.

46. Lee, S. H., and Rao, K. C. V. G. *Cranial Computed Tomography.* New York: McGraw-Hill, 1983.

47. Leeds, W. M., Morley, T. F., Zappasodi, S. J., et al. Computed tomography for diagnosis of tracheoesophageal fistula. *Crit. Care Med.* 14:591, 1986.

48. Levisman, J. A., and Abbasi, A. A. Abnormal motion of the mitral valve with pericardial effusion: Pseudo prolapse of the mitral valve. *Am. Heart J.* 91:18, 1976.

49. Levitsky, S. New insights in cardiac trauma. *Surg. Clin. North Am.* 55:43, 1975.

50. Lois, J. F., Gomes, A. S., Brown, K., et al. Magnetic resonance imaging of the thoracic aorta. *Am. J. Cardiol.* 60:358, 1987.

51. McLaughlin, M. J., Weisbrod, G., Wise, D. J., et al. Computed tomography in congenital anomalies of the aortic arch and great vessels. *Radiology* 138:399, 1981.

52. McNeil, B. J., Holman, B. L., and Adelstein, S. J. The scintigraphic definition of pulmonary embolism. *J.A.M.A.* 227:753, 1974.

53. Magnetic Resonance Imaging—Consensus Conference. *J.A.M.A.* 259:2132, 1988.

54. Mann, T., McLaurin, L., Grossman, W., et al. Assessing hemodynamic severity of acute aortic regurgitation due to infective endocarditis. *N. Engl. J. Med.* 293:108, 1975.

55. Miller, D. P., Burns, R. J., Gill, J. B., and Ruddy, T. D. (eds.). *Clinical Cardiac Imaging.* New York: McGraw-Hill, 1988.

56. Miller, S. W., Feldman, L., Palacios, I., et al. Compression of the superior vena cava and right atrium in cardiac tamponade. *Am. J. Cardiol.* 50:1287, 1982.

57. Mintz, G. S., Victor, M. F., Kotler, M. N., et al. Two-dimensional echocardiographic identification of surgically correctable complications of acute myocardial infarction. *Circulation* 64:91, 1981.

58. Miyatke, K., Izumi, S., Okamoto, M., et al. Semiquantitative grading of severity of mitral regurgitation by real-time two-dimensional Doppler flow imaging technique. *J. Am. Coll. Cardiol.* 7:82, 1986.

59. Moothart, R. W., Spangler, R. D., and Blount, S. G., Jr. Echocardiography in aortic root dissection and dilatation. *Am. J. Cardiol.* 36:11, 1975.

60. Nanda, C., Gramiak, R., and Shah, P. M. Diagnosis of aortic root dissection by echocardiography. *Circulation* 48:506, 1973.

61. Norwood, S. H., and Civetta, J. M. Abdominal CT scanning in critically ill surgical patients. *Ann. Surg.* 202:166, 1985.
62. Omoto, R. (ed.) *Color Atlas of Real-Time Two-Dimensional Doppler Echo-cardiography* (2nd ed.). Tokyo: Shindan-To-Chiryosha Co. Philadelphia: Lea & Febiger, 1987.
63. Osborn, A. G. Computed tomography in neurologic diagnosis. *Ann. Rev. Med.* 30:189, 1978.
64. Panidis, I. P., Ross, J., and Mintz, G. S. Normal and abnormal prosthetic valve function as assessed by Doppler echocardiography. *J. Am. Coll. Cardiol.* 8:317, 1986.
65. Parisi, A. F., and Tow, D. E. *Noninvasive Approaches to Cardiovascular Diagnosis.* New York: Appleton, 1979.
66. Parker, M. M., Cunnion, R. E., and Parillo, J. E. Echocardiography and nuclear cardiac imaging in the critical care unit. *J.A.M.A.* 254:2935, 1985.
67. Parkey, R. W., Bonte, F. J., Buja, M. L., and Willenson, J. T. *Clinical Nuclear Cardiology.* New York: Appleton, 1979.
68. Perez, L. A. Clinical experience: Technetium 99 labeled phosphate myocardial imaging. *Clin. Nucl. Med.* 1:2, 1976.
69. Perry, G. J., and Nanda, N. C. Recent advances in color Doppler evaluation of valvular regurgitation. *Echocardiography* 4:503, 1987.
70. Perry, G. J., Helmicke, F., Nanda, N. C., et al. Evaluation of aortic insufficiency by Doppler color flow mapping. *J. Am. Coll. Cardiol.* 9:952, 1987.
71. Pohost, G. M., Zir, L. M., Moore, R. H., et al. Differentiation of transient ischemia from infarcted myocardium by serial imaging after a single dose of thallium 201. *Circulation* 55:294, 1977.
72. Pohost, G. M., and Camby, R. C. Nuclear resonance imaging: Current applications and future prospects. *Circulation* 75:88, 1987.
73. Ramsey, R. G. *Computerized Tomography of the Brain: With Clinical Angiographic and Radionuclide Correlation.* Philadelphia: Saunders, 1977.
74. Raval, B., Steinberg, R., and Rauschkolb, E. Artifact-free computed tomography of the chest and abdomen in the severely ill patient. *J. Comput. Tomogr.* 9:9, 1988.
75. Robinson, J. G., and Pollack, T. W. Computed tomography in the diagnosis and localization of intra-abdominal abscesses. *Am. J. Surg.* 145:136, 1983.
76. Roche, J. Effectiveness of computed tomography in the diagnosis of intra-abdominal abscesses. *Med. J. Aust.* 25:85, 1981.
77. Roy, P., Tajik, A. J., Giuliani, E. R., et al. Spectrum of echocardiographic findings in bacterial endocarditis. *Circulation* 53:474, 1976.
78. Sahn, D. J. Real-time two-dimensional Doppler echocardiographic flow mapping. *Circulation* 71:849, 1985.
79. Saini, S., Kellum, J. M., O'Leary, M. O., et al. Improved localization and survival in patients with intra-abdominal abscesses. *Am. J. Surg.* 145:136, 1983.
80. Sheedy, P. F., Stephens, D. H., Hattery, R. R., Brown, L. R., and MacCarty, R. L. Computed tomography of the abdominal organs. *Adv. Intern. Med.* 24:455, 1979.
81. Singh, S., Wann, L. S., Schuchard, G. H., et al. Right ventricular and right atrial collapse in patients with cardiac tamponade—A combined echocardiographic and hemodynamic study. *Circulation* 70:966, 1984.
82. Sipponen, J. T., Sepponen, R. E., and Sivula, A. Chronic subdural hematoma: Demonstration by magnetic resonance. *Radiology* 150:79, 1984.
83. Stephens, P. H., Williamson, B., Sheedy, P. F., Hattery, R. R., and Miller,

W. E. Computed tomography of the retroperitoneal space. *Radiol. Clin. North Am.* 15:377, 1977.

84. Strauss, H. W., Harrison, K., Langan, J. K., Lebowitz, E., and Pitt, B. Thallium 201 for myocardial imaging—Relation of thallium 201 to regional perfusion. *Circulation* 51:641, 1975.

85. Strauss, H. W., and Pitt, B. Thallium 201 as a myocardial imaging agent. *Semin. Nucl. Med.* 7:49, 1977.

86. Switzer, D. F., and Nanda, N. C. Color Doppler evaluation of valvular regurgitation. *Echocardiography: A Review of Cardiovascular Ultrasound* 2:533, 1985.

87. Ter-Pogossian, M. M. Computerized cranial tomography: Equipment and physics. *Semin. Roentgenol.* 12:13, 1977.

88. Ter-Pogossian, M. M., Phelps, M. E., Brownell, G. L., et al. *Reconstruction Tomography in Diagnostic Radiology and Nuclear Medicine.* Baltimore: University Park Press, 1977.

89. Ter-Pogossian, M. M., Phelps, M. E., Hoffman, E. J., and Mullani, N. A. Positron-emission transaxial tomograph for nuclear imaging (PETT). *Radiology* 114:89, 1975.

90. Tow, D. E., and Simon, A. L. Comparison of lung scanning and pulmonary angiography in the detection and follow-up of pulmonary embolism: The urokinase pulmonary embolism trial experience. *Prog. Cardiovasc. Dis.* 17:239, 1975.

91. Usher, B. W., and Popp, R. L. Electrical alternans: Mechanisms of pericardial effusion. *Am. Heart J.* 83:459, 1972.

92. Vandenbossche, J. L., and Englert, M. Doppler color flow mapping demonstration of diastolic mitral regurgitation in severe acute aortic regurgitation. *Am. Heart J.* 114:889, 1987.

93. van Dongen, K. J., Braakman, R., and Gelpke, G. J. Prognostic value of computerized tomography in comatose head injured patients. *J. Neurosurg.* 59:951, 1983.

94. Victor, M. F., Mintz, G. S., Kotler, M. N., et al. Two-dimensional echocardiographic diagnosis of aortic dissection. *Am. J. Cardiol.* 48:1155, 1981.

95. Visser, C. A., Kan, G., David, G. K., et al. Echocardiographic-cineangiographic correlation in detecting left ventricular aneurysm: A prospective study of 422 patients. *Am. J. Cardiol.* 50:337, 1982.

96. Wackers, F. J. T., Becker, A. E., Samson, G., et al. Location and size of acute transmural myocardial infarction estimated from thallium 201 scintiscan: A clinicopathological study. *Circulation* 56:72, 1977.

97. Wann, L. S., Dillon, J. C., Weyman, A. E., et al. Echocardiography in bacterial endocarditis. *N. Engl. J. Med.* 295:135, 1976.

98. Weisberg, L. A. Computed tomography in the diagnosis of intracranial disease. *Ann. Intern. Med.* 91:87, 1979.

99. Whitley, N. O., and Shatley, C. H. Diganosis of abdominal abscesses in patients with major trauma: The use of computed tomography. *Radiology* 147:179, 1982.

100. Willerson, J. T., Parkey, R. W., Bonte, F. J., Meyer, S. L., and Stokely, E. M. Acute subendocardial myocardial infarction in patients; its detection by Tc-99m stannous pyrophosphate myocardial scintigrams. *Circulation* 51:436, 1975.

101. Willerson, J. T., Parkey, R. W., Bonte, F. J., Stokely, E. M., and Breja, L. M. Technetium stannous pyrophosphate myocardial scintigraphy: A new method of proven value for the diagnosis and localization of proven value

infarcts and for the detection of infarct extension in patients. *Tex. Med.* 72:51, 1976.

102. Willerson, J. T., Parkey, R. W., Buja, L. M., Lewis, S. E., and Bonte, F. J. Causes of necrosis other than infarction; myocardial trauma. In R. W. Parkey (ed.), *Clinical Nuclear Cardiology.* New York: Appleton, 1979. Pp. 209–224.
103. Zimmerman, R. A., Bilaniuk, L. A., Generalli, T., Bruce, D., Dolinskas, C., and Uzell, B. Cranial computed tomography in diagnosis and management of acute head trauma. *A.J.R.* 131:27, 1978.

Hemodynamic Monitoring

Albert Joseph Varon
Joseph M. Civetta

The critically ill patient represents a major challenge to the physician. The "traditional" clinical evaluation, usually the initial assessment tool, is often unreliable. There may be major changes in cardiovascular function that are not accompanied by obvious clinical findings.

Invasive hemodynamic monitoring at the bedside permits the acquisition of information concerning cardiorespiratory performance and the effects of therapy. However, it is of paramount importance that the gathered data be accurate and that the clinician use this information in an appropriate manner.

In this chapter we will review the monitoring equipment, the indications and information obtained from arterial and pulmonary artery catheterization, and the techniques of insertion and the complications of arterial catheterization. We will also discuss the relevance of the cardiopulmonary profile and the utility of continuous mixed venous oximetry.

The techniques of insertion and the complications of the pulmonary artery catheter are discussed in Chapter 15, and noninvasive hemodynamic monitoring is reviewed in Chapter 5.

MONITORING EQUIPMENT

Characteristics of a Pressure Monitoring System

The generation of waveforms in a monitor is a complex physical process. The pulsatile flow created by cardiac contraction is accomplished by episodic injection of the stroke volume into the elastic vascular system. This pulsatile flow creates a to-and-fro fluid movement in the intravascular catheter. When the catheter is connected to a transducer, the fluid motion in the vascular system is transformed into an electrical signal. The transducer is an electromechanical device (Fig. 6-1) in which a fluid-filled dome is applied to a sensitive diaphragm. Because fluid is not compressible, the to-and-fro motion of the fluid is directly transmitted to the diaphragm and results in periodic motion. On the undersurface of the diaphragm, a strain gauge, which is a system of variable resistances, is connected to an elec-

89

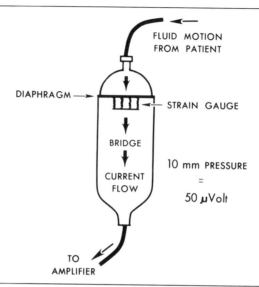

FLUID MOTION
FROM PATIENT

DIAPHRAGM ——→

STRAIN GAUGE

BRIDGE

CURRENT
FLOW

10 mm PRESSURE
=
50 μVolt

TO
AMPLIFIER

Fig. 6-1. Diagrammatic representation of a blood pressure transducer. The transducer changes energy of one form into another. In this instance, the energy generated by the pulsatile flow against the transducer diaphragm is transformed into an electrical current. (From J. M. Civetta, Pulmonary Artery Catheter Insertion. In C. L. Sprung (ed.), *The Pulmonary Artery Catheter, Methodology and Clinical Application.* Rockville, Md.: Aspen Publishers, 1983. Reproduced by permission.)

trical component called a *Wheatstone bridge.* When motion is imparted to the diaphragm by fluid flow, the variable resistances in this component change, inducing an electrical current that is delivered to an amplifying circuit in the monitor. Solid-state disposable electronic transducers, a recent development, maintain a linear pressure response and virtually eliminate baseline drift. They are, however, more expensive. Finally, the monitor creates a visible tracing on the screen.

There are four major considerations with the intravascular catheter, connecting tubing, transducer, and electronic monitor: frequency response, relative natural frequency, damping, and catheter whip artifact [20, 40].

1. *Frequency response.* Biologic signals are composed of many different waveforms that are described by the number of cycles per second, or hertz. The pressure tracings visible in the oscilloscope represent the sum of at least 1 to 10 cycle/sec variations. Since the heart rate commonly reaches at least 120/min (2 beats/sec), the system must be able to respond accurately to at least 20 cycles/sec (20 Hz)—the 10 cycles per heartbeat times the 2 beats/sec—to display all the variations produced by the cardiac contraction. If the heart rate increased to 180/min, the monitor should be able to reproduce 30 Hz. When the system's frequency response is inadequate, the displayed pressure will be lower than the true physiologic signal, because

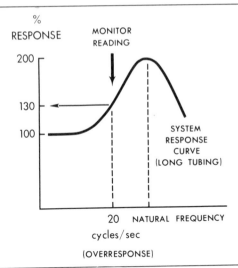

Fig. 6-2. Natural frequency and response relationship of a pressure monitoring system. When an excessively long piece of connecting tubing is used, the system response curve is shifted to the left, so that, at 20 hertz, there is already overresponse, or "ringing," in the system. (From J. M. Civetta, Pulmonary Artery Catheter Insertion. In C. L. Sprung (ed.), *The Pulmonary Artery Catheter, Methodology and Clinical Application*. Rockville, Md.: Aspen Publishers, 1983. Reproduced by permission.)

the highest frequencies will not be reproduced. This will be found most frequently when heart rates are rapid and the waveform is particularly steep: that is, in the rigid cardiovascular system of elderly patients with hypertension and arteriosclerosis.

2. *Natural frequency.* Each fluid-filled system has a natural frequency, at which amplification of the applied signal occurs. When the vibrations in the system approach the natural frequency, an increment in the amplitude of the power signal results. The resulting amplification created by the overresponse of the amplifier circuit causes the displayed pressure to exceed the true physiologic signal. The overall natural frequency relationships are displayed in Figure 6-2. One of the major determinants of natural frequency of a monitoring system is the length of the tubing connecting the catheter to the transducer. As the length of the tubing increases, the natural frequency decreases. Thus, an excessive length of tubing can make the natural frequency of the system occur in the physiologic range. As long as the natural frequency occurs outside the range necessary to faithfully reproduce the biologic signal (20 hertz) the monitor reading will display the correct pressure. If an excessively long piece of connecting tubing is used, however, the system response curve is shifted to the left, so that, at 20 hertz, there is already overresponse, or "ringing," in the system. This potential must be considered if the tubing is longer than 4 feet.

3. *Damping.* The damping coefficient refers to how quickly the system

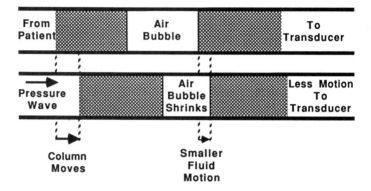

Fig. 6-3. The effect of an air bubble in the transmission tubing is depicted. Because the air is compressible, some of the fluid motion generated by pulsatile flow is lost in compressing the air bubble. Thus, the motion that is transmitted to the diaphragm of the transducer is less than that generated by the pulsatile flow. (From J. M. Civetta, Pulmonary Artery Catheter Insertion. In C. L. Sprung (ed.), *The Pulmonary Artery Catheter, Methodology and Clinical Application*. Rockville, Md.: Aspen Publishers, 1983. Reproduced by permission.)

comes to rest. Overdamping represents loss of physiologic signal in the transmission system. The most common artifact that causes overdamping is an air bubble in the circuit. Part of the energy of the fluid motion coming from the vessel is used to compress the air bubble (Fig. 6-3), and less is present in the transducer diaphragm. Less movement of the diaphragm produces a less-powerful electronic signal, and the displayed pressure is, therefore, lessened. Another example is when compliant (soft) plastic tubing is utilized to connect the catheter to the transducer. In this case, some of the to-and-fro motion will be lost in expanding the plastic tubing. When a system is overdamped, the waveform may have a slower rate of rise to systolic pressures and fall to diastolic pressure, blunting of the pressure peak, and loss of the dicrotic notch; in this case the systolic pressure will be underestimated (Fig. 6-4). When a system is underdamped the waveform may have a narrow, high-peak systolic curve with a low but prominent dicrotic notch; in this case the systolic pressure will be overestimated (Fig. 6-4). Whether the system is over- or underdamped, the diastolic pressure will also be affected, but it is much more tolerant of dynamic response inadequacies. Also, the electronic mean pressure is affected little by the dynamic response of the system. Recording the mean pressure, rather than the systolic and diastolic pressures, will minimize dynamic response artifact. However, for calculation of derived variables—i.e., rate-pressure

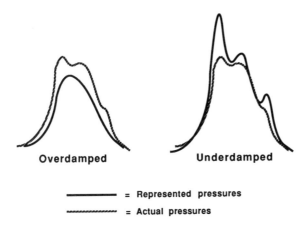

Overdamped   **Underdamped**

———————— = **Represented pressures**

~~~~~~~~~~~ = **Actual pressures**

Fig. 6-4. Graphic representation of damping in the arterial pressure waveform. When a system is overdamped, the waveform has a slower rate of rise to systolic pressures and fall to diastolic pressure, blunting of the pressure peak, and loss of the dicrotic notch. When a system is underdamped, the waveform has a narrow, high peak systolic curve with a low but prominent dicrotic notch.

product or coronary perfusion pressure—it is important to have accurate systolic and diastolic pressures.

4. *Catheter whip artifact.* This occurs in the pulmonary artery circulation as a result of the mechanical forces of acceleration of the heart generated during its contraction. This contraction imparts an acceleration to the catheter sitting within the pulmonary artery. This is a high-frequency artifact and can be handled effectively by incorporating a filter into the system.

Catheter-transducer systems used in intensive care can be described as "underdamped, second-order dynamic systems" [40]. Specification of the natural frequency and damping coefficient will completely characterize the system dynamics. The ability to excite the system with a rapid closure of the fast-flush valve permits measurement of natural frequency and damping coefficient. This can be performed simply by using a fast-flush test and recording the pressure waveform. Detailed discussion of these measurements and interpretation can be found in an excellent review by Gardner [40].

The pressure monitoring systems with the best dynamic response are those which have a high natural frequency (determined by the fast-flush method). A system with a natural frequency less than 10 Hz will be marginal.

To minimize factors known to lead to errors in measurement, use transparent tubing and fluid pathways, so that air bubbles can be easily seen and removed; keep the system simple, with the fewest number of components; use only low-compliance pressure tubing and as short a length as possible (less than 4 feet).

The digital display of pressures can lead to errors in interpretation, particularly in the pulmonary circulation, because the numbers displayed may represent an average of some seconds to avoid a constantly changing display. However, positive and negative artifacts induced by breathing will then be included in the calculation of the displayed number. To minimize these errors, the pressure to be recorded should be obtained from a calibrated oscilloscope or a strip recorder, if there is difficulty in interpretation [72].

Components of a Pressure Monitoring System

The clinical pressure monitoring system consists of three component groups: the intravascular catheters, connecting tube, and flush system; the electromechanical transducer; and the electronic amplifier and display. The assembled external components are displayed in Figure 6-5.

In an extensive review of infection control practices related to pressure monitoring devices, Keeler [58] noted that some procedures—such as aseptic technique during assembly and manipulation of components, disinfection of transducer heads between patients, tubing system arrangements eliminating the static fluid column, use of closed-flush systems, and use of heparinized normal saline instead of glucose solutions—are now generally accepted practice. Other variables have not been adequately supported by research.

Calibration of Equipment

Balancing

Balancing consists in the introduction of a zero reference point to the monitoring system. The zero reference signal is usually chosen to be the midpoint of the cardiac chambers. The patient's midaxillary line is the reference point most commonly used. Although it is often suggested that the diaphragm of the transducer be adjusted to this level and atmospheric pressure introduced by opening a stopcock on the transducer dome, this is not necessary or desirable. Leaving the transducer in a stationary position may avoid damage to this delicate instrument. The entire system is assembled and filled with fluid. The transducer is closed completely, and the unconnected tip of the transmission tubing is placed at the zero reference point and the balance control of the monitor adjusted. The secured and *stationary* transducer need never be moved to compensate for changes in the position of the patient or the height of the bed. It is only necessary to rebalance by disconnecting the end of the transmission tubing and adjusting it to the proper level.

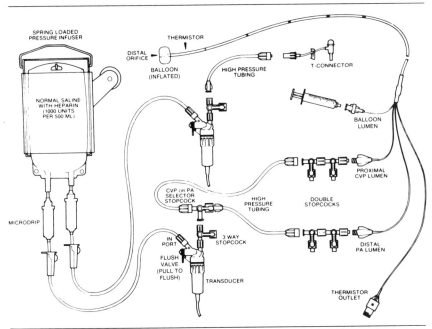

Fig. 6-5. External components of a pressure monitoring system. A single pressure infuser can be used to power the infusion devices in both arterial and pulmonary artery catheters. The use of a double stopcock enables one transducer to serve both the proximal and distal lumens of the pulmonary artery catheter. Additional components are identified in the drawing. (From J. M. Civetta, Pulmonary Artery Catheter Insertion. In C. L. Sprung (ed.), *The Pulmonary Artery Catheter, Methodology and Clinical Application.* Rockville, Md.: Aspen Publishers, 1983. Reproduced by permission.)

Calibrating

Calibrating consists in creating an electrical signal to represent a known pressure. This can be done through internal or external calibration.

Internal calibration is provided in most monitors. It involves activation of the calibration control, which introduces an electrical signal to the monitor "as if" that calibration pressure had been applied to the transducer itself. Although the transducers are supposed to be accurate to within 5 percent, in practice this accuracy is rarely achieved with reusable transducers [18]. Internal calibration is a satisfactory method with single-use disposable transducers.

A simple external calibration system that tests the transmission tubing, transducer, and monitor seems desirable with reusable transducers. An actual physical signal representing a known pressure is applied to the transducer diaphragm. To calibrate a system for a pulmonary artery catheter, a column of water equivalent to 20 mm Hg pressure is externally applied to the transducer. Because mercury weighs approximately 13.4 times

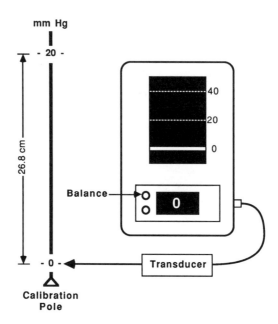

Fig. 6-6. External calibration using the introduction of a known signal. The first step is to attach the end of the pressure tubing to the 0 point on the calibration pole. The monitor itself is then adjusted so that this 0 reference pressure is displayed. (Modified from J. M. Civetta, Pulmonary Artery Catheter Insertion. In C. L. Sprung (ed.), *The Pulmonary Artery Catheter, Methodology and Clinical Application.* Rockville, Md.: Aspen Publishers, 1983. With permission.)

as much as water, this would require introduction of a water column 26.8 cm (268 mm H_2O). This can be easily accomplished using an IV pole as a calibration tool. An alligator clip is fastened to the zero point and the second clip is fastened at a measured distance of 26.8 cm above the zero reference point. The free end of the transmission tubing is attached to the zero clip and the monitor is balanced to this zero level (Fig. 6-6). The end of the tubing is then elevated to the 26.8 cm (20 mm Hg) reference point, and the gain or calibration control is adjusted so that 20 mm Hg is displayed on the monitor (Fig. 6-7). The free end of the tubing is then placed at the selected level on the patient's chest wall and the zero reference control readjusted (rebalanced). The tip of the transmission tubing is then reattached to the monitoring catheter. To calibrate a system for arterial blood pressure monitoring, the same steps are performed; however, a column of water of 134 cm, equivalent to 100 mm Hg, is used.

The new generation of solid-state disposable pressure transducers appears to be extremely accurate and stable over time. Although the elimination of balancing, mechanical calibration, and fluid movement in the

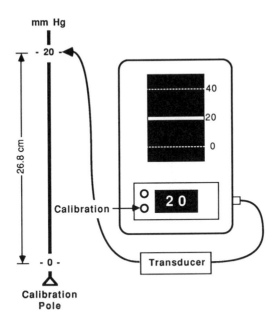

Fig. 6-7. Introduction of the actual pressure signal. The end of the tubing is then elevated to a preselected point corresponding to 20 mm Hg (26.8 cm above the 0 reference point). The monitor is then adjusted to reflect this signal. (Modified from J. M. Civetta, Pulmonary Artery Catheter Insertion. In C. L. Sprung (ed.), *The Pulmonary Artery Catheter, Methodology and Clinical Application.* Rockville, Md.: Aspen Publishers, 1983. With permission.)

transducer has diminished the potential for contamination and error in measurement, occasional confirmation of accurate calibration seems prudent.

The Centers for Disease Control recommend replacing the disposable dome and delivery system of invasive monitoring devices every 48 hours [15], although some reports have indicated that the "safe" interval may be extended to 72 hours [51] with the reusable transducers and up to 96 hours [66] when using the new disposable transducers.

ARTERIAL CATHETERIZATION

Indications

It is widely accepted that an arterial indwelling catheter is indicated whenever there is a need for continuous monitoring of blood pressure and/or frequent sampling of arterial blood in critically ill patients [19, 43, 78, 81].

States in which precise and continuous blood pressure data are necessary include acute hypertensive crises, shock of any etiology, use of potent vasoactive or inotropic drugs, hypotensive anesthesia, high levels of respiratory support (high intrathoracic pressures)—indeed, any situation in which any of the factors affecting cardiac function is rapidly changing. This is particularly true in patients with shock, because indirect measurement of blood pressure by a cuff has been shown to be inaccurate [24].

Sequential analysis of blood gas tensions and pH is necessary in any acute illness involving cardiovascular or respiratory dysfunction, or when hyperventilation is instituted in patients with CNS injuries. The preanalytic error—that which occurs prior to arrival of the sample in the lab—has been noted to be higher in "single-stick" samples than in samples obtained from indwelling cannulas, especially in patients with unstable cardiac or respiratory status [94].

Inserting arterial lines is a relatively safe and inexpensive procedure. There are no absolute contraindications to arterial catheterization per se, although bleeding diathesis and anticoagulant therapy may increase the risk of hemorrhagic complications. Severe occlusive arterial disease with distal ischemia, the presence of a vascular prostheses, and local infection are contraindications to specific sites of catheterization.

Information Obtained

With an indwelling arterial catheter and monitoring system, the systolic (SBP), diastolic (DBP), and mean (MAP) pressures will be continuously displayed. The pulse rate can be calculated from the arterial tracing when the electrocardiogram (ECG) is not available (i.e., during electrocautery use in surgery).

The shape of the arterial pressure tracing represents a particular stroke volume ejected at a particular state of myocardial contractility. Qualitative interpretation may be made in a hypovolemic patient with a small stroke volume, which will thus create a smaller pressure wave. If myocardial contractility is diminished, the rate of increase in aortic pressure will diminish, and the upslope of the arterial pressure tracing will decrease. Although quantitation of stroke volume has been attempted (using computers to solve the equations necessary to relate the shape of the arterial pressure tracing to actual stroke volume ejected [112]) critical illness introduces too many variables to make this measurement reliable. The location of the dicrotic notch on the arterial waveform has also been advocated as an indicator of the systemic vascular resistance; however, Gerber [41] was unable to demonstrate any statistically significant correlation.

An indwelling arterial catheter can provide ready access for arterial blood gas sampling and other samples necessary to chart the progression of multisystemic illness. Removal of an adequate discard volume (4 ml) before sampling has been suggested [23] for reliable tests. On the other hand, conflicting data [55, 82] exist about the accuracy of coagulation studies obtained through these catheters.

Techniques of Insertion

Various techniques and sites have been used to access the arterial circulation for continuous monitoring. Insertion can be accomplished using direct puncture with over-the-needle catheters or using the modified Seldinger technique (see below). The superficial temporal, axillary, brachial, radial, ulnar, femoral, and dorsalis pedis arteries have all been used. The selection of anatomic site remains a "parochial" issue [19] depending basically on its availability and the experience of the clinician. Although the technique of insertion varies depending on the anatomic site chosen, some general principles can be applied [73].

1. The percutaneous approach is preferred over direct surgical exposure of the vessel, to minimize both vascular trauma and the risk of infection.
2. Proper positioning of the anatomic site is of major importance for localization and fixation of the vessel and for the comfort of the operator.
3. It is prudent to confirm collateral blood flow by a modified Allen's test (for radial and ulnar sites), or by the presence of distal pulses (for axillary and femoral sites) and other pulses (posterior tibial pulse for dorsalis pedis artery). Confirmation will not guarantee prevention of ischemia, but it would be risky to proceed without it.
4. Meticulous sterile technique, using gloves, mask, wide antiseptic skin prep, and proper draping, should lower the incidence of local infection.
5. Proper selection of catheter size (the smaller the better) and design (nontapered) will decrease thrombotic and hemorrhagic complications.
6. Atraumatic catheter insertion and proper fixation to the skin may lessen the risk of thrombosis, infection, bleeding, and dislodgement.
7. Aseptic dressing changes at appropriate intervals (48 hours) will minimize infectious complications.
8. Continuous infusion of small volumes of heparinized (2 units/ml) saline will help to maintain catheter patency.
9. Repeated careful inspection of the insertion site for redness, tenderness, or drainage and of the distal extremity for ischemic changes will allow early detection of complications, so that the catheter may be promptly removed.

Radial Artery
The dual blood supply to the hand and the superficial location of the vessel make the radial artery the most commonly used site for arterial catheterization. Cannulation is technically easy, as is securing the catheter in place, and there is a low incidence of complications.

Most authors [43, 73, 81, 97] recommend assessing the adequacy of collateral circulation before cannulation of the radial artery. The most commonly used test is the modified Allen test [33], which differs from the original description by Allen in 1929 [1]. In this modification, the patient is instructed to elevate the hand and clench the fist firmly, thus squeezing the blood from the vessels of the hand. After the examiner simultaneously compresses both the radial and ulnar arteries, the patient lowers and opens the hand in a relaxed fashion (carefully, so as not to overextend it). The examiner then releases the pressure over the ulnar artery, and the time for return of color is noted. It is considered normal if the capillary blush of the hand is complete within 6 seconds. Other methods, such as ultrasonic Doppler technique [71], plethysmography [10], and pulse oximetry [84], have also been used to assess the adequacy of the collateral arterial supply.

Of interest, Slogoff [98] challenged the use of the Allen test after he studied 1699 cardiovascular surgical patients. He noted that in the *absence* of peripheral vascular disease, the Allen test was not a predictor of ischemia of the hand during or after radial artery cannulation, that decreased or absent radial artery flow following cannulation was of no clinical conse-

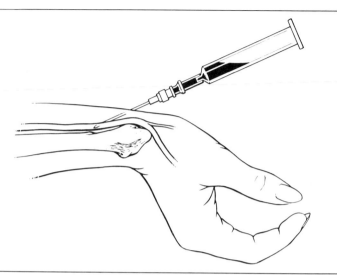

Fig. 6-8. Technique for radial artery cannulation. The arm should also be draped to create a sterile field. (From B. Sabo and R. B. Smith, A tiny adjunct to arterial cannulation. *Anesthesiology* 64:534, 1986. Reproduced by permission.)

quence, and that radial artery cannulation was a low-risk, high-benefit monitoring technique. Since more than 88 percent of the arteries in this study were cannulated less than 36 hours, these data should not be extrapolated to critically ill patients, especially those who have prolonged low-flow states and are receiving high doses of vasoactive drugs.

The wrist should be stabilized and hyperextended by fixing the forearm and arm to a board. Locate the radial artery just proximal to the head of the radius. After cleansing the area with povidone-iodine solution [6] and draping, infiltrate with 1% lidocaine *without* epinephrine. Insert a 20-gauge, 1.5 in. Teflon catheter needle device attached to a 3-ml syringe (without plunger) [90] at a 30-degree angle to the surface of the skin and advance (Fig. 6-8). After the artery is punctured and a flash appears in the hub, while the continual backflow is observed in the empty syringe, the needle is advanced to ensure that the catheter has also entered the lumen of the artery. *If* free flow continues, the catheter is advanced while the needle is held in the fixed position. The artery can also be cannulated after transfixation, in which the posterior wall is deliberately punctured, the needle is removed, and the catheter is retracted and then threaded when pulsatile blood flow is obtained. No significant difference in the incidence of thrombus formation after decannulation has been noted between the direct threading or transfixation techniques [26, 53]. Recently, some catheter devices have included a small guidewire to facilitate catheter threading after successful artery puncture. The catheter is then connected to the pressure monitoring system and the waveform examined. Finally, the catheter should be fixed to the skin with sutures and covered with povidone-iodine ointment [6] and a sterile dressing.

In an alternative approach to radial artery catheterization [83], the radial artery is cannulated on the dorsum of the hand, where it emerges from the anatomic snuffbox. Advantages claimed are preservation of the palmar branch of the radial artery (which is an important contributor to the superficial palmar arch) and a possible decrease in the incidence of digital ischemia. However, this procedure was successful in only 78 percent of patients.

Axillary Artery
The axillary artery has been recommended as suitable for long-term direct arterial pressure monitoring. Its use has been associated with relatively few complications and no reported permanent sequelae. The major advantages include its larger size, freedom for the patient's hand, and placement in close proximity to the aorta with better representation of the pressure waveform [11, 12, 105]. Pulsation and pressure are maintained even in the presence of shock with marked peripheral vasoconstriction. Also, because of the extensive collateral circulation that exists between the thyrocervical trunk of the subclavian artery and the subscapular artery (which is a branch of the distal axillary artery), thrombosis of the axillary artery will not lead to compromised flow in the distal arm. The arm is abducted and externally rotated more than 90 degrees. Cannulation is then performed using a modified Seldinger technique. The needle is inserted into the artery as high as possible. Once free arterial flow is obtained, a guidewire is passed through the needle. The needle is then removed and a 19- or 20-gauge Teflon catheter 16-cm-long is inserted over the wire. Aseptic technique and fixation procedures similar to the above described should be followed. Major disadvantages are its rather deep location and mobility, which increase the technical difficulty for insertion.

Femoral Artery
The femoral artery has also been utilized for continuous blood pressure monitoring. Major advantages are its superficial location and large size, making it easy to cannulate [45]. The femoral artery should be identified and a site approximately 2 cm below the inguinal ligament chosen for insertion. The skin and artery are entered at a 45-degree angle, and a 16-cm-long, 19- or 20-gauge Teflon catheter is introduced using the modified Seldinger technique. The major disadvantages are associated with maintaining a clean dressing in the presence of draining abdominal wounds and ostomies in surgical patients. It would seem prudent to avoid the femoral route whenever abdominal sepsis and/or advanced peripheral vascular disease are present. In spite of these potential disadvantages, studies have failed to demonstrate a higher complication rate in patients with femoral artery catheters [89, 105].

Other Sites
The dorsal pedal arteries have no significant cannulation hazards if collateral flow can be demonstrated to the remainder of the foot through the posterior tibial artery. This can be done by occluding the dorsalis pedis artery, blanching the great toe by compressing the toenail for several sec-

onds, and then releasing the toenail while observing the return of color [52]. The artery is cannulated in a fashion similar to that used with the radial. Major disadvantages are the artery's relatively small size and problems relating to ambulation.

The superficial temporal artery has been extensively used in infants and in some adults for continuous pressure monitoring. However, because of its small size and tortuousity, surgical exposure is required for cannulation. Furthermore, a very small but worrisome incidence of neurologic complications has been reported in infants [13, 96].

Although the brachial artery has been successfully used for short-term monitoring, there is little evidence to support the use of prolonged brachial artery monitoring, and its use has been discouraged [19]. If collateral circulation is inadequate, obstruction of the brachial artery may be catastrophic, leading to loss of the forearm and hand.

Complications

Ischemic

The most significant catheter-related complications include partial or complete thrombosis and infarction. Most of the reports that have described the complications following radial artery cannulation have stressed the high incidence (25–38%) of early radial artery occlusion and the rarity of late ischemic damage [8, 98]. Recannulation of the occluded artery generally occurs but may take several weeks [8]. The incidence of radial artery thrombosis has progressively declined as a result of the understanding of the effects of different catheter size (20 gauge is better than 18 gauge) and material (Teflon is better) and of the use of continuous heparin flow instead of intermittent flushing [97]. Several risk factors have been associated with ischemic complications [115]: female sex, low cardiac output states, use of vasoconstrictor drugs, multiple attempts or hematoma formation, small size of radial artery or small wrist circumference, severe peripheral vascular disease, and increased duration of cannulation. Reports of permanent ischemic damage attributed solely to radial artery cannulation are apparently few, but aggressive management—brachial plexus or stellate ganglion block or surgical exploration—may be required to avoid permanent necrosis if arterial occlusion causes any sign of ischemia.

Infectious

Infections related to arterial catheterization were studied by Band and Maki [6], who found an 18 percent local infection rate and a 4 percent incidence of catheter-related septicemia. Important features associated with infection of arterial cannulas are placement of the catheter for more than 4 days, insertion by surgical cutdown rather than percutaneously, and local inflammation—although the absence of this sign should not be used to exclude consideration of catheter-related infection. Most cases of catheter-related infection respond to removal of the catheter with or without additional antibiotics. Rarely, an abscess can follow cannulation of the radial artery [65].

Other
Common problems associated with arterial catheterization are hematoma formation and disconnection from the monitoring system with bleeding. Other possible complications include cerebral embolization (when flushing catheters), aneurysms, arteriovenous fistulas, and compression neuropathy secondary to hematoma in anticoagulated patients. Finally, inadvertent injection of vasoactive drugs or other agents into an artery can cause severe pain, distal ischemia, and tissue necrosis.

CENTRAL VENOUS CATHETERIZATION
Indications
The most common indications for central venous catheterization in the critically ill are for fluid therapy, drug infusions, or parenteral nutrition, and for central venous pressure (CVP) monitoring. Central venous catheters have also been used to aspirate air in case of embolism during neurosurgical procedures in the sitting position, for placement of cardiac pacemakers or inferior vena cava filters, and for hemodialysis access. There are no absolute contraindications for CVP catheter placement, although coagulopathies, thrombocytopenia, and anticoagulant or thrombolytic therapy are factors that increase the risk of hemorrhagic complications. Thrombosed vessels and areas with local infection or inflammation should be avoided.

Information Obtained
Although central venous lines are placed primarily for venous access, useful information occasionally can be obtained by measuring the CVP. The CVP may be useful in a hypotensive trauma patient to differentiate a pericardial tamponade from hypovolemia [78].

The CVP can be measured with accuracy if the tip of the catheter is in any large intrathoracic vein or in the right atrium itself [46]. The catheter should be attached to a transducer monitor system, since water manometric measurements are unreliable [19, 109].

A properly placed catheter can be used to measure right atrial pressure, which, in the absence of tricuspid valve disease, will reflect the right ventricular end-diastolic pressure. CVP, therefore, can give information about the relationship between intravascular volume and *right* ventricular function but cannot be used to assess either of these factors independently. CVP cannot be used to assess left ventricular function in critically ill patients, since ventricular disparity and independence of right and left atrial pressures have been confirmed repeatedly in these patients [2, 9, 21, 38, 107]. Furthermore, CVP is only a single parameter, in contradistinction to the more complete information concerning pressures, flow, and venous gas measurements available with pulmonary artery catheters (see below).

Techniques of Insertion and Complications
The techniques of insertion and the complications of central venous catheterization are discussed in Chapter 25.

PULMONARY ARTERY CATHETERIZATION

Indications

Investigators have reported that in patients with acute myocardial infarction, clinical criteria were predictive of cardiac index and pulmonary artery (PA) occlusion pressure in 81 percent and 85 percent of the subjects, respectively [37]. In patients with uncomplicated myocardial infarction, clinical and radiologic criteria are sufficient to monitor the majority. This is not the case in critically ill patients.

In a series of critically ill patients without myocardial infarction [25], ICU physicians correctly predicted the pulmonary artery occlusion pressure only 42 percent of the time (within a broad clinical range), and the cardiac index only 44 percent of the time. Even when three or more physicians concurred, overall accuracy was not improved. In another study [32], the pulmonary artery occlusion pressure was correctly predicted 30 percent of the time, and cardiac output and systemic vascular resistance were correctly predicted only 50 percent of the time. Therefore, clinical estimates were similar to or worse than those that could have been obtained by flipping a coin! Not surprisingly, as a result of the information obtained by pulmonary artery catheterization, the planned therapy was changed in almost 50 percent of the cases in both studies.

Although the pulmonary artery catheter permits a more accurate hemodynamic assessment and therapy may be modified as a result, this does not prove that knowledge of this data and alteration of the therapy improves overall patient outcome. The use of the pulmonary artery catheter has been criticized as unproven and dangerous; some authors believe a moratorium and a clinical trial are necessary [86, 108]. However, others have expressed doubt that effectiveness can be proven by a randomized trial [104].

In a recent community-wide study of the use of pulmonary artery catheters in patients with acute myocardial infarction [44], the use of the catheter was associated with a higher mortality and increased length of hospital stay. However, the authors recognized the retrospective nature of the study and acknowledged a possible selection bias, because the medical record was used as the primary data source. It was not possible to determine if the sicker patients with acute myocardial infarction were chosen for a PA catheter—which might be postulated, since clinicians were not participating in a study but rather choosing care for patients individually.

Yet on the basis of this study, Robin [87] expressed fear that "masses of patients have been harmed or died" from the use of the PA catheter and urged a moratorium on the use of this device.

The use of this catheter cannot be expected in and of itself to improve outcome, as if it were an amulet. Clearly, there is a clinical process of many steps linking a device with an outcome: physicians do select only certain patients to be monitored, the monitoring system must produce accurate numbers, abnormal values need to be recognized, pathophysiologic causes have to be identified, the need for therapy must be appreciated, a specific form of therapy must be selected and administered appropriately, the pa-

Table 6-1. Indications for pulmonary artery catheterization

I. Surgical
  A. Preoperative cardiovascular assessment and perioperative management of high-risk patients undergoing extensive surgical procedures
  B. Postoperative cardiovascular complications
  C. Multisystem trauma
  D. Assessment of the effect of intravascular volume on cardiac function
  E. Shock unresponsive to perceived adequate fluid therapy
  F. Delineation of cardiovascular contribution to multiple organ system dysfunction
II. Pulmonary
  A. To differentiate noncardiogenic ("ARDS") from cardiogenic pulmonary edema
  B. To assess effects of high levels of ventilatory support on cardiovascular status
III. Cardiac
  A. Complicated myocardial infarction
  B. Unstable angina requiring intravenous nitroglycerin therapy
  C. Congestive heart failure unresponsive to conventional therapy, to guide preload and afterload therapy
  D. Pulmonary hypertension, for diagnosis and monitoring during acute drug therapy

---

tient must respond, and this response must improve the clinical condition sufficiently to augment survival.

Complete hemodynamic monitoring, including pulmonary artery catheterization, is indicated whenever precise information can replace the uncertainty of clinical impressions [19]. Table 6-1 represents the indications most often noted in the medical literature [16, 43, 91, 100]. There are no specific contraindications to PA catheterization, but the same cautions as those attached to central venous access apply.

Information Obtained

The pulmonary artery catheter has provided a "quantum leap" in the physiologic information available for the management of critically ill patients [19]. The information that can be obtained includes central venous pressure, pulmonary artery diastolic pressure (PADP), systolic (PASP) and mean (MPAP) pressures, pulmonary artery occlusion pressure (PAOP), cardiac output (CO) by thermodilution, mixed venous blood gases by intermittent sampling, and continuous mixed venous oximetry. Also, right ventricular pressures and oxygen saturation can be measured during catheter insertion and removal. On the basis of this information, a multitude of derived parameters (see below) can also be obtained.

Pressures

Pressure measurements are affected by the respiratory variations; therefore, they should be performed at end-expiration. Use of the analog rather than the digital readings can prevent errors in measurement [92]. Recently, various algorithms have been incorporated into monitors to decrease the effect of these artifacts [35, 68].

The central venous and PA pressures can be displayed continuously, and the PAOP is obtained by inflating the balloon intermittently. To determine if the catheter is in the "wedge" position, the waveform needs to be inspected. When there is doubt, aspiration of capillary blood from the wedge position can confirm the position, since at this level the O_2 tension and pH are higher and the CO_2 tension lower than the arterial [69].

The PAOP reflects the relationship between intravascular volume and left ventricular function. When the balloon is inflated (1.5 cc), the blood flow in a distal segment of the pulmonary artery is occluded, creating a conduit through which left atrial pressure (LAP) can be measured. The PAOP is a reliable index of the LAP even in the presence of elevated pulmonary vascular resistance [64]. The PA diastolic pressure has also been used as an index of LAP. However, it is not as reliable, particularly in the presence of tachycardia, or increased pulmonary vascular resistance or during rapid infusion of blood [61].

The PAOP represents the LAP as long as this conduit (proximally occluded segment) is patent to the left atrium [56]. This may not be so if the catheter is positioned in an area of the lung where the alveolar pressure exceeds pulmonary venous pressure (zone 2 as described by West [113]) or both pulmonary artery and venous pressures (West's zone 1), causing intermittent or continuous collapse of the pulmonary capillaries. This is particularly important when the patient has low pulmonary vascular pressure and/or high positive end-expiratory pressure (PEEP). Fortunately, since the PA catheter is "flow directed," it is most likely to pass into lung segments with high blood flow (West's zone 3), where both pulmonary artery and venous pressures exceed alveolar pressure, so that there is a continuous column of blood between the distal lumen of the catheter and the left atrium. A lateral chest x-ray can be used to determine the location of the catheter tip in relation to the left atrium; if the tip of the catheter is at or below this chamber, zone-3 conditions will exist even if high levels of end-expiratory pressure are used [88, 106].

In the absence of mitral valve disease, the left atrial pressure reflects the left ventricular end-diastolic pressure (LVEDP), and if there are no alterations in the left ventricular compliance, LVEDP will reflect left ventricular end-diastolic volume (LVEDV). In the intact ventricle, LVEDV reflects the end-diastolic stretch of the muscle fiber, which represents the true preload.

Raising the intrathoracic pressure introduces an artifact that affects all intrathoracic pressures to an extent that depends on the state of pulmonary compliance [49]. In patients with acute respiratory insufficiency, the PEEP artifact should usually not excced 1 mm Hg for every 5 cm H_2O of PEEP applied. A greater discrepancy can be seen if the patient is hypovolemic or if the catheter is malpositioned as described above [19]. When high levels of intrathoracic pressure are used, more-accurate "transmural" PAOP readings may be obtained by subtracting the intrapleural pressures, which can be measured with a catheter or by an esophageal balloon. Methods of calculating transmural pressures, however, have many technical limitations. Another method is brief, cautious removal of PEEP. Hypoxemia is avoided by using a high inspired oxygen concentration and manual bag ventilation during the measurement [28]. This procedure need only be performed a few times a day to document how much of the PEEP is transmitted to the PAOP.

The PAOP does not always equate with preload, probably because of abnormalities in left ventricular compliance in the critically ill [14, 47, 85]. Therefore, the use of the pulmonary artery catheter demands knowledge of the assumptions involved and of the factors mentioned above for proper interpretation.

Cardiac Output

The thermodilution technique is used for measurement of the cardiac output. Thermodilution represents an application of the indicator dilution principle in which a change in the heat content of the blood is induced at one point of the circulation and the resulting change in temperature is detected at a point downstream [39]. This change is produced by a rapid injection of a known volume of fluid at a known temperature (colder than the body), into the right atrium via the proximal port of the PA catheter. The change in temperature is registered by a thermistor embedded in the catheter wall approximately 4 cm from the tip of the catheter. This lowered temperature decreases the electrical resistance of the thermistor and results in a thermodilution curve. If for any reason the fluid bolus cannot be injected through the atrial port of the catheter (i.e., obstructed lumen), it can be administered through the side port of the introducer [63, 110].

The measurement of the cardiac output is based on a modification of the Stewart-Hamilton equation [7, 31, 39].

$$CO = \frac{V_I(T_B - T_I)K_1K_2}{\int_0^x \Delta T_B(t)dt}$$

where

CO = cardiac output
V_I = injectate volume
T_B = blood (PA) temperature
T_I = injectate temperature
K_1 = density factor (injectate/blood)
K_2 = computation constant
$\int \Delta T_B(t)dt$ = change in blood temperature as a function of time

The "numerator variables" are selected by the operator before the actual injection: the volume (V_I) and type of injectate solution (K_1) are chosen; the computation constant (K_2) for the catheter in use is entered in the computer; and the injectate temperature (T_I) and the blood temperature (T_B) are monitored by the reference probe and the catheter thermistor, respectively.

The remaining variable, the denominator of the equation, is the thermodilution curve produced by the injection of the indicator. The computer integrates the area under this curve and the resulting calculation is displayed as the cardiac output in liters per minute. The area under the curve is inversely proportional to cardiac output: that is, the larger the area under the curve, the lower the cardiac output. In actuality, right ventricular output is being measured: in the absence of intracardiac shunting, right and left ventricular cardiac outputs are equivalent [7].

The injectate solution can be either 5% D/W or normal saline, since the density factor (K_1) for each solution is similar [39]. Both iced and room temperature injectates have been shown to be accurate and to produce reproducible cardiac output determinations in critically ill patients [34, 74, 80]. Possible advantages of room temperature injectate include immediate availability, convenience of use, stability of injectate temperature, and avoidance of dysrhythmias [48]. The volume most commonly used is 10 ml; smaller volumes may decrease reproducibility of the results [34, 80] unless iced injectate is used [34]. The volume of injectate used must be quantified accurately, because the amount of change in injectate volume creates a linear error in the measured value.

The computation constant (K_2) corrects for differences in units of measurement, injection or proximal lumen dead space, heat transfer, injection rate, and volume and temperature of injectate. This constant will differ for each manufacturer, computer, catheter model, and injectate temperature and volume and must be determined and adjusted prior to measurement [7]. The thermodilution cardiac output measured by different computers may differ [67].

Because PA blood temperature varies during the ventilatory cycle, the baseline temperature for the thermal curve varies according to the phase of ventilation at which the measurement is initiated [116]. Also, there may be changes of the stroke volume at different phases of the ventilatory cycle. Most authors recommend timing the injections with a specific phase of the respiratory cycle—i.e., injecting at end-inspiration, rather than at random [3, 102]. The measurement protocol should be consistent, and triplicate measurements should be done, since a single measurement is not reliable [54]. The injections should be smooth and completed within 4 seconds.

Potential sources of error include injectate temperature different from the temperature used to determine the computation constant or that of the fluid being monitored by the reference probe; delivered volume less than the one chosen for the computation; incorrect computation constant; infusion of intravenous fluids via the introducer, proximal, or distal lumens during measurements; faulty catheter lumens [62, 69]; improperly positioned catheter (i.e., if the catheter is in the "wedge" position or if the proximal lumen is above the atrium or within the introducer sheath [27, 103]); and presence of intracardiac shunts or tricuspid regurgitation [7].

Another source of error is baseline temperature fluctuation caused by peripheral infusions; therefore, rapid volume infusions should be either maintained at a constant rate or discontinued for at least 30 seconds prior to the measurement of cardiac output [114].

Venous Blood Gases

The pulmonary artery catheter can also be used to obtain true mixed venous blood samples for analysis or to measure mixed venous oxygen saturation ($S\bar{v}O_2$) continuously (see below). Sampling technique is important. Blood should be withdrawn from the most proximal pulmonary artery location possible, and at a very slow rate. A fast rate of blood withdrawal or a malpositioned catheter (distal migration or wedging) may cause a falsely elevated mixed venous oxygen tension ($P\bar{v}O_2$). This is due to "contamination" of the mixed venous blood with arterialized pulmonary capillary blood. Shapiro et al. [95] have identified contaminated samples by comparing the CO_2 tensions in blood obtained from systemic ($PaCO_2$) and pulmonary ($P\bar{v}CO_2$) arteries. A $P\bar{v}CO_2$ equal to or lower than a simultaneous $PaCO_2$ suggests contamination of pulmonary arterial blood by pulmonary capillary blood.

Techniques of Insertion and Complications

The pulmonary artery catheter is most commonly placed percutaneously into a central vein. This procedure has been facilitated by the use of introducer assemblies. Once the catheter attains central venous location and the balloon is inflated, it usually passes through the right ventricle and into the appropriate pulmonary artery position rapidly. Maneuvers often employed to facilitate passage through the pulmonary valve include elevating the head of the bed and increasing ventricular ejection in low output states by the administration of calcium chloride or other inotropic drugs.

PA catheters should be removed as soon as they are no longer needed. If continued monitoring is necessary, the catheter should probably be changed after 4 days in "clean" patients and 3 days in patients with a known source of infection. If there are no signs of local infection, the catheter can be changed once over a guidewire, provided that the catheter tip and the intracutaneous segment of the introducer are cultured semiquantitatively. If culture results are positive the next day (more than 15 colonies), the replaced catheter should be removed and a new insertion site selected [50]. We have noticed that second guidewire changes are used infrequently and have a high incidence of positive catheter cultures [22]; therefore, they should probably be avoided. A new silver impregnated collagen sleeve (Vitacuff[1]) can be placed over the introducer and positioned subcutaneously. In preliminary studies, the rate of positive cultures does not increase over at least a 2-week period. Preliminary calculations show a lower cumulative rate with the original catheter protected with the sleeve than that associated with using guidewires initially and then switching sites after a specified duration (3 or 4 days).

The techniques of insertion and the complications of pulmonary artery catheterization are discussed in Chapter 15.

DERIVED CARDIOPULMONARY PARAMETERS

Although rate, blood pressure, and respiratory rate may provide an overview of the "stability" of intensive care unit patients, traditional vital signs

[1]Vitaphore Corp., San Carlos, Calif.

do little to suggest therapy in these patients. The derived hemodynamic parameters aid the clinician by quantitating the relationships among heart rate, filling pressures, resistance, contractility, and cardiac output. The parameters derived from gas analysis help the physician to estimate the adequacy of oxygen delivery and pulmonary function. The collection of the measured and derived cardiopulmonary parameters is known as the cardiopulmonary profile (CPP). Normal values can be seen in Table 6-2. Calculation of these parameters has been greatly simplified by the use of programmable calculators and microcomputers [17, 59].

Hemodynamic Parameters

The first parameter usually derived from the measured hemodynamic parameters is the mean pressures (MP). Mean pressures may be measured electronically by the bedside monitor or calculated from the systolic (SP) and diastolic (DP) pressures by the formula

$$MP = DP + \frac{(SP - DP)}{3}$$

Often, mean pressures, rather than systolic and diastolic pressures, are recorded because they are less influenced by the dynamic response of the monitoring system.

An index is a method used to eliminate the effect of body size and provide "normal" ranges. Dividing a parameter by the body surface area (BSA) is one of the accepted methods. The BSA may be obtained using a height-weight nomogram or by using the classic Du Bois formula [30]:

$$BSA(m^2) = 0.007184 \times ht(cm)^{0.725} \times wt(kg)^{0.425}$$

A simpler formula is a modification of an equation by Gehan and George [70]:

$$BSA(m^2) = \sqrt{\frac{ht(cm) \times wt(kg)}{3600}} \ or \ BSA(m^2) = \sqrt{\frac{ht(in) \times wt(lb)}{3131}}$$

Cardiac index (CI) is then equal to the cardiac output (CO) divided by the body surface area. Similar indices have been used for systemic and pulmonary vascular resistance, right and left ventricular stroke work, and stroke volume.

Cardiac output is the sum of all stroke volumes ejected in a given time. It is usually represented as the product of average stroke volume (SV) and heart rate (HR; beats per minute), where stroke volume is the amount of blood ejected by the heart with each contraction. When cardiac output and HR are known, SV is the quotient of CO divided by HR.

The primary determinants of stroke volume are the ventricular preload, afterload, and contractility.

Preload is the muscle fiber length of the ventricle prior to systole and therefore is not usually measured directly in critically ill patients. On the

Table 6-2. Measured and derived cardiopulmonary parameters

Parameter	Unit	Normal range
Systolic blood pressure (SBP)	mm Hg	100–140
Diastolic blood pressure (DBP)	mm Hg	60–90
Mean arterial blood pressure (MAP)	mm Hg	70–105
Pulmonary artery systolic pressure (PASP)	mm Hg	15–30
Pulmonary artery diastolic pressure (PADP)	mm Hg	4–12
Mean pulmonary artery pressure (MPAP)	mm Hg	9–16
Right ventricular systolic pressure (RVSP)	mm Hg	15–30
Right ventricular end-diastolic pressure (RVEDP)	mm Hg	4–12
Central venous pressure (CVP)	mm Hg	0–8
Pulmonary artery occlusion pressure (PAOP)	mm Hg	2–12
Cardiac output (CO)	liters/min	*
Stroke volume (SV)	ml/beat	*
Cardiac index (CI)	liters/min/m²	2.8–4.2
Stroke index (SI)	ml/beat/m²	30–65
Left ventricular stroke-work index (LVSWI)	gm × m/m²	43–61
Right ventricular stroke-work index (RVSWI)	gm × m/m²	7–12
Systemic vascular resistance (SVR)	dyne × sec × cm⁻⁵	900–1400
Pulmonary vascular resistance (PVR)	dyne × sec × cm⁻⁵	150–250
Arterial oxygen tension (PaO$_2$)	mm Hg	70–100
Arterial oxygen saturation (SaO$_2$)	(fraction)	0.93–0.98
Arterial oxygen content (CaO$_2$)	ml O$_2$/dl blood	16–22
Mixed venous oxygen tension (P$\bar{v}$O$_2$)	mm Hg	36–42
Mixed venous oxygen content (C$\bar{v}$O$_2$)	ml O$_2$/dl blood	12–17
Arteriovenous oxygen content difference C(a-v)O$_2$	ml O$_2$/dl blood	3–5
Oxygen delivery (DO$_2$)	ml/min	640–1400
Oxygen consumption (VO$_2$)	ml/min	180–280
Oxygen utilization (O$_2$ util)	(fraction)	0.22–0.30
Pulmonary venous admixture ($\dot{Q}_s/\dot{Q}_t$)	(fraction)	0.03–0.05

*Varies with size.

basis of the work by Otto Frank and others, Starling described the relationship between the resting fiber length of the myocardium and ventricular work [101]. As resting fiber length increases, there is an increase in work performed upon subsequent contraction. Beyond a certain point, however, further increases in fiber length will not increase external mechanical work, and work may, in fact, decrease—a description of cardiac failure. The end-diastolic fiber length determines the end-diastolic volume of the ventricle (LVEDV). For a given compliance (the relationship between pressure and volume), end-diastolic volume is proportional to end-diastolic pressure. "Starling curves" have been constructed by plotting stroke volume, cardiac output, or stroke work as a function of left ventricular end-diastolic pressure, or PAOP. Although this is helpful, it is not absolutely correct or accurate. Therefore, caution should be taken in the interpretation of the PAOP as the sole measure of left ventricular preload, because of compliance changes in critically ill patients.

The second determinant of stroke volume is afterload. Afterload is the wall stress faced by the myocardium during left ventricular ejection; therefore, it depends on a complicated relationship of left ventricular size, shape, pressure, and wall thickness. Afterload, however, can be thought as the impedance to left ventricular ejection, which, in the absence of aortic stenosis, depends on the distensibility of the large arteries and the systemic vascular resistance (SVR). Changes in vascular resistance usually reflect altered blood viscosity or vascular tone. The SVR does not necessarily reflect left ventricular loading conditions, since the true measure of ventricular afterload must consider the interaction of factors internal and external to the myocardium [60]. Although it is not physiologically correct to speak of afterload in terms of SVR, it is clinically useful to relate changes in SVR to changes in ventricular afterload. Resistance may be calculated by using an analogy derived from Ohm's law, which relates voltage, current flow, and resistance in electrical circuits. We substitute the pressure differential across the system for voltage and cardiac output for current flow, then calculate resistance according to the following formulas. For the left ventricle (systemic vascular resistance):

$$\text{SVR (dyne} \times \text{sec} \times \text{cm}^{-5}) = \frac{\text{MAP} - \text{CVP}}{\text{CO}} \times 80$$

For the right ventricle (pulmonary vascular resistance):

$$\text{PVR (dyne} \times \text{sec} \times \text{cm}^{-5}) = \frac{\text{MPAP} - \text{PAOP}}{\text{CO}} \times 80$$

Since the sympathetic control of the circulation mediated by peripheral baroreceptors is designed to maintain blood pressure within relatively narrow limits, CO is inversely proportional to SVR, whenever this control is functioning. However, in the human circulatory system, additional factors are so often present that this relationship should not be assumed to be a substitute for measurement and calculation.

Contractility, the final determinant of stroke volume, may be estimated in the laboratory by the maximum velocity of contraction of the cardiac muscle fibers. At the bedside, we only have inferences based on the stroke work performed by the ventricle as filling pressure ("preload") changes. Plotting the work done by the ventricle for each beat—the left or right ventricular stroke work index (LVSWI or RVSWI)—against an estimate of preload and comparing that point with a normal range may be a useful means of assessing ventricular function in the intensive care unit. Work is equal to force times distance, and when fluids are involved, the units are pressure change and volume:

$$\text{LVSWI (gm} \times \text{m/m}^2) = \frac{\text{SV} \times (\text{MAP} - \text{PAOP})}{\text{BSA}} \times 0.0136$$

$$\text{RVSWI (gm} \times \text{m/m}^2) = \frac{\text{SV} \times (\text{MPAP} - \text{CVP})}{\text{BSA}} \times 0.0136$$

"Ventricular function curves" are affected by alterations in preload, but they are also influenced importantly by afterload and therefore do not reflect true contractility [36]. Recently, a new group of measures, the end-systolic indices, have been proposed for the evaluation of myocardial contractility. These indices are derived from plotting left ventricular volume against pressure and appear to be sensitive to changes in contractility. Thus, plotting PAOP and stroke work against normal curves is an appropriate use of data currently available in the ICU, but the underlying physiology is often better understood if it is considered in terms of the ventricular pressure-volume relation.

Other derived hemodynamic parameters often used are the rate-pressure product (RPP) and the coronary perfusion pressure (CPP). The goal of most cardiopulmonary interventions is to increase peripheral oxygen delivery at minimal cost in terms of myocardial oxygen consumption. However, the effect of interventions on the balance between myocardial oxygen delivery and consumption must be considered. Although no currently available measurement is suitable for routine bedside assessment of myocardial oxygen consumption, the RPP is proportional in certain laboratory preparations and can be used to estimate changes caused by our interventions:

$$\text{RPP} = \text{HR} \times \text{SBP}$$

Similarly, myocardial oxygen delivery cannot be directly measured, but since coronary blood flow (in patients with fixed coronary vascular resistance due to occlusive disease) is pressure-dependent, the change in CPP may be inferred to represent the most likely direction of change in coronary blood flow resulting from an intervention:

$$\text{CPP} = \text{DBP} - \text{PAOP}$$

The measured and derived data can be used to formulate a plan of intervention designed to improve oxygen delivery relative to myocardial and

Table 6-3. Formulas derived from blood gas analysis

Arterial O_2 content	$CaO_2 = (Hb \times SaO_2 \times 1.39) + (0.0031 \times PaO_2)$
Mixed venous O_2 content	$C\bar{v}O_2 = (Hb \times S\bar{v}O_2 \times 1.39) + (0.0031 \times P\bar{v}O_2)$
Pulmonary capillary O_2 content	$CcO_2 = (Hb \times 1.39)^* + (0.0031 \times PaO_2)$
Alveolar O_2 tension	$PAO_2 = FiO_2 (PB - PH_2O) - \dfrac{PaCO_2}{RQ}$
Arteriovenous content difference	$C(a - v)O_2 = CaO_2 - C\bar{v}O_2$
Respiratory quotient	$RQ = \dfrac{\dot{V}CO_2}{\dot{V}O_2}$
O_2 consumption	$\dot{V}O_2 = C(a - v)O_2 \times CO \times 10$
O_2 delivery	$\dot{D}O_2 = CaO_2 \times CO \times 10$
O_2 utilization	$O_2 \text{ util} = \dfrac{\dot{V}O_2}{\dot{D}O_2} = \dfrac{C(a - v)O_2 \times CO}{CaO_2 \times CO} = \dfrac{C(a - v)O_2}{CaO_2}$
Venous admixture	$\dot{Q}_s/\dot{Q}_t = \dfrac{CcO_2 - CaO_2}{CcO_2 - C\bar{v}O_2}$

Hb = hemoglobin concentration; SaO_2 = arterial O_2 saturation; PaO_2 = arterial O_2 tension; $S\bar{v}O_2$ = mixed venous oxygen saturation; $P\bar{v}O_2$ = mixed venous O_2 tension; PB = barometric pressure; PH_2O = partial pressure of water vapor (47 mm Hg at 37°C); CO = cardiac output; FiO_2 = inspired O_2 fraction; $\dot{V}CO_2$ = CO_2 production.
*Assumes 100% Hb saturation.

systemic oxygen needs. This analysis is a dynamic process that evolves as new data are obtained and appropriate therapy instituted.

Parameters Based on Analysis of Blood Gases

Just as the derived hemodynamic parameters can be used to evaluate the choice and effects of hemodynamic interventions, parameters derived from blood gases yield information regarding the adequacy of cardiopulmonary function in meeting the tissue demands for oxygen. Blood gas values are usually reported in terms of directly measured partial pressures (PO_2 or PCO_2) and calculated saturations (SO_2). Saturations may also be measured directly in a cooximeter or continuously by using transmission or reflectance spectrophotometry. The formulas for the calculation of these parameters are reviewed in Table 6-3. A detailed discussion of the evaluation of oxygen transport can be found in Chapter 9.

MIXED VENOUS OXIMETRY

The function of the cardiorespiratory system is to deliver enough oxygen to satisfy the oxygen demands of the tissues. Failure of adequate oxygen delivery results in tissue hypoxemia, acidosis, multiple organ failure, and eventually, death. Measurement of the mixed venous oxygen saturation ($S\bar{v}O_2$) is helpful in assessment of the oxygen supply-demand relationship

Fiberoptic catheter oximetry in vivo

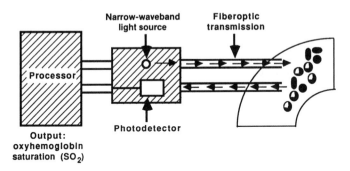

Fig. 6-9. Principle of reflection spectrophotometry used by the continuous in vivo oximeter. (Reprinted with permission from Abbott Laboratories.)

in critically ill patients [93]. The use of improved fiberoptic oximetry systems in conventional pulmonary artery catheters has now permitted continuous monitoring of the $S\bar{v}O_2$ and made practical the bedside application of this relationship.

Technical Considerations

Continuous $S\bar{v}O_2$ monitoring is based on the principle of reflection spectrophotometry (Fig. 6-9). Oxyhemoglobin and reduced hemoglobin have characteristic absorption patterns of certain wavelengths of red and infrared light. Fiberoptic bundles capable of transmitting and receiving this light have been incorporated into the pulmonary artery catheter. The light is generated by an optic module that is attached to the hub of the catheter. In this system, light-emitting diodes send alternating pulses of two or three different wavelengths that travel through a single optical fiber to illuminate the blood flowing past the catheter tip. This illuminating light is absorbed, refracted, and reflected by the red blood cells, depending on its constituents. The reflected light is collected by a second fiber and returned through the catheter to a photodetector in the optical module. Using the relative intensities of the signals representing the light levels at the various wavelengths, a computer calculates the oxygen saturation and the average for the preceding 5 seconds is displayed.

This system can be calibrated by standardization prior to insertion or by obtaining a mixed venous blood sample, measuring the $S\bar{v}O_2$ with a cooximeter and entering this value into the processor. Ease of insertion of the currently manufactured fiberoptic thermodilution catheters is comparable to that of standard nonfiberoptic thermodilution pulmonary artery catheters.

The reliability of $S\bar{v}O_2$ data is excellent, as confirmed by numerous correlations of in vivo and in vitro measurements [5, 76, 111]. However, it has been noted recently that the three-wavelength method is more accurate than that using just two wavelengths [42].

Definition of Mixed Venous Blood

Mixed venous blood is a mixture of all blood that has traversed the capillary beds capable of extracting oxygen. This venous effluent is thoroughly mixed, so that the oxygen saturation is a flow-weighted representation of blood with different oxygen saturations from different vascular beds. Therefore, $S\bar{v}O_2$ measurements will reflect the *total body balance* between oxygen delivery and current oxygen consumption of *perfused* tissues [77]. Sampling of this blood can only be accurately performed at the proximal pulmonary artery.

Determinants of Mixed Venous Oxygen Saturation ($S\bar{v}O_2$)

The $S\bar{v}O_2$ can be derived from the Fick equation, which relates cardiac output, oxygen consumption, and arterial-venous oxygen content difference. When the Fick equation is solved for $S\bar{v}O_2$ [77] (Table 6-4), it becomes apparent that as long as SaO_2 is maintained close to 1 (100%), the $S\bar{v}O_2$ will be determined by the ratio of oxygen consumption ($\dot{V}O_2$) to oxygen delivery ($\dot{D}O_2$), also known as the oxygen utilization coefficient. The determinants of oxygen delivery are the cardiac output (CO) and the arterial oxygen content (CaO_2); the determinants of arterial oxygen content are hemoglobin (Hb), arterial saturation (SaO_2), and to a very small degree, arterial oxygen tension (PaO_2). These determinants may be represented as follows:

$$S\dot{v}O_2 \approx 1 - \frac{\dot{V}O_2}{\dot{D}O_2} \qquad S\bar{v}O_2 \approx 1 - \frac{\dot{V}O_2}{CO \times 10 \times CaO_2}$$
$$(Hb \times SaO_2 \times 1.39 + PaO_2 \times 0.003)$$

Interpretation of Changes in Mixed Venous Oxygen Saturation

There are no good correlations between $S\bar{v}O_2$ and any single component of the equation ($\dot{V}O_2$, CO, SaO_2, Hb)—as would be expected, since there are four separate determinants.

With the above formula in mind, it is easy to understand that the $S\bar{v}O_2$ will decrease when there is an imbalance between oxygen consumption and delivery caused by a decrease in CO, Hb, or SaO_2 or an increase in $\dot{V}O_2$.

The normal range for $S\bar{v}O_2$ is 0.60 to 0.80 [93]. A rapid or prolonged fall from this level is indicative of a significant deterioration in the patient's clinical condition [29]. A decrease in $S\bar{v}O_2$ of greater than 0.10 is likely to be of significance regardless of the initial value [77]. Values below the normal range may be associated with increased oxygen consumption due to fever, shivering, seizures, exercise, and agitation or associated with decreased oxygen delivery due to low cardiac output states, anemia, or arterial oxygen desaturation. Values of about 0.53 correspond to a $P\bar{v}O_2$ of about 28 mm Hg; values at or below this level have been often associated

Table 6-4. Derivation of $S\bar{v}O_2$ from Fick Equation

$\dot{V}O_2 = C(a - v)O_2 \times CO \times 10$	Fick equation
$\dfrac{\dot{V}O_2}{CO \times 10} = C(a - v)O_2$	Divide by $(CO \times 10)$
$\dfrac{\dot{V}O_2}{CO \times 10} = CaO_2 - C\bar{v}O_2$	Substitute $CaO_2 - C\bar{v}O_2$ for $C(a - \bar{v})O_2$
$\dfrac{\dot{V}O_2}{CO \times 10} - CaO_2 = -C\bar{v}O_2$	Subtract CaO_2
$C\bar{v}O_2 = CaO_2 - \dfrac{\dot{V}O_2}{CO \times 10}$	Multiply by -1
$\dfrac{C\bar{v}O_2}{CaO_2} = 1 - \dfrac{\dot{V}O_2}{CO \times 10 \times CaO_2}$	Divide by CaO_2
$\dfrac{C\bar{v}O_2}{CaO_2} = 1 - \dfrac{\dot{V}O_2}{\dot{D}O_2}$	Substitute $\dot{D}O_2$ for $CO \times 10 \times CaO_2$
$\dfrac{C\bar{v}O_2}{CaO_2} \approx \dfrac{S\bar{v}O_2}{SaO_2}$	Substitution of saturation for content (disregard dissolved oxygen)
$S\bar{v}O_2 \approx 1 - \dfrac{\dot{V}O_2}{\dot{D}O_2}$	If $SaO_2 = 1$, it can be canceled out
$S\bar{v}O_2 \approx 1 - O_2$ utilization	Definition of O_2 utilization

SaO_2 = arterial O_2 saturation; $S\bar{v}O_2$ = mixed venous O_2 saturation; CaO_2 = arterial O_2 content; $C\bar{v}O_2$ = mixed venous O_2 content; $C(a - v)O_2$ = arteriovenous O_2 content difference; $\dot{D}O_2$ = O_2 delivery; CO = cardiac output; $\dot{V}O_2$ = oxygen consumption.

with anaerobic metabolism, lactic acidosis, and death [57]. However, a recent study was unable to identify the critical level of $S\bar{v}O_2$ associated with lactic acidosis in patients with sepsis or acute myocardial infarction [4].

Values above the normal range indicate an increase in oxygen delivery relative to consumption and are associated with the hyperdynamic phase of sepsis, cirrhosis, peripheral left-to-right shunting, general anesthesia (when $\dot{V}O_2$ is low), cellular poisoning such as cyanide toxicity (rare), marked arterial hyperoxia, or a technical malfunction of the system (i.e., wedged catheter).

Normal or high values do not ensure that the oxygen supply-demand balance is satisfactory since, as mentioned above, $S\bar{v}O_2$ is a "flow-weighted" average of all the end-capillary oxygen contents of the body. Also, accurate interpretation assumes intact and consistent vasoregulation, which is not the case in some disease states (i.e., sepsis).

Clinical Utility of Continuous $S\bar{v}O_2$ Monitoring

Continuous $S\bar{v}O_2$ monitoring serves three major functions. First, it is an indicator of the adequacy of the oxygen supply-consumption balance of perfused tissues. In clinically stable patients, a normal and stable $S\bar{v}O_2$ may be considered an additional assurance of cardiopulmonary stability. Further assessment of CO and arterial and mixed venous blood gas analysis in this case could be eliminated. Second, continuously measured $S\bar{v}O_2$

may function as an early warning signal of untoward events. In this situation, although an alert has been given, the cause of the change in $S\bar{v}O_2$ is not necessarily clear, since the change in $S\bar{v}O_2$ is sensitive but not specific. It may be necessary to measure CO, SaO_2, and Hb in this setting to identify the etiology of the $S\bar{v}O_2$ change. Third, continuously monitored $S\bar{v}O_2$ may improve the efficiency of the delivery of critical care by providing immediate feedback as to the effectiveness of therapeutic interventions.

Cost Effectiveness
With continuous venous oximetry, the potential of cost savings lies in the decreased use of other modes for assessing oxygen transport balance—i.e., CO measurements and venous blood gas analysis. The savings in some institutions exceed the price of the catheter, and this technique has been judged cost effective [75, 79].

CONCLUSIONS
Hemodynamic monitoring is an integral part of the diagnosis and management of critically ill patients. The monitoring devices are not amulets that by themselves protect the patient. There must be a clinical process linking the device to outcome: physicians must select the correct patients to be monitored, the monitoring system must produce accurate numbers, abnormal values need to be recognized, pathophysiologic causes have to be identified, the need for therapy must be appreciated, an appropriate form of therapy must be selected and administered in a timely fashion and correctly, the patient must respond, and this response must improve the clinical condition sufficiently to improve survival. The sequence still is based, we believe, upon the clinician's knowledge, but unless hemodynamic monitoring is initiated, the potential for improvement in outcome can never be realized.

REFERENCES
1. Allen, E. V. Thromboangiitis obliterans: Methods of diagnosis of chronic occlusive arterial lesions distal to the wrist with illustrative cases. *Am. J. Med. Sci.* 178:237, 1929.
2. Ansley, D. M., et al. The relationship between central venous pressure and pulmonary capillary wedge pressure during aortic surgery. *Can. J. Anaesth.* 34:594, 1987.
3. Armengol, J., et al. Effects of the respiratory cycle on cardiac output measurements: Reproducibility of data enhanced by timing the thermodilution injections in dogs. *Crit. Care Med.* 9:852, 1981.
4. Astiz, M. E. Relationship of oxygen delivery and mixed venous oxygenation to lactic acidosis in patients with sepsis and acute myocardial infarction. *Crit. Care Med.* 16:655, 1988.
5. Baele, P. L., et al. Continuous monitoring of mixed venous saturation in critically ill patients. *Anesth. Analg.* 61:513, 1982.
6. Band, J. D., and Maki, D. G. Infections caused by arterial catheters used for hemodynamic monitoring. *Am. J. Med.* 67:735, 1979.
7. Banner, T., and Banner, M. J. Cardiac Output Measurement Technology. In J. M. Civetta, R. W. Taylor, and R. R. Kirby, *Critical Care.* Philadelphia: Lippincott, 1988. Pp. 361–376.

8. Bedford, R. F., and Wollman, H. Complications of percutaneous radial artery cannulation: An objective prospective study in man. *Anesthesiology* 38:228, 1973.

9. Berglund, E. Balance of left and right ventricular output: Relation between left and right atrial pressures. *Am. J. Physiol.* 178:381, 1954.

10. Brodsky, J. B. A simple method to determine patency of the ulnar artery intraoperatively prior to radial artery cannulation. *Anesthesiology* 42:626, 1975.

11. Brown, M., et al. Intravascular monitoring via the axillary artery. *Anaesth. Intensive Care* 13:38, 1984.

12. Bryan-Brown, C. W., et al. The axillary artery catheter. *Heart Lung* 12:492, 1983.

13. Bull, M. J., et al. Neurologic complications following temporal artery catheterization. *J. Pediatr.* 96:1071, 1980.

14. Calvin, J. E., et al. Does the pulmonary capillary wedge pressure predict left ventricular preload in critically ill patients? *Crit. Care Med.* 9:437, 1981.

15. Centers for Disease Control. *National Nosocomial Infections Study Report, Annual Summary 1979.* March 1982.

16. Civetta, J. M., and Gabel, J. C. Flow directed-pulmonary artery catheterization in surgical patients: Indications and modifications of technique. *Ann. Surg.* 176:753, 1972.

17. Civetta, J. M. Cardio-pulmonary calculations: A rapid, simple and inexpensive technique. *Intensive Care Med.* 3:208, 1977.

18. Civetta, J. M. Clinical utilization of monitoring equipment. Part 2. *NEREM 71 Record.* Newton, Mass.: IEEE Press, 1971. Pp. 18–25.

19. Civetta, J. M. Invasive Catheterization. In W. C. Shoemaker and W. L. Thompson (eds.), *Critical Care: State of the Art,* vol. 1, section B. Fullerton, Calif.: Society of Critical Care Medicine, 1980. Pp. 1–47.

20. Civetta, J. M. Pulmonary Artery Catheter Insertion. In C. L. Sprung (ed.), *The Pulmonary Artery Catheter, Methodology and Clinical Application.* Rockville, Md.: Aspen Publishers, 1983. Pp. 21–71.

21. Civetta, J. M., et al. Disparate ventricular function in surgical patients. *Surg. Forum* 22:136, 1971.

22. Civetta, J. M., et al. Utility and efficacy of guidewire changes. *Crit. Care Med.* 15:380, 1987.

23. Clapham, M. C. C., et al. Minimum volume of discard for valid blood sampling from indwelling arterial cannulae. *Br. J. Anaesth.* 59:232, 1987.

24. Cohn, J. N. Blood pressure measurement in shock. *J.A.M.A.* 199:972, 1967.

25. Connors, A. F., et al. Evaluation of right heart catheterization in the critically ill patient without acute myocardial infarction. *N. Engl. J. Med.* 308:263, 1983.

26. Cronin, K. D., et al. Radial artery cannulation. The influence of method on blood flow after decannulation. *Anaesth. Intensive Care* 14:400, 1986.

27. Curley, J., et al. Erroneous cardiac output determination due to pulmonary artery catheter proximal port dysfunction. *Anesthesiology* 64:662, 1986.

28. De Campo, T., and Civetta, J. M. The effect of short-term discontinuation of high level PEEP in patients with acute respiratory failure. *Crit. Care Med.* 7:47, 1979.

29. Divertie, M. B. and McMichan, J. C. Continuous monitoring of mixed venous oxygen saturation. *Chest* 85:423, 1984.

30. Du Bois, D., and Du Bois, E. F. A formula to estimate the approximate surface area if height and weight be known. *Arch. Intern. Med.* 17:863, 1916.

31. Ehlers, K. C., et al. Cardiac output measurements. A review of current techniques and research. *Ann. Biomed. Eng.* 14:219, 1986.

32. Eisenberg, P. R., et al. Clinical evaluation compared to pulmonary artery catheterization in the hemodynamic assessment of critically ill patients. *Crit. Care Med.* 12:489, 1984.

33. Ejrup, B., et al. Clinical evaluation of blood flow to the hand: The false positive Allen Test. *Circulation* 33:778, 1966.

34. Elkayam, U., et al. Cardiac output by thermodilution technique: Effect on injectate's volume and temperature on accuracy and reproducibility in the critically ill patient. *Chest* 84:418, 1983.

35. Ellis, D. M. Interpretation of beat-to-beat blood pressure changes in the presence of ventilatory changes. *J. Clin. Monit.* 1:65, 1985.

36. Fifer, M. A. and Braunwald, E. End-systolic pressure-volume and stress-length relations in the assessment of ventricular function in man. *Adv. Cardiol.* 32:36, 1985.

37. Forrester, J. S., et al. Correlative classification of clinical and hemodynamic function after acute myocardial infarction. *Am. J. Cardiol.* 39:137, 1977.

38. Forrester, J. S., et al. Filling pressures in the right and left sides of the heart in acute myocardial infarction. *N. Engl. J. Med.* 285:190, 1971.

39. Ganz, W., and Swan, H. J. C. Measurement of blood flow by thermodilution. *Am. J. Cardiol.* 29:241, 1972.

40. Gardner, R. M. Direct blood pressure measurements—Dynamic response requirements. *Anesthesiology* 54:227, 1981.

41. Gerber, M. J., et al. Arterial waveforms and systemic vascular resistance: Is there a correlation? *Anesthesiology* 66:823, 1987.

42. Gettinger, A., et al. In vivo comparison of two mixed venous saturation catheters. *Anesthesiology* 66:373, 1987.

43. Goldenheim, P. D., and Kazemi, H. Cardiopulmonary monitoring of critically ill patients. Part two. *N. Engl. J. Med.* 311:776, 1984.

44. Gore, J. M., et al. A community-wide assessment of the use of pulmonary artery catheters in patients with acute myocardial infarction. *Chest* 92:721, 1987.

45. Gurman, G. M., and Kriemerman, S. Cannulation of big arteries in critically ill patients. *Crit. Care Med.* 13:217, 1985.

46. Guyton, A. C., and Jones, C. E. Central venous pressure: Physiological significance and clinical implications. *Am. Heart J.* 86:431, 1973.

47. Hansen, R., et al. Poor correlation between pulmonary arterial wedge pressure and left ventricular end-diastolic volume after coronary artery bypass graft surgery. *Anesthesiology* 64:764, 1986.

48. Harris, A. P., et al. The slowing of sinus rhythm during thermodilution cardiac output determination and the effect of altering injectate temperature. *Anesthesiology* 63:540, 1985.

49. Hasan, F., et al. Influence of lung injury on pulmonary wedge-left atrial pressure correlation during positive end-expiratory pressure ventilation. *Am. Rev. Respir. Dis.* 131:246, 1985.

50. Hudson-Civetta, J. A., Civetta, J. Clean and aseptic technique at the bedside. In J. M. Civetta, R. W. Taylor, and R. R. Kirby. *Critical Care.* Philadelphia: Lippincott, 1988. Pp. 183–195.

51. Hudson-Civetta, J. A., et al. Risk and detection of pulmonary artery catheter related infection in septic surgical patients. *Crit. Care Med.* 15:29, 1987.

52. Johnstone, R. E., and Greenhow, D. E. Catheterization of the dorsalis pedis artery. *Anesthesiology* 39:654, 1973.

53. Jones, R. M., et al. The effect of method of radial artery cannulation on postcannulation blood flow and thrombus formation. *Anesthesiology* 55:76, 1981.

54. Kadota, L. Reproducibility of thermodilution cardiac output measurements. *Heart Lung* 15:618, 1986.
55. Kajs, M. Comparison of coagulation values obtained by traditional venipuncture and intra-arterial line methods. *Heart Lung* 15:622, 1986.
56. Kane, P., et al. Artifacts in the measurement of pulmonary artery wedge pressure. *Crit. Care Med.* 6:36, 1978.
57. Kasnitz, P., et al. Mixed venous oxygen tension and hyperlactemia. *J.A.M.A.* 236:570, 1976.
58. Keeler, C, et al. A review of infection control practices related to intravascular pressure monitoring devices (1975–1985). *Heart Lung* 16:201, 1987.
59. Krasner, J. K., and Marino, P. L. The use of a pocket computer for hemodynamic profiles. *Crit. Care Med.* 11:826, 1983.
60. Lang, M., et al. Systemic vascular resistance: An unreliable index of left ventricular afterload. *Circulation* 74:1114, 1986.
61. Lappas, D., et al. Indirect measurement of left-atrial pressure in surgical patients. Pulmonary-capillary wedge pressure and pulmonary-artery diastolic pressures compared with left-atrial pressure. *Anesthesiology* 38:394, 1973.
62. Latson, T., and Maruschak, G. A faulty lumen resulting in erroneous thermodilution cardiac output measurement. *J. Clin. Monit.* 1:213, 1985.
63. Lee, D. W. and Stevens, G. H. Comparison of thermodilution cardiac output measurements by injection of the proximal lumen versus side port of the Swan-Ganz catheter. *Heart Lung* 14:126, 1985.
64. Levin, R. I., and Glassman, E. Left atrial-pulmonary wedge pressure relation: Effect of elevated pulmonary vascular resistance. *Am. J. Cardiol.* 55:856, 1985.
65. Lindsay, S. L., et al. Abscess following cannulation of the radial artery. *Anaesthesia* 42:654, 1987.
66. Luskin, R. L., et al. Extended use of disposable pressure transducers. A bacteriologic evaluation. *J.A.M.A.* 255:916, 1986.
67. Matthew, E. B., and Vender, J. Comparison of thermodilution cardiac output measured by different computers. *Crit. Care Med.* 15:989, 1987.
68. Mitchell, M. M., et al. Accurate, automated, continuously displayed pulmonary artery pressure measurement. *Anesthesiology* 67:294, 1987.
69. Morris, A. H., and Chapman, R. H. Wedge pressure confirmation by aspiration of pulmonary capillary blood. *Crit. Care Med.* 13:756, 1985.
70. Mosteller, R. D. Simplified calculation of body-surface area. *N. Engl. J. Med.* 317:1098, 1987.
71. Mozersky, D. J., et al. Ultrasonic evaluation of the palmar circulation. *Am. J. Surg.* 126:810, 1973.
72. Naloy, L. Monitoring systemic arterial blood pressure: Strip chart recording versus digital display. *Heart Lung* 15:627, 1986.
73. Nelson, L. D., and Civetta, J. M. Surgical intensive care and perioperative monitoring. In A. P. Monaco, R. S. Jones, P. Ebert, R. Simmons (eds.), *Textbook of Surgery*. New York, Macmillan. In press.
74. Nelson, L. D., and Anderson, H. B. Patient selection for iced versus room temperature injectate for thermodilution cardiac output determinations. *Crit. Care Med.* 13:182, 1985.
75. Nelson, L. D. Application of venous saturation monitoring. In J. M. Civetta, R. W. Taylor, and R. R. Kirby. *Critical Care*. Philadelphia: Lippincott, 1988. Pp. 327–334.
76. Nelson, L. D. Continuous venous oximetry in surgical patients. *Ann. Surg.* 203:329, 1986.
77. Nelson, L. D. Mixed venous oximetry. In J. V. Snyder and M. R. Pinsky (eds.),

Oxygen Transport in the Critically Ill. Chicago: Year Book, 1987. Pp. 235–248.

78. Nelson, L. D. Monitoring and measurement in shock. In J. Barrett and L. M. Nyhus, *Treatment of Shock. Principles and Practice.* Philadelphia: Lea & Febiger, 1986. Pp. 35–55.
79. Orlando, R. Continuous mixed venous oximetry in critically ill surgical patients: "High-tech" cost-effectiveness. *Arch. Surg.* 121:470, 1986.
80. Pearl, R. G., et al. Effect of injectate volume and temperature on thermodilution cardiac output determination. *Anesthesiology* 64:798, 1986.
81. Pierson, D. J., and Hudson, L. D. Monitoring hemodynamics in the critically ill. *Med. Clin. North Am.* 67:1343, 1983.
82. Pryor, A. C. The intra-arterial line: A site for obtaining coagulation studies. *Heart Lung* 12:586, 1983.
83. Pyles, S. T., et al. Cannulation of the dorsal radial artery: A new technique. *Anesth. Analg.* 61:876, 1982.
84. Raju, R. The pulse oximeter and the collateral circulation. *Anaesthesia* 41:783, 1986.
85. Raper, R., and Sibbald, W. J. Misled by the wedge? The Swan-Ganz catheter and left ventricular preload. *Chest* 89:427, 1986.
86. Robin E. D. The cult of the Swan-Ganz catheter. Overuse and abuse of pulmonary flow catheters. *Ann. Intern. Med.* 103:445, 1985.
87. Robin, E. D. Death by pulmonary artery flow-directed catheter. Time for a moratorium? *Chest* 92:727, 1987.
88. Roy, R., et al. Pulmonary wedge catheterization during positive end-expiratory pressure ventilation in the dog. *Anesthesiology* 46:385, 1977.
89. Russell, J. A., et al. Prospective evaluation of radial and femoral artery catheterization sites in critically ill adults. *Crit. Care Med.* 11:936, 1983.
90. Sabo B., and Smith, R. B. A tidy adjunct to arterial cannulation. *Anesthesiology* 64:534, 1986.
91. Savino, J. A., and Del Guercio, L. R. M. Preoperative assessment of high-risk surgical patients. *Surg. Clin. North Am.* 65:763, 1985.
92. Schmitt, E. A., and Brantigan, C. O. Common artifacts of pulmonary artery and pulmonary artery wedge pressures: Recognition and interpretation. *J. Clin. Monit.* 2:44, 1986.
93. Schweiss, J. F. Mixed venous hemoglobin saturation: Theory and application. *Int. Anesthesiol. Clin.* 25:113, 1987.
94. Shapiro, B. A. Monitoring gas exchange in acute respiratory failure. *Respir. Care* 28:605, 1983.
95. Shapiro, H. M., et al. Errors in sampling pulmonary arterial blood with a Swan-Ganz catheter. *Anesthesiology* 40:291, 1974.
96. Simmons, M. A., et al. Serious sequelae of temporal artery catheterization. *J. Pediatr.* 92:284, 1978.
97. Sladen, A. Complications of invasive hemodynamic monitoring in the intensive care unit. In M. M. Ravitch (ed.), *Current Problems in Surgery,* vol. 25:12. Chicago: Year Book, 1988.
98. Slogoff, S. On the safety of radial artery cannulation. *Anesthesiology* 59:42, 1983.
99. Spackman, T. N. Low thermodilution cardiac output due to an intracatheter septal defect. *Anesth. Analg.* 63:962, 1984.
100. Sprung, C. L., and Jacobs, L. J. Indications for pulmonary artery catheterization. In C. L. Sprung (ed.), *The Pulmonary Artery Catheter, Methodology and Clinical Application.* Rockville, Md.: Aspen Publishers, 1983. Pp. 7–19.

101. Starling, E. H. *The Linacre Lecture on the Law of the Heart.* Presented at Cambridge. 1915. London: Longmans, Green, 1918.
102. Stevens, J. H., et al. Thermodilution cardiac output measurement: Effects of the respiratory cycle on its reproducibility. *J.A.M.A.* 253:2240, 1985.
103. Stoller, J., et al. Spuriously high cardiac output from injecting thermal indicator through an ensheathed port. *Crit. Care Med.* 14:1064, 1986.
104. Swan, H. J. C., and Ganz, L. O. Hemodynamic measurement in clinical practice: A decade in review. *J. Am. Coll. Cardiol.* 1:103, 1983.
105. Thomas, F., et al. The risk of infection related to radial versus femoral sites for arterial catheterization. *Crit. Care Med.* 11:807, 1983.
106. Tooker, J., et al. The effect of Swan-Ganz catheter height on the wedge pressure-left atrial pressure relationship in edema during positive pressure ventilation. *Am. Rev. Respir. Dis.* 117:721, 1978.
107. Toussaint, G. P., et al. Central venous pressure and pulmonary wedge pressure in critical surgical illness. *Arch. Surg.* 109:265, 1974.
108. Tuchschmidt, J., and Sharma, O. P. Impact of hemodynamic monitoring in a medical intensive care unit. *Crit. Care Med.* 15:840, 1987.
109. Verweij, J., et al. Comparison of three methods for measuring central venous pressure. *Crit. Care Med.* 14:288, 1986.
110. Vicari, M., and Ogle, V. Comparison of measurements of cardiac output from the side port versus the proximal lumen of the Swan-Ganz catheter: Follow-up study. *Heart Lung* 16:379, 1987.
111. Waller, J. L., et al. Clinical evaluation of a new fiberoptic catheter during cardiac surgery. *Anesth. Analg.* 61:676, 1982.
112. Warner, H. R., et al. Computer-based monitoring of cardiovascular function in postoperative patients. *Circulation* 37:68, 1968.
113. West, J. B., et al. Distribution of blood flow in isolated lung: Relation to vascular and alveolar pressures. *J. Appl. Physiol.* 19:713, 1964.
114. Wetzel, R. C., and Latson, T. W. Major errors in thermodilution cardiac output measurement during rapid volume infusion. *Anesthesiology* 62:684, 1985.
115. Wilkins, R. G. Radial artery cannulation and ischemic damage: A review. *Anaesthesia* 40:896, 1985.
116. Woods, M., et al. Practical considerations for the use of a pulmonary artery thermistor catheter. *Surgery* 79;469, 1976.

Respiratory Monitoring

Howard S. Nearman
James E. Sampliner

Respiratory monitoring provides the basis for the establishment of guidelines for the initiation of oxygen therapy, the use of mechanical ventilatory support, and the discontinuation of these respiratory support techniques. Assessment of the pulmonary status in the critically ill patient can be divided into three major categories comprising methods of evaluating (1) the adequacy and efficiency of oxygen exchange, (2) the adequacy of ventilation, and (3) respiratory mechanics and ventilatory reserve. The various methods available for obtaining and interpreting data in these categories are presented in this chapter.

Patients with significant respiratory dysfunction require and benefit from monitoring of pulmonary status. Equally important, however, is respiratory function monitoring in patients admitted to the intensive care unit (ICU) for problems other than pulmonary insufficiency. In these patients, careful surveillance of respiratory function status can often allow early recognition of respiratory impairment and thereby often avoid the morbidity and mortality associated with florid pulmonary insufficiency.

ARTERIAL BLOOD GASES

Since arterial blood gas parameters provide the foundation for the assessment of respiratory function, a review of basic chemical principles and of technical aspects of analysis, interpretation, and reliability of results is warranted.

Blood gas measurements can provide information regarding oxygen transport, the efficiency of gas exchange, acid-base status, and the adequacy of alveolar ventilation. They can also be used in the calculation of parameters that aid in the determination of pulmonary shunting and cardiac output (by the Fick method). The importance of blood gases cannot be overemphasized. However, one must not rely solely on them, or on any other single measurement, in the care of the critically ill.

Theoretical Considerations

Barometric Pressure

The molecules present in the earth's atmosphere have weight and exert a force on the earth that is great enough to support a column of mercury 760 mm high at sea level. This is termed the *atmospheric (barometric) pressure.*

Dalton's Law

The earth's atmosphere is composed of several gases, the major ones being nitrogen and oxygen. Dalton's law states that the total atmospheric pressure is the sum of the individual gas pressures and that each of these partial pressures is as though that gas alone occupied the space. Dry air is composed of 79.03 percent nitrogen, 20.93 percent oxygen, and 0.04 percent carbon dioxide.

To determine the partial pressure of any gas, one multiplies the fractional concentration of the gas by the barometric pressure (P_B).

Example

To determine the partial pressure of oxygen in room air:

Barometric pressure = 760 torr
Fractional concentration of O_2 (F_IO_2) = 20.93%
$$PO_2 = 760 \times 0.2093$$

The PO_2 is then calculated as 159 torr.

Henry's Law

The amount of gas that will dissolve in a liquid at a given temperature is directly proportional to the partial pressure of that gas in the gas phase. However, this law applies only to that fraction of the gas physically dissolved in the liquid and not to the fraction of gas that is combined chemically with either the liquid or a solute within the liquid. Both carbon dioxide and oxygen dissolve physically in plasma. Carbon dioxide, however, also reacts chemically with water, and both carbon dioxide and oxygen react chemically with hemoglobin. Henry's law applies only to the physically dissolved fractions of these two gases. Therefore, only the physically dissolved gas, and not the gas that is chemically combined, exerts a partial pressure in the plasma.

When the partial pressure in the liquid is equal to the partial pressure of the gas that is chemically combined, the two phases are in equilibrium. A change in either will disrupt this equilibrium and cause a corresponding change in the opposite phase until equilibrium is reestablished.

The amount of carbon dioxide and oxygen that is physically dissolved in plasma is dependent on the solubility coefficient for the gas, the temperature, and the partial pressure of the gas. At 37°C, the solubility coefficient of oxygen is 0.0031 vol%/torr and that of carbon dioxide is 0.063 vol%/torr. For example, to determine the partial pressure of oxygen dissolved in plasma when the arterial PO_2 is 215 torr, one multiplies 215 torr by 0.0031 vol%/torr, which equals 0.6665 vol%. As one can see, the amount of gas physically dissolved will be relatively small except at extremely high partial pressures of a given gas (i.e., inhalation of 100% oxygen, and especially hyperbaric oxygen).

In review:

1. The total volume of gas in a solution is equal to the sum of the volume of physically dissolved gas plus that volume of gas chemically combined with other solutes (i.e., hemoglobin).
2. The total concentration of oxygen and carbon dioxide in blood is much greater than the concentration of physically dissolved oxygen and carbon dioxide.
3. The partial pressure of a gas in solution is proportional only to the amount of gas that is physically dissolved and not to the total concentration of the gas.
4. The chemical reactions, as well as the physiologic properties, of gases depend on the partial pressure of those gases rather than on their total concentration in solution.

Water Vapor Pressure
The importance of water vapor pressure (P_{H_2O}) lies in its effect on diluting gases in dry air. By the time inspired air reaches the bronchioles, the effect of P_{H_2O} is to lower the partial pressure of oxygen by approximately 100 torr. P_{H_2O} varies directly with changes in temperature.

Technical Aspects of Blood Gas Analysis
The actual measurement of blood gases is extremely important, since the results often serve as a guide to therapy. Therefore, a brief explanation of how the determinations are made follows.

pH
The glass pH electrode contains an inner chamber in which a solution of a "known" pH is sealed. The electrical potential generated between the outside of the electrode and the inner, "known," solution is then read directly by the blood gas machine as the pH of the blood.

PCO_2
PCO_2 is measured by dissolving carbon dioxide in the blood in an aqueous medium. Acid is then formed, and this changes the pH of the electrolyte contained within the electrode. The Severinghaus electrode measures the change in pH of the electrolyte due to the flow of carbon dioxide through a gas-permeable membrane that covers the electrode. This pH value is then converted electronically by the blood gas machine into the corresponding PCO_2 value.

PO_2
The Clark electrode is used to measure PO_2 and is referred to as an oxygen electrode. Inside the electrode is a platinum wire. Oxygen molecules are broken down rapidly on this surface, causing a change in ionic current that is then measurable as a change in current flow between the silver cathode and the platinum anode. This electrical current is read by the blood gas machine and converted into a corresponding PO_2 value.

Bicarbonate

In most institutions, the bicarbonate that is reported with the blood gas results is a standard bicarbonate, as opposed to an actual bicarbonate. It is based on pH and PCO_2 and is calculated by the Henderson-Hasselbalch equation.

It is important to remember that bicarbonate represents the major blood base.

Percent Saturation

Percent saturation (SO_2) is obtained in one of two ways: by calculation, using a special slide rule based on PO_2 and pH, or by a reading on an oximeter (i.e., spectrophotometrically). The latter method is more accurate, since it involves direct reading of the percent oxyhemoglobin saturation. There are many instances in which the spectrophotometric method has distinct advantages over the calculated determination—for example, in the patient with a shifted oxyhemoglobin dissociation curve, or in the patient with a high blood level of carboxyhemoglobin.

Clinical Interpretation of Blood Gases

The increased clinical use of blood gas determinations has led to the proliferation of publications dealing with measurement and interpretation. The material presented in this section is not intended to replace these references and will not add significantly to what has already been contributed. Rather, our goal is to provide a review for quick reference.

As with most tests, there are "normal" values for blood gases. However, these should not be overemphasized, since the patient's previous pulmonary status often has not been normal. Whenever possible, baseline or preoperative blood gas values should be obtained, especially when the patient is having major surgery. Also, when indicated, a complete pulmonary function workup can be invaluable for preoperative preparation, anesthesia evaluation, and postoperative management.

Representative blood gas values for arterial and mixed venous blood are listed in Table 7-1. In any comparison with these values, however, the patient's age and previous pulmonary status both must be taken into account, and it must be kept in mind that normal values for mixed venous blood gases are more variable than are those for arterial blood gases.

pH

The pH determines the patient's acid-base status (see Chapter 24). An arterial pH less than 7.35 indicates acidemia: an arterial pH greater than 7.45 indicates alkalemia.

The pH allows one to determine whether or not acidemia or alkalemia exists or, if both are present, which is predominant. The pH is defined as the negative log of the hydrogen ion concentration. The Henderson-Hasselbalch equation is the mathematical statement of pH and is written as follows:

pH = pK + log (base/acid)

Table 7-1. Normal blood gas values

Blood gas	Arterial	Mixed venous
pH	7.40 (7.35–7.45)	7.36 (7.31–7.41)
PCO$_2$	35–45 torr	41–51 torr
PO$_2$	80–100 torr	35–40 torr
HCO$_3^-$	22–26 mEq/liter	22–26 mEq/liter
SO$_2$ (% saturation)	95 or greater	75 (70–75)
Base excess	−2 to +2	−2 to +2

The pK is defined as the pH at which a substance is half-dissociated and half-undissociated. The pK of blood under physiologic conditions is 6.1. In the Henderson-Hasselbalch equation, the base is bicarbonate (HCO$_3^-$), and the acid is carbonic acid. The normal ratio between bicarbonate and carbonic acid is 20 : 1. This is an important relationship to keep in mind. One may determine the value for carbonic acid by multiplying the PCO$_2$ by 0.03.

PaCO$_2$

The partial pressure of arterial carbon dioxide (PaCO$_2$) is the parameter that allows one to assess the adequacy of alveolar ventilation. In addition, the arteriovenous carbon dioxide difference is primarily determined by the metabolic rate. Therefore, the PaCO$_2$ is a reflection of the adequacy of the alveolar ventilation in relation to the metabolic rate.

PaCO$_2$ may be normal, increased (hypercapnia), or decreased (hypocapnia). A normal PaCO$_2$ means normal alveolar ventilation; an increased PaCO$_2$ can occur as compensation for metabolic disturbances, as well as primarily on a respiratory basis.

PaCO$_2$ also has an effect on pH. As previously stated, the pH is the result of the ratio of plasma bicarbonate to plasma carbonic acid, normally 20 : 1. Assuming that HCO$_3^-$ remains within the normal range, a relationship between pH and H$_2$CO$_3$ results. This represents the pH change that is secondary to changes in alveolar ventilation (i.e., changes in acid-base status due to respiration). The relationship is inverse and nearly linear. Because of this, the following guideline can be put forth: for every acute increase of 10 torr in PaCO$_2$, the pH will decrease by 0.08 units; and for every acute decrease of 10 torr in PaCO$_2$, the pH will increase by 0.08 units.

PaO$_2$

The arterial oxygen tension (PaO$_2$) by itself provides little physiologic information beyond indicating the adequacy of arterial oxygenation. However, if the PaO$_2$ and FiO$_2$ are considered together, information relative to the efficiency of oxygen exchange is obtained.

It is important to remember that PaO$_2$ will be affected by the presence of preexisting lung disease as well as by age, and that both must be taken into account in interpreting a patient's PaO$_2$. Large degrees of variability in PaO_2 exist within individual patients; changes up to 45 torr have been reported in stable ICU patients [10].

Bicarbonate
The normal value for HCO_3^- is 22 to 26 mEq/liter (with a mean value of 24 mEq/liter). As the $PaCO_2$ is referred to as the respiratory parameter, the HCO_3^- can be called the metabolic parameter. As such, HCO_3^- is primarily a function of the kidneys (this, of course, is somewhat of an oversimplification).

As the kidneys are the prime regulators of HCO_3^-, changes in this parameter are slow (24–36 hr) in comparison with changes in $PaCO_2$, which can occur within minutes. Plasma HCO_3^-, however can be manipulated artificially (e.g., by administration of sodium bicarbonate or ammonium chloride) and thereby quickly changed.

Bicarbonate represents the primary blood base. Strictly speaking, an increase in bicarbonate will cause a metabolic alkalosis, whereas a decrease in bicarbonate or an accumulation of acid (e.g., lactic or β-hydroxybutyric acid) will cause a metabolic acidosis. However, whether an alkalosis or acidosis is actually present depends on the respiratory compensation for the underlying process (see Chapter 24).

Percent Oxygen Saturation
Oxygen saturation is equal to the oxygen content (minus the physically dissolved oxygen) divided by the oxygen capacity (minus the physically dissolved oxygen). In general, an arterial oxygen saturation equal to 90 percent or greater is considered acceptable. This saturation roughly corresponds to a PaO_2 of 60 torr. When dealing with venous blood, an acceptable value for mixed venous oxygen saturation is 75 percent, which corresponds approximately to a PO_2 of 40 torr.

Interpretation and Reliability

The Concept of In Vitro
One factor often overlooked when interpreting blood gas results is that these measurements have been made in vitro and not in vivo. Probably one of the most significant variables in in vitro measurement of blood gases is the effect of temperature. All blood gas machines are equipped so that the specimen is brought to a given temperature (usually 37°C) either before or during the analysis. PO_2 and PCO_2 vary directly with temperature at the following rates: 4 percent per degree centigrade for PCO_2 and 7 percent per degree centigrade for PO_2.

Although in most cases the fact that blood gases are measured at 37°C in the laboratory is not significant, there are situations in which this fact could assume real importance (e.g., operations performed under controlled hypothermia). Any corrections for these temperature factors must be made by the physician, since most laboratories do not correct blood gases for temperature. It should also be pointed out that other factors can be corrected for in blood gases (in particular, the effect of

Table 7-2. Effect of time and temperature on blood gas parameters

Parameter	37°C	20°C
pH	0.01/10 min	0.001/10 min
PaCO$_2$	1 torr/10 min	0.1 torr/10 min
PaO$_2$	0.5 vol%/10 min	0.05 vol%/10 min

pH on percent saturation). Again, this is not done by the laboratory, but various nomograms are available for use in these situations (see Appendix 3).

The Reliability of Results

The key question about any laboratory report is whether or not the results are correct. Often, physicians may take the attitude that if the result is what they expected, it is correct. This is a dangerous assumption. Others may take the attitude that results that come from their laboratory must be correct. This, too, is fallacious. One must scrutinize all laboratory results with a critical eye, and when a significant question of accuracy arises, the test must be repeated.

The method in which the sample is collected and transported also may influence the accuracy of the measured variables.

When blood is drawn for blood gas analysis, it is essential to ensure that the specimen is adequately anticoagulated. Adequate anticoagulation can be easily achieved with sodium heparin; neither ammonium heparin nor edetate (EDTA) should be used, since both significantly affect pH readings. However, too much sodium heparin can change pH to the acidotic side. A general rule is not to use more than 0.05 ml of sodium heparin for each milliliter of blood sample drawn.

Although plastic containers absorb oxygen, this process appears to be insignificant in blood gas analysis when the PaO$_2$ is in the normal range. However, with a high PaO$_2$ (i.e., greater than 160 torr), diffusion of oxygen from the syringe into the atmosphere may be hastened by the use of a plastic syringe.

Frequently, air enters the syringe when a blood gas specimen is being drawn. It is important to remember that these air bubbles should be removed before the specimen is analyzed. The most dangerous air bubbles are the small ones; because of their increased surface area, they have the greatest effect upon the reading. CO$_2$ from the blood is lost into the bubbles, while the effect on PO$_2$ depends on its value with respect to that of air.

Blood is living tissue that continues to consume oxygen and produce carbon dioxide even after being placed in a syringe. Table 7-2 shows the effect of time on blood gas values when the syringe is kept at body temperature. In view of this effect, the sample should immediately be iced, so that the temperature will not rise above 20°C. When this is accomplished, the changes in PaCO$_2$ and pH will be insignificant even over several hours.

EVALUATING THE EFFICIENCY AND ADEQUACY OF OXYGENATION

Arterial Oxygen Tension

The arterial oxygen tension remains the standard for assessing the adequacy of oxygenation. However, the measurement of PaO_2 is invasive, intermittent, and expensive. In addition, it is also an insensitive indicator of the efficiency of oxygen exchange in the lungs. Many patients in the early stage of acute respiratory failure will be able to maintain adequate oxygenation.

Oximetry

Pulse oximetry monitoring makes use of the fact that oxyhemoglobin and reduced hemoglobin have different light absorption spectra. A pulsating arterial vascular bed is placed between a two-wavelength light-emitting diode source and a sensor. The transmission of light varies with the pulsatile arterial flow, using the changing transmittance ratio between the two wavelengths of light to calculate the arterial oxygen saturation (SaO_2). The probe may be placed on the lobe of the ear, tip of the finger, or toe, as long as a good pulse waveform is detected.

Numerous studies have documented the accuracy and reproducibility of this continuous, noninvasive monitoring technique in the critically ill patient [7, 12]. Accordingly, pulse oximeters have gained widespread clinical application in the operating room, intensive care unit, and during patient transport. Limitations do exist, however. Inaccurate readings may occur with hypoperfusion (hypotension, use of vasoconstrictors), with lower SaO_2 values (<50%), with external light interference (fluorescent light, sunlight, heating lamps), and in the presence of jaundice or intravenous dyes (methylene blue, fluorescein). Since oximeters are not capable of distinguishing between oxyhemoglobin and abnormal hemoglobin species, elevated levels of carboxyhemoglobin or methemoglobin will usually lead to an overestimation of SaO_2. Oximetry is not a sensitive guide to changes in PaO_2 values above 90 torr, due to the flattening of the oxyhemoglobin dissociation curve in that region. In spite of these limitations, pulse oximetry may be very helpful in continuous monitoring of trends in oxygenation.

Transcutaneous Oxygen Monitoring

There is normally a large oxygen gradient between arterial blood and the skin surface. This gradient may be lowered by heating the skin to a temperature greater than 40°C, causing hyperemia of the underlying capillary bed and increasing the diffusion of oxygen. Transcutaneous oxygen tension ($PtcO_2$) is measured using a heated Clark polarographic electrode mounted on the skin. A number of factors affect the correlation between $PtcO_2$ and PaO_2, including sensor location, skin thickness, patient age, and anesthetic agents. Even more important, however, is the effect of blood flow. When skin perfusion is maintained, $PtcO_2$ follows PaO_2; if a low-flow state occurs, $P_{TC}O_2$ does not track PaO_2, but rather reflects cardiac output [11]. Although this form of oxygen monitoring seems to be successful in the neonate, its use in critically ill adults requires an understanding of the inherent limitations of the measurement and is therefore less useful. Other shortcomings include lengthy warm-up time and calibration, delayed response, and the need to rotate sites every 6 hours to avoid burns.

Transconjunctival oxygen ($P_{CJ}O_2$) monitoring avoids some of the pitfalls of transcutaneous oxygen monitoring, since the epithelial layer separating the capillary network from the electrode surface is only 2 to 4 cells thick and no external heating is necessary. However, flow considerations are similar to those discussed above, and significant individual variations in the $P_{CJ}O_2/PaO_2$ ratio exist [5].

Derived Oxygenation Indices

Alveolar-Arterial Oxygen Gradient
One of the first indices suggested for evaluating the efficiency of oxygen exchange in the lungs is the alveolar-arterial oxygen gradient [$P(A-a)O_2$]. The $P(A-a)O_2$ may be measured at any given FIO_2; however, it is most commonly determined with the patient inhaling 100% oxygen ($FIO_2 = 1.0$).

When the patient is on an FIO_2 of 1.0, the oxygen tension is the same in all ventilated alveoli (i.e., the partial pressure of oxygen in all ventilated alveoli is the same). The PO_2 in the alveolus is abbreviated as PAO_2. Under these circumstances ($FIO_2 = 1.0$), the $P(A-a)O_2$ is a reflection of physiologic shunting in the lung—i.e., of alveoli that are perfused but not ventilated. It must be noted that the calculation of the $P(A-a)O_2$ at $FIO_2 = 1.0$ carries with it the possibility of complications and/or erroneous results. The concern is that inhalation of 100% oxygen, even for short periods of time, can cause absorption atelectasis, with a resultant increase in shunt. In this situation, flow of oxygen out of the alveolus occurs rapidly because of the large diffusion gradient between PAO_2 and $P\bar{v}O_2$. After the oxygen has left the alveolus, only the pressure due to PCO_2 and PH_2O remains, because the nitrogen normally present has been washed out. With the nitrogen "splint" gone, there may be insufficient pressure to maintain the alveolus in an open state. When absorption atelectasis occurs, it may be difficult to reopen the alveolus, because of the surface tension of such small units. Clinically, it may require high inspiratory pressures to open these atelectatic units [6, 14].

CALCULATION OF THE $P(A-a)O_2$ AT FIO_2 OF 1.0. The patient should be placed on 100% oxygen for 20 minutes. During this period of time the patient must not be disconnected from the ventilator, and physical activity should be held to a minimum. Arterial blood gases are drawn and the corrected barometric pressure (PB) obtained.

Example
Arterial blood gas (FIO_2 1.0) = pH, 7.48; $PaCO_2$, 39 torr; PaO_2, 325 torr; HCO_3^-, 28 mEq/liter; SaO_2, 99.7%. The barometric pressure reading = 752 torr. Using these values, the calculation is made as follows [2, 3]:

P_B	752	torr
P_{H_2O}	−47	

Corrected P_B	705
P_ACO_2	−39

P_AO_2	666
PaO_2	−325

$P(A-a)O_2$	341	torr

CALCULATION OF THE $P(A-a)O_2$ AT AN FIO_2 LESS THAN 1.0. When the FIO_2 is reduced below 1.0, the calculation of the $P(A-a)O_2$ becomes slightly more complex. The P_AO_2 can be estimated using a modified alveolar air equation [2] as follows:

$$P_AO_2 = (P_B - P_{H_2O}) \times FIO_2 - \frac{P_ACO_2}{R}$$

where

P_B = barometric pressure
P_{H_2O} = water vapor pressure (47 torr)
FIO_2 = fractional inspired oxygen concentration
P_ACO_2 = partial pressure of carbon dioxide in the alveolus (can be assumed to be the same as $PaCO_2$)
    R = respiratory quotient (ratio of the volume of carbon dioxide produced to the volume of oxygen consumed, usually 0.8)

The $P(A-a)O_2$ is most reliable in stable patients breathing room air. In addition, its value changes unpredictably with changes in FIO_2 and varies independently with changes in oxygen consumption and arterial oxygen saturation [9]. Therefore, its clinical applicability in critically ill patients is somewhat limited.

Arterial-Alveolar Oxygen Tension Ratio
The arterial-alveolar oxygen tension ratio (PaO_2/P_AO_2) remains relatively stable with varying levels of FIO_2. It is most reliable with FIO_2 levels less than 0.55 or when PaO_2 is less than 100 torr with the patient's FIO_2 greater than 0.3 [4]. Its value in predicting pulmonary shunting in critically ill patients is slightly better than that of the alveolar-arterial oxygen gradient [1]. The lower limit of normal is 0.8; values less than 0.55 imply a significant degree of pulmonary shunting [8].

Arterial–Inspired-Oxygen Ratio
Since the alveolar air equation requires some assumptions that may not hold true in the unstable patient, the arterial–inspired-oxygen ratio (PaO_2/FIO_2) has been suggested as a simple index to approximate the degree of venous admixture. The reliability of this measurement is similar to that of

the arterial-alveolar oxygen tension ratio [1]. Values less than 300 represent a significant shunt, correlating with a $\dot{Q}_s/\dot{Q}_t$ of approximately 15 percent or greater.

The Percent of Pulmonary Shunt

The percent of pulmonary shunt ($\dot{Q}_s/\dot{Q}_t$) (i.e., the right-to-left shunt) is defined as that portion of the cardiac output ($\dot{Q}_t$) (pulmonary blood flow) that is perfusing unventilated alveoli ($\dot{Q}_s$). Thus, measuring the shunt enables one to quantitate the percentage of cardiac output that returns to the left heart unoxygenated, with a PO_2 equal to that of the mixed venous blood. This is also referred to as pulmonary venous admixture. There are four causes of total pulmonary shunting: (1) impaired diffusion, (2) ventilation-perfusion inequalities, (3) anatomic shunts (e.g., in the normal person, this is due to blood returning to the left heart via the bronchial and thebesian veins), and (4) alveolar collapse (i.e., where the $\dot{V}_A/\dot{Q} = 0$). In the normal person, $\dot{Q}_s/\dot{Q}_t$ is in the range of 3 to 5 percent; however, in the critically ill patient, a shunt of 15 percent is not at all uncommon.

Of all the derived indices, $\dot{Q}_s/\dot{Q}_t$ is clearly the most reliable in assessing and following efficacy of oxygenation in the acutely ill patient. The major drawbacks are that calculation of it is somewhat complex and that a pulmonary artery catheter is necessary to obtain a mixed venous blood sample.

The $\dot{Q}_s/\dot{Q}_t$ can be measured with the patient on either 100% oxygen or a lesser oxygen concentration. There are, however, certain advantages to measuring the percent of shunt on an FIO_2 of 1.0. When the patient is breathing 100% oxygen, the calculation of the $\dot{Q}_s/\dot{Q}_t$ is simplified, because the calculation of the $P(A-a)O_2$, which is required in the shunt equation, is simplified. In addition, when the patient is on an FIO_2 of 1.0, the causes of total pulmonary shunting are reduced to only anatomic shunting and alveolar collapse. However, although placing the patient on an FIO_2 of 1.0 simplifies the calculation of $\dot{Q}_s/\dot{Q}_t$ and reduces the causes of shunting, one must remember the effect that an FIO_2 of 1.0 alone may have on alveoli (i.e., absorption atelectasis) [15].

CALCULATION OF $\dot{Q}_s/\dot{Q}_t$. To calculate the percent of pulmonary shunt ($\dot{Q}_s/\dot{Q}_t$), one must have the following information: (1) the PAO_2 (alveolar PO_2), (2) the PaO_2 (arterial PO_2), (3) the arteriovenous oxygen content difference (a-$\bar{v}DCO_2$) (the calculation of which also requires that one know the patient's hemoglobin).

The patient is placed on 100% oxygen for 20 minutes, and then arterial and mixed venous blood gases are obtained, along with the measurement of hemoglobin. The $\dot{Q}_s/\dot{Q}_t$ is then calculated from the following formula. The only additional requirement for calculating the shunt is that the PaO_2 must be at least 150 torr (at this level, hemoglobin is fully saturated with oxygen, and any further increases in PaO_2 only affect the amount of dissolved oxygen in plasma). If the PaO_2 is less than 150, another formula must be used.

CALCULATION OF THE $\dot{Q}_s/\dot{Q}_t$ WHEN THE PaO_2 IS AT LEAST 150 TORR. When the PaO_2 is at least 150 torr, the $\dot{Q}_s/\dot{Q}_t$ is calculated as follows:

$$\dot{Q}_S/\dot{Q}_T = \frac{(P_AO_2 - PaO_2) \times 0.0031}{a\text{-}\bar{v}DCO_2 + (P_AO_2 - PaO_2) \times 0.0031}$$

where

$\dot{Q}_s$ = unventilated alveoli
$\dot{Q}_t$ = cardiac output
P_AO_2 = partial pressure of oxygen in the alveolus
PaO_2 = partial pressure of oxygen in arterial blood
0.0031 = solubility coefficient (Bunsen) for oxygen dissolved in plasma
$a\text{-}\bar{v}DCO_2$ = arteriovenous oxygen content difference

The P_AO_2 is calculated in the same way as previously described. The arteriovenous oxygen content difference is calculated as follows:

$$a\text{-}\bar{v}DCO_2 = CaO_2 - CvO_2$$

where

CaO_2 = $(Hb \times 1.39)$ SaO_2 + $(PaO_2 \times 0.0031)$
$C\bar{v}O_2$ = $(Hb \times 1.39)$ $S\bar{v}O_2$ + $(P\bar{v}O_2 \times 0.0031)$
CaO_2 = the oxygen content of arterial blood
$C\bar{v}O_2$ = the oxygen content of mixed venous blood
Hb = hemoglobin concentration in gm/100 ml
1.39 = ml of oxygen capable of being carried by 1 gm of hemoglobin (theoretical)
SaO_2 = oxyhemoglobin saturation of arterial blood
$S\bar{v}O_2$ = oxyhemoglobin saturation of mixed venous blood
PaO_2 = partial pressure of oxygen in arterial blood
$P\bar{v}O_2$ = partial pressure of oxygen in mixed venous blood
0.0031 = solubility coefficient for oxygen physically dissolved in solution

CALCULATION OF THE $\dot{Q}_s/\dot{Q}_t$ WHEN THE PaO_2 IS LESS THAN 150 TORR. If the PaO_2 is less than 150 torr, calculation of the $\dot{Q}_s/\dot{Q}_t$ is as follows:

$$\dot{Q}_s/\dot{Q}_t = \frac{CcO_2 - CaO_2}{CcO_2 - C\bar{v}O_2}$$

where

$\dot{Q}$ = total pulmonary blood flow
CaO_2 = oxygen content of arterial blood
$C\bar{v}O_2$ = oxygen content of mixed venous blood
CcO_2 = oxygen content of pulmonary capillary blood

In this equation, CaO_2 and $C\bar{v}O_2$ are calculated as described previously. The calculation of CcO_2, however, requires one to assume that this would be the oxygen content that arterial blood would have if fully equilibrated with alveolar air. This assumption is necessary because of the inaccessibility of pulmonary capillary blood for direct measurement. For example, a patient with an FIO_2 of 0.5 has the following values: Hb = 15 gm/100 ml, PaO_2 = 105 torr, SaO_2 = 99.2%. The values for mixed venous blood are $P\bar{v}O_2$ = 40 torr and $S\bar{v}O_2$ = 75%. Before calculating the $\dot{Q}_s/\dot{Q}_t$, it is necessary to determine the PAO_2 (see page 134). In this case, the PAO_2 was calculated to be 650 torr. Now that all the necessary information for the calculation of $\dot{Q}_s/\dot{Q}_t$ has been obtained, one can proceed with the calculation of CcO_2, CaO_2, and $C\bar{v}O_2$.

$$CcO_2 = (Hb \times 1.39)\, SaO_2 + (PAO_2 \times 0.0031)$$

Note
Because the PO_2 of alveolar air on 100% oxygen will always exceed 150 torr, one can assume that the saturation of blood exposed to alveolar air (i.e., pulmonary capillary blood) will be 100%.

$$CcO_2 = (15 \times 1.39) + (650 \times 0.0031)$$
$$CcO_2 = 22.86 \text{ vol}\%$$
$$CaO_2 = (15 \times 1.39)\, 0.992 + (105 \times 0.0031)$$
$$CaO_2 = 21.00 \text{ vol}\%$$
$$C\bar{v}O_2 = 15.76 \text{ vol}\%$$

The calculation of $\dot{Q}_s/\dot{Q}_t$ is now completed as follows:

$$\dot{Q}_s/\dot{Q}_t = \frac{22.86 - 21.00}{22.86 - 15.76}$$

$$\dot{Q}_s/\dot{Q}_t = 0.26$$

Note
This value is then converted to a percentage by multiplying by 100.

$$\dot{Q}_s/\dot{Q}_t = 26\%$$

EVALUATING THE ADEQUACY OF VENTILATION
Arterial Carbon Dioxide Tension
The $PaCO_2$ as measured from the arterial blood gas determines the adequacy of ventilation. Unlike the arterial oxygen tension, the $PaCO_2$ is a specific and sensitive indicator. However, it shares the problems of being invasive, intermittent, and expensive.

Capnography
Capnography is the measurement of end-tidal carbon dioxide partial pressure ($PETCO_2$). In normal patients, the plateau value of $PETCO_2$ is usually 1

to 5 torr below the $PaCO_2$ and thus provides a continuous, noninvasive assessment of ventilatory adequacy. Two common techniques are available to the clinician for measuring $PetCO_2$: infrared absorption and mass spectrometry.

Infrared CO_2 analyzers operate by emitting a source of infrared radiation through a chamber containing the gas mixture to be analyzed, measuring the PCO_2 by detection of the reduction in intensity of the absorbed light. Mainstream infrared CO_2 analyzers place the infrared source and detector on opposite sides of the main gas stream, usually between the endotracheal tube and the Y-piece in the ventilator circuit. Resistance is low with this configuration, and secretions are rarely a problem. The analyzer is heavy and must be heated—a potential danger, since it is in close proximity to the patient. Sidestream infrared CO_2 analyzers aspirate gas from the main respiratory circuit through a small-bore tubing to a remote analyzer. Little weight or dead space is added to the circuit; however, response time is slower and clogging of the sample tubing does occur.

Mass spectrometry measures CO_2 (as well as other respiratory and anesthetic gases) by ionization and separation of the constituent molecules, picking up each gas on a separate detector electrode. These machines are large and quite expensive, making them impractical for use as single-patient–dedicated units. Consequently, the sampling and response times depend upon the location and number of patients utilizing the monitoring system.

Patients with an uneven distribution of ventilation will have an increased $PaCO_2$-$PetCO_2$ gradient, on the order of 10 to 20 torr. Although under these conditions $PetCO_2$ is no longer a reliable approximation of $PaCO_2$ [16], if cardiopulmonary function is stable, the relationship is sufficiently constant to be helpful in monitoring changes in ventilatory status. The use of capnography is considered routine practice in the operating room, with spillover into the ICU also occurring.

Transcutaneous Carbon Dioxide Monitoring

Most of the same theoretical and technical difficulties that limit the practicality of transcutaneous oxygen monitoring also apply to transcutaneous carbon dioxide ($PtcCO_2$) monitoring. In patients with adequate perfusion, $PtcCO_2$ exceeds $PaCO_2$ by a relatively constant and sizable gradient (approximately 20 torr); when perfusion is poor, $PtcCO_2$ changes inversely with cardiac index and correlates poorly with $PaCO_2$ [13].

Tidal Volume

Tidal volume (V_T), defined as the volume of air moved in or out of the lungs in any single breath, may readily be measured at the bedside using a hand-held respirometer. If the tidal volume is depressed, the patient may have difficulty in both oxygenation and ventilation.

V_D/V_T (Physiologic Dead Space)

Frequently, the critically ill patient will hyperventilate, yet the $PaCO_2$ will be normal. This is because of increased physiologic dead space—that portion of the tidal volume that does not exchange with pulmonary blood. Although this may be obvious in some patients, in others this observation is not so easily made. In these situations, the measurement of V_D/V_T may prove useful. The normal value for V_D/V_T is from 0.2 to 0.4. The formula that is used clinically is derived from Bohr's equation and is as follows:

$$V_D/V_T = \frac{PaCO_2 - P\bar{E}CO_2}{PaCO_2}$$

where

$\quad V_D$ = dead space
$\quad V_T$ = tidal volume
$PaCO_2$ = arterial carbon dioxide tension
$P\bar{E}CO_2$ = mean expired carbon dioxide tension

The classic case in which one finds an increased V_D/V_T is pulmonary embolism. In this situation, there are areas of lung that are ventilated but not perfused. Changes in V_D/V_T also occur following shock and in pulmonary insufficiency. The V_D/V_T will vary with changes in either anatomic or alveolar dead space or tidal volume. However, V_D/V_T does not differentiate anatomic from alveolar dead space, nor does it differentiate dead-space change from ventilation-perfusion inequalities.

The clinical measurement of V_D/V_T is primarily of value when the tidal volume is greater than normal and when the increased tidal volume is relatively consistent. These conditions are met by most patients on mechanical ventilatory assistance.

The following are some situations in which one can observe an increased V_D/V_T:

1. In nonperfusion of a ventilated alveolus (e.g., a pulmonary embolus).
2. In hypotension, in which gravity and a low pulmonary artery pressure promote a redistribution of blood volume and flow, favoring the dependent portion of the lung, so that many alveoli are ventilated but not perfused.
3. When there is an increase in mean airway pressure, occurring in some alveoli to the extent that the capillary perfusion during the respiratory cycle causes a redistribution of blood flow to the remainder of the lung. In the presence of refractory atelectasis, a portion of this redistributed blood flow will go to atelectatic areas. As a result, both V_D/V_T and $\dot{Q}_s/\dot{Q}_t$ are increased.

EVALUATING RESPIRATORY MECHANICS AND VENTILATORY RESERVE

In addition to the evaluation of oxygenation and ventilation, it is necessary to consider the mechanics and work of breathing. Abnormalities in pulmonary mechanics are common in critically ill patients, and their measurement provides useful information concerning need for mechanical ventilatory assistance. Vital capacity, inspiratory force, functional residual capacity (FRC), and compliance are parameters that can be followed.

Vital Capacity

Vital capacity is defined as a maximal expiration following a maximal inspiration. Normally, vital capacity should be in the range of 60 to 70 ml/kg. Although vital capacity can be readily measured in the intensive care unit, its value is quite dependent upon patient cooperation. Patients who are on ventilatory assistance can be considered ready for weaning when their vital capacity is at least 10 ml/kg. When the vital capacity reaches 15 ml/kg, the patient will probably be able to tolerate being off the ventilator permanently.

Maximal Inspiratory Force

Inspiratory force is measured as the maximal pressure below atmospheric pressure that a patient can exert during a period of 10 to 20 seconds against a completely occluded airway. This measurement is less dependent on the cooperation of the patient and is particularly useful with unconscious or anesthetized patients. The normal value for inspiratory force is -75 to -100 cm H_2O. The measurement of inspiratory force requires only the following: a face mask or a connector to an endotracheal or tracheostomy tube and a manometer capable of registering pressure below atmospheric pressure.

This measurement serves as a rough indicator of global respiratory muscle strength. Experience has shown that the muscular power needed to generate a vital capacity of 15 ml/kg produces a negative inspiratory force of more than -25 cm H_2O within 20 seconds.

Functional Residual Capacity

Functional residual capacity (FRC) is defined as the gas remaining in the lung following a normal expiration. Patients with pulmonary insufficiency have decreased FRC; the use of positive end-expiratory pressure (PEEP) has been found to increase FRC. Routine clinical determinations of FRC are rarely done at the bedside.

Compliance

Compliance is defined as the forces resisting expansion of the lung. There are a variety of methods available to measure compliance, but the discussion here will be confined to the measurement of so-called effective dynamic compliance (EDC).

Compliance is measured as volume change per pressure change (ml/cm H_2O). Effective dynamic compliance measurement should not be confused with static compliance measurement (i.e., when no air is moving). EDC only indicates change in lung compliance (i.e., the stiffness of the lungs).

The interpretation of EDC is not without problems, since it is affected by high airway pressures and the distensibility of the tubing used on the respirator. Despite these problems, we have used it to indicate a trend. As EDC increases, the lung is becoming less stiff; conversely, as EDC decreases, the lung is becoming stiffer: That is to say, as EDC increases, it takes less pressure to produce a given tidal volume. A sudden decrease in EDC may be an indicator of a blocked airway, and this cause should be ruled out before assuming that the lung has become stiffer.

To measure EDC, one divides the tidal volume by the plateau airway pressure minus any positive end-expiratory pressure the patient may be receiving.

EDC = tidal volume (ml)/plateau airway pressure − PEEP (cm H_2O)

Values less than 50 ml/cm H_2O indicate increasing lung dysfunction.

ANCILLARY TECHNIQUES
Although the sophisticated respiratory monitoring techniques described above are essential in the evaluation of the patient with (or at risk for developing) pulmonary insufficiency, one should never abandon the routine, clinical assessments of observation, auscultation, and chest roentgenography.

Observation
Increased respiratory rate, recruitment of accessory respiratory muscles, and asynchronous, paradoxical motion of the rib cage and abdomen are all evidence of increasing respiratory distress. In the spontaneously breathing patient, these signs may point to the need for institution of mechanical ventilatory support. If these observations are noted in the patient being weaned from the ventilator, it is likely that such weaning will not be successful.

Auscultation
A physician would not be a physician without a stethoscope, and even though auscultatory changes come very late in pulmonary insufficiency, the physician must frequently auscultate the patient's chest to detect gross changes. For example, a pneumothorax may develop in a patient on PEEP, and in this instance the stethoscope and chest roentgenogram will prove useful (blood gases would probably also reveal a deterioration in PaO_2).

Chest Roentgenograms
Chest roentgenograms are routinely taken in patients with pulmonary insufficiency. However, roentgenographic changes often lag behind clinical changes in such patients.

FUTURE DIRECTIONS
Technological advances will enhance the ability of the physician to monitor the respiratory status of the critically ill patient. The efficiency and accuracy of noninvasive monitoring techniques will be improved, so that their use will become more clinically relevant. Methodology for continuous invasive measurement of arterial PO_2 and PCO_2 now exists; its routine use will enable uninterrupted observation of the unstable patient and immediate feedback on the effects of interventional therapeutic maneuvers.

Adherence to a defined monitoring program provides the physician with data to support the clinical findings in the making of critical decisions regarding initiation and discontinuance of respiratory support care (see Table 7-3 and Chapters 10 and 11).

Table 7-3. Guidelines for the institution and discontinuation of mechanical ventilatory support in patients with pulmonary insufficiency

Parameter	Normal range	Indication for ventilatory assistance	Indication for weaning
Mechanics			
Respiratory rate	12–20	>35	<30
Vital capacity (ml/kg of body weight)[a]	65–75	<15	12–15
Inspiratory force (cm H_2O)	75–100	>25	>25
Oxygenation			
PaO_2 (mm Hg)	100–75 (room air)	<70 (on mask O_2)	—[b]
$P(A-a)O_2$ ($FiO_2 = 1.0$) (mm Hg)[c]	25–65	450	<400
Ventilation			
$PaCO_2$ (mm Hg)	35–45	>55[d]	—[e]
V_D/V_T	0.25–0.40	>0.60	<0.58

[a]Patient's ideal weight is used if weight appears grossly abnormal.

[b]When the physician is deciding to wean the patient, the $P(A-a)O_2$ ($FiO_2 = 0.50$ or 1.0) serves as a better criterion than any given PaO_2.

[c]The $P(A-a)O_2$ is measured after the patient has been on an $FiO_2 = 1.0$ for 10 to 20 min (in the nonemphysematous patient 10 min is adequate). *Note:* It was mentioned earlier that there are certain problems associated with measuring the $P(A-a)O_2$ at an FiO_2 of 1.0. If, however, it must be measured at 1.0, the patient should be sighed (i.e., the lungs hyperinflated) with nitrogen-containing mixtures following the discontinuation of the 100% oxygen.

[d]Except in patients with chronic hypercapnia.

[e]Since $PaCO_2$, while the patient is on the ventilator, is a function of the respirator settings as well as the patient's lungs, it is not a useful measurement for assessing readiness for weaning.

Note: The temptation to rely on a list of objective criteria as the definitive ruling on intubation and weaning is great. However, it should be kept in mind that the trend of values is more important than any given value alone, and that clinical correlation is of major consideration.

Source: Modified from R. S. Wilson and H. Pontoppidan. Acute respiratory failure. *Crit. Care Med.* 2:293, 1974.

REFERENCES

1. Cane, R. D., et al. Unreliability of oxygen tension-based indices in reflecting intrapulmonary shunting in critically ill patients. *Crit. Care Med.* 16:1243, 1988.
2. Comroe, J. H., et al. *The Lung: Clinical Physiology and Pulmonary Function Tests* (2nd ed.). Chicago: Year Book, 1962. Pp. 15–19.
3. Comroe, J. H., et al. *The Lung: Clinical Physiology and Pulmonary Function Tests* (2nd ed.). Chicago: Year Book, 1962. Pp. 339–341.
4. Gilbert, R., et al. Stability of the arterial/alveolar oxygen partial pressure ratio. Effects of low ventilation/perfusion regions. *Crit. Care Med.* 7:267, 1979.
5. Hess, D., et al. The relationship between conjunctival PO_2 and arterial PO_2 in 16 normal persons. *Resp. Care* 31:191, 1986.
6. McAslan, T. C., et al. Influence of 100% oxygen in intrapulmonary shunt in severely traumatized patients. *J. Trauma* 13:811, 1973.
7. Mihm, F. G., and Halperin, B. D. Noninvasive detection of profound arterial desaturations using a pulse oximetry device. *Anesthesiology* 62:85, 1985.
8. Peris, L. V., et al. Clinical use of the arterial-alveolar oxygen tension ratio. *Crit. Care Med.* 11:88, 1983.
9. Pontoppidan, H., et al. Acute respiratory failure in the adult. *N. Engl. J. Med.* 287:745, 1972.
10. Thorson, S. H., et al. Variability of arterial blood gas values in stable patients in the ICU. *Chest* 84:14, 1983.
11. Tremper, K. K., and Shoemaker, W. C. Transcutaneous oxygen monitoring of critically ill adults, with and without low flow shock. *Crit. Care Med.* 9:706, 1981.
12. Tremper, K. K., et al. Accuracy of a pulse oximeter in the critically ill adult: Effect of temperature and hemodynamics. *Anesthesiology* 63(3A):A175, 1985.
13. Tremper, K. K., et al. Transcutaneous PCO_2 monitoring on adult patients in the ICU and the operating room. *Crit. Care Med.* 9:752, 1981.
14. West, J. B. Pulmonary gas exchange in the critically ill patient. *Crit. Care Med.* 2:171, 1974.
15. West, J. B. *Respiratory Physiology: The Essentials* (3rd ed.). Baltimore: Williams & Wilkins, 1987.
16. Yamanaka, M. K., and Sue, D. Y. Comparison of arterial-end-tidal PCO_2 difference and dead space/tidal volume ratio in respiratory failure. *Chest* 92:832, 1987.

SELECTED READINGS

Brown, M., and Vender, J. S. Noninvasive oxygen monitoring. *Crit. Care Clin.* 4:493, 1988.

Kelleher, J. F. Pulse oximetry. *J. Clin. Monit.* 5:37, 1989.

Moore, F. D., et al. *Post-Traumatic Pulmonary Insufficiency: Pathophysiology of Respiratory Failure and Principles of Respiratory Care After Surgical Operations, Trauma, Hemorrhage, Burns and Shock.* Philadelphia: Saunders, 1969.

Nochomovitz, M. L., and Cherniack, N. S. *Noninvasive Respiratory Monitoring.* New York: Churchill-Livingstone, 1986.

Pontoppidan, H., et al. *Acute Respiratory Failure in the Adult.* Boston: Little, Brown, 1973.

Shapiro, B. A. *Clinical Application of Blood Gases* (4th ed.). Chicago: Year Book, 1989.

Stock, M. C. Noninvasive carbon dioxide monitoring. *Crit. Care Clin.* 4:511, 1988.

Suter, P. M., et al. Shunt, lung volume and perfusion during short periods of ventilation with oxygen. *Anesthesiology* 43:617, 1975.

Tobin, M. J. Respiratory monitoring in the intensive care unit. *Am. Rev. Respir. Dis.* 138:1625, 1988.

8

In Situ Monitoring of Organs

Klaus Frank
Manfred Kessler
Klaus Appelbaum

Josef Zündorf
Hans-Peter Albrecht
Günther Siebenhaar

Remission spectra from biologic pigments located within capillaries and cells provide us with information concerning basic mechanisms of tissue function.

The first precise measurements of transmission spectra from suspended mitochondria were performed by Chance [4–6], using a double-beam technique.

For a long time the systematic application of tissue photometry was restricted to completely immobilized organs, because the measuring optical systems available could only be adapted by the use of lenses that had to be focused. The decisive breakthrough in the field of tissue spectroscopy, made by Chance [7, 18, 19], was achieved with the use of highly flexible micro–lightguides, which solved the problem of optimal adaptation of the optical instrument to the surfaces of organs in man and mammals.

A rapid micro-lightguide spectrometer (EMPHO I) of high sensitivity has been constructed in order to record spectra of high quality in moving organs. This instrument enables quantitative measurements of light signals originating from small catchment volumes of tissue [8].

The adaptation of the lightguides to the surface of intact organs—and thereby, quantitative spectroscopy—enables the noninvasive measurement of the following local and functional parameters from a few capillaries and surrounding cells [9–12].

1. Intracapillary hemoglobin oxygenation
2. Intracapillary hemoglobin concentration
3. Local oxygen-uptake rate
4. Local capillary blood flow
5. Size changes of subcellular particles
6. Permeability of capillary walls, when exogenous dyes of different molecular weight are injected

Monitoring of these parameters in the skin or skeletal muscle during an operation or in the critical care unit provides the clinician with early warning information. These parameters, unlike control parameters, are sensitive to the beginning of pathophysiologic changes within the patient. Centralization effects, for example, can be observed at an early stage before changes in global parameters develop.

The distribution of the oxygen supply in conjunction with functional tests of the organ during surgical interventions enable the assessment of the regulatory state, the functional reserves, the severity of the pathologic disturbance, and the success of the surgical procedure.

METHODOLOGY
EMPHO I

A schematic drawing of the EMPHO I is shown in Figure 8-1. The light of the xenon arc lamp (1) is collimated by a lens system (2) and focused onto the incident plane of the illuminating micro-lightguide fiber (3). The light is transmitted by a single micro-lightguide fiber to the tissue surface. The remitted light is collected by surrounding micro-lightguide fibers (4) and led to the detection unit.

The light, transmitted by the detection micro-lightguide, passes through a rotating interference bandpass filter disk (5), which is mounted on the axle of a micromotor (6). A filter disk that covers the spectral domain from 502 to 620 nm is installed in the EMPHO I. A wheel (7) for the decoding of the angular position of the filter disk, also mounted on the axle of the driving motor, triggers the data acquisition.

The monochromated light is transmitted to a photomultiplier tube (8). The output of the photomultiplier tube is current to voltage converted and amplified by a cascade amplifier.

The signal is digitalized by an analog-to-digital converter that is triggered by the impulses from the decoder wheel.

The data are then processed, stored, and displayed by an IBM AT–compatible computer.

Data Acquisition and Evaluation

A schematic drawing of the data acquisition system is shown in Figure 8-2. The analog to digital conversion is triggered by a decoder system containing an EPROM. The trigger impulses are assigned to the corresponding wavelength using values from a calibration curve that are stored in the EPROM.

The program for the data acquisition and the online data evaluation is written in MODULA II. This programming language enables parallel processing of four different program lines:

1. The data acquisition
2. The data storage
3. The online evaluation
4. The display of the data on the computer screen

No assembler routines were necessary for the data acquisition system [2].

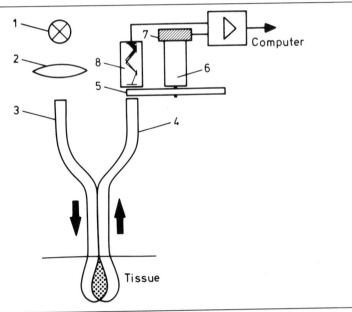

Fig. 8-1. Schematic drawing of the EMPHO I. 1. Xenon high-pressure arc lamp. 2. Lens system. 3. Illuminating micro-lightguide fiber. 4. Detecting micro-lightguide. 5. Interference filter disk. 6. Driving micromotor. 7. Decoder wheel. 8. Photomultiplier tube.

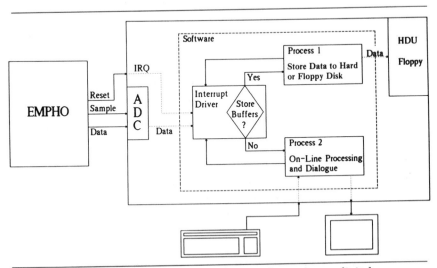

Fig. 8-2. Scheme of the data acquisition system. The analog-to-digital conversion of the signal coming from the EMPHO I is triggered by the sample impulses. The reset signal indicates the start of the data acquisition for one spectrum. The spectra are plotted on the computer screen by process 2. When process 1 is activated, the data are also stored on the hard disc.

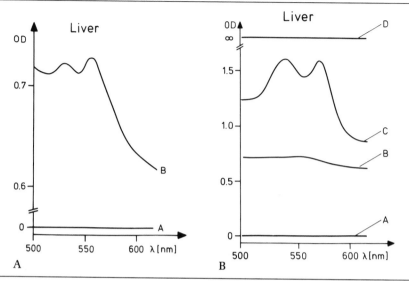

Fig. 8-3. Spectra of isolated perfused rat liver. A. Remission spectrum of incident light intensity. B. Basic remission spectrum of hemoglobin-free perfused liver. C. Remission spectrum of hemoglobin-perfused liver. D. Zero light curve.

Basic Remission Spectra of Tissue Before and After the Addition of Hemoglobin

The isolated perfused rat liver [17] was used for the determination of basic tissue spectra, and superimposed hemoglobin spectra were obtained by the addition of erythrocytes to the perfusate.

Figure 8-3 shows the remission spectrum (A) of the incident light, obtained as the remission spectrum of the white standard $BaSO_4$. This spectrum is required for the calibration of the measuring system. Spectrum B represents the so-called basic remission function of liver tissue [10], which is composed of the remission spectrum of scattered light superimposed by the absorption by the intramitochondrial enzymes (cytochromes b, c, aa_3) and other tissue pigments of lower concentration.

When erythrocytes are added to the perfusate in a concentration of 3.4 g%, a typical tissue hemoglobin spectrum (C) appears, characterizing the intrasinusoidal hemoglobin oxygenation.

Curve D represents the zero light curve obtained for infinite optical density. This latter curve is also needed for the calibration of the measuring system [8].

FUNCTIONAL PRINCIPLES OF OXYGEN SUPPLY TO TISSUE

Capillary populations of different lengths and diameters with various capillary flow rates are found in all tissues of humans and mammals. The oxygen consumption of the respiring cells produces gradients of intracap-

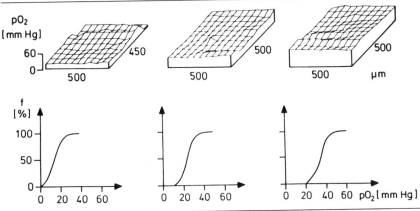

Fig. 8-4. PO$_2$ topograms and corresponding cumulative histograms of the skeletal muscle, indicative of three different capillary supply units.

illary hemoglobin oxygenation along each capillary, as well as oxygen diffusion gradients from the capillaries into the tissue.

Even though all these different parameters produce great heterogeneities in the distribution patterns of microflow, intracapillary HbO$_2$, and cellular pO$_2$, common functional structures are found in all tissues.

A recent and interesting finding is that capillary units supplied by one terminal arteriole reveal relatively homogeneous distribution patterns, whereas pronounced heterogeneities exist between different supply units [14–16, 20, 21].

As shown by Harrison [13] a few of the supply units show very high flow rates and thus provide shunt channels for the circulating flow reserve found in all organs. The reserves manifested by the topograms of different oxygenation and the shunt channels can only be mobilized by modulation of the vascular tone of the terminal arterioles, thus rapidly providing more homogeneous patterns of supply to the tissue [13].

Typical pO$_2$ topograms of different oxygenation levels in the resting skeletal muscle are shown in Figure 8-4. They are representative of local oxygen of the final measurable supply parameter transported by the complex and highly regulated convective and diffusive chain that provides the mass transfer from the atmosphere to the mitochondria [3, 21].

MEASUREMENTS IN HUMAN SKIN AND HEART

Skin

Intracutaneous spectra of the skin can be recorded at any surface location of the human body. However, a highly suitable area for placement of the micro-lightguide of the EMPHO I is the hand, which is easily accessible, and has a relatively high capillarization and blood flow.

A pseudo–three-dimensional plot of intracapillary HbO$_2$ spectra measured on the back of the hand of a healthy human volunteer is shown in

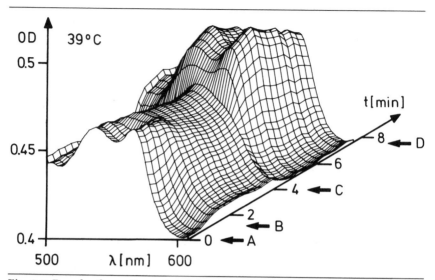

Fig. 8-5. Pseudo–three-dimensional drawing of hemoglobin spectra from human skin during an occlusion reaction. A–B. control. B–C. perfusion stop induced by inflation of a pressure cuff. C–D. reactive hyperemia.

Figure 8-5. On the abscissa the wavelength is given in nanometers. The ordinate corresponds to the light intensity [optical density (OD) = $\log(I_0/I)$] and the z-axis to the time scale in minutes. The spectra were measured in an area where the skin temperature was raised to 39°C by local heating.

The time course of the intracapillary hemoglobin oxygenation and concentration, evaluated from the spectra depicted in Figure 8-5, are shown in Figures 8-6 and 8-7. Well-oxygenated control spectra with two peaks are plotted from A to B. The quantitative evaluation resulted in oxygenation values of 71 percent, with small oscillations of ±5 percent. A perfusion stop was induced at time B by inflating a pressure cuff. Due to the oxygen uptake rate of the skin, a complete deoxygenation of the intracapillary hemoglobin developed within 2 minutes. Immediately after the beginning of reperfusion (C), there was a rapid rise in hemoglobin oxygenation, which subsequently returned to the initial range. The very pronounced increase in the amplitudes of the spectra corresponded to a 170 percent increase in intracapillary hemoglobin concentration, which is also indicative of a higher capillary blood flow.

Due to the fact that hemoglobin oxygenation and concentration are recorded simultaneously, the cellular oxygen uptake rate of the skin can be calculated by use of the formula

$$O_2 \text{ uptake rate} = (dHbO_2)/dt \times Hb(t)/Hb(t = O)$$

The results are shown in Figure 8-8 based on the curves of Figures 8-6 and 8-7. During an initial period down to a hemoglobin oxygenation of 31

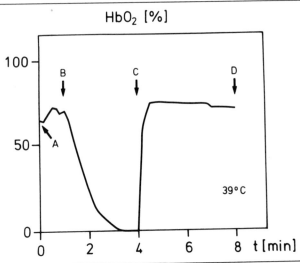

Fig. 8-6. Intracapillary hemoglobin oxygenation measured during occlusion reaction in human skin. Changes in oxygen uptake rate cause the deviation of the curve from linearity.

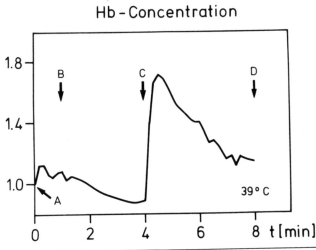

Fig. 8-7. Intracapillary hemoglobin concentration measured during occlusion reaction in human skin.

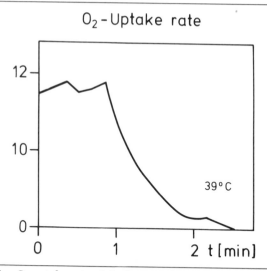

Fig. 8-8. Relative O_2 uptake rate of the human skin at a temperature of 39°C during perfusion stop. The oxygen uptake rate remains fairly constant during the first minute after perfusion stop. At an HbO_2 value of 31 percent, the O_2 uptake rate diminishes exponentially. Two minutes after perfusion stop, at HbO_2 1.2 percent, the O_2 uptake rate decreases further, changing the reaction kinetics.

percent, the O_2 uptake rate remains constant. Below this value an exponential decay is observed, revealing a steady decrease in O_2 uptake rate. At an HbO_2 of 1.2 percent, which may be equivalent to the critical mitochondrial PO_2 values, a change in the exponential slope is observed.

Heart

Recently, systematic spectroscopic investigations were performed in coronary bypass patients during open heart surgery [12]. The measurements were performed in the subepicardial layers of the beating heart by use of a "light pen" gently held by hand at the surface of the myocardium. The short sampling time of 10 msec for each spectrum and the fast movements of the beating myocardium allowed 100 spectra per second to be recorded from different locations of the tissue. Because of the high frequency of the recording, it took only 2 seconds to gain enough HbO_2 values (n = 200) for the computer construction of a cumulative histogram determined within an area of 2.25 cm^2. The preoperative diagnostic test comprised the measurement of histograms in 16 such areas.

Typical examples of two series of spectra obtained in one local area of the myocardium before and after bypass surgery are shown in the Figures 8-9 and 8-10. In both figures, 50 of 200 spectra are plotted.

Before the therapeutic intervention was made, very poor tissue oxygenation combined with low hemoglobin concentration was observed at the 50 different points depicted in Figure 8-9. After the opening of the bypass

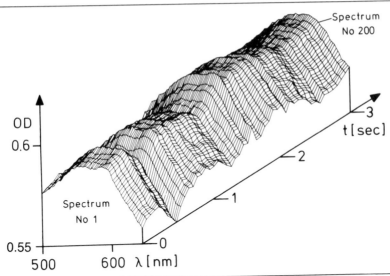

Fig. 8-9. Typical intracapillary hemoglobin remission spectra measured during open heart surgery in one patient suffering from a three-vessel disease, with an occlusion of the LAD, in a 2.25-cm² area of the anterior wall of the left ventricle before bypass surgery.

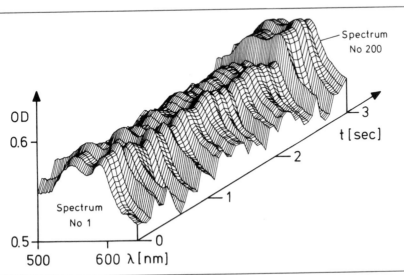

Fig. 8-10. Typical intracapillary hemoglobin remission spectra measured during open heart surgery of the same patient in the same area of the anterior wall of the left ventricle after bypass surgery.

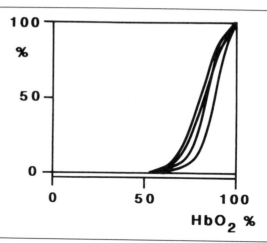

Fig. 8-11. Four normal cumulative histograms of intracapillary HbO$_2$ measured in one area of the myocardium in a 64-year-old patient before bypass surgery.

the spectra recorded at the various local spots of the beating heart revealed an impressive improvement in tissue oxygenation and hemoglobin concentration (Fig. 8-10).

When the measured HbO$_2$ values are grouped into different classes, cumulative HbO$_2$ histograms can be constructed. Figure 8-11 shows four histograms recorded in an area of the human myocardium with normal tissue oxygenation. As can be seen, the lowest values of intracapillary hemoglobin oxygenation from the venous end of the capillaries are found to lie around 50 percent.

In a 70-year-old female patient with severe three-vessel disease and stable angina, a dramatically left-shifted cumulative HbO$_2$ histogram with very low values was observed preoperatively, as shown in Figure 8-12. Under such conditions, critical PO$_2$ values below 5 mm Hg are always found in the poorly perfused myocardium [1]. Such conditions of local oxygen supply of the tissue characterize an absolute borderline situation that is always associated with the existence of pronounced hypokinetic zones. As shown by the histogram No. 2, recorded after the opening of the bypass, surgical intervention led to a normalization of the local oxygenation.

The results of HbO$_2$ measurements performed in a 50-year-old patient with unstable angina are depicted in Figure 8-13. The preoperative histogram shows a distinct bulging and a so-called tail of a small percentage of values lying in the range of 40 to 0 percent saturation. In this patient, too, a complete normalization of tissue oxygenation was observed after coronary bypass surgery.

A relatively moderate pathophysiologic situation is depicted in Figure 8-14, which shows cumulative HbO$_2$ histograms found in one of 16 areas of the anterior wall of a 60-year-old patient suffering from three-vessel dis-

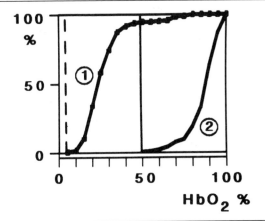

Fig. 8-12. Cumulative histograms of intracapillary HbO_2 measured in a 70-year-old patient suffering from stable angina caused by three-vessel disease with occlusion of the LAD. The HbO_2 curve No. 1, characteristic of a borderline situation, was recorded before operation; No. 2 shows the result after opening of the bypass.

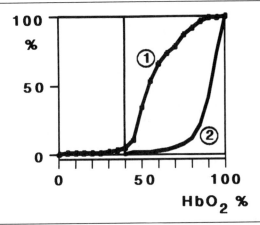

Fig. 8-13. Cumulative histograms of intracapillary HbO_2 measured in a 50-year-old patient suffering from unstable angina caused by three-vessel disease. The protective situation corresponds to a moderate pathophysiologic state of tissue oxygenation.

ease. These histograms are typical for the early stage of a local disturbance caused by coronary sclerosis.

Analysis of these tail-type disturbances resulted in the finding that early warning topograms with low capillary perfusion rates must exist in all tissues. When regional oxygen supply is reduced critically, the oxygen sensors within the supply areas represented by these topograms cause an

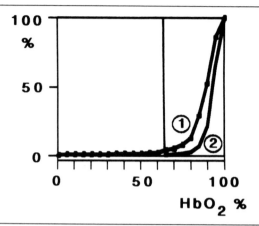

Fig. 8-14. Cumulative histograms of intracapillary HbO_2 measured in a 60-year-old patient suffering from unstable angina caused by three-vessel disease.

alarm that activates the protective mechanisms of the endangered tissue. In the critically perfused myocardium, hypokinetic zones are induced, thus producing a decrease in O_2 uptake rate.

As shown in Figure 8-15, this decrease in energy metabolism causes a shift in the cumulative histogram toward normal values. The fact that the higher oxygenation values increase but the low ones do not in the early warning topograms (tailed region) gives evidence that such situations of early hypokinesia induce not only shifts of the HbO_2 curves, but also alterations in the distribution of the microflow patterns. The positive effect of such regulation, which moves the oxygenation back toward a physiologic state with more heterogeneity between the topogram structures, is that the early warning topogram remains at a low HbO_2 level, close to the regulatory threshold of the cellular oxygen sensors. Thus, the hypokinetic state can be maintained despite a high oxygenation level, with 95 percent of local HbO_2 values exceeding the critical level.

CONCLUSIONS
The application of micro-lightguide spectroscopy has proved to be a most valuable tool for obtaining precise diagnostic information about intracapillary hemoglobin oxygenation.

The cellular oxygen uptake rate can be reduced by the action of a local regulatory and protective system. The measurement of cumulative intracapillary HbO_2 histograms, together with determination of the oxygen uptake rate, enables monitoring of the degree to which these protective mechanisms have been activated. This improves the quality of information in a most decisive way.

This new technique for tissue monitoring opens up two main fields of application:

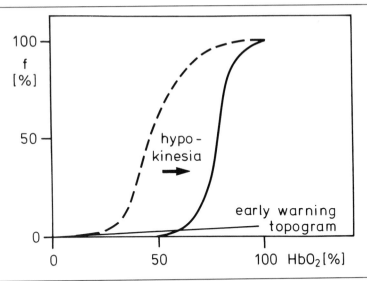

Fig. 8-15. Curve A shows the recorded actual HbO_2 values. The early warning topogram reveals a steep HbO_2 gradient starting at arterial HbO_2 values and ending at borderline hypoxic values. Curve B would exist without down-regulation of local myocardial wall motion.

1. Routine and continuous monitoring of disturbances of the local tissue supply and drainage in all human organs.
2. The possibility of gaining information about early global disturbances of tissue perfusion in the human organism, induced by hypovolemia. The best organs for the monitoring of disturbances due to centralization caused by a decrease of cardiac output are the skin and the skeletal muscle, because they show early signs of decompensation.

These two tissues can characterize protective changes in the following parameters:

1. A decrease in intracapillary hemoglobin oxygenation.
2. Induction of a more homogeneous distribution of intracapillary hemoglobin oxygenation of the various arteriolar supply units caused by utilization of capillary flow reserves. This mechanism is stimulated by cellular oxygen sensors (type-1 signal oxidases).
3. A decrease in local oxygen uptake rate when the regional microflow reserves fall to critical HbO_2 values (Fig. 8-8), also induced by activation of cellular oxygen sensors (type-2 signal oxidases).
4. A decrease in intracapillary hemoglobin concentration.
5. Changes in capillary vasomotion.

The fact that not only relative spectroscopic measurements, but also true quantitative tissue spectroscopy providing absolute readings, have become possible means that a new dimension of patient monitoring at the level of capillaries and living cells has been opened.

REFERENCES

1. Anderer, W. Lokale Sauerstoffversorgung und mechanische Funktion der Vorderwand des linken Ventrikels beim Hund. Diss., Friedrich Alexander Universität, Erlangen-Nürnberg, 1989.
2. Appelbaum, K. Entwicklung eines rechnergestützten Aufnahme-und Auswertesystems für photometrische Meßdaten. Studienarbeit, Friedrich Alexander Universität, Erlangen-Nürnberg, 1987.
3. Beier, I. Die Verteilung des Sauerstoffpartialdruckes an der Oberfläche des musculus gracilis der Ratte. Diss., Friedrich Alexander Universität, Erlangen-Nürnberg, 1987.
4. Chance, B. Rapid and sensitive spectrophotometer. I. The accelerated and stopped-flow method for the measurement of the reaction kinetics and spectra of unstable compounds in the visible region of the spectrum. *Rev. Sci. Instr.* 22:619, 1951.
5. Chance, B., and Lagallain, V. Rapid and sensitive spectrophotometer. II. A stopped flow method for a stabilized quartz spectrophotometer. *Rev. Sci. Instr.* 22:627, 1951.
6. Chance, B. Rapid and sensitive spectrophotometry. III. A double beam apparatus. *Rev. Sci. Instr.* 22:634, 1951.
7. Chance, B., et al. Basic principles of tissue oxygen determination from mitochondrial signals. *Adv. Exp. Med. Biol.* 37:277, 1974.
8. Frank, K. H., et al. The erlangen micro-lightguide spectrophotometer EMPHO I. *Phys. Med. Biol.* In press, 1989.
9. Frank, K. H., et al. Measurements of angular distributions of Rayleigh and Mie scattering events in biological models. *Phys. Med. Biol.* In press, 1989.
10. Frank, K. H., et al. Theoretical aspects of light scattering in living tissues of mammals and men. Submitted to *Phys. Med. Biol.,* 1988.
11. Frank, K. H., et al. Spectroscopic Measurements of Patients Undergoing Open Heart Bypass Surgery—A Pilot Study. In M. Kessler, B. Chance, A. Mayevsky, K. H. Frank, and D. K. Harrison (eds.), *Quantitative Spectroscopy in Tissue.* Berlin, Heidelberg, New York, Tokyo: Springer-Verlag. In preparation.
12. Frank, K. H., et al. Measurements of myocardial oxygenation during bypass surgery. Submitted to *Cardiology,* 1989.
13. Harrison, D. K., et al. The role of high flow capillary channels in the local supply to skeletal muscle. *Adv. Exp. Med. Biol.* 222:623, 1988.
14. Harrison, D. K., et al. Regulation of capillary blood flow: A new concept. *Adv. Exp. Med. Biol.* In press, 1989.
15. Harrison, D. K., et al. Regulation of capillary blood flow and oxygen supply in skeletal muscle in dogs during hypoxemia. Submitted to *J. Physiol.* (Lond.), 1989.
16. Harrison, D. K., et al. Local O_2 supply and blood flow regulation in the contracting muscle in dogs and rabbits. In preparation, 1989.
17. Höper, J., and Kessler, M. Constant pressure perfusion on the isolated rat liver: Local oxygen supply and metabolic function. *Int. Microcirc. J. Clin. Exp.* 7:155, 1988.
18. Ji, S., et al. Some Quantitative Aspects of Micro-Light Photometry of Biological tissues. In B. Ryback (ed.), *Proceedings of NATO Advanced Science Institute.* Paris: 1978.
19. Ji, S., and Chance, B. Micro–light guides: A new method for measuring tissue fluorescence and reflectance. *Am. J. Physiol.* 79:144, 1979.

20. Kessler, M., et al. Tissue oxygen measurement techniques. In C. H. Baker and W. F. Nastuk (eds.), *Microcirculatory Technology*. New York: Academic Press, 1986. Pp. 391–425.
21. Kessler, M., et al. Die Bedeutung der lokalen O_2 Versorgung für das Entstehen hypokinetischer Myokardareale. In J. Grote (ed.), *Funktionsanalyse biologischer Systeme 18*. Stuttgart, New York: Gustav Fischer Verlag, 1988. Pp. 215–223.

9

Oxygen Transport and the Oxyhemoglobin Dissociation Curve

Christopher W. Bryan-Brown

Oxygen transport ($\dot{D}O_2$) is one of the determinants of survival in the critically ill patient. When deficits occur in the delivery system, the normal adaptive mechanism may be sufficient to compensate. It is therefore essential to try to correct, as quickly as possible, any disorder that interferes with the efficiency of tissue oxygenation. A measure of adequacy is the achievement of a $\dot{D}O_2$ that will increase oxygen uptake or utilization ($\dot{V}O_2$) to a level sufficient to meet metabolic needs. In acute illness and high-risk surgery and following major trauma, this will be a supranormal value [3, 14, 15]. One of the hallmarks of acute illness and recovery is that an inefficiency develops in the oxygen delivery system. The ratio of $\dot{V}O_2 : \dot{D}O_2$ (extraction ratio) declines, so that $\dot{D}O_2$ has to be increased by even more than would be predicted from increased metabolism [17].

The normal responses to a greater bodily need for oxygen are an increased ventilation and cardiac output [19] and a redistribution of the circulation from tissues such as skin and resting muscle (supply-independent) to tissues such as brain and myocardium (supply-dependent). These responses will acutely direct the oxygen to where it is most needed [5]. Unfortunately, over a longer term this rerouting may be detrimental to other organ systems (e.g., hepatic, splanchnic, and renal), especially when these areas may already have some compromise at the cellular or even mitochondrial level [4, 8].

Eventually, other mechanisms may also come into play, such as a decreased affinity of oxygen for hemoglobin and increased blood volume and erythropoietin. Anaerobic metabolism is not a viable alternative to aerobic metabolism for some tissues, especially those of the central nervous system. With current management, neurons reduced to anaerobiasis sufficient to produce a marked lactic acidosis appear "destined to die" (Britton Chance) even if some recovery takes place. The cells of striated muscle can survive and even perform work under conditions of almost total oxygen lack. Therefore, oxygen transport and organ failure will differ from system to system with an acute oxygen deficit.

161

NORMAL PHYSIOLOGY

The components of oxygen transport are mechanisms for loading the blood with oxygen and for allocating it to areas where it is needed and at a sufficient tension to diffuse at the necessary rate to keep up with aerobic metabolism in the mitochondria. The physiology of this process consists of adjustments in ventilation, cardiac output, oxygen capacity of the blood, and of distribution of flow and the affinity of hemoglobin for oxygen (see Table 9-1).

Ventilation

Under basal conditions, ventilation and perfusion in the lungs are matched, so that about 2.8 liters/M^2 (body surface area) of alveolar ventilation is adjusted to 3.5 liters/M^2 of cardiac output ($\dot{V}/\dot{Q} = 0.8$). This allows for the most efficient transfer of 140 ml/min/M^2 of oxygen from the atmosphere to the blood. The physiologic mechanism that governs ventilation normally is not oxygen deprivation; rather, it is a positive feedback system that reacts to arterial carbon dioxide tension ($PaCO_2$) and hydrogen ion concentration on the central nervous system chemoreceptors. Thus, the response to both respiratory and nonrespiratory acidosis is an increase in ventilation that is governed by minute changes in $PaCO_2$ or pH [19].

The response to hypoxemia is small until there has been a fall in arterial oxygen tension (PaO_2) to at least 50 torr. The sensors (the carotid and aortic bodies) follow reductions in hemoglobin saturation. This is because of a local cytochrome that has a hemoglobinlike affinity to oxygen [2]. Under normal conditions, hemoglobin is 85 percent saturated at this level, and the delivery to the tissues is only marginally less efficient. The effect of the increased ventilation on pulmonary function is small: a reduction of the amount of lung with a subnormal $\dot{V}/\dot{Q}$ ratio, an increase of wasted (dead space) ventilation, and a slight reciprocal increase in alveolar oxygen tension due to the washout of carbon dioxide. The consequent respiratory alkalosis temporarily improves the loading of oxygen into the erythrocytes because of the increased affinity of hemoglobin. This may have an adverse effect on the unloading of oxygen in the tissues. During strenuous exercise in the trained athlete, the lung can oxygenate five to six times the basal cardiac output, with a 15-fold increase in oxygen uptake.

Cardiac Output

Cardiac output does not respond directly to moderate changes in oxygen tension or content. The "available oxygen" or "arterial oxygen transport" ($\dot{D}O_2$) is the product of cardiac output and arterial oxygen content. Various compensatory mechanisms can adjust oxygen delivery in the tissues, except when the oxygen level is inadequate to maintain normal metabolism.

Hypoxemia

Hypoxemia increases sympathetic tone, but this begins to have a marked effect on cardiac output only when the PaO_2 falls to 50 torr. The effect of an increasing metabolism in any tissue is to lower the oxygen tension. There is a greater diffusion of oxygen from the smaller arterioles, diminishing the oxygen tension in the distal part of the arteriolar system and

Table 9-1. Oxygen transport: responses to demand

Responses	Mechanisms
	Time constant: seconds
Ventilation ↑	PaCO$_2$ or [H$^+$] acting on CNS respiratory centers Severe hypoxia
Cardiac output ↑	Increased venous return due to vasodilation in the tissues with increased metabolism, by hypoxia, elevated [H$^+$] (carbonic or lactic acid), or vasodilator substances (e.g., adenosine) Reflex increase in sympathetic tone on capacitance vessels, raising cardiac filling pressure Sympathetic stimulation of the myocardium
Redistribution of blood flow to tissues with maximum oxygen extraction	Autoregulation; vasodilation in tissues with greater metabolic activity (see below) Increased sympathetic tone, elevating vascular resistance to tissues with low oxygen extraction
Affinity of hemoglobin for oxygen ↓, P$_{50}$ ↑	[H$^+$] ↑ in severe hypoxia (Bohr effect)
	Time constant: hours
Affinity of hemoglobin for oxygen ↓, P$_{50}$ ↑	Increase in red cell [2,3-DPG] Unsaturated hemoglobin binds more 2,3-DPG, increasing synthesis Unsaturated hemoglobin buffers more [H$^+$]; PFK activity ↑, glycolysis ↑ [H$^+$] ↓, respiratory alkalosis induced by hypoxic drive to respiration
Adjustment of hemodynamics to cope with changed red cell mass, or hypovolemia	Plasma volume expansion from ECF, reducing blood viscosity and returning flow characteristics toward normal Adjustment of vascular resistance to control increased cardiac output due to blood volume and viscosity change Water and sodium retention adjusted by antidiuretic hormone and aldosterone secretion
	Time constant: weeks
Increased red cell mass	Bone marrow stimulated by increased erythropoietin production by hypoxic kidney

[H$^+$] = hydrogen ion concentration; ↓ = decreased; ↑ = increased; CNS = central nervous system; ECF = extracellular fluid; PFK = phosphofructokinase; 2,3-DPG = 2,3-diphosphoglycerate.

thereby causing vasodilatation. This increases the amount of blood flowing through the tissue and so increases the oxygen delivery and the venous return. Thus, by a system of autoregulation, the cardiac output keeps pace with metabolic activity. Potassium, hydrogen ion (derived from lactic or carbonic acid), and adenosine also have a concomitant vasodilator activity [4].

Redistribution of Blood Flow
Redistribution of blood flow for required oxygen delivery enables the body to compensate for an increase of 50 percent in oxygen utilization by a decrease in arteriolar tone in regions where metabolism is increased. If oxygen delivery is diminished, sympathetic activity increases. The initial effect is an increase in the tone of capacitance vessels and increased cardiac filling and output with some tachycardia. Subsequently, the arteriolar tone increases [13]. However, diminished oxygen supply has less effect on autoregulatory tissues: blood is redistributed to the heart and brain, while tissues with a low oxygen requirement, such as skin and resting muscle, get a reduced supply. The splanchnic and renal circulations are markedly reduced, particularly with severe limitations of oxygen supply.

The myocardium has the greatest oxygen extraction of the body's tissues. Normally, it has an arteriovenous oxygen content difference $[C(a - v)O_2]$ of 11 ml of oxygen/100 ml of blood. The coronary sinus blood usually has an oxygen tension of 20 to 25 torr. The heart is working very near hypoxia at all times, and coronary blood flow is increased with the slightest increase in myocardial metabolism. It is controlled by oxygen requirement. The heart receives about 5 percent of cardiac output and 10 percent of oxygen uptake. The brain has a $C(a - v)O_2$ of about 8 ml/100 ml of blood and a venous oxygen tension of 32 to 35 torr. The cerebral circulation is not very sensitive to reduced oxygen tension unless it is below 50 torr. Regulation is mainly by carbon dioxide and adenine [12]. Under basal conditions, the brain gets about 20 percent of the oxygen uptake and 15 percent of the cardiac output.

During hypoxic states, flow is diverted from tissues that have a low oxygen consumption to those that use more. When severe deficits in oxygen delivery occur, they may seriously compromise tissues that normally have a moderate oxygen extraction. In the splanchnic area, the pancreas frequently has a proportionately greater reduction in blood flow, which may cause lysosomes to break down and release myocardial depressant factor. The kidneys may undergo the syndrome of acute vasomotor nephropathy (i.e., acute tubular necrosis).

Hematocrit
Hematocrit is related to blood viscosity; normally, blood has about twice the viscosity of pure water. In anemia, the oxygen-carrying capacity of the blood diminishes and the viscosity falls, decreasing the resistive forces to cardiac output and allowing an easier venous return. Cardiac output increases, partially compensating for the decreased arterial blood oxygen content. In the experimental setting, if half the normal red cells are re-

placed with cells filled with methemoglobin (which alter the viscosity but not the oxygen-carrying capacity), the cardiac output increases a trivial amount. If half the red cell mass is replaced by a plasma expander (dextran) the cardiac output may nearly double [16]. On the other hand, normovolemic polycythemia greatly increases the resistance to venous return and can reduce cardiac output and arterial oxygen transport [9].

The ideal hematocrit is far from constant in all conditions. Maximum oxygen delivery to the brain occurs with hematocrits in the range of 45 to 47 percent. Because of reduced viscosity, the health of an ischemic limb may be best served by a hematocrit of 30 percent. Patients in acute respiratory failure have been shown to have a better outcome if the hematocrit is in excess of 40 percent, but other studies have shown that patients with trauma, major surgery, and sepsis may have a lower mortality rate when the hematocrit is in the range of 33 percent. From the point of view of myocardial work, the most efficient oxygen delivery for oxygen uptake occurs when the hematocrit is in the range of 40 to 44 percent. In conditions of nonpulsatile blood flow and reduced temperature, such as occurs in extracorporeal bypass, a lower-than-normal hematocrit improves oxygen delivery. At present, the best that can be offered the critically ill patient with multisystem failure is monitoring of oxygen delivery in relation to hematocrit by testing the system with blood transfusion if the hematocrit is low [4].

Blood Volume
Blood volume deficits impair oxygen delivery by decreasing mean circulatory pressure, reducing flow in supply-independent tissues, and increasing the resistance to venous return, thus reducing the cardiac output. $\dot{V}O_2$ and $\dot{D}O_2$ and utilization can be increased by increasing the blood volume.

In healthy individuals, the hemodynamic changes are adjusted toward normal by changes in peripheral vascular resistance, which keep a balance between the effects of changes in blood volume and viscosity. The blood volume enlarges after normovolemic polycythemia is induced; the plasma volume expands and the viscosity is reduced, returning the flow characteristics and cardiac output toward normal.

Neurohumoral Sympathetic Control
Neurohumoral sympathetic control of cardiac output increases the force of contraction and cardiac rate. The nervous control of redistribution of blood flow has the least effect on the organs with high oxygen consumption. Skin normally gets about 2 percent of the oxygen uptake and a little less than 10 percent of the cardiac output. When the body needs to lose more heat, blood flow is increased through the skin, due to a reflex loss of vasomotor tone. In cardiac failure, strong sympathetic activity can decrease skin blood flow to one-tenth of normal; in cardiogenic shock, with severely reduced myocardial function, gangrene of the extremities can even develop. The difference between the skin and core temperature has been used to assess the adequacy of cardiac output [10].

Hemoglobin Concentration

Hemoglobin concentration is increased when there is a decrease in arterial blood oxygen content, a reduction of hemoglobin concentration, or an increased affinity of hemoglobin for oxygen. This is sensed in the kidney, which produces erythropoietin when the renal oxygen supply is decreased relative to metabolic demand. Provided there are adequate iron stores, the rate of production of erythrocytes may be doubled. This is too slow an increase to have much relevance for the treatment of the critically ill. In hypoxic states, when the P_{50} rises (P_{50} = PO_2 at which hemoglobin is half-saturated with oxygen), the production of erythropoietin may decline.

Hemoglobin Affinity for Oxygen

Hemoglobin affinity for oxygen is altered by various factors, summarized in Table 9-2. The actions of most of these factors combine to maintain a normal oxyhemoglobin dissociation, provided oxygen transport is adequate. Thus, in acute acidosis, hemoglobin unloads more oxygen at a given oxygen tension (PO_2). The higher red-cell hydrogen ion concentration decreases phosphofructokinase (PFK) activity, and glycolysis is reduced. Synthesis and concentration of 2,3-diphosphoglycerate (2,3-DPG) fall, and the hemoglobin affinity for oxygen increases toward normal. When there is hypoxia from arterial hypoxemia, anemia, or low cardiac output, the affinity of hemoglobin for oxygen becomes less, thereby facilitating a greater unloading of oxygen at a given PO_2 [1]. Although much research has gone into manipulating oxyhemoglobin dissociation, there has been virtually no telling evidence of the clinical efficacy of this maneuver in the critically ill [11].

OXYHEMOGLOBIN DISSOCIATION

The relation of PO_2 to hemoglobin oxygen saturation (SO_2) is described by the oxyhemoglobin dissociation curve (see Figs. 9-1 and 9-3–9-6). The characteristics of this curve ensure that at the wide range of oxygen tensions found in the pulmonary capillary circulation, the hemoglobin will be easily saturated with oxygen. At the oxygen tensions found in metabolically active tissue capillaries (e.g., heart, 23 torr; brain, 32 torr), a slight fall in oxygen tension will release a large amount of oxygen. This property of normal hemoglobin determines the ability of the oxygen transport system to deliver adequate oxygen from the blood to the tissues.

Dissociation Curve Analysis

Dissociation curve analysis is done either by describing the whole curve or by deriving the PO_2 at which the hemoglobin is half-saturated with oxygen (P_{50}). An analysis can refer to the relationship under the conditions of the pH, temperature (T), and base excess (BE) of the patient (i.e., in vivo P_{50}, or P_{50iv}) or under conditions in which pH is 7.4, T is 37°C, and BE is zero (i.e., "standard" P_{50}, or $P_{50(7.4)}$).

The factors used to convert between in vivo P_{50} and standard P_{50} are interdependent variables. An increase in temperature will decrease the effect of hydrogen ion and 2,3-DPG on the hemoglobin molecule and increase the effect of carbon dioxide. Increased 2,3-DPG concentration will increase the effect of hydrogen ion but decrease the effect of carbon dioxide, with which it competes directly as a ligand [18]. Fortunately for purposes of calculation, the factors are nearest constant in the midsaturation range (30–70%). The Severinghaus factors are frequently used to make approximate in vitro conversions:

$$\log PO_2 = \begin{array}{l} -0.48\ \Delta pH \\ 0.024\ \Delta T \\ 0.0013\ BE \end{array}$$

Thus, for a given saturation (e.g., 50%), if the blood-sample-measured pH was 7.10 and the PO_2 was 37.1 torr, the PO_2 at a pH of 7.40 would be 26.6 for the same saturation (see Fig. 9-4). If the temperature of a patient was 39.0°C and the sample was found to have a PO_2 of 26.6 torr at 37.0°C, the PO_2 that would give the same saturation at the patient's temperature would be 29.2 torr. Further, if the same blood sample had a base excess of +10 mEq/liter, and the base excess was corrected to zero, the PO_2 and 37°C would be changed only to 26.8 torr. This last, minor correction makes up for changes in oxyhemoglobin dissociation due to carbon dioxide. The P_{50iv} gives information about the adequacy of oxygen transport in the patient, whereas the standard P_{50} tells of changes irrespective of acid-base alterations. Ideally, the red cell pH should be intracellular. Normally, this is 0.2 pH units less than whole blood pH, but it may be highly variable in disease states [5].

Hill Equation
Various forms of the Hill equation can be used to linearize the oxyhemoglobin dissociation curve for easier analysis. Although more-complicated formulas can give an accurate fit to the whole curve, the Hill equation is acceptable for clinical purposes. The approximation is reasonably accurate between saturation values of 20 to 80 percent (see Fig. 9-1).

$$\log\frac{y}{100 - y} = A(\log x) + B$$

where

$$y = SO_2 \text{ and } x = PO_2$$

$$P_{50} = \text{antilog } \frac{-B}{A}$$

A, the slope of the curve, is often given a value of 2.7. If this value is used to calculate P_{50} from a single PO_2, the error is usually less than 1 torr if the SO_2 is between 30 and 70 percent. This is probably as much accuracy as can be achieved in most clinical laboratories by trying to establish the slope from several samples with different oxygen tensions using polarographic oximetry.

Table 9-2. Factors affecting hemoglobin affinity for oxygen (P_{50})

P_{50} ↑	P_{50} ↓	Time constant	Comment
$[H^+]$ ↑	$[H^+]$ ↓	Stat	Bohr effect.
$[K_i^+] + [Na_i^+]$ ↑ $+ [Cl_i^-]$ ↑	$[K_i^+] + [Na_i^+]$ ↓ $+ [Cl_i^-]$ ↓	Stat	Salt effect; related to intraerythrocyte ion concentration.
T ↑	T ↓	Stat	Carbaminohemoglobin has less O_2 affinity.
PCO_2 ↑	$\begin{cases} PCO_2 ↓ \\ \text{Carbon monoxide} \end{cases}$	Stat / Stat	Carbaminohemoglobin has less O_2 affinity. Carboxyhemoglobin has very high O_2 affinity.
$[H^+]$ ↓	$[H^+]$ ↑	Hr	PFK activity inhibited by acidosis; glycolysis and 2,3-DPG synthesis. MCHC related to $[H^+]$.
Hypoxia or anemia	Hyperoxia	Hr, days	[2,3-DPG] ↑ when PO_2 ↓. More 2,3-DPG bound to deoxyhemoglobin; activation of PGM; 2,3-DPG synthesis. Reaction reduced if compensatory respiratory alkalosis absent. Deoxyhemoglobin buffers H^+; PFK activated.

MCHC ↑	MCHC ↓	Stat	?Intraerythrocyte hemoglobin buffers $[H^+]$.
Plasma inorganic phosphate ↑	Plasma inorganic phosphate ↓	Hr, days	Substrate for ATP and 2,3-DPG. [ATP], [2,3-DPG], and $[K_i^+]$ ↓.
	Storage at 4°C	Days	[2,3-DPG] 20% in 10 days ACD storage. CPD storage slows ATP and 2,3-DPG loss.
Nucleic acids		Min	Substrate for ATP and 2,3-DPG. Inosine used in vivo. Inosine + adenine used in vitro.
Methylprednisolone sodium succinate (high dose)		Min	Mechanisms not established: Subnormal $[K_i^+]$ ↑ in minutes. $[H_i^+]/[H_p^+]$ increased over 30 min. No constant change of [2,3-DPG] observed. Effect lasting.

$[H^+]$ = hydrogen ion concentration; $[H_p^+]$ = hydrogen ion concentration in plasma; $[Cl_i^-]$, $[K_i^+]$, and $[Na_i^+]$ = intraerythrocyte ion concentrations (hydrogen, chloride, potassium, and sodium); 2,3-DPG = 2,3-diphosphoglycerate; PFK = phosphofructokinase; MCHC = mean corpuscular hemoglobin concentration; ATP = adenosine triphosphate; ACD = acid citrate dextrose; CPD = citrate-phosphate-dextrose.

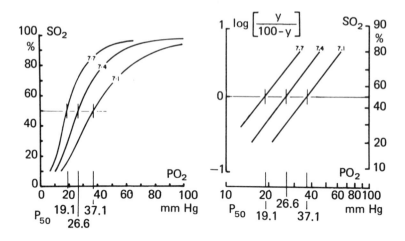

Fig. 9-1. Hill plot. This is a linear approximation, which has fair accuracy for SO₂ values of between 20 and 80 percent. It is frequently used in estimating position of oxyhemoglobin dissociation curve. Comparison with P_{50} values is given, demonstrating standard curves for three pH values and their linearized versions.

The position of the oxyhemoglobin dissociation curve can be analyzed with the Hill equation:

1. Single-point analysis from PO_2 and SO_2.
2. Multiple-point analysis (requires special calibration of PO_2 electrode for accuracy).
3. Tonometry with calibrating gases to get accurate PO_2 values. Tonometry gases: oxygen, 2.5 to 5.5 percent (PO_2, → 18–39 torr); carbon dioxide, 5.6 percent (PCO_2, 40 torr); → nitrogen, balance.

Saturation and pH are measured on 2 to 4 samples of blood tonometered with oxygen mixtures with PO_2 values that straddle the P_{50}, and corrections are made on each PO_2 to standardize the pH and base excess. Values for A and B can be calculated by least-squares fit in a linear regression analysis of the data in the Hill equation. From this can be calculated the standard P_{50} and curve positions for any values of pH, base excess, and temperature for calculation of the P_{50iv}.

Dissociation Curve Analyzers

Dissociation curve analyzers are made for plotting the whole curve. The sample of blood is deoxygenated with nitrogen containing 5% carbon dioxide. This process is sometimes not complete within 30 minutes, which can lead to baseline error. The PO_2 is then recorded while the blood is being saturated with oxygen with 5% carbon dioxide.

Radiometer DCA records on an X-Y-Y' plotter the PO_2 in a sealed chamber above deoxygenated blood and the PO_2 in the sample as it is saturated with oxygen. The fall in pressure in the gas is proportional to the amount of gas moving into the blood sample. The points for SO_2 values of 0 and 100 percent are the X positions at the beginning of the measurement and where the pressure no longer falls in the gas phase. Y is plotted as the PO_2 of the blood and Y' as pH, so that points can be corrected or standardized.

A curve analysis takes 45 minutes to 1 hour to perform. When the hemoglobin is saturated, it becomes more acid. As the system is closed, the PCO_2 will rise, but usually less than 1 torr—not enough to lead to appreciable error.

Blood can be saturated with increasing oxygen tensions and either continuous or multiple measurements of SO_2, PO_2, and pH plotted.

Samples of blood can be deoxygenated with nitrogen containing 5% carbon dioxide and saturated with 21% oxygen containing 5% carbon dioxide. The deoxygenated and saturated samples are then mixed in precisely measured proportions and the PO_2 is measured. The oxygen content of the mixture is known, since it was all provided by the saturated sample, so the SO_2 can be calculated and a point on the curve established [20].

Bellingham Formula

The Bellingham formula [18] calculates the P_{50iv} from most of the factors that are known to be of clinical importance.

$$\log P_{50iv} = \log [26.6 + 0.5 \,(MCHC - 33) + 0.69 \,(2,3\text{-}DPG - 14.5)] + 0.0013 \, BE + 0.48 \,(pH - 7.4) + 0.024 \,(T - 37)$$

where 2,3-DPG is measured in μmole/gm Hb, MCHC = mean corpuscular hemoglobin concentration, and Hb = hemoglobin.

In Vivo Temperature Correction Factors

In vivo temperature correction factors should be used to convert the patient's acid-base data measured at 37°C to in vivo values.

The temperature corrections for pH can be approximated by

$$pH = -0.0146 \,\Delta T$$

A closer value is obtained if the decrease in temperature coefficient as the pH falls is taken into account:

$$pH = [0.0065 \,(7.4 - pH_{37}) - 0.0146] \,\Delta T, \text{ when the pH is measured at 37°C.}$$

The change in PCO_2 for a change in temperature is approximated by

$$\Delta \log PCO_2 = 0.019 \,(T - 37), \text{ when } PCO_2 \text{ is measured at 37°C}$$

Correction factors of oxygen data generally become less accurate when the saturation is high. The normal factor for temperature change is as follows:

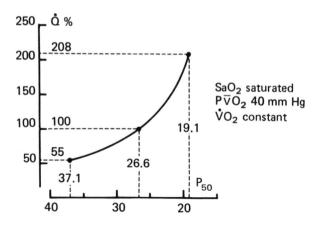

Fig. 9-2. Change of cardiac output plotted against P_{50}. As P_{50} decreases, a greater cardiac output is needed to maintain $P\bar{v}O_2$ at 40 torr.

$$\Delta\log PO_2 = 0.031\ \Delta T$$

When the saturation is greater than 80 percent, the temperature coefficient of oxygen solubility in blood begins to influence the result. If the PO_2 is above 250 torr, $PO_2/\Delta T$ is directly related to it. For saturations above 80 percent, changes can be approximated by the following:

$$\Delta\log PO_2 = \frac{3130\ -\ 62.5\ \text{Sat}\ +\ 0.312008\ \text{Sat}^2}{100,000\ -\ 1993\ \text{Sat}\ +\ 9.931\ \text{Sat}^2} \times \Delta T$$

Oxygen Delivery

The need for oxygen delivery is altered by changes in hemoglobin affinity for oxygen. Figure 9-2 shows the changes in cardiac output needed to maintain a mixed venous PO_2 of 40 torr. The arterial blood is saturated and the oxygen utilization is constant. The changes in P_{50} could be produced by acute pH changes of 7.1 ($P_{50} = 37.1$ torr) and 7.7 ($P_{50} = 19.1$ torr) from the normal values of 7.4 ($P_{50} = 26.6$ torr). A P_{50} value of 19.1 torr could also occur if the 2,3-DPG concentration was 3.7 μmole/gm Hb. This sort of value can be found in patients after massive transfusions of stored acid citrate dextrose blood.

Under normal circumstances the arteriovenous oxygen saturation difference is about 25 percent. Figure 9-3 shows the advantages of a high P_{50} in hypoxic states. The $P_{50} = 37.1$ torr curve shows an ability to drop 25 percent of SO_2 at a higher PO_2 when loaded at PO_2 of 60 torr than does a normal curve when loaded at 80 torr. This advantage would be lost at a loading PO_2 of 50 torr.

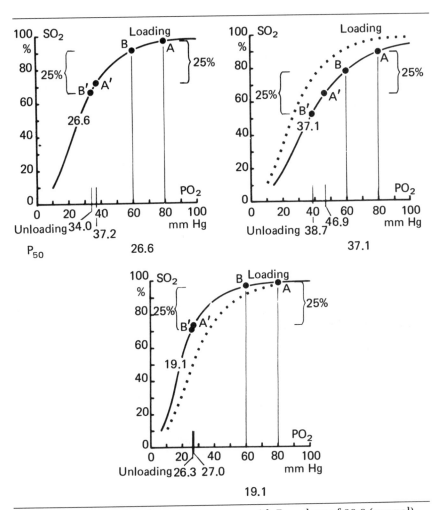

Fig. 9-3. Oxyhemoglobin dissociation curves with P_{50} values of 26.6 (normal), 37.1, and 19.1 torr (normal curve indicated on latter two graphs by dotted line). Effect of a 25 percent decrease in saturation is compared at loading tensions of 80 and 60 torr (A and B) and unloading tensions at A' and B'. Note that curve of a P_{50} of 37.1 is able to unload at a higher tension, even when loaded at 60 torr, than the others loaded at 80 torr. Also note that an increase in PO_2 from 60 to 80 torr makes no significant change in unloading tension in curve of a P_{50} of 19.1 torr.

The three graphs of Figure 9-3 show that there is a marked difference in PO_2 unloading, with the higher PO_2 value (80 torr) of loading only when the P_{50} is high. When the P_{50} is low, an increase of cardiac output is the only way to make a significant increase in oxygen delivery, since raising the loading tension in the lungs has a relatively small effect.

In experimental conditions, the coronary blood flow has been related to increasing hemoglobin affinity for oxygen. Since the coronary circulation initially dilates to the stimulus of hypoxia, it is not surprising to find the flow increasing when the hemoglobin requires lower-than-normal PO_2 levels to release oxygen [7]. Various other, less well-substantiated clinical data would suggest that the response to increased oxygen demand can be a reduction of saturation as well as an increased cardiac output in persons with a high P_{50}. Those with a low P_{50} can respond only with increased cardiac output and have limited exercise tolerance. In various experimental hemodynamic and septic shock models, a high P_{50} is associated with greater survival.

When oxygen delivery becomes less efficient, P_{50iv} is found to increase. It has been difficult to show the clinical relevance of changes of the affinity of hemoglobin for oxygen in terms of morbidity or mortality.

Factors Affecting the Oxyhemoglobin Relationship
The factors affecting the oxyhemoglobin relationship are summarized in Table 9-2.

Hydrogen Ion Concentration
Hydrogen ion concentration has a direct effect on the hemoglobin molecule. Oxygen affinity decreases as the hydrogen ion concentration increases (Bohr effect). Figure 9-4 shows three oxyhemoglobin dissociation curves plotted for both saturation and content. An acute pH change from 7.4 (normal) to 7.1 will increase the amount of oxygen released at a PO_2 of 20 torr from two-thirds to over four-fifths, thereby increasing the consumable oxygen. If there is an acute alkalemia to a pH of 7.7, less than half the oxygen will be released at this point.

Sodium and Potassium
Sodium, potassium, and chloride ions increase the bonds bridging the chains of the hemoglobin molecule, reducing oxygen affinity (salt effect). Restoration of normal red cell cation concentration causes a rise in P_{50}.

Temperature
Temperature increase lowers hemoglobin oxygen affinity.

Carbon Dioxide
By forming carbaminohemoglobin, carbon dioxide increases the P_{50}. This is shown whenever blood is acidified by carbon dioxide rather than by direct acidification; the curve shift is about 25 percent greater than that for pH change alone.

Carbon Monoxide
Carbon monoxide has an affinity for hemoglobin 280 times that of oxygen. The occupation of the hemoglobin molecule by carbon monoxide (carboxyhemoglobin) causes both a severe loss of oxygen-carrying capacity and a marked increase in the hemoglobin's affinity for oxygen. Fifty percent carboxyhemoglobin has a P_{50} of 13.3 torr (see Fig. 9-5). This would require over six times the cardiac output required in an anemia with half

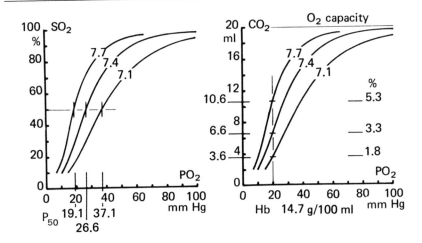

Fig. 9-4. Oxyhemoglobin dissociation curves plotted for different pH values. Note that at PO_2 of 20 torr, curve 7.7 has over half the oxygen content still bound to hemoglobin (normal 33%). The 7.1 curve has less than one-fifth of oxygen capacity utilized, showing how an increased right shift of curve causes more oxygen to be released at given PO_2.

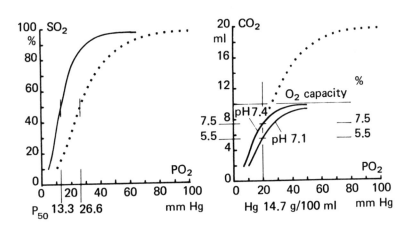

Fig. 9-5. Oxyhemoglobin dissociation curves (normal, *dotted lines*; 50% carboxyhemoglobin, *solid lines*). Note far left shift of curve ($P_{50} = 13.3$) and decreased oxygen capacity. Also notice that acute acidosis of pH 7.1 will increase oxygen available at 20 torr (consumable oxygen) by 2 ml/100 ml blood, or 80 percent. This indicates danger of overzealous treatment of acidosis in carbon monoxide poisoning.

the normal hemoglobin concentration! The consumable oxygen in the content graph is 2.5 ml at pH 7.4; in a normal man at the absolute limits of hypoxia compatible with survival, this would require at least a 10-liter cardiac output to deliver a minimum of oxygen.

Patients with severe carbon monoxide poisoning are usually hypoxic enough to become acidotic. At a pH of 7.1, the theoretical minimum cardiac output could be reduced by about 45 percent. The correction of acidosis in this type of patient might prove fatal. Alterations of PCO_2 do not affect oxygen affinity with carboxyhemoglobin.

Indirect Effect of Hydrogen Ion Concentration

Hydrogen ion concentration also has an indirect effect, which may be related to most of the processes that result in an increased 2,3-DPG concentration. PFK activity is reduced by increasing amounts of hydrogen ion. This inhibition of glycolysis decreases 2,3-DPG synthesis. It has also been found that the MCHC is reduced in acidosis, which also reduces the P_{50}. Thus, after a few hours of acidosis, the oxyhemoglobin dissociation curve can return almost to normal. In alkalosis, there is a reciprocal relation with hydrogen ion concentration and 2,3-DPG production, leading to a normalization of the P_{50}. In the critically ill patient, 2,3-DPG formation may be slowed down, leaving oxygen transport deranged for days.

Hypoxia and Anemia

Hypoxia and anemia both produce a similar response, causing a right shift of the curve. The reason for this is an increase in 2,3-DPG concentration. Figure 9-6 shows a typical change that might be seen in severe anemia with half the normal hemoglobin concentration. The dissociation curve has become shifted to the left in chronic anemia, with an increase in P_{50} to 31.9 torr, brought about by a 54 percent increase in 2,3-DPG concentration. If the oxygen content (CO_2) versus tension (PO_2) graph is considered, the amount of oxygen available at a PO_2 of 20 torr (consumable oxygen) [5] is 1.2 ml/100 ml, or 12 percent more than the oxygen capacity of chronic anemia. If the arterial blood is fully saturated, this would allow for a 10 percent decrease in cardiac output for oxygen delivery at a PO_2 of 40 torr. The graphs in Figure 9-6 are not corrected for arteriovenous acid-base and carbon dioxide changes.

In anemia, there is less hemoglobin to buffer respiratory acid, so the Bohr effect is increased, releasing even more oxygen to the tissues. The increase in 2,3-DPG may be due to the greater affinity of deoxyhemoglobin for 2,3-DPG. Phosphoglyceromutase (PGM) activity is inhibited by 2,3-DPG. As there is less free 2,3-DPG, PGM can convert more 1,3-DPG to 2,3-DPG (Rapaport-Luebering shunt), so that the more time the red cell spends in a low oxygen tension environment, the more the red cell concentration is increased. The problem with this theory is that the 2,3-DPG concentration does not rise as much if the hypoxia-induced respiratory alkalosis is corrected or the patient is given acetozolamide to slow down the rate of breakdown of carbonic acid. The increase in 2,3-DPG may therefore be due to increased glycolysis, since PFK is activated by the lower hydrogen

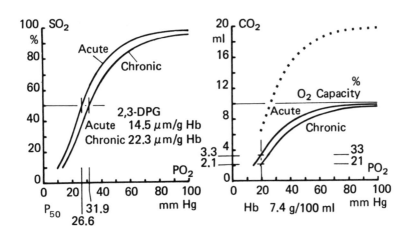

Fig. 9-6. Oxyhemoglobin dissociation curves plotted for anemia. Increase in 2,3-DPG occurring in chronic anemia has shifted curve to right. In capacity graph (CO_2), hemoglobin affinity for oxygen is decreased 18 percent at 20 torr, indicating additional release of "consumable" oxygen of 1.2 ml/100 ml of blood.

ion concentration. Also, deoxyhemoglobin is a weaker acid than oxyhemoglobin and may buffer more red cell hydrogen ion. Adult patients with chronic respiratory or cardiac failure and children with cyanotic heart disease have high red cell 2,3-DPG concentrations.

Mean Corpuscular Hemoglobin Concentration

Mean corpuscular hemoglobin concentration is associated with a decreased hemoglobin affinity for oxygen. This could be due to the increased concentration of intracellular buffer, reducing hydrogen ion concentration, and this would increase 2,3-DPG synthesis. Mean corpuscular hemoglobin concentration and 2,3-DPG concentration rise and fall together in chronic alkalosis and acidosis.

Plasma Inorganic Phosphate Concentration

Plasma inorganic phosphate concentration influences the synthesis of red cell 2,3-DPG and adenosine triphosphate (ATP). This is probably because it is a substrate in the elaboration of these compounds.

Effect of Blood Storage

Storage of blood in conventional blood banks has long been associated with an increase in hemoglobin affinity for oxygen. This is found in patients who have large transfusions of stored blood (Valtis and Kennedy effect). The normal storage of acid citrate dextrose blood at 4°C reduces the 2,3-DPG level to 20 percent of normal in 10 to 14 days. This by itself would reduce the P_{50} to 18.6 torr, which would require a more than doubled cardiac output to maintain normal oxygen delivery. The levels of ATP and potassium are also reduced. The use of citrate phosphate dextrose has enabled blood to maintain a more normal oxygen affinity longer. Inosine and adenine are also added to blood for storage for this purpose ("Adsol").

If the respiratory function of stored blood is to be maintained, the red cells have to be deep frozen in glycerol solutions.

Nucleic Acids

Inosine and adenine can be used to restore and even give supranormal levels of 2,3-DPG in red cells. If the outdated cells are incubated in a medium containing pyruvate, inosine, glucose, and phosphate (PIGP) and then resuspended in a suitable medium for transfusion, this can be achieved (these techniques are still under investigation). If adenine is added to the PIGP, further improvement in respiratory function is marginal, but the ATP concentration is further increased. Work now suggests that if glucose is not included in the incubating solution, a greater decrease in oxyhemoglobin dissociation occurs [18]. On a preliminary basis, inosine infusions have been used in man.

Methylprednisolone

Methylprednisolone sodium succinate has been demonstrated to decrease the affinity of hemoglobin for oxygen, especially when it is abnormally high. In high dosage (15–30 mg/kg of body weight), it markedly increases the P_{50} over a half-hour to an hour, and the change persists. In patients who have a low red cell potassium concentration, the P_{50} is restored in a few minutes. The red cell pH decreases relative to that of the whole blood for half an hour [5, 6]. High doses of steroids have now been shown not to increase survival in shock patients.

Arterial Oxygen Tension

PaO_2 cannot give an adequate picture of hypoxia. It can be normal when the delivery to the tissues is defective because of an inadequate cardiac output, anemia, or the increased affinity of hemoglobin for oxygen. In addition, particularly in hypovolemia, many tissues are poorly perfused due to redistribution.

Mixed Venous Oxygen Tension

Mixed venous oxygen tension is a more appropriate measure of oxygen delivery than is PaO_2, since it reflects the overall oxygen tension of the blood leaving the tissues. Blood flow through tissues usually varies in relation to metabolism. In pathologic states, the greatest contribution to the mixed venous blood is from the best perfused tissues, and the deficits of other regions with inadequate oxygen may be masked. Since their contribution to the overall amount is small, only a markedly low mixed venous oxygen tension is significant. However, a minor reduction may be masking considerable regional hypoxia. Mixed venous oxygen saturation can now be accurately monitored continuously through fiberoptic pulmonary artery catheters (see Chapter 6).

Lactate

Lactate measurements may also indicate the adequacy of oxygen transport. A rise in the lactate level may be due to increased anaerobic metabolism. As a measurement of oxygen transport, however, lactate concentration suffers from the same drawback as mixed venous oxygen tension, in that poorly perfused tissues will not add much to the circulation, and regional hypoxia will not necessarily be detected. The drawback of the lactate-pyruvate ratio is that the levels of both substances rise in the circulation when glycolysis increases. Thus, with β-adrenergic stimulation, lactate and pyruvate appear in greater quantity in the blood; and in β-blockade, lactate levels decrease. Even so, serial lactate levels are a good way to observe a patient's progress. The normal is less than 2 mM/liter. Levels of 10 mM/liter are associated with very high mortality.

Other Signs of Hypoxia

2,3-DPG and P_{50iv} increase when the oxygen delivery is poor and may represent an index of prolonged deficit in oxygen delivery. The change is best seen in nondepleted shock patients or in patients with primary cardiopulmonary disease. It may take several days for the P_{50iv} to be spontaneously restored in sick, septic, and acidotic patients.

Clinical evaluation of cerebral function, especially by staff continually at a patient's bedside, may pick up the early changes of cerebral hypoxia (e.g., disorientation, forgetfulness, torpor, confusion, and restlessness). The kidneys may not be able to concentrate urine, and ventricular cardiac arrhythmias may occur.

CLINICAL IMPLICATIONS

The clinical management of the patient with pulmonary and cardiovascular insufficiency and in shock states is dealt with in other chapters. The alteration of the affinity of hemoglobin for oxygen has not been conclusively shown to benefit the outcome of a patient who is critically ill. On the other hand, the efficiency of the circulation in delivering oxygen at a given oxygen tension is decreased when the affinity increases. It is readily inferred that correction of this portion of the oxygen delivery system might add a margin for survival to the patient who would otherwise die because other compensatory mechanisms were inadequate. The clinical implications are therefore largely putative.

Some helpful therapeutic maneuvers should be mentioned. Massive blood transfusions will improve oxygen delivery if the blood contains either fresh or rejuvenated red cells. Patients with low-flow states who require blood replacement and patients on extracorporeal perfusion might best be treated with fresh blood or rejuvenated red cells. Acidosis, unless very acute, should be corrected slowly, to allow the P_{50iv} to be maintained. The addition of phosphate to the correction of diabetic ketoacidosis greatly speeds the restoration of red cell 2,3-DPG. Chronic respiratory acidosis should be reduced slowly, once the pH is above 7.3. Plasma phosphate levels should be maintained in all patients on total parenteral nutrition, as 2,3-DPG synthesis is dependent on an adequate phosphate concentration. The major resuscitative maneuvers when oxygen uptake is less than is needed for optimal survival value seem to be the correction of hypoxic hypoxia and increasing cardiac output to supranormal levels [15].

REFERENCES

1. Bellingham, A. J., Detter, J. C., and Lenfant, C. Regulatory mechanisms of hemoglobin oxygen affinity in acidosis and alkalosis. *J. Clin. Invest.* 50:700, 1971.
2. Berger, A. J., Mitchell, R. R., and Severinghaus, J. W. Regulation of respiration. *N. Engl. J. Med.* 297:92, 138, 194, 1977.
3. Bland, R. D., Shoemaker, W. E., Abraham, E., Cobo, J. C. Hemodynamic and oxen transport patterns in surviving and nonsurviving patients. *Crit. Care Med.* 13:85, 1985.
4. Bryan-Brown, C. W. Blood flow to organs. Parameters for function and survival in critical illness. *Crit. Care Med.* 16:170, 1988.
5. Bryan-Brown, C. W., Baek, S. M., Makabali, G., Shoemaker, W. C. Consumable oxygen: Availability of oxygen in relation to oxyhemoglobin dissociation. *Crit. Care Med.* 1:17, 1973.
6. Bryan-Brown C. W., Makabali, G., Baek, S. M., Shoemaker, W. C. Hemodynamic Responses and Oxygen Delivery After Methylprednisolone Sodium Succinate. In T. M. Glen (ed.), *Steroids and Shock.* Baltimore: University Park Press, 1974. Pp. 361–375.
7. Duvelleroy, M. A., Mehmel, H. C., and Laver, M. B. The hemoglobin-oxygen equilibrium and coronary blood flow: An analog model. *J. Appl. Physiol.* 35:480, 1973.
8. Gutierrez, G., Lund, N., and Bryan-Brown, C. W. Cellular Oxygen Utilization During Multiple Organ Failure. In M. R. Pinsky (ed.), *Multiple Systems Organ Failure*, Critical Care Clinics, 5:2. Philadelphia: *Saunders*, 1989.
9. Guyton, A. C., and Richardson, T. Q. Effect of hematocrit on venous return. *Circ. Res.* 9:157, 1961.
10. Joly, H., and Weil, M. H. Temperature of the great toe as an indication of the severity of shock. *Circulation* 39:131, 1969.
11. Kloche, R. A. Oxygen Transfer from Red Cell to Mitochondria. In C. W. Bryan-Brown and S. M. Ayres (eds.), *New Horizons II. Oxygen Transport and Utilization.* Fullerton, Calif.: Society of Critical Care Medicine, 1987. Pp. 239–270.
12. Kontos, H. A. Regulation of the Cerebral Microcirculation in Hypoxia and Ischemia. In C. W. Bryan-Brown and S. M. Ayres (eds.), *New Horizons II. Oxygen Transport and Utilization.* Fullerton, Calif.: Society of Critical Care Medicine, 1987. Pp. 311–326.
13. Rowell, L. B. *Human Circulation: Regulation During Physical Stress.* New York: Oxford University Press, 1986.
14. Shoemaker, W. C., Appel, P. L., and Kram, H. B. Tissue oxygen debt as determinant of lethal and nonlethal postoperative organ failure. *Crit. Care Med.* 16:1117, 1988.
15. Shoemaker, W. C., Appel, P. L., Kram, H. B. Waxman, K., Lee, T-S. Prospective trial of supranormal values of survivors as therapeutic goals in high-risk surgical patients. *Chest* 94:1176, 1988.
16. Siesjö, B. K. Critical Degrees of Hypoxia and Ischemia When Cerebral Function and Metabolism Are Perturbed. In C. W. Bryan-Brown and S. M. Ayres (eds.), *New Horizons II. Oxygen Transport and Utilization.* Fullerton, Calif.: Society of Critical Care Medicine, 1987. Pp. 293–310.
17. Taylor A. E., Hernandez, L., Perry, M., Smith, M., Womack, W. Overview of

Tissue Oxygen Utilization. In C. W. Bryan-Brown and S. M. Ayres (eds.), *New Horizons II. Oxygen Transport and Utilization.* Fullerton, Calif.: Society of Critical Care Medicine, 1987. Pp. 13–24.

18. Valeri, C. K., Bryan-Brown, C. W., and Altshule, M. (eds.). Symposium on function of red blood cells. *Crit. Care Med.* 7:357, 1979.

19. Wasserman, K. Coupling of external to internal respiration. *Am. Rev. Respir. Dis.* 129:S21, 1984.

20. Wolson, R. S., and Laver, M. B. Oxygen analysis. *Anesthesiology* 37:112, 1972.

SELECTED READINGS

Bryan-Brown, C. W., and Ayres, S. M. (eds.). *New Horizons II. Oxygen Transport and Utilization.* Fullerton, Calif.: Society of Critical Care Medicine, 1987.

Perutz, M. F. Hemoglobin structure and respiratory transport. *Sci. Am.* 239:92, 1978.

Pinsky, M. R. (ed.). *Multiple Systems Organ Failure,* Critical Care Clinics, 5:2. Philadelphia: Saunders, 1989.

Snyder, J. V. *Oxygen Transport in the Critically Ill.* Chicago: Year Book, 1987.

Wade, O. L., and Bishop, J. M. *Cardiac Output and Regional Blood Flow.* Oxford: Blackwell, 1962.

Ventilatory Management of the Critically Ill Patient

Hillary F. Don

Failure of gas exchange in the lung is common in critically ill patients, regardless of the underlying primary disease. In a majority of patients, it is impossible to identify the exact reason for this failure.

Chief among the predisposing factors is sepsis, where the focus of infection is outside the lung. This is associated with increase in pulmonary vascular resistance, prevention of pulmonary arterial vasoconstriction in response to hypoxia, and pulmonary edema. Other diseases specifically associated with alteration in lung function are heart failure, uremia, hepatic cirrhosis, acute pancreatitis, nonthoracic trauma, central nervous system diseases, and thoracic cage abnormalities.

Instituted treatments may also have associated respiratory complications—for example, immunosuppressive medications predispose to pulmonary infection or may have a direct toxic effect. Finally, major additional factors are the patient's degree of mobility and level of mental obtundation. Inability to move freely or to sit up and decreased cough obviously predispose to the development of atelectasis and pulmonary infections. This is particularly true in the obese patient or the patient with preexisting pulmonary disease.

EARLY DETECTION OF RESPIRATORY DISEASE

The possibility of the development of lung dysfunction dictates the need for close monitoring to detect its onset. In conscious patients, this may be heralded by dyspnea, cough, or chest pain. Auscultation and percussion of the chest, recording of respiratory rate, assessment of intercostal retraction, and tracheal tug are also important.

Analysis of arterial blood for partial pressure of oxygen (PaO_2), carbon dioxide ($PaCO_2$), and pH is an essential guide in the critically ill patient. Arterial oxygen tension must be interpreted with these factors in mind: (1) the inspired oxygen fraction (FiO_2), (2) the alveolar oxygen tension (PAO_2), and (3) the alveolar-to-arterial oxygen tension gradient [$P(A-a)O_2$].

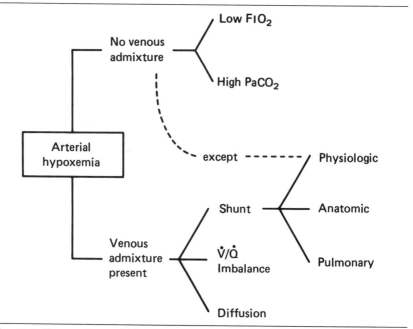

Fig. 10-1. Causes of arterial hypoxemia. In the figure the dashed line indicates that even in healthy young subjects, a small amount of venous admixture is present.

The FiO_2 is difficult to assess in the patient who is breathing through the normal airway. With a face mask, where delivered oxygen fraction is 1.0, the inspired oxygen fraction may range from 0.3 to 0.6. It can be measured from gas samples taken from the posterior pharynx.

The alveolar oxygen tension is influenced by two major factors: the inspired oxygen tension and alveolar carbon dioxide tension. Alveolar carbon dioxide is approximately equal to $PaCO_2$, and alveolar oxygen tension can be assessed by a simplified form of the alveolar gas equation:

$$PAO_2 = PiO_2 - \frac{PaCO_2}{R}$$

where PiO_2 is inspired oxygen tension in moist gas and R is the respiratory quotient. Elevation of $PaCO_2$—for example, by drug overdose—will necessarily cause a decrease in alveolar, and therefore arterial, PO_2, unless inspired oxygen tension is increased.

The alveolar-arterial oxygen tension gradient reflects the presence of venous admixture due to shunt, areas of low ventilation-perfusion ratio, or diffusion (Fig. 10-1). The normal or physiologic shunt increases with age, which is an important determinant of PaO_2, such that, in the supine position:

$PaO_2 = 100 - \frac{1}{2}$ (age in years) torr

If $P(A-a)O_2$ is increased due to lung disease, arterial oxygen tension may be normal due to compensatory hyperventilation, with lowering of $PaCO_2$ and elevation of PAO_2. Hypocapnia is therefore a frequent early indicator of the development of lung disease.

The chest x-ray is useful but has limited value in the early detection of lung disease. In a reported series, 7 percent of patients with acute respiratory disease had a normal chest x-ray [21]. Equally, a supine portable antero-posterior chest x-ray taken at a small inspiratory lung volume in a normal subject may resemble that of a patient with pulmonary vascular congestion and atelectasis.

In certain disease states, interval measurement of simple pulmonary function may be an appropriate monitor—for example, in a patient with central neurologic disease, peripheral neuropathy, myasthenia gravis, or cervical cord injury. The vital capacity measures the resultant difference between the amount of work that can be done and that needed to be done to inflate and deflate the lungs. A reduction in vital capacity in a patient with myasthenia gravis indicates either a decline in muscle strength or the development of pulmonary parenchymal disease, such as atelectasis. Vital capacity is also impaired by changes in the patient's mental state and level of cooperation.

CAUSES OF RESPIRATORY DISEASE

When lung disease is detected, the cause can be placed in one or more of the following categories.

Central Control of Respiration

In the absence of chronic lung disease or other factors such as narcotic administration, elevation of $PaCO_2$ is rarely seen in the early stages of acute lung disease. Hypercapnia therefore necessitates a search for a central or peripheral cause (Table 10-1). In the absence of dyspnea, tachypnea, or marked hypoxemia, central depression of ventilation is commonly found.

A frequent cause is the use of narcotic analgesia; depression of breathing for up to 6 days following administration of morphine in anuric patients and a similar effect in patients with normal renal and hepatic function after the use of methadone have been shown [46]. Naloxone, a narcotic antagonist with no inherent respiratory effect, can be used with relative safety to test for the presence of narcotics. Nausea, vomiting, cardiac arrhythmias, and marked systemic hypertension may, however, follow the administration of naloxone.

Metabolic alkalosis, particularly if produced by nasogastric suctioning, frequently causes hypercapnia. Obesity may be associated with an elevation of $PaCO_2$. The term *Pickwickian* is used to describe the syndrome of obesity, hypercapnia, hypoxemia breathing room air, hypersomnolence,

Table 10-1. Causes of Hypercapnia

A. Lung disease present
B. No lung disease present but
    1. Organic disease of the brain
    2. Functional depression
       a. Sleep
       b. Drugs
       c. Oxygen
       d. Metabolic alkalosis
    3. Ventilatory apparatus abnormal
       a. Muscle weakness
       b. Upper or lower airway obstruction
       c. Mechanical deformation of chest wall
    4. Obesity
    5. Ondine's curse
    6. Primary idiopathic hypoventilation

polycythemia, twitching, periodic breathing, and right ventricular hypertrophy or failure. This syndrome may be associated with upper airway obstruction. Different syndromes of sleep apnea have been described, in which repeat episodes of apnea lasting more than 10 seconds occur during sleep. This condition is frequently associated with upper airway obstruction and is relieved by endotracheal intubation or tracheostomy. A central cause is also described.

Ondine's curse was first described following bilateral cervical cordotomy, with hypercapnia attributed to deafferentation of the reticular activating mechanism. It has been seen following unilateral cordotomy, cervical laminectomy, and surgery on the bodies of the upper cervical vertebrae. Occurring from 1 hour to 1 week after surgery, it usually resolves spontaneously.

Mechanical Failure of Ventilatory Pump
In the presence of normal central control of breathing, the ventilatory pump may fail owing to a defect of any link of the chain of spinal cord, anterior horn cell, peripheral nerve, neuromuscular junction, respiratory muscles, thoracic cage (including abdomen), and pleural space. The cause may be obvious—for example, trauma to the chest—or subtler, as in hypophosphatemia. Hypophosphatemia depletes cellular energy stores and impairs oxygen delivery to the tissues due to a shift to the left of the oxygen dissociation curve. Phosphorus levels below 1.0 mg/dl can result in muscle weakness severe enough to produce respiratory arrest. Similarly, semistarvation or hypomagnesemia can cause ventilatory muscle weakness [44].

Upper Airway Obstruction
Obstruction of the airway is commonly due to collapse of the soft tissues of the upper airway—for example, the tongue or posterior pharynx. Infection of the tonsils, adenoids, or epiglottis may produce supraglottic ob-

struction. Acute pharyngotracheitis may cause subglottic obstruction. Spasm or edema of the vocal cords may occur due to reflex stimulation or in association with anaphylactic reaction. A variety of foreign bodies may obstruct the upper airway. The lumen of the airway may also be narrowed by tumor. Extrinsic compression of the airway may occur—for example, with hemorrhage, tumor, or subfascial air.

Lower Airway Obstruction

The causes of lower airway obstruction are similar to those of upper airway obstruction. Edema, secretions, or spasm of bronchiolar smooth muscle are additional causes of lower airway obstruction. Smooth-muscle spasm may be caused by drug administration; beta-blocking agents can cause increased airway resistance even in the absence of a history of asthma or chronic obstructive pulmonary disease [8].

Lung Disease

Acute disease involving the lung parenchyma predominantly causes hypoxemia rather than hypercapnia; in the early stages, hypocapnia is usual. The following types of lung disease can be identified, although considerable overlap exists.

Infection

In the critically ill patient, defense mechanisms are impaired, and uncommon agents may infect the lung. Additionally, the use of immunosuppressive medications may lead to the development of opportunistic infections with unusual bacteria, fungi, viruses, mycoplasma, rickettsiae, and the protozoan *Pneumocystis carinii*. The last-named organism has been shown to be common [59], but the spectrum of causative organisms is ever-increasing [45]. Examination of the sputum by stain and culture is mandatory, but the diagnosis is frequently elusive. For example, daily acid-fast stain may not uncover mycobacteria, and the diagnosis may be established only by biopsy of bone marrow. The present pandemic of acquired immunodeficiency syndrome (AIDS) has caused widespread interest in the diagnosis and management of opportunistic pneumonias. Pneumonia due to *Pneumocystis carinii* can be diagnosed by indirect immunofluorescence assay of induced sputum [34].

Fiberoptic instrumentation has made bronchoscopy relatively easy and safe, even for critically ill patients on mechanical ventilation [12, 56]. Transtracheal aspiration may be helpful [11], but this procedure is associated with cardiac arrhythmias and hypoxemia. Open lung biopsy, with endotracheal intubation and insertion of a chest tube, is perhaps the safest and most fruitful technique for diagnosis of pulmonary infection in the critically ill patient [37, 55], although, as noted above, special techniques of examining induced sputum are reliable tests in some diseases.

High-Pressure Pulmonary Edema

In high-pressure pulmonary edema, pulmonary extravascular lung water is increased due to an elevation in left atrial pressure. This, in turn, may be due to cardiac arrhythmia, mitral or aortic valvular disease, cardiomyopathy, myocardial ischemia, pericardial tamponade, left atrial myxoma, and expanded intravascular volume.

Suggested by physical examination, the diagnosis is established securely only by measurement of left atrial pressure [22]. Although occasionally directly measured by means of a left atrial catheter inserted during cardiac surgery, left atrial pressure is usually assessed by balloon occlusion of a branch of a pulmonary artery using a flotation catheter. The consequent occlusion, or wedge pressure (PCWP) is elevated if it exceeds 15 torr. Interpretation of the wedge pressure is confused by changes in pleural pressure. During spontaneous breathing, PCWP should be measured at the end of exhalation, but it may be artificially elevated in the presence of increased expiratory resistance, since pleural pressure remains positive to maintain expiratory gas flow. Positive end-expiratory pressure during mechanical ventilation will also elevate pleural pressure, usually by about one-third to one-quarter of the applied pressure. In these circumstances, an elevated PCWP may be misinterpreted as indicating increased cardiac filling when the reverse may be true [38]. Thorough assessment of the indication for, and careful insertion and maintenance of, pulmonary artery catheters are essential, since pulmonary complications, such as infarction or pulmonary arterial rupture, have been associated with their use [23, 27].

Low-Pressure Pulmonary Edema

Low-pressure pulmonary edema is diagnosed if arterial blood gas tensions and chest x-ray films suggest pulmonary edema, but PCWP is normal or low. Newer methods of measurement of extravascular lung water—for example, by double indicators—are becoming helpful in establishing the diagnosis [30].

The causes of this type of edema fall into five categories: (1) circulating toxins (e.g., severe burns, sepsis, acute pancreatitis), (2) hypoproteinemia, (3) damage through the airway (e.g., smoke inhalation, aspiration of gastric contents), (4) neurogenic, and (5) antigen-antibody reaction.

An increase in lung water is a thread running through the pathologic diagnosis in many cases of acute respiratory failure [5]. The title adult respiratory distress syndrome (ARDS) has been applied to the syndrome of the acute onset of dyspnea, tachypnea, severe hypoxemia, small functional residual capacity, reduced lung compliance, and bilateral infiltrate on chest x-ray. At postmortem, each lung may be increased to 200 to 300 percent of normal weight. The syndrome is established only when specific causes of this clinical picture (e.g., infection) are excluded. The causes of ARDS remain obscure [54].

Pulmonary Embolism by Blood Clot

The accurate diagnosis of pulmonary embolism is important, because the treatment results in a significant decrease in mortality; equally, the danger of bleeding from the use of heparin requires that it not be incorrectly diagnosed.

Pulmonary embolism can present one of four overlapping clinical pictures [15]: (1) dyspnea with normal chest x-ray; (2) pulmonary infarction with chest pain, dyspnea, and hemoptysis; (3) acute cor pulmonale, with elevation of pulmonary arterial and right atrial pressures when more than 60 percent of the pulmonary vasculature is obstructed (shock may predominate); and (4) unexplained increase in prior left ventricular failure.

The symptoms in one report [4] included chest pain in 88 percent, dyspnea in 84 percent, cough in 53 percent, and hemoptysis in 30 percent of patients with documented pulmonary embolism. The associated clinical signs were a respiratory rate above 16 per minute in 92 percent, rales in 58 percent, pulse rate above 100 per minute in 44 percent, and temperature above 37.8°C in 43 percent of patients. Predisposing factors included current venous disease, immobilization, congestive heart disease, chronic lung disease, a history of a recent surgical procedure, obesity, diabetes mellitus, hypertension, and malignant neoplasm.

Combined ventilation and perfusion scans constitute a useful screening test, and objective assessment of venous thrombosis provides further information [32]. However, the definitive diagnosis of pulmonary embolism is made only by pulmonary angiogram.

Fat Embolism

The triad of neurologic dysfunction, respiratory insufficiency, and petechiae that follows trauma, particularly that involving long-bone fractures, is imperfectly understood. This syndrome of fat embolism is also found in association with drug overdosage, severe infection, diabetes mellitus, and burns. The diagnosis is supported by the finding of fat globules in the retina and the urine. Stained neutral fat droplets may be identified in rapidly frozen clotted blood [36].

Amniotic-Fluid Embolism

The diagnosis of amniotic-fluid embolism is usually based on presumptive evidence. However, a smear of aspirated right heart blood may reveal lanugo and fetal squamous cells, confirming the diagnosis of amniotic-fluid embolism.

Aspiration of Gastric Contents

There is no discrete clinical picture of aspiration. Acute asphyxia may occur due to obstruction of the larynx or trachea with gastric contents. Obstruction of lobar or segmental airways may result in localized collapse. The syndrome of aspiration of acid gastric secretions (pH < 2.4) is associated with the development of pulmonary edema.

The diagnosis of aspiration is usually based on the clinical history but may occur silently in the elderly, the sick, or the obtunded patient.

The use of corticosteroids and antibiotics has been advocated, but there is no evidence of a decrease in morbidity when these are employed following aspiration.

Pulmonary Hemorrhage

Pulmonary hemorrhage is usually, but not always, accompanied by hemoptysis. The causes include (1) bleeding diathesis, (2) acute infection, (3) tumor, (4) trauma, (5) cardiac disease, (6) thromboembolic disease, (7) idiopathic pulmonary hemosiderosis, (8) pulmonary-renal syndrome (e.g., Goodpasture's syndrome), (9) aspiration of foreign body, and (10) chronic lung disease.

Disseminated intravascular coagulation (DIC) is among the causes of bleeding diathesis. DIC is associated with disseminated cancer, localized ischemia, hypoxia, childbirth, acute infections, burns, trauma, and cardiopulmonary bypass.

Disease Due to Immunologic Reaction in the Lung

The acute onset of pulmonary infiltrates on chest x-ray film, dyspnea, fever, and eosinophilia can occur as a hypersensitivity reaction to drugs (Table 10-2) and industrial and animal exposures (Table 10-3) [39]. Hypersensitivity reactions may also occur with radiation. Some drugs may cause a dose-related toxicity that is not a hypersensitivity reaction; these include bleomycin, cyclophosphamide, and, probably, amiodarone. Obviously, it is important to identify the presence of a drug, animal, or vegetable effect on the lung, since withdrawal of the cause will aid resolution of the problem.

Other causes of immunologic pulmonary disorders associated with vasculitis include serum sickness, glomerulonephritis, periarteritis nodosa, and systemic lupus erythematosus.

MANAGEMENT OF RESPIRATORY DISEASE

The foregoing discussion indicates a variety of causes for acute respiratory disease, with varying degrees of difficulty in establishing a precise diagnosis. Even when the diagnosis is established, effective therapy may not exist. In a majority of patients, respiratory care is, unfortunately, solely supportive—sustaining life while the body itself, or instituted treatment, can repair the damage of the disease process. Manipulation of these supportive modalities to minimize overall toxicity lies at the heart of respiratory care.

Oxygen Administration

The first indication for increasing inspired oxygen fraction is to maintain a life-supporting PaO_2. The level of PaO_2 below which the function of the body is threatened is approximately 40 torr. In order to provide a safety margin in the event of sudden further deterioration, it is probably safer to maintain a level greater than 60 torr, unless there is a relative contraindication, such as chronic lung disease. Correction of low PaO_2 will also reverse pulmonary vasoconstriction.

The second indication is where a higher-than-normal PaO_2 is necessary. In the presence of myocardial ischemia, increased FiO_2 has been shown to reduce infarct size in dogs [43]. In contrast, another study demonstrated that the administration of 40 percent oxygen appears to promote myocardial injury after coronary ligation in dogs [7]. It is possible that wound healing is hastened.

Finally, an augmented FiO_2 is indicated as a preventive measure against the development of hypoxemia, for example, in the postoperative period.

Table 10-2. Drugs associated with pulmonary infiltrates

WITH EOSINOPHILIA

Aminosalicylic acid	Isoniazid
Aspirin	Mephenesin carbamate
Carbamazepine	Nitrofurantoin
Chlorpropamide	Penicillin
Cromolyn sodium	Pituitary snuff
Furazolidone	Sulfonamides
Imipramine	

WITHOUT EOSINOPHILIA

Amitriptyline	Methotrexate
Azathioprine	Narcotics (heroin, methadone)
Cyclophosphamide	Paraquat
Erythromycin	Pentolinium
Hexamethonium	Dextran 40
Hydrochlorothiazide	Blood transfusions
Indomethacin	Ethchlorvynol
Phenylbutazone	Busulfan
Procarbazine	Mecamylamine
Propoxyphene	

Table 10-3. Vegetable and animal products associated with hypersensitivity pneumonitis

Disease	Source
VEGETABLE PRODUCTS	
Farmer's lung	Moldy hay
Bagassosis	Moldy pressed sugarcane
Sequoiosis	Contaminated wood dust
Humidifier lung	Contaminated home humidifier
Tobacco grower's lung	Tobacco plants
Grain measurer's lung	Cereal grains
Mushroom worker's disease	Moldy compost
Byssinosis	Cotton
ANIMAL PRODUCTS	
Pigeon breeder's disease	Pigeon droppings
Duck fever	Bird feathers

Source: From M. Lopez and J. Salvaggio, Hypersensitivity pneumonitis: Current concepts of etiology and pathogenesis. *Ann. Rev. Med.* 27:453, 1976.

Hazards of Oxygen
The hazards of oxygen are

1. Combustion.
2. Suppression of respiratory drive, particularly in patients with chronic lung disease, asthma, obesity, kyphoscoliosis, metabolic alkalosis, and central nervous system disease and in the presence of respiratory depressant drugs.
3. Infection owing to a contaminated delivery system.

4. Mechanical failure, providing the patient with either too little or too much oxygen.
5. Drying effect if the gas is not adequately humidified.
6. Retrolental fibroplasia. Although primarily a disease of the premature infant, this entity has been claimed to occur in adults.
7. Lung oxygen toxicity. Scant data are available on the effect of high inspired-oxygen tensions on human diseased lungs, and results from animal experiments require careful interpretation. Oxygen toxicity is modified by species variations, administered drugs, increased resistance of diseased lungs, and attenuation of toxicity by slow increase in FIO_2 up to 1.0. Consequently, the time-dose relationship of oxygen toxicity in the diseased human lung is not known. Life-threatening hypoxemia should not be tolerated, because of the fear of oxygen toxicity. In the adult, it is probable that 100 percent oxygen can be tolerated by the sick lung for at least 36 hours. An FIO_2 below 0.6 is probably safe for more prolonged periods (2–3 weeks).
8. Atelectasis owing to the greater solubility of oxygen compared with nitrogen. Studies of this effect have shown conflicting data. Results of the effect of 100 percent inspired oxygen show that the production of trapped gas or loss of functional residual capacity is no greater compared with that at FIO_2 0.3 [17]. Studies on the acute effect of breathing FIO_2 1.0 have demonstrated both an increase and a decrease in venous admixture, depending on the initial shunt [51]. The changes in shunt could be attributed to alterations in the distribution of pulmonary perfusion.

Methods of Delivery of Oxygen

NASAL PRONGS. The advantages of nasal prongs are that they are well tolerated by patients and can be worn while eating. They also provide a low, controlled inspired oxygen fraction and can be used in addition to a face mask to increase FIO_2 further.

Inspired oxygen fractions from 0.22 to approximately 0.35 can be provided by varying the delivered oxygen flow from 0.25 to 6 liters per minute. Higher flows dry the nasal mucosa, producing discomfort and nasal hemorrhage. Nasal prongs can be used whether the patient breathes through the nose or the mouth.

VENTURI MASK. Venturi masks produce a high flow of gas at a known constant oxygen concentration. A flow of 4 to 8 liters per minute enters the device through a narrow orifice. Lateral negative pressure so produced entrains room air. The usual delivered oxygen concentrations are 0.4, 0.35, 0.28, or 0.24. The volumes of air entrained for each liter flow of oxygen are 3, 5, 10, or 20 liters, respectively. Additional humidity can be added by a collar attached around the entrainment ports.

AEROSOL MASK OR FACE TENT. Wide-bore tubing connecting the mask or face tent to a nebulizer allows delivery of humidity and an increaseed FIO_2. The usual delivered inspired oxygen fraction (FDO_2) is 0.21, 0.4, 0.7, and 1.0. The use of an oxygen-air mixing device to supply the nebulizer gas flow enables any FDO_2 from 0.21 to 1.0 to be delivered.

In the absence of a reservoir of gas, inspired oxygen will be less than FDO_2 whenever the patient's inspiratory flow rate exceeds the flow rate of the delivered gas. An FIO_2 greater than 0.7 is rarely achieved with an aerosol mask delivering an oxygen fraction of 1.0. The difference between FDO_2 and FIO_2 must be taken into account when assessing the severity of defect in gas exchange. If necessary, FIO_2 can be measured by aspirating a gas sample from the oropharynx.

PARTIAL REBREATHING MASK. Narrow-bore tubing connects the partial rebreathing mask to an oxygen flowmeter. The system is designed so that the first portion of the exhaled tidal volume, which is similar to delivered oxygen and carbon dioxide tensions, enters a plastic, collapsible reservoir, to be rebreathed with the next inhalation. It is not designed to rebreathe carbon dioxide. Inspired oxygen fractions of 0.8 may be achieved.

Humidity

In patients breathing through an endotracheal tube, the presence of moist inspired gas is essential to prevent the accumulation of dry secretions, with the danger of airway obstruction. Whether added humidity aids pulmonary toilet by liquefying secretions is disputed. Although few data support its use, it is frequent clinical experience that patients will produce more secretions when given added moisture by the airway. Water can be added either as vapor or as particles. Nebulized water may irritate the airway, provoking bronchospasm. Other hazards are the spread of infection, overheating the inspired gas, and adding excessive water, particularly if an ultrasonic nebulizer is used in children.

Pulmonary Physiotherapy

Breathing exercises, postural drainage, percussion, and vibration should be used to provide better expansion of the lungs, improving the mobilization of secretions and creating more effective cough. The effectiveness of physiotherapy in the resolution of pneumonia has been challenged, although mechanical vibration physiotherapy has been shown to improve arterial oxygenation [31].

Nasotracheal suctioning may be indicated to stimulate a cough and to aid pulmonary toilet. This mode of therapy is associated with arterial desaturation during the procedure and may provoke cardiac arrhythmia, nasal hemorrhage, or vomiting, with the danger of aspiration.

Intermittent Positive Pressure Breathing (IPPB)

The utilization of IPPB has diminished dramatically during the past decade. The objective of the treatment is to increase lung volume during inhalation, opening otherwise closed airways, reexpanding collapsed parts of the lung, and aiding pulmonary toilet. IPPB is helpful if vital capacity is less than 20 ml/kg body weight, when abdominal or thoracic pain limits the willingness of the patient to inhale deeply, or when the patient is fatigued.

An absolute contraindication to the use of IPPB is the presence of pneumothorax without a chest tube in place. Complications of IPPB include insufflation of gas into the gastrointestinal tract, lung disruption, and hyperventilation with hypoxemia when IPPB is stopped.

The procedure of IPPB must be performed with clear objectives and with stated mechanisms for recognizing the achievement of these goals.

Incentive Spirometry

The encouragement of deep inhalation by the use of an incentive spirometer is indicated when vital capacity is greater than 20 ml/kg body weight and the patient's motivation and level of cooperation are judged adequate.

Endotracheal Intubation

The first indication for endotracheal intubation is to allow positive-pressure ventilation. Mechanical ventilation using an iron lung, cuirass or "rain coat" ventilator, or a rocking bed does not require the presence of an endotracheal tube. These types of ventilators are unsatisfactory for acute lung disease, in which positive pressure ventilation is used, necessitating the insertion of an endotracheal tube.

Other indications for endotracheal intubation are to maintain a patent airway, to protect the airway from aspiration, and to facilitate pulmonary toilet. Finally, an endotracheal tube may be used to guarantee an FIO_2 or to apply continuous pressure during exhalation.

Desirable Features of an Endotracheal Tube

The tube should be of clear, plastic material, certified for tissue compatibility by animal implantation tests. The material must not irritate mucous membranes and should be smooth and sufficiently flexible to conform to the patient's anatomy. However, the tube should not kink at small radius or flatten due to the pressure of the cuff or the walls of the upper airway. A radiopaque marker must be present at the distal end of the tube. A side hole should also be present. The cuff should be firmly bonded to the tube and should have a high residual volume with high compliance when inflated.

Hazards of Endotracheal Intubation

The substitution of an artificial airway for the patient's own is a potentially lethal alteration. The complications of endotracheal intubation include

1. At the time of insertion, hypoxemia, reflex cardiac arrhythmia, and vomiting with possible aspiration may occur. Trauma to the mucosa or hemorrhage may be caused by the nasal route.
2. The endotracheal tube will introduce infection and break the continuity of the patient's natural lung clearance mechanisms.
3. The tube may be incorrectly placed into the esophagus or a main-stem bronchus. There has been at least one report of a patient swallowing an endotracheal tube. A tracheostomy tube may be accidentally placed in the subcutaneous tissues of the neck.
4. The endotracheal tube may become obstructed by kinking, by an overinflated cuff compressing the tube or evaginating over the end of the tube, or by materials such as blood clot or secretions within the lumen.
5. Erosion of the trachea may occur, with development of a tracheomediastinal or -esophageal fistula. Tracheotomy, in particular, may cause erosion of the innominate artery.

6. Following removal of a translaryngeal tube, laryngeal problems such as airway obstruction or hoarseness may occur for a variable length of time. Stenosis of the trachea may also be found.

Choice of Route of Tracheal Intubation

Three routes are available: nasotracheal, orotracheal, or tracheotomy. The initial route of tracheal intubation in the critically ill patient should be through the nose. The advantages of this technique are that it can usually be inserted during maintained spontaneous breathing without many drugs, it is easy to secure once inserted, and it is more comfortable for the patient than the oral route. The disadvantage of this approach is that the oral route accommodates a shorter tube of wider diameter. A nasal tube can also cause nasal hemorrhage and can be obstructed by pressure from the walls of the nasal passages. Paranasal sinusitis is also common, occurring in about 25 percent of patients [47]. In an emergency situation, oral intubation aided by neuromuscular blockade with succinylcholine is probably the preferred route [20].

Tracheostomy is employed initially only if intubation through the nose or mouth is impossible. The decision to perform tracheostomy in a patient with an existing oral or nasal tube is made to increase the patient's comfort, to allow easier mobilization, to allow short periods of talking if possible, and to permit easier swallowing of food.

The disadvantages of tracheostomy include trauma and hemorrhage at the time of tracheotomy. Pulmonary infection has been shown to be increased, as compared with nasal intubation, in children with burns. Following extubation, tracheal stenosis is much more common following tracheostomy and may approach 30 percent of patients, compared with probably less than 5 percent by the translaryngeal route. The maximum length of time that translaryngeal intubation should be allowed before tracheostomy is performed is not known. In a study of adult burn patients, it was recommended that initial tracheal intubation be through the nose for periods up to 3 weeks [40].

Procedure for Nasotracheal Intubation

The procedure for nasotracheal intubation must be meticulously planned and prepared. The patient is informed of what is to be done and is connected to a cardiac monitor. The following drugs and equipment must be at the bedside: atropine (0.4 mg); succinylcholine (100 mg); suction apparatus; a hand-ventilating device with appropriate face mask and oxygen supply; endotracheal tubes of the selected size and one size smaller; laryngoscope and blade; Magill forceps; and oral airway.

The nasal mucosa is sprayed with cocaine (4%) to produce topical anesthesia and to shrink the mucosa. The lubricated endotracheal tube is inserted into the nostril and advanced slowly and firmly. Through a feeding tube inserted to the distal end of the endotracheal tube, 1% lidocaine (maximum 10 ml) is injected in front of the tube. The tube is advanced, using audible or visible (by water condensation) guides, through the larynx. The tube is secured, and its position relative to the nares is noted. Auscultation of the chest checks the position of the tube. A chest x-ray is mandatory, however, since auscultation is an unreliable guide.

The equipment and preparation are similar for oral intubation. Topical anesthesia (1% lidocaine) is applied to the tongue, epiglottis, and larynx with direct laryngoscopy before tracheal intubation. Neuromuscular blockade with succinylcholine can be instituted prior to intubation if necessary.

Safeguarding the position and patency of the endotracheal tube is a high priority. The endotracheal tube is anchored by adhesive tape passed around the patient's neck. The distance from the end of the endotracheal tube to the lip or nose is measured and recorded every 2 hours. Warmed humidified gases are always used, to prevent accumulation and drying of secretions within the lumen of the tube.

The endotracheal tube is not changed unless a mechanical defect develops, such as a leak in the cuff.

The cuff is inflated just enough to prevent a leak during positive-pressure inflation. The necessary volume is recorded every 8 hours. A hand-ventilating device and an endotracheal tube one size smaller than in use are kept at the bedside.

Removal of the Endotracheal Tube
The first criterion for extubation is that the indication for intubation has been corrected. Second, the patient should be conscious and want the tube removed. Coma or an obtunded mental state do not indicate that extubation is impossible, however. In this situation, the ability of the patient to protect the airway can be assessed by whether the patient (1) coughs when a catheter is inserted through the endotracheal tube, (2) gags when the pharynx is stimulated with a tongue depressor, (3) swallows water poured into mouth, and (4) has good tone in the muscles of the jaw.

Extubation of the trachea must be carefully planned, and all the equipment for reintubation must be instantly available. The patient is informed of the plan and must be connected to an electrocardiac monitor. Secretions are aspirated from the trachea and mouth. The patient's lungs are hyperinflated with 100 percent oxygen, and the endotracheal tube cuff is deflated. The tube is withdrawn during exhalation from full inhalation. The patient is provided with humidified oxygen. Laryngeal obstruction is treated with added airway humidity and racemic epinephrine (Vaponefrin) by inhalation.

Mechanical Ventilation
Mechanical ventilation by intermittent positive pressure (IPPV) will, first, circulate gas in and out of the lungs, increasing minute ventilation (unless dead space increases equally). Hence, impaired minute ventilation can be corrected, and the work normally performed by the patient for spontaneous breathing is taken over by the machine. Second, mechanical ventilation will inflate and deflate the lungs and may increase mean lung volume, improving the distribution of ventilation, decreasing shunt, and allowing clearance of the lung through previously closed airways. Third,

mechanical ventilation increases alveolar pressure, which in itself might have an effect on ventilatory and hemodynamic function.

Indications for Mechanical Ventilation

FAILURE TO MAINTAIN ADEQUATE ALVEOLAR VENTILATION. Treatable causes of hypercapnia must first be sought, such as narcotic overdosage or partial neuromuscular block due to the residual effect of relaxant drugs. An elevated $PaCO_2$ is not in itself an absolute indication for IPPV. Some patients with chronic lung disease will tolerate $PaCO_2$ greater than 80 torr, remaining awake, comfortable, and cooperative. An arterial pH below 7.1 is usually considered an indication for mechanical ventilation, however.

RAISED INTRACRANIAL PRESSURE. Deliberate hypocapnia by IPPV may be indicated to lower raised intracranial pressure, in diseases such as Reye's syndrome.

HYPOXEMIA [18]. Perhaps the most frequent indication for mechanical ventilation in the ICU, a life-threatening PaO_2 will usually be increased by IPPV, probably because the increased tidal volume, provided mechanically, increases mean lung volume. The specific criteria indicating the need for mechanical ventilation are, approximately, (1) PaO_2 less than 40 torr on maximal inspired oxygen; (2) increasing obtundation of the patient's mental state, with loss of ability to cooperate with treatments and to communicate changes in symptoms; (3) rapidly progressing respiratory disease; (4) the appearance of intercostal indrawing and tracheal tug during inhalation, indicating increased work of breathing; and (5) elevation of $PaCO_2$.

PROPHYLAXIS. In certain situations, such as in the face of hemodynamic instability, mechanical ventilation may be instituted to maintain ventilatory function.

INCREASED WORK OF BREATHING. Increased work of breathing is disputed as an indication for IPPV, since simply diverting cardiac output from the respiratory muscles to more useful areas of the body is not of great advantage. The increase in the work of breathing might indicate impeding respiratory failure.

POSSIBLE THERAPEUTIC BENEFITS. Positive-pressure ventilation stabilizes the chest wall of patients with injuries such as flail chest. It may be true that pulmonary collapse and atelectasis benefit physically from IPPV, and normal lung function is more quickly restored.

Choice of Mechanical Ventilator

Since the fundamental purpose of a ventilator is to deliver tidal volume, the cycling from inhalation to exhalation is most effectively achieved by a volume or time mechanism. Pressure-cycled ventilators will fail to deliver the desired tidal volume in the face of changes in airway resistance or lung and chest wall compliance. However, when using uncuffed endotracheal tubes, which will have a variable leak, pressure-cycled ventilators may produce a more constant tidal volume.

The onset of the inspiratory phase should be time-cycled, with the option of the assist mode by pressure. Synchronization of the intermittent mandatory ventilation (IMV) with the patient's spontaneous breath is desirable.

The power source of most ventilators is electricity, but the availability of a ventilator driven by compressed gas allows safer transportation of patients on mechanical ventilation.

The ventilator should be as small and simple as is compatible with its function. It must be reliable and be backed by enthusiastic service. It should have a range of tidal volume suitable for the patient population, from 100 to 2500 ml. The ventilatory frequency should be from 1 to 60 breaths per minute. The inspiratory flow should be adjustable from 5 to 100 liters/min. An infinitely adjustable range of FIO_2 from 0.21 to 1.0 must be standard. The peak airway pressure must be at least 150 cm H_2O, and the output of the ventilator should vary little at that back pressure.

The patient circuit must be easily sterilizable. Bacterial filters in both the inspiratory and expiratory limbs of the circuit may be advantageous.

A parallel breathing circuit with the same FIO_2 as the ventilator must be available, to allow spontaneous breathing between the mechanical breaths. In the event of failure of the gas supply to the ventilator, a fail-safe device must allow spontaneous breathing of room air. Positive end-expiratory pressure up to 50 cm H_2O should be incorporated.

Alarms for high- and low-pressure limits, FIO_2, tidal volume, and inspired gas temperature are mandatory.

Hazards of Mechanical Ventilation

MECHANICAL PROBLEMS. Possibly the greatest hazard with the ventilator and its circuitry is mechanical. In one report, mechanical problems occurred in 103 out of 354 separate episodes of acute respiratory failure [68].

DEPRESSION OF CARDIAC OUTPUT. During a spontaneous inhalation, pleural pressure becomes increasingly negative. Positive pressure, on the other hand, creates increasingly less negative pleural pressure and, in fact, may become positive. This increase in pleural pressure increases intrathoracic venous pressure—which, in turn, may reduce venous return, with consequent depression of cardiac output. Pulmonary vascular resistance is also increased.

The rise in venous pressure may increase venous bleeding and elevate the back pressure in the hepatic and renal circulations.

Although cardiac filling may be decreased due to the more positive pleural pressure, it is possible that left ventricular function is aided, since the positive pressure tends to reduce afterload [9].

INTRACRANIAL PRESSURE. Intracranial pressure may increase, but since cerebrospinal fluid pressure rises equally in the closed cranium, the distending pressure across the brain does not increase. The rise in pressure can be minimized in the head-up position. A decrease in cardiac output or systemic mean pressure may cause marked cerebral vasodilatation and an increase in intracranial pressure.

LUNG DISRUPTION. Lung disruption is not infrequent. Air can track from the bronchovascular bundle to the mediastinum, the subcutaneous tissues, and the pleural space. It may track into the retroperitoneum and may appear as free air in the peritoneal space, mimicking the x-ray film of a ruptured abdominal viscus. The incidence of pneumothorax varies from less than 1 to 15 percent [14]. Finally, lung disruption may result in vascular air embolism.

HYPERINFLATION. Hyperinflation, either of both lungs or of discrete areas in the lungs, may occur. This is presumably due to a ball-valve effect aggravated by limited expiratory time.

FLUID RETENTION. Increases in both antidiuretic hormone [35] and aldosterone [13] have been attributed to positive-pressure ventilation.

Adjustment of Tidal Volume
Tidal volume (V_T) is initially set at approximately 15 ml/kg. A high tidal volume is chosen to maintain mean lung volume and to prevent the development of atelectasis. Total compliance has been shown to increase as tidal volume is changed from 5 to 15 ml/kg [64].

Reduction of the size of tidal volume is indicated in patients with chronic lung disease or asthma, where hyperinflation and a markedly positive pleural pressure may develop. An alteration in tidal volume of as little as 100 to 200 ml may lower pleural pressure and increase cardiac output. Gas trapping is detected if initially exhaled volume is less than the volume inhaled. With a time- or volume-cycled ventilator, this is seen as an initial stepwise increase in exhaled volume. Prolonged exhalation following disconnection of the ventilator provides further evidence.

A reduction in tidal volume is also indicated in the presence of low chest wall compliance. In this circumstance, the positive pleural pressure on inhalation is accentuated, impending venous return.

Adjustment of Inspiratory Waveform
Alterations of inspiratory waveform have been shown to alter the distribution of ventilation and gas exchange [3, 16]. The clinical significance of these findings is not clear. The inspired flow rate should be adjusted to maintain a ratio of inhalation to exhalation of approximately 1 : 1.5.

Adjustment of Ventilator Frequency
With the tidal volume fixed, the frequency of ventilation is adjusted to maintain $PaCO_2$ at approximately 35 torr. The initial frequency in an adult is between 8 and 14 breaths per minute, and in a child, between 15 and 40 breaths per minute.

Hypocapnia has the hazards of potentiating the effects of digitalis, reducing cerebral blood flow, increasing airway resistance, shifting the oxygen dissociation curve to the left, and causing retention of hydrogen ion by the kidney. If $PaCO_2$ is too low in the presence of satisfactory V_T and frequency, mechanical dead space should be inserted in the ventilator circuit.

A modifying factor in the choice of frequency is patient acceptance. Dyspnea can sometimes be relieved by instituting a rapid respiratory rate. A slow rate might be used in the presence of increased airway resistance, promoting more even distribution of inhaled gas. A guide to the appropriate length of exhalation is to ensure that prior to inhalation the exhalation is complete, by watching the spirometer on the ventilator.

Two major modifications of ventilator frequency have been introduced. The first of these is mechanical ventilation at high frequency. At frequencies above 60 per minute, respiration-synchronous variation in blood pressure and flow is eliminated, and spontaneous ventilation usually ceases. This technique appears to simplify the process of mechanical ventilation [60].

The second method is a departure from conventional therapy: the production of high-frequency (15 Hz) sine wave oscillation at the airway, with no bulk flow of gas. Elimination of carbon dioxide is normal in human subjects using this technique [10]. Its role is not yet defined [24].

Inspired Oxygen Fraction

Optimal FIO_2 is that which maintains PaO_2 at approximately 60 torr. Comparative dangers of different levels of FIO_2 are unknown in sick human lungs, but oxygen toxicity is unlikely when FIO_2 is less than 0.6.

Sedation

Adequate medication should be given to provide sedation or narcosis. Spontaneous ventilation need not be totally suppressed, since the negative pleural pressure may aid venous return.

The choice of drugs is arbitrary. Intravenous morphine sulfate (0.05 mg/kg) or diazepam (0.05 mg/kg) is usually satisfactory. In babies and infants, the use of drugs that block the neuromuscular junction, such as pancuronium (0.05 mg/kg), may be necessary. These drugs have a prolonged effect in patients with impaired hepatic or renal function. The actions of pancuronium and morphine are pharmacologically reversible, however. In adults, neuromuscular blockade may occasionally improve oxygenation by reducing oxygen consumption. However, in this circumstance the patient must be protected from inadequate sedation.

Discontinuation of Mechanical Ventilation

ASSESSMENT OF PATIENT. The criteria for commencing weaning from mechanical ventilation, and its successful accomplishment, have received considerable attention in the literature. No simple factors or combination of factors has been shown to cover all aspects of weaning from mechanical ventilation. The rigid application of criteria based on physiologic variables is inappropriate and probably leads to unnecessarily prolonged periods of mechanical ventilation. Although the management of weaning is tailored to an individual patient, the following represent guidelines.

The initiating indication for mechanical ventilation has been eliminated or modified.

The defect of gas exchange is assessed. In acute lung disease, the usual defect is an increase in venous admixture, $\dot{Q}_s/\dot{Q}_t$, and in the alveolar to arterial oxygen tension difference, $P(A-a)O_2$. The latter can be assessed by the measurement of PaO_2 following the inhalation of 100 percent oxygen for 30 minutes. A $P(A-a)O_2$ of greater than 300 torr is said to be associated with difficulty in weaning. However, in a series of 80 patients, we found that successful weaning occurred with $P(A-a)O_2$ as large as 580 mm Hg. In fact, improvement in gas exchange may follow tracheal extubation, because the patient's own cough may provide a more effective pulmonary toilet.

Assessment of $P(A-a)O_2$ on FIO_2 1.0 is helpful, because it presents a wider range of PaO_2 and can be accurately assessed throughout a patient's period of deterioration and recovery. Gas exchange can also be assessed by measuring the $P(A-a)O_2$ on lower inspired-oxygen fractions. Data using these values have not been well documented, however. The advantage of using an FIO_2 less than 1.0 is the possibility that 100 percent oxygen itself causes an increase in the shunt [52]. The defect so produced is probably caused by the effect of high FIO_2 on the distribution of pulmonary blood flow.

The use of the alveolar-arterial oxygen tension difference does not take into account the influence of alterations of mixed venous oxygen content on gas exchange. A more accurate assessment is to calculate venous admixture using measured mixed venous oxygen content. This equation takes into account alterations in cardiac output, oxygen consumption, hemoglobin, and the position of the oxygen dissociation curve.

The measurement of $P(A-a)O_2$ or venous admixture on FIO_2 1.0 is normally of limited value in patients with acute exacerbations of chronic lung disease, unless they have superimposed acute pneumonia or pulmonary edema.

The functional state of the lung also can be assessed by measurement of total effective compliance, which should be greater than 20 ml/cm H_2O; by measurement of the fraction of tidal volume (V_T) that is dead space (V_D), which should be less than 0.6; and by measurement of functional residual capacity, which should be greater than 50 percent of predicted.

The mechanical properties of the lung and chest wall are assessed by first temporarily disconnecting the patient from the ventilator and observing a maximum inhalation. There should be no intercostal indrawing or tracheal tug. The presence of either of these motions indicates partial neuromuscular blockade, upper or lower airway obstruction, or decreased lung compliance. Conversely, the movement of the abdomen should be noted. Failure of the abdomen to move outward during the maximum inhalation suggests unilateral or bilateral diaphragmatic paralysis, which may follow surgery in the chest or neck.

Measured vital capacity should exceed 12 ml/kg, but values as low as 5 ml/kg are compatible with successful weaning. Maximum inspiratory pressure generated against a closed glottis should be less negative than -20 cm H_2O.

The control of breathing is assessed first by the mental state of the patient. If the patient is alert and responding appropriately, mechanical ventilation is discontinued and spontaneous breathing of 100 percent oxygen allowed. A lower FiO_2 should be used when indicated—for example, in the presence of chronic lung disease. An obtunded mental state does not contraindicate a trial of spontaneous breathing, but the effect of any depressant drugs, such as narcotics, previously administered should be reversed, and the trial should be approached more cautiously.

After 30 minutes of spontaneous breathing, $PaCO_2$ should be less than 46 torr. If it is higher, but less than 50 torr, the trial of spontaneous breathing is continued; if $PaCO_2$ remains below 50 torr, extubation can be considered. If it is higher than 50 torr, and pH is below 7.30, further attempts at weaning should be modified (see below) or postponed.

If judged not to need mechanical ventilation, the patient is then assessed for the need for endotracheal intubation, and the endotracheal tube removed, if appropriate.

TECHNIQUES OF WEANING. Should the patient be judged as still needing mechanical ventilation, the following options for management are available.

Mechanical ventilation is continued with testing at intervals of 12 to 24 hours to judge possibility of weaning. If the factor influencing the decision is the amount of venous admixture, positive end-expiratory pressure (PEEP) may be added to the exhalation limb of the ventilator.

Alternatively, using a parallel breathing circuit, the frequency of mechanical breaths is decreased at appropriate intervals. This technique of intermittent mandatory ventilation (IMV) allows maintenance of safe arterial gas tensions, while providing an increasing amount of spontaneous breathing. The rate of reduction of mechanical breaths is judged from alterations in arterial blood gas tensions, and the symptoms and signs of respiratory distress shown by the patient. This technique is safe, easy to institute, and minimizes mechanical accident and bacterial contamination.

Some patients, particularly those with chronic lung disease, may not tolerate IMV but accept increasing periods of spontaneous breathing interrupted by short periods of mechanical ventilation.

Spontaneous breathing with continuous positive airway pressure (CPAP) may improve the ability of patients with chronic lung disease to breathe spontaneously, presumably by maintaining airway patency during exhalation. Caution should be exercised, since the resultant increase in functional residual capacity may impede both hemodynamic and ventilatory function.

A more recent method of weaning patients from mechanical ventilation is pressure support ventilation, which provides adjustable positive pressure during inspiration. Its role in accelerating or accomplishing weaning has not been defined [42].

Continuous Positive Pressure

Although the technique of PEEP breathing dates back more than 40 years, its modern application to the management of acute respiratory disease was described by Ashbaugh et al. in 1969 [1]. The interpretation of the acronyms used to identify different forms of positive-pressure breathing varies: for the present description, CPPV (continuous positive-pressure ventilation) indicates the maintenance of positive airway pressure throughout the inspiratory and expiratory phases of a mechanical tidal volume; CPPB (continuous positive-pressure breathing) refers to spontaneous breathing with positive pressure maintained during both inhalation and exhalation; and EPPB (expiratory positive-pressure breathing) indicates spontaneous breathing with positive pressure at the airway only during the expiratory phase.

Positive-pressure breathing has its effect presumably by increasing functional residual capacity (FRC), which, in turn, improves the matching of ventilation to perfusion and allows better lung clearance.

Although it has been disputed, the positive pressure itself may improve hemodynamic function through reduction of preload [28] and, possibly, of left ventricular afterload [9].

Intrinsic PEEP may occur if expiratory time does not allow lung volume to return to initial resting levels. This will be found when expiratory time is too brief or airway obstruction is present [48].

Indications for PEEP

The role of PEEP in the management of patients with acute lung disease is still not clearly defined [50]. There are five basic categories of indications for the use of PEEP:

1. When arterial oxygen tension is sufficiently low to threaten life in the face of maximum inspired-oxygen fraction. PaO_2 less than 40 torr, with hemodynamic instability, altered mental state, and the development of metabolic acidosis fulfill this criterion. The addition of PEEP usually increases PaO_2.
2. When life-supporting PaO_2 is maintained only by a potentially life-threatening FiO_2. The use of PEEP will allow reduction of FiO_2, creating an optimal environment for recovery of pulmonary function. However, the relative toxicity of high inspired-oxygen fraction compared with PEEP cannot be defined. The judgment, for example, that PEEP of 10 cm H_2O plus FiO_2 0.4 is less harmful to the lung than PEEP of 0 cm H_2O plus FiO_2 0.8 is arbitrary.
3. When it is thought that PEEP will actually treat the lung disease. That the actual disease process, and not merely the arterial blood gas, is improved by the use of PEEP is disputed [61]. Although it is probably true that atelectasis or collapse may resolve more quickly when treated with PEEP, it is well established that lung water is not diminished by the addition of PEEP to ventilatory support.
4. Some patients, particularly those with chronic lung disease, may benefit from PEEP during spontaneous breathing. This is presumably the equivalent of breathing with pursed lips. This technique may be assessed in patients who experience difficulty while weaning from mechanical ventilation.
5. Prophylaxis. The newborn, with a chest wall of high compliance, maintains FRC by creating increased laryngeal resistance to flow during exhalation. This

is prevented by the presence of an endotracheal tube, and PEEP is indicated in this age group to maintain lung volume and prevent atelectasis. The adult does not usually have a dynamically determined FRC, and the prophylactic use of PEEP is not indicated. The age at which PEEP is no longer advantageous is not identified, but is possibly at approximately 3 years. The early application of PEEP in high-risk patients has no effect on the incidence of the adult respiratory distress syndrome [49].

Hazards of PEEP

A false sense of security may be the first hazard of PEEP. An improvement in gas exchange following institution of PEEP may not reflect any real change in the amount of lung disease, but might reduce the impetus for a careful and thorough search for the underlying cause of the pulmonary deficit.

An increased risk of lung disruption may be produced. It has been claimed, however, that the risk of pneumothorax even with high levels is no greater than if mechanical ventilation were used without PEEP [33].

Cardiac output may be unchanged or may change in either direction. The determinants of the effect of PEEP on hemodynamics include the blood volume and cardiac status of the patient. In the presence of hypovolemia, cardiac output may fall. If congestive heart failure is present, cardiac output may increase [28]. The benefits of PEEP to hemodynamics in this situation can be through preload or afterload reduction [9]. The presence of decreased lung compliance will attenuate the transmission of positive alveolar pressure to the pleural space [38]. Usually, about one-third of PEEP applied at the airway is seen as changes in pleural pressure. Oxygen transport may decrease, therefore, since an increase in arterial oxygen content may be offset by a decline in cardiac output.

Systemic blood pressure may decrease but is frequently maintained, even in the presence of a fall in cardiac output. Left atrial diastolic pressure, assessed by measurement of pulmonary capillary wedge pressure, is almost invariably elevated when PEEP is added. This does not imply that atrial filling pressure has increased, because pleural pressure may rise equally. In this situation, a decrease in filling pressure may accompany a rise in pulmonary capillary wedge pressure (PCWP). Simultaneous measurements of esophageal pressure allow interpretation of changes in filling pressures [38], but the clinical utility of this technique, in the supine position, has not been established. The changes in right atrial pressures are similar to those in the left atrium.

Pulmonary vascular resistance (PVR) may increase with PEEP, although this is not a universal finding [62]. The change in PVR may cause a decrease in cardiac output. In the presence of an unequal distribution of lung disease, the increase in resistance will be felt primarily by well-ventilated lung, causing a shift of pulmonary blood flow away from well-ventilated areas. In the presence of an intracardiac defect, right-to-left shunt may be increased. The increase in intrathoracic venous pressure caused by the rise in pleural pressure may increase intracranial pressure, but this is not invariable; an increase in intracranial pressure is most in evidence if mean systemic pressure falls.

The amount of venous admixture is usually diminished by PEEP. The dead space fraction (VD) of tidal volume is usually not altered.

Renal function may be impaired, but probably only as a function of a decrease in cardiac output. Intravenous dopamine will usually correct this alteration in kidney perfusion [29]. An increase in antidiuretic hormone and aldosterone may also occur during therapy with PEEP.

The work of breathing is usually not increased during CPPB, so long as the pressure at the airway does not decrease significantly during spontaneous inhalation. If airway pressure decreases to ambient pressure during inhalation (EPPB), the work of breathing increases linearly to as much as 100 percent with the application of 20 cm H_2O of end-expiratory pressure [26].

Functional residual capacity usually increases with PEEP, although this may not be seen with EPPB [26]. In the adult, the change in FRC is in the order of 100 ml/cm H_2O PEEP. The increase in FRC may be deleterious in a patient with preexisting elevation of FRC or total lung capacity, such as is found in pulmonary emphysema.

Correct Levels of PEEP

Although many authors have struggled for the answer, identification of the optimum level of PEEP is not possible at present. It has been stated that the optimum level of PEEP to be applied is that which reduces the amount of venous admixture to near normal [33, 63]. A second published view is that the objective is to maximize oxygen transport [66]. None of these reports, however, has asked the key question, What level of PEEP is associated with the greatest return of pulmonary function in the shortest time and with the least toxicity to the organ systems of the body? The published reports quoted above are concerned with the immediate, short-term effects of PEEP. Looking at the long-term goals of PEEP, one nonrandomized, retrospective study concluded that an improvement in PaO_2 and decrease in shunt fraction following a trial of PEEP portends a favorable outcome, but its continued use appears to prolong life for a few days without affecting hospital mortality [61].

The answer to the question of how PEEP should be optimally used is therefore not apparent at this time. The effect of PEEP must be studied in each individual patient. One system is to apply PEEP when PaO_2 on FIO_2 1.0 has declined to approximately 100 torr. PEEP is added to increase PaO_2 to over 150 torr, allowing FIO_2 to be reduced to 0.8, with PaO_2 at least 60 torr. Acutely deleterious hemodynamic effects of PEEP are sought by measurement of mixed venous oxygen content ($C\bar{v}O_2$), metabolic acidosis, urine output, blood pressure, electrocardiogram, and cardiac output. Central nervous system changes are also assessed. Infusion of fluid or vasopressor agents such as dopamine may be used to offset these harmful effects of PEEP. The trend of the amount of pulmonary disease is then assessed at intervals of 2 to 24 hours, depending on the severity of the defect. If oxygen exchange is further impaired after the initial improvement, PEEP is increased in steps of 3 or 5 cm H_2O to reverse this downward trend. An inspired oxygen of less than 0.6 should be achieved within 24 hours if possible.

Technique of Applying PEEP

PEEP should be achieved with a threshold, rather than a flow, resistor. The safest apparatus is probably wide-bore expiratory tubing inserted to the appropriate depth under water. Continuous positive-pressure breathing compared to CPPV has a less depressant effect on cardiac output and a lower tendency to produce lung disruption; it has been used successfully in adult patients both with [66] and without endotracheal intubation. We have found the latter technique too difficult and traumatic to the patient's face, for prolonged use.

CPPB is probably preferable to EPPB, because the hemodynamic and ventilatory advantages are approximately the same, but the work of breathing is less.

The use of the assist mode for cycling the beginning of a mechanical breath has been shown to have no advantage over controlled ventilation [19].

A continuous negative chest wall pressure has been used in both children and adults as an alternative to PEEP. A sustained improvement in oxygenation has been reported without need for endotracheal intubation [57].

Reducing PEEP

Premature withdrawal of PEEP in the face of an improvement in gas exchange may result in significant deterioration in oxygenation, which may persist even if the previous level of PEEP is restored [41]. It is our practice not to reduce PEEP within 12 hours of establishing a given level. Control measurements of venous admixture or $P(A-a)O_2$ on FiO_2 1.0 are then made before and after reduction in PEEP by 3 to 5 cm H_2O. If a significant increase in $P(A-a)O_2$ (i.e., more than 75 torr) occurs, the initial PEEP is restored.

Extracorporeal Membrane Oxygenation

Prolonged extracorporeal membrane oxygenation (ECMO) has been shown to be practical, and survivors are reported [67].

Indications for ECMO

The first indication for ECMO is when a life-supporting PaO_2 cannot be maintained with maximum FiO_2, mechanical ventilation, and PEEP. If a potentially reversible lung condition is suspected, ECMO will usually support life, so that perhaps time, and instituted treatments, will effect recovery.

The second indication is that the alternative support modalities (FiO_2, positive airway pressure) can be reduced to a less toxic range. This supposes that the added burden of ECMO is less harmful than the morbidity of the reduced alternative supports.

The third indication is the conjecture that venoarterial bypass will reduce pulmonary blood flow and pulmonary capillary and venous pressures, hence improving pulmonary edema and facilitating recovery of normal lung structure. Certainly, ECMO will allow safe therapeutic regimens, such as suctioning or lung lavage, should these not be possible without the support.

Methods of ECMO
Three routes are available. The most popular is venoarterial bypass, which may improve oxygenation by three mechanisms: mixing in the aorta of oxygenator's effluent blood with left ventricular output, increased mixed venous oxygen content, and decrease of venous admixture in the lung by vascular decompression. If the improvement in PaO_2 is only by the first of these mechanisms, coronary arterial blood may be significantly desaturated.

The second route is venovenous bypass, which has the disadvantage that the oxygenator may scavenge already oxygenated blood. Additionally, the technique does not provide hemodynamic support, and pulmonary blood flow is not reduced.

The third route is the arteriovenous, which has the features of maintaining the load on the left ventricle and providing limited oxygenator flow.

Management During ECMO
The major hazards of ECMO are sepsis and hemorrhage due to the need to heparinize the patient's blood. During bypass, the FIO_2 is reduced to a point compatible with safe oxygenation. An FIO_2 of 0.6 should be achieved. The tidal volume and PEEP should probably be reduced. If, however, PEEP is in fact therapeutic in keeping airways open and allowing lung clearance, the latter move might be detrimental.

Future of ECMO
The published results of a multicenter randomized study conducted by the NIH showed that mortality of patients supported with or without ECMO was 9.5 and 8.3 percent, respectively [67]. The failure of ECMO to improve survival indicates that the support was instituted too late, that it is equally as damaging to the lung as FIO_2 and PEEP, or that without more specific treatment, merely buying time with support does not improve salvageability. It was of interest that the incidence of pneumothorax was 45 percent in both groups of patients. There was also no difference in the incidence of septicemia. In the management of the patients described in the report, and with the criteria for selection described, it was concluded that the use of ECMO is not justified until a therapy to produce or accelerate lung healing is available. A more recent, uncontrolled study has revived the suggestion that low-flow venovenous bypass is an effective alternative to conventional methods of treatment in patients with severe acute respiratory failure [25].

Lung Transplantation
Improvements in immunosuppression and surgical techniques have prolonged survival following lung transplantation. One study reported continued survival at 14 months and 24 months after the procedure [65]. The first indication for transplantation is in the presence of permanent destruction

of lung tissue to an extent incompatible with a reasonable quality of life. Second, transplantation has been thought of as providing a temporary, safer, long-term "membrane oxygenator."

Other Aspects of Management

Bronchodilating Agents

Detected increased lower airways resistance should be treated with bronchodilating agents. Initial route of choice is by inhalation, where lower blood levels are associated with similar therapeutic levels in the smooth muscles of the airway. The more specific beta-2 stimulants such as terbutaline (0.75–1.5 mg every 3 hr) should be used. Inhaled atropine (0.05–0.1 mg/kg) can also be used should the beta-2 agents fail to improve airway resistance. Where lung clearance is a problem, inhaled bronchodilators should be used even in the absence of expiratory rhonchi.

Persistent bronchospasm should be treated with the continuous infusion of aminophylline. A bolus of 5 mg/kg is initially given over 20 minutes. A continuous infusion of 0.7 mg/kg/hr is then maintained. Drug dosage is reduced by one-third in the presence of hepatic disease, congestive heart failure, and metabolic acidosis. Dosage is regulated by measuring plasma theophylline levels, which should be between 10 and 20 µg/ml. One study, however, reported that intravenous aminophylline increases the toxicity, but not the efficacy, of inhaled beta-adrenergic therapy in acute exacerbations of asthma [53, 58].

Corticosteroids

Corticosteroids are of undoubted value in the management of severe asthma. Their use in other forms of acute pulmonary disease is more questionable. A recent study has shown that in patients with established ARDS due to sepsis, aspiration, or a mixed cause, high-dose methylprednisolone does not affect outcome [6]. Two functions are attributed to the use of steroids: restoring or maintaining capillary wall integrity when this defect is thought to cause pulmonary edema, and aiding regeneration of surfactant production.

Nutrition

Nutrition is obviously essential in the care of critically ill patients. Nasogastric tube feeding or hyperalimentation should be started as appropriate within 3 days of hospitalization, if possible. The administration of lipids, rather than carbohydrates, as the primary energy source will decrease the respiratory quotient and carbon dioxide production, possibly facilitating the weaning of patients from mechanical ventilation.

Phosphorus and Magnesium Therapy

Hypophosphatemia impairs the contractile properties of the diaphragm in patients with acute respiratory failure. The maintenance of normal serum inorganic phosphate levels is therefore important in the care of such patients [2]. Similarly, the correction of hypomagnesemia with intravenous magnesium has been shown to improve ventilatory muscle power [44].

Monitoring the Progress of Pulmonary Disease

The essential question of whether the lung disease is improving, getting worse, or staying the same must be assessed at appropriate intervals. If the answer is that improvement is occurring, it is probably as well to leave the ventilatory support basically unchanged. Should the status be deteriorating, the support or treatment modalities must be reexamined and altered. It is essential, for any particular patient, to examine at intervals the factors that follow changes in pathophysiology most accurately. The more precise the understanding of the abnormalities, the fewer guides are necessary.

The following parameters may be helpful:

1. Simple pulmonary function tests. Measurement of vital capacity (3–5 consecutive measurements) should be made at intervals in cases of muscle weakness (e.g., myasthenia gravis). Forced expiratory volume in 1 second should also be measured in patients with chronic lung disease or asthma.
2. Alveolar-arterial oxygen tension difference while breathing F_{IO_2} 1.0 for 20 minutes can be measured at intervals. The advantages of this measurement are that it measures the predominant defect in most patients with acute lung disease, it can be used throughout the patient's course and provides easy comparisons of day-to-day alterations, groups of patients can also be easily compared, the range of PaO_2 measured (50–650 torr) allows for accurate interpretation of changes, and the F_{IO_2} is usually accurate. The disadvantage is that an F_{IO_2} 1.0 may increase the shunt and for that reason is less commonly used. The increase in shunt is usually immediately reversible on resuming a lower F_{IO_2} and is probably due to an alteration in pulmonary perfusion distribution [52].
3. Measurement of venous admixture by the application of the equation

$$\frac{\dot{Q}_s}{\dot{Q}_t} = \frac{CcO_2 - CaO_2}{CcO_2 - C\bar{v}O_2}$$

   where $\dot{Q}_s$ is that portion of total cardiac output ($\dot{Q}_t$) which perfuses unventilated alveoli, CcO_2 is capillary oxygen content, CaO_2 is arterial oxygen content, and $C\bar{v}O_2$ is mixed venous oxygen content.

   The use of this equation takes account of alterations in $C\bar{v}O_2$, which will increase $P(A\text{-}a)O_2$ in the presence of a constant amount of venous admixture. Mixed venous oxygen content is reduced by a decrease in cardiac output (oxygen consumption being unchanged) or hemoglobin or by a shift of the oxygen dissociation curve to the right.
4. Quantification of the fraction of a tidal breath that is dead space. Measurement of the carbon dioxide tension of mixed expired gas ($P\bar{E}CO_2$) and the tension in arterial blood ($PaCO_2$) allows calculation of dead space ventilation by the Enghoff modification of the Bohr equation:

$$\frac{V_D}{V_T} = \frac{PaCO_2 - P\bar{E}CO_2}{PaCO_2}$$

5. Mixed venous oxygen partial pressure. Interval monitoring of mixed venous oxygen partial pressure and saturation, with calculation of oxygen content, is a useful indicator of the appropriateness of oxygen delivery to the tissues. A value below 35 torr is an indication of tissue hypoxia.

6. Total effective compliance [tidal volume divided by (peak inspiratory pressure minus positive end-expiratory pressure)] is a guide to improvement of acute lung disease, where either lung compliance is reduced or airway resistance is increased.

7. Functional residual capacity is markedly reduced to less than 50 percent of predicted in many forms of acute lung disease.

8. Pulmonary artery pressure and calculated pulmonary vascular resistance are usually increased in the presence of acute parenchymal lung disease. The increase in PVR may become a primary cause of the development of systemic hypoperfusion as the pulmonary disease progresses. The use of vasodilating agents (e.g., sodium nitroprusside) to increase pulmonary blood flow is monitored by measurement of pulmonary artery pressure and cardiac output.

9. Measurement of PCWP is an essential guide to the management of high-pressure pulmonary edema. It is also of value in the management of fluid balance in acute lung disease where maintenance of low PCWP (< 10 torr) may minimize low pressure edema.

REFERENCES

1. Ashbaugh, D. G., et al. Continuous positive-pressure breathing (CPPB) in adult respiratory distress syndrome. *J. Thorac. Cardiovasc. Surg.* 57:31, 1969.

2. Aubier, M., et al. Effect of hypophosphatemia on diaphragmatic contractility in patients with acute respiratory failure. *N. Engl. J. Med.* 313:420, 1985.

3. Baker, A. B., et al. Effects of varying inspiratory flow waveform and time in intermittent positive pressure ventilation. II. Various physiological variables. *Br. J. Anaesth.* 49:1221, 1977.

4. Bell, W. R., et al. The clinical features of submassive and massive pulmonary emboli. *Am. J. Med.* 62:355, 1977.

5. Bergofsky, E. H. Pulmonary insufficiency after non-thoracic trauma: Shock lung. *Am. J. Med. Sci.* 264:93, 1972.

6. Bernard, G. R., et al. High-dose corticosteroids in patients with the adult respiratory distress syndrome. *N. Engl. J. Med.* 317:1565, 1987.

7. Borgia, J. F., et al. Persistent myocardial ischemia following chronic hyperoxia in conscious dogs. *J. Thorac. Cardiovasc. Surg.* 86:710, 1983.

8. Broquetas, J., et al. Oxprenolol-induced life-threatening bronchospasm. *Chest* 87:555, 1985. (Letter.)

9. Buda, A. J., et al. Effect of intrathoracic pressure on left ventricular performance. *N. Engl. J. Med.* 301:453, 1979.

10. Butler, W. J., et al. Ventilation of humans by high frequency oscillation. *Anesthesiology* (Suppl.) 51:S368, 1979.

11. Chamarro, H, et al. Tracheobronchial studies via transcricothyroid approach. *J.A.M.A.* 227:631, 1974.

12. Chastre, J., et al. Prospective evaluation of the protected specimen brush for the diagnosis of pulmonary infections in ventilated patients. *Am. Rev. Respir. Dis.* 130:924, 1984.

13. Cox, J. R., et al. The effect of positive pressure respiration on urinary aldosterone excretion. *Clin. Sci.* 24:1, 1963.

14. Cullen, D. J., and Caldera, D. L. The incidence of ventilator-induced pulmonary barotrauma in critically ill patients. *Anesthesiology* 50:185, 1979.

15. Dalen, J. E. (ed.). *Pulmonary Embolism.* New York: Medcom, 1972.

16. Dammann, J. F., et al. Optimal flow pattern for mechanical ventilation of the lungs. 2. The effect of a sine versus square wave flow pattern with and without an end-expiratory pause on patients. *Crit. Care Med.* 6:293, 1978.

17. Don, H. F., et al. The effect of anesthesia and 100% oxygen on the functional residual capacity of the lungs. *Anesthesiology* 32:521, 1970.
18. Don, H. F. Hypoxemia. In H. F. Don (ed.), *Decision Making in Critical Care.* Toronto: Decker, 1985.
19. Downs, J. B., et al. Comparison of assisted and controlled mechanical ventilation in anesthetized swine. *Crit. Care Med.* 7:5, 1979.
20. Dronen, S. C., et al. A comparison of blind nasotracheal and succinylcholine-assisted intubation in the poisoned patient. *Ann. Emerg. Med.* 16:650, 1987.
21. Dyck, D. R., et al. Acute respiratory distress in adults. *Radiology* 106:497, 1973.
22. Fein, A. M., et al. Is pulmonary artery catheterization necessary for the diagnosis of pulmonary edema? *Am. Rev. Respir. Dis.* 129:1006, 1984.
23. Foote, G. A., et al. Pulmonary complications of the flow-directed balloon-tipped catheter. *N. Engl. J. Med.* 290:927, 1974.
24. Froese, A. B., and Bryan, A. C. High frequency ventilation. *Am. Rev. Respir. Dis.* 135:1363, 1987.
25. Gattinoni, L., et al. Low-frequency positive pressure ventilation with extracorporeal CO_2 removal in severe acute respiratory failure. *J.A.M.A.* 256:881, 1986.
26. Gherini, S., et al. Mechanical work on the lungs and work of breathing with positive end-expiratory pressure and continuous positive airway pressure. *Chest* 76:251, 1979.
27. Gore, J. M., et al. A community-wide assessment of the use of pulmonary artery catheters in patients with acute myocardial infarction. *Chest* 92:721, 1987.
28. Greenbaum, D. M. Positive end-expiratory pressure, constant positive airway pressure, and cardiac performance. *Chest* 76:248, 1979.
29. Hemmer, M., and Suter, P. M. Treatment of cardiac and renal effects of PEEP with dopamine in patients with acute respiratory failure. *Anesthesiology* 50:399, 1979.
30. Hill, S. L., et al. Changes in lung water and capillary permeability following sepsis and fluid overload. *Crit. Care Med.* 7:137, 1979. (Abstract.)
31. Holody, B., and Goldberg, H. S. The effect of mechanical vibration physiotherapy on arterial oxygenation in acutely ill patients with atelectasis or pneumonia. *Am. Rev. Respir. Dis.* 124:372, 1981.
32. Hull, R. D., et al. Diagnostic value of ventilation-perfusion lung scanning in patients with suspected pulmonary embolism. *Chest* 88:819, 1985.
33. Kirby, R. R., et al. High level positive end expiratory pressure (PEEP) in acute respiratory insufficiency. *Chest* 67:156, 1975.
34. Kovacs, J. A., et al. Diagnosis of *Pneumocystis carinii:* Improved detection in sputum with use of monoclonal antibodies. *N. Engl. J. Med.* 318:589, 1988.
35. Kumar, A., et al. Inappropriate response to increased plasma ADH during mechanical ventilation in acute respiratory failure. *Anesthesiology* 40:215, 1974.
36. Lahiri, B., and ZuWallack, R. The early diagnosis and treatment of fat embolism syndrome: A preliminary report. *J. Trauma* 17:956, 1977.
37. Leight, G. S., Jr., et al. Open lung biopsy for the diagnosis of acute, diffuse pulmonary infiltrates in the immunosuppressed patient. *Chest* 73:477, 1978.
38. Loeber, N. V., and Don, H. F. Effect of lung, chest wall, and total static compliance on pleural pressure changes during mechanical ventilation with PEEP. In Abstracts of Scientific Papers, for the Annual Meeting of the American Society of Anesthesiologists, 1978. P. 449.

39. Lopez, M., and Salvaggio, J. Hypersensitivity pneumonitis: Current concepts of etiology and pathogenesis. *Ann. Rev. Med.* 27:453, 1976.

40. Lund, T., et al. Upper airway sequelae in burn patients requiring endotracheal intubation or tracheostomy. *Ann. Surg.* 201:374, 1985.

41. Luterman, A., et al. Withdrawal from positive end-expiratory pressure. *Surgery* 83:328, 1978.

42. MacIntyre, N. R. Respiratory function during pressure support ventilation. *Chest* 89:677, 1986.

43. Maroko, P. R., et al. Reduction of infarct size by oxygen inhalation following acute coronary occlusion. *Circulation* 52:360, 1975.

44. Molloy, D. W., et al. Hypomagnesemia and respiratory muscle power. *Am. Rev. Respir. Dis.* 129:497, 1984.

45. Myerowitz, R. L., et al. Opportunistic lung infection due to "Pittsburgh pneumonia agent." *N. Engl. J. Med.* 301:953, 1979.

46. Norris, J. V., and Don, H. F. Prolonged depression of respiratory rate following methadone analgesia. *Anesthesiology* 45:361, 1976.

47. O'Reilly, M. J., et al. Sepsis from sinusitis in nasotracheally intubated patients. *Am. J. Surg.* 147:601, 1984.

48. Pepe, P. E., and Marini, J. J. Occult positive end-expiratory pressure in mechanically ventilated patients with airflow obstruction. *Am. Rev. Respir. Dis.* 126:166, 1982.

49. Pepe, P. E., et al. Early application of positive end-expiratory pressure in patients at risk for the adult respiratory-distress syndrome. *N. Engl. J. Med.* 311:281, 1984.

50. Petty, T. L. The use, abuse, and mystique of positive end-expiratory pressure. *Am. Rev. Respir. Dis.* 138:475, 1988.

51. Quan, S. F., et al. Changes in venous admixture with alterations of inspired oxygen concentration. *Anesthesiology* 52:477, 1980.

52. Quan, S. F., et al. The effect of varying inspired oxygen concentrations on calculated intrapulmonary shunt. Abstracts of Scientific Papers for the Annual Meeting of the American Society of Anesthesiologists, 1978. P. 453.

53. Rebuck, A. S. Nebulized anticholinergic and sympathomimetic treatment of asthma and chronic obstructive airways disease in the emergency room. *Am. J. Med.* 82:59, 1987.

54. Rinaldo, J. E., and Rogers, R. M. Adult respiratory distress syndrome: changing concepts of lung injury and repair. *N. Engl. J. Med.* 306:900, 1982.

55. Rossiter, S. J., et al. Open lung biopsy in the immunosuppressed patient. Is it really beneficial? *J. Thorac. Cardiovasc. Surg.* 77:338, 1979.

56. Sackner, M. A., et al. Applications of bronchofiberoscopy. *Chest* (Suppl.) 62:70S, 1972.

57. Sanyal, S. K., et al. Continuous negative chest-wall pressure therapy in management of severe hypoxemia due to aspiration pneumonitis: A case report. *Respir. Care* 24:1022, 1979.

58. Siegel, D., et al. Aminophylline increases the toxicity but not the efficacy of an inhaled beta-adrenergic agonist in the treatment of acute exacerbations of asthma. *Am. Rev. Respir. Dis.* 132:283, 1985.

59. Singer, C., et al. Diffuse pulmonary infiltrates in immunosuppressed patients. Prospective study of 80 cases. *Am. J. Med.* 66:110, 1979.

60. Sjöstrand, U. Pneumatic systems facilitating treatment of respiratory insufficiency with alternative use of IPPV/PEEP, HFPPV/PEEP, CPPB or CPAP. *Acta Anaesth. Scand.* (Suppl.) 64:123, 1977.

61. Springer, R. R., and Stevens, P. M. The influence of PEEP on survival of patients in respiratory failure. A retrospective analysis. *Am. J. Med.* 66:196, 1979.

62. Sturgeon, C. L., et al. PEEP and CPAP: Cardiopulmonary effects during spontaneous ventilation. *Anesth. Analg.* 56:633, 1977.
63. Suter, P. M., et al. Optimum end-expiratory airway pressure in patients with acute pulmonary failure. *N. Engl. J. Med.* 292:284, 1975.
64. Suter, P. M., et al. Effect of tidal volume and positive end-expiratory pressure on compliance during mechanical ventilation. *Chest* 73:158, 1978.
65. Toronto Lung Transplant Group. Unilateral lung transplantation for pulmonary fibrosis. *N. Engl. J. Med.* 314:1140, 1986.
66. Venus, B., et al. Treatment of the adult respiratory distress syndrome with continuous positive airway pressure. *Chest* 76:257, 1979.
67. Zapol, W. M., et al. Extracorporeal membrane oxygenation in severe acute respiratory failure. *J.A.M.A.* 242:2193, 1979.
68. Zwillich, C. W., et al. Complications of assisted ventilation. *Am. J. Med.* 57:161, 1974.

Oxygen Administration

Robert L. Smith

One of the most important functions of the lungs is to supply oxygen to the mixed venous blood passing through the pulmonary capillary bed. The proper oxygenation of blood in the lungs depends on many factors that may be affected by disorders of the lungs. Whenever the normal matching of ventilation and blood flow in the myriad of peripheral lung units is disturbed by disease, hypoxemia is a regular consequence. Also, hypoxemia results when the barrier for diffusion of oxygen from the alveoli to the capillaries is increased by diseases such as pulmonary fibrosis. Finally, even though ventilation and blood flow are evenly matched and diffusion is normal, a decrease in the overall level of alveolar ventilation can reduce the partial pressure of oxygen in the alveoli and lead to hypoxemia.

Hypoxemia and the resulting alterations in oxygen delivery to the peripheral tissues can have serious effects on the function of vital organs, including the brain and the heart. Even moderate degrees of brain hypoxia may produce muscular discoordination, restlessness, and confusion. Inadequate oxygen delivery to the heart can eventually result in bradycardia and hypotension. However, hypoxemia and its consequences can be relieved even in the presence of severe lung disorders by the administration of supplemental oxygen.

At sea level, atmospheric air contains 20.93 percent oxygen and has a partial pressure (PO_2) of about 159 mm Hg. As inspired air passes over the upper respiratory tract, it is heated and humidified and its water vapor pressure increases. Because of the uptake of oxygen from the alveoli and the transfer of carbon dioxide from the mixed venous blood into the alveoli, the partial pressure of oxygen in the alveolar air (P_AO_2) is only about 100 to 110 mm Hg. Normally, the arterial PO_2 is about 80 to 90 mm Hg, depending on age, but this value will be reduced by disorders of the lung that result in a mismatching of ventilation and blood flow or produce a diffusion defect. Regardless of impairments in lung functions, the alveolar PO_2 and, consequently, the arterial PO_2 can be altered by increasing the concentration of oxygen in the inspired air.

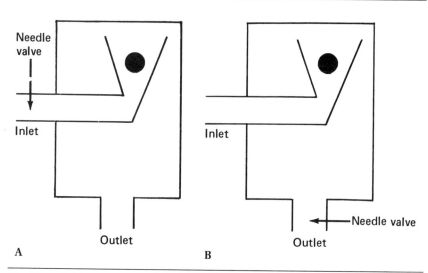

Fig. 11-1. A. Non–pressure-compensated flowmeter. B. Pressure-compensated flowmeter.

FLOWMETERS

The flow of oxygen from either wall or cylinder sources is indicated by a flowmeter. The flowmeter produces a pressure drop from 50 ψ at the gas inlet to atmospheric pressure at the outlet. A needle valve that controls the flow of oxygen is regulated by an adjusting wheel, and the rate of gas flow is indicated by the level of a ball float suspended in the airstream within the flow tube. The float is suspended in the airstream because of the difference in pressure on either side of the float.

In non–pressure-compensated systems, the needle valve is placed between the gas inlet and the ball float. Normally, the pressure at the gas outlet is at atmospheric levels, but with any narrowing or partial obstruction at the gas outlet, the pressure difference across the float and, consequently, the position of the float will change even though the rate of airflow may be maintained.

The commonly used flowmeters are pressure compensated. The needle valve is located downstream between the ball and the gas outlet, so that even with a blockage at the flowmeter outlet, the position of the ball float will accurately reflect the rate of gas flow (Fig. 11-1).

HUMIDIFICATION

Continuous oxygen flow from both wall and cylinder sources is dry. Even in patients breathing in the usual manner through the nose and mouth, the gas must be humidified or it will produce drying and irritation of the mucous membranes of the upper respiratory tract.

Humidifiers

Adequate humidification of oxygen delivered at low-to-medium flow rates to patients breathing by mouth or nose can be achieved with a simple humidifier. The most commonly used type is the bubble humidifier. From the flowmeter, oxygen passes down a tube and through a porous head submerged under water, forming small bubbles that return to the surface. As the bubbles rise through the water, the pressure of vaporization forces water vapor into the oxygen. Further vaporization occurs at the water surface when the bubbles break.

The efficiency of the bubble humidifier will depend on a number of factors. Smaller bubbles promote better humidification by increasing the surface area of gas exposed to water. Also, the length of time of contact of gas and water is important in promoting humidification. The humidifier jar must be properly filled, to ensure that the bubbles of oxygen pass through as much water as possible.

Oxygen passing through a bubble humidifier is only about 40 percent saturated with water vapor at body temperature; complete humidification is achieved by some water loss from the upper respiratory tract.

METHODS OF OXYGEN ADMINISTRATION

The basic objective of oxygen administration is to increase the concentration of oxygen in the inspired air. This can be accomplished in a variety of ways, depending on the required degree of oxygen enrichment of inspired air and the need for humidification.

Supplemental oxygen is most commonly administered through a nasal cannula, simple face mask, or face mask with reservoir bag, using low rates of oxygen flow from a tank or wall source.

In some circumstances, when the concentration of oxygen in the inspired air must be accurately and tightly controlled, a high-airflow system with oxygen enrichment, using a jet-mixing or Venturi apparatus, is employed.

In patients with endotracheal tubes or tracheostomies, medium- and high-flow systems using a Briggs adaptor or tracheostomy mask are used to ensure not only supplemental oxygen delivery, but also proper humidification of inspired air.

Nasal Cannula

The nasal cannula (Fig. 11-2) consists of two short plastic prongs that fit into the external nares and are connected to the oxygen supply. Because of its comfort and simplicity, the nasal cannula is the preferred method of administration of low-to-moderate concentrations of supplemental oxygen.

The continuous flow of oxygen through the cannula displaces air in the nasal passages, pharynx, and larynx and creates an oxygen reservoir in this area. When the contents of the pharynx and larynx are added to room air during inspiration, an increase in the concentration of oxygen in the inspired air is achieved.

At a flow rate of 1 liter/min the inspired-oxygen concentration increases

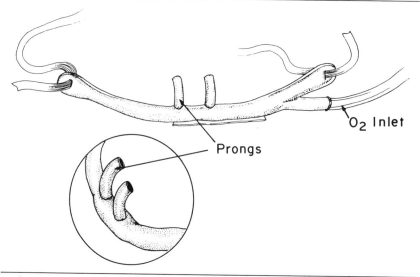

Fig. 11-2. Nasal cannula.

to approximately 24 percent. At flow rates of 6 to 8 liter/min the reservoir in the nasopharynx and larynx generally is optimally filled with oxygen, and the inspired-oxygen concentration rises to about 40 to 45 percent. Further increases in oxygen flow produce little additional increase in the inspired oxygen concentration.

The effect of a given flow of oxygen through the nasal cannula on the overall inspired-oxygen concentration will also depend on the size of the tidal volume and the volume of ventilation. If ventilation falls but the oxygen flow is maintained, the inspired-oxygen concentration will rise.

Because of variations in the level of ventilation, precise regulation of the inspired-oxygen concentration is not possible with a nasal cannula.

In order that oxygen administered by nasal cannula be effective in raising the inspired-oxygen concentration, it is clearly important that the nasal passages be patent. However, nasally administered oxygen is as effective in raising the inspired-oxygen concentration in mouth breathers as it is in nose breathers.

The major advantages of the nasal cannula are its simplicity, its comfort, and the fact that oxygen administration does not have to be discontinued during eating or coughing.

Recently developed alternatives for administering supplemental oxygen with enhanced conservation benefits include the reservoir cannulae, pulsed oxygen delivery, and transtracheal oxygen delivery.

Transtracheal oxygen administration is a new mode of delivering continuous oxygen directly to the lower airways via a small catheter inserted into the trachea at the base of the neck [7].

The most commonly reported advantages of transtracheal oxygen administration are decreased oxygen flow rates, increased patient mobility, avoidance of nasal and ear irritation, improved patient compliance, provision of an alternative for treating refractory hypoxemia, and a more acceptable appearance. In addition, restoration of normal sleep, reduced dyspnea, and improved ability to smell and taste, as well as improved appetite, are occasionally observed.

Disadvantages of transtracheal procedure include bleeding, subcutaneous emphysema, abscess, pneumothorax, bronchospasm, respiratory failure, and pneumonia.

Pulse oxygen devices deliver oxygen only during inspiration. These devices, while using less oxygen, provide results (PaO$_2$ and %Hb Sat) [1] equivalent to results obtainable with continuous-flow oxygen systems in conjunction with a nasal cannula. Further, supplemental humidification is not required for flow rate setting (1–6 liter/min) with nasal cannula [3, 5].

Face Mask

A common alternative method of administering supplemental oxygen is by face mask. Oxygen face masks are shown in Figures 11-3, 11-4 and 11-5. The mask has side ports and may be equipped with a reservoir bag.

Depending on the presence of a reservoir bag and whether or not the ports are fitted with directional valves, the inspired-oxygen concentration can be increased to about 40 to 90 percent using a face mask. The face mask is somewhat less comfortable than the nasal cannula, but the major disadvantage is that the mask must be removed for eating, drinking, coughing, and expectoration.

Simple Mask

Oxygen from a wall or cylinder source passes through the flowmeter and humidifier directly into the mask (Fig. 11-3), displacing air and creating a small oxygen reservoir. During inspiration, the oxygen in the mask is inhaled. In addition, some room air is entrained through the ports and through the spaces between the mask and the face, so that the inspired-oxygen concentration is considerably less than 100 percent. The extent to which the inspired-oxygen concentration can be increased is dependent on the volume of the oxygen reservoir, determined by the size of the mask. Even the simple face mask can provide inspired-oxygen concentrations that are higher than can be achieved with the nasal cannula. Generally, oxygen flow rates of 6 to 10 liters/min through a simple face mask raise the inspired-oxygen concentration to 35 to 55 percent.

Mask with Reservoir Bag

Further increases in inspired-oxygen concentration can be provided by the addition of a reservoir bag to the face mask (Fig. 11-4), thus enlarging the potential reservoir of oxygen. Inspired gas is made up primarily of the oxygen in the mask and reservoir bag, with smaller amounts of room air passing through the ports of the mask.

During exhalation, most of the expired air passes out through the ports, but some expired air returns to the reservoir bag. This undesirable dead space effect results in a fall of the PO$_2$ and a rise in the PCO$_2$ in the bag and must be avoided by ensuring a sufficiently high rate of oxygen flow to keep

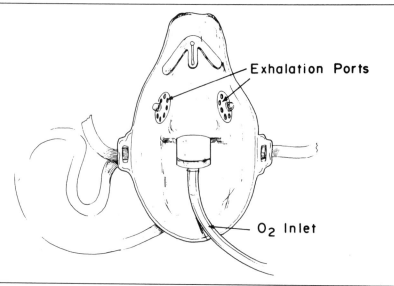

Fig. 11-3. Simple mask.

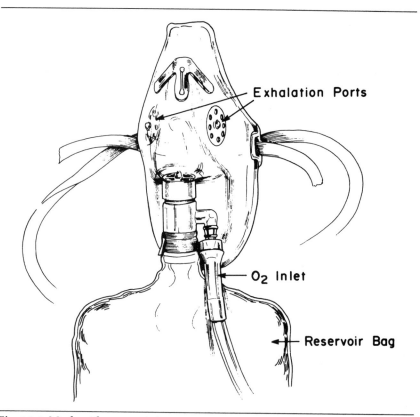

Fig. 11-4. Mask with reservoir bag.

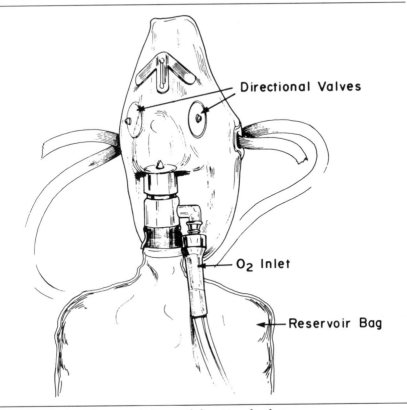

Fig. 11-5. Mask with reservoir bag and directional valves.

the bag washed out. Oxygen flow rates of 8 to 10 liter/min are commonly used with the mask and reservoir bag; this provides an inspired-oxygen concentration of between 50 and 80 percent. However, the rate of oxygen flow must be adjusted such that inspiration empties the reservoir bag by no more than a half.

Mask with Reservoir Bag and Directional Valves
The flow of room air into the face mask through the side ports during inspiration can be completely prevented by covering the side ports with directional valves (Fig. 11-5). The entire volume of the breath during inspiration, with the exception of the small amount of air that passes between the mask and face, will then be made up of oxygen from the mask and reservoir bag. When directional valves are employed, it is critical that the rate of oxygen flow be high—in the range of 12 to 15 liter/min. In this manner, the inspired-oxygen concentration can be raised to as high as 90 to 95 percent.

Since virtually all of the inspired gas comes from the mask and bag, it is critically important that adequate oxygen flows be maintained. If the res-

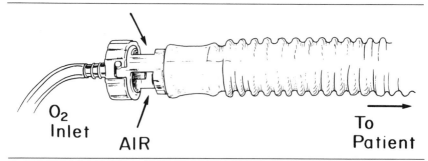

Fig. 11-6. Diagram of high-airflow system with oxygen enrichment.

ervoir bag is inadvertently allowed to empty, asphyxia may occur, particularly in the debilitated patient.

During exhalation, the port valves open, and expired air passes out of the mask to the atmosphere. The passage of expired air back into the reservoir bag may also be prevented by a directional valve situated between the mask and the bag.

HIGH-AIRFLOW SYSTEMS WITH OXYGEN ENRICHMENT
High-airflow systems with oxygen enrichment (Fig. 11-6) employ the principle of air entrainment with constant-pressure jet mixing.

A jet of oxygen from a wall or tank source is passed through a precision orifice and results in the entrainment of room air through ports in the surrounding cylinder. The amount of entrainment and the final oxygen concentration of the gas in the mask can be varied by using different sizes of orifices and different rates of oxygen flow.

Commercially available high-flow systems are designed to deliver oxygen concentrations of 24 to 50 percent.

Data regarding oxygen flow, air/oxygen dilution, and total gas flow are shown in Tables 11-1 and 11-2.

The major advantages of the high-airflow systems with oxygen enrichment are that the total gas flow is maintained at high levels and that the concentration of inspired oxygen is kept constant even over a fairly wide range of oxygen flow rates and is independent of the size of the tidal volume and the minute volume of ventilation. This is particularly important in patients with chronic obstructive pulmonary disease and alveolar hypoventilation, who tend to hypoventilate progressively as the arterial oxygen tension is increased.

NEBULIZER
Greater humidifying and warming of inspired air are required in patients in whom the normal heating and humidifying mechanisms of the upper respiratory tract are bypassed by a tracheostomy or endotracheal tube.

Large amounts of humidification can be achieved with a nebulizer (Fig. 11-7), a device that produces a suspension of fine water droplets. Basically, a nebulizer is made up of an inlet tube, an attached perpendicular draw

Table 11-1. Obtainable oxygen concentrations with low
flow oxygen administration devices

Device	Oxygen flow (liter/min)	Oxygen concentration
Nasal cannula	6–8	40–45%
Simple mask	6–10	35–55%
Mask with reservoir	8–12	50–80%
Mask with reservoir and directional valves	10–15	90–95%

Table 11-2. High-airflow systems with oxygen enrichment

Oxygen concentration (%)	Oxygen flow (liter/min)	Air/oxygen ratio	Total gas flow (liter/min)
24	4	25/1	104
28	4–6	10/1	44–66
31	6–8	7/1	48–64
35	8–10	5/1	48–60
40	8–12	3/1	32–48
50	12	1.75/1	33

tube partly submerged in water, and a baffle. Oxygen passes through the
narrow inlet tube at a high flow rate, causing the pressure at the end of the
draw tube to fall below atmospheric pressure, according to Venturi's principle. Consequent to the pressure drop within the draw tube, water moves
up the tube into the stream of gas and is propelled against the baffle, where
the liquid is broken up into a suspension of fine drops, generally ranging
in size from 0.5 to 5.0 μ.

The oxygen leaving the nebulizer may be fully saturated at ambient temperature, but the water in the nebulizer must be heated to ensure full humidification at body temperature. By incorporating a heater into the nebulizer, the water can be heated to a level about 10° to 15°C greater than
body temperature to compensate for temperature loss as the gas passes
along the tubing to the patient (tubing 3–5 ft in length with ¾ in. inside
diameter).

When inspired gas is heated and humidified by means of a nebulizer,
water loss from the airways can be completely eliminated.

DEVICES FOR THE DELIVERY OF HIGHLY HUMIDIFIED GAS MIXTURES

Warmed and highly humidified gas mixtures must be provided to patients
with tracheostomies and endotracheal tubes, in order to avoid drying out
of the tracheal and bronchial mucosa. Humidified gas mixtures may also

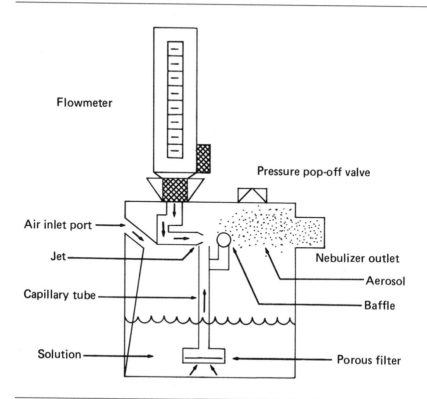

Flowmeter

Pressure pop-off valve

Air inlet port

Jet

Nebulizer outlet

Aerosol

Capillary tube

Baffle

Solution

Porous filter

Fig. 11-7. Diagram of mechanical nebulizer.

be administered to patients following extubation and to patients with thick tracheobronchial secretions.

Humidification is provided with a nebulizer. In patients with tracheostomies and endotracheal tubes, the nebulizer is also heated, although in individuals breathing through the mouth and nose, heating of the gas mixture may not be necessary. Some find the heated gas mixtures to be quite uncomfortable.

Aerosol Mask

This device (Fig. 11-8) consists of a plastic mask with open side ports. The mask is connected to a large-bore delivery tube for the delivery of humidified gas.

Face Tent

The face tent (Fig. 11-9) is a plastic wraparound half-mask that is positioned around the chin and cheeks. The humidified oxygen mixture is delivered from the bottom of the unit while expired air passes out through the open upper portion.

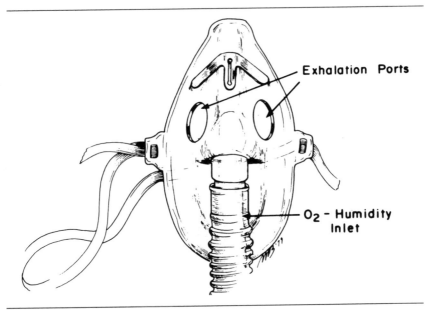

Fig. 11-8. Aerosol mask.

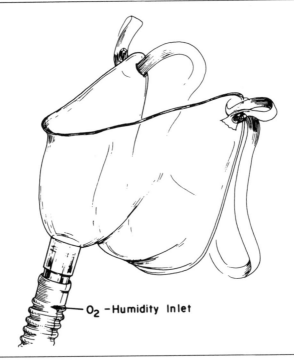

Fig. 11-9. Face tent.

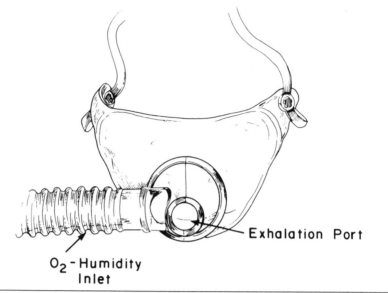

Exhalation Port

O_2-Humidity
Inlet

Fig. 11-10. Tracheostomy mask.

Tracheostomy Mask

This consists of a soft, small plastic mask positioned over a tracheostomy tube or stoma (Fig. 11-10). The major disadvantage of this apparatus is that patients are able to breathe unheated and poorly humidified room air around the mask.

Briggs Adaptor

The use of a Briggs adaptor (Fig. 11-11) or T piece in patients with an endotracheal or tracheostomy tube ensures that inspired gas consists only of the prescribed heated oxygen mixture. This large bore T-shaped apparatus is fitted directly onto the endotracheal or tracheostomy tube. The heated, nebulized gas mixture is delivered through one limb of the T, while expired air leaves by the other. An additional length of tubing fitted to the expiratory limb of the T-piece can serve as a reservoir when the patient's inspiratory flow rate exceeds the rate of flow of the gas mixture from the source.

HAZARDS AND PRECAUTIONS

The administration of supplemental oxygen is clearly important in the management of patients with hypoxemia. However beneficial it may be, oxygen administration is not without risk and potential dangers.

Inspired gas must be properly humidified in order to avoid drying of the mucous membranes of the tracheobronchial tree. Improper humidification, particularly with high-airflow systems and in patients with tracheos-

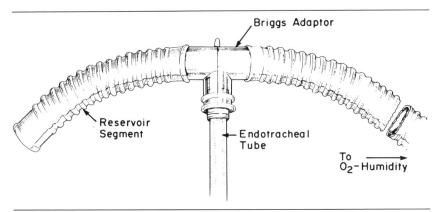

Fig. 11-11. Briggs adaptor.

tomies and endotracheal tubes, can interfere with mucociliary clearance mechanisms and result in drying and inspissation of airway secretions.

The prolonged administration of high concentrations of supplemental oxygen can produce toxic effects on the lung. The likelihood of this occurrence can be significantly reduced by ensuring that no more oxygen is given than that required to achieve a normal arterial PO_2.

In patients with chronic obstructive pulmonary disease, alveolar hypoventilation, and chronic arterial hypercapnia, respiratory responses to hypercapnia are blunted, and respiratory stimulation occurs solely as a consequence of hypoxemia. The administration of excessive supplemental oxygen in these patients has a tendency to promote increasing hypoventilation, with a resulting progressive rise in PCO_2. It is particularly important to maintain the inspired-oxygen concentration at a fixed, unvarying level by using a high-airflow system with oxygen enrichment and to aim to achieve an arterial PO_2 no greater than 55 to 60 mm Hg.

All parts of any oxygen delivery system must be checked on a regular basis. Flowmeters must reliably reflect the rate of supplemental oxygen delivery. Water in humidifiers and particularly in heated nebulizers may become contaminated with bacteria that can be transmitted to the patient's respiratory tract. Thus, these pieces of equipment must be changed at least daily. All connections must be tight, and kinking and obstructions due to condensation accumulation in tubing must be avoided.

Finally, oxygen administration should be monitored carefully. The use of arterial blood gases, pulse oximetry, and transcutaneous oxygen monitoring will provide substantial information for evaluating the effectiveness of supplemental oxygen administration.

REFERENCES

1. Brooks, C. J., et al. Performance of a demand oxygen saver system during rest, exercise, and sleep in hypoxemic patients. Kansas City Pulmonary Clinic and Research Medical Center, Kansas City, Missouri. Presented at the American Thoracic Society, May 1986.

2. Egan, D. F. *Fundamentals of Respiratory Therapy* (3d ed.). St. Louis: Mosby, 1977.
3. Floreani, A., Kerby, G. R., Pingelton, S. K., Whitman, R. A., and Shippy, M. B. Evaluation of a demand flow oxygen delivery device. *Chest* 89:484S, 1986.
4. Heimlich, H. J. Respiratory rehabilitation with transtracheal oxygen system. *Ann. Otol. Rhinol. Laryngol.* 91:643, 1982.
5. Kerby, G. R., and O'Donohue, W. Comparison of continuous and pulse flow oxygen in hospital patients. The University of Kansas Medical Center, Kansas City, Kansas and AMI St. Joseph Hospital at Creighton University, Omaha, Nebraska. 1987.
6. McPherson, S. P. *Respiratory Therapy Equipment*. St. Louis: Mosby, 1977.
7. Scacci, R. Air entrainment masks: Jet mixing is how they work; the Bernoulli and Venturi principles are how they don't. *Respir. Care* 24:928, 1979.
8. Shapiro, B. A., Harrison, R. A., and Walton, J. R. *Clinical Application of Blood Gases* (2d ed.) Chicago: Year Book, 1977.
9. Spofford, B. T., Christopher, K. C., McCarty, D. C., and Goodman, J. R. Scoop transtracheal oxygen therapy—A guide for the Respiratory Therapist. *Respir. Care* 32:345, 1987.

12

Physiologic Diagnosis and Management of Acute Pulmonary Insufficiency in the Adult Respiratory Distress Syndrome

John H. Siegel and Joan C. Stoklosa

ETIOLOGIC FACTORS IN THE ADULT RESPIRATORY DISTRESS SYNDROME

The development of the adult respiratory distress syndrome (ARDS) following traumatic injury or sepsis represents one of the most serious and often fatal complications of injury or major infection [75, 79, 99]. Its incidence has been shown to be approximately 7 percent in critically ill [36, 37] or injured [44] patients. However, the presence of acute aspiration has been shown to increase the chance of the development of ARDS to more than 35 percent, and posttrauma patients having two or more major-system injuries in association with soft-tissue trauma, chest injury, and shock have been demonstrated to have an incidence in excess of 40 percent as a consequence of the interaction of these types of complex injuries. Despite present methods of cardiovascular and ventilatory support, the ARDS mortality rate remains high, ranging from 41 percent in a large series of blunt trauma patients [44] to nearly 65 percent in a general series of ICU patients in whom a variety of intercurrent diseases were also present [36, 37]. In the early phase of ARDS the major problem appears to be respiratory insufficiency, which is due to acute inflammation of the alveolar capillary endothelium and interstitium with invasion of neutrophils, monocytes, and fibroblasts [3, 21, 63, 74]. This stage often progresses to a state of acute and chronic respiratory failure related to a combination of hypoxemia, nosocomial pneumonia, and fibrosis [8, 73, 125]. However, ARDS in the late phase of the disease is frequently a component of what has been known as the multiple organ failure syndrome (MOFS) and may indeed be the initial event in the sequence of fatal organ failures characterizing this poorly understood pathophysiologic process [8, 29, 73, 75, 99].

The Role of Mediators in the Evolution of ARDS

The etiologic factors in the development of human ARDS are not fully established. However, a number of important relationships have been elucidated. These appear related to the initiation of the major cascade of complement activation secondary to the primary insult, such as soft-tissue injury with hemorrhage, that initiates the coagulation and Hageman factor sequence [51, 52], or the defense mechanisms initiated by bacterial sepsis, especially those associated with endotoxin-producing bacteria [8]. An early mediator in this process appears to be related to the appearance of the C5a by-product of complement activation sequence. [49, 117] This may initiate early aspects of the neutrophil response that is a prominent feature of this disease process. The neutrophils play an important role in the evolution of ARDS through their ability to release a variety of enzymes, such as elastase, lysozymes, cathepsins, collagenase, and myeloperoxidase, that can attack and degrade the integrity of the alveolar capillary basement membrane [29, 121]. In addition, the neutrophils, when appropriately stimulated, have the capability of generating toxic oxygen radicals known as superoxides, which can produce direct injury to the lung capillary endothelium [117, 121, 123].

Several other major sequences have been suggested as initiating or priming events in the evolution of ARDS. These appear related to the two major pathways (cyclooxygenase and lipoxygenase) of arachidonic acid metabolism when that compound is freed from membrane phospholipids [51, 65]. This sequence may be initiated by a number of events. However, an apparently important factor in the mobilization of this sequence, which begins with membrane phospholipase A2 activation, is the release of platelet-activating factor (PAF). This has been implicated in a number of key biologic reactions related to the initiation of the ARDS process: platelet aggregation, neutrophil aggregation, and the induction of the cyclooxygenase and lipoxygenase pathways resulting from the arachidonic acid release [51, 52, 65]. The activation of these two pathways, resulting in the prostaglandin end products and the leukotrienes from the cyclooxygenase and lipoxygenase sequences, respectively, appear to have major effects as mediators of the ARDS process. The two major eicosanoid factors resulting from the cyclooxygenase pathway are thromboxane A_2, which produces vascular smooth-muscle constriction and platelet aggregation, and prostacyclin $PGF_1\alpha$, which tends to counteract the thromboxane action by vasodilatation, membrane stabilization, and platelet deaggregation [27, 51]. Other important prostaglandins released by this pathway are PGE_2, which is thought to have an immune suppressant effect; and $PGF_2\alpha$, which, like thromboxane A_2, is also a potent vasoconstrictor [29, 52]. The vasoconstrictor cyclooxygenase mediators, especially thromboxane A_2, are felt to be responsible for the acute pulmonary hypertension and microvascular thrombus formation that are features of the early aspects of the ARDS syndrome. The other arachidonic acid pathway, that of lipoxygenase, induces the formation of a variety of leukotrienes from the HPETE sequence [29, 31, 51, 65]. These substances, especially LTC_4, D_4, and E_4, produce additional pulmonary vasoconstriction [31]. Leukotriene B_4 (LTB_4) appears to augment neutrophil endothelial adherence, and increase capillary permeability, and it may play a role in the induction of the leukocyte respiratory burst with resultant superoxide formation that is felt to be a major causative factor in ARDS lung damage [29, 65, 117, 121].

A poorly understood but apparently very important set of factors comprises those released from the macrophages (monocyte activation). These appear to be a somewhat later phenomenon than the initial events previously described. The inflammatory modulators (monokines) include interleukin 1 (IL1) and tumor necrosis factor (TNF). Both of these play an important role in initiating the hypermetabolic and catabolic states seen in sepsis and in ARDS, and they also may be related to the induction of the later multiple organ failure syndrome [29]. However, with regard to ARDS, IL1 appears to have an important attractant effect on neutrophils and monocytes and may be related to the induction of neutrophil degranulation and endothelial adherence by this class of white cell [29, 121, 123, 126]. TNF has been implicated in the permeability changes that are characteristic of the ARDS syndrome [111]. The altered alveolar capillary permeability is most related to the abnormal respiratory gas exchange. This is manifested in the increase in the alveolar-arterial oxygen gradient and to the decrease in the compliance of the lung parenchyma. Several other factors, such as histamines and serotonins, have also been implicated in the ARDS process, although their present roles are not so clearly defined as they were once thought to be.

The importance of these factors in the evolution of this disease process lies in the potential for the development of specific pharmacologic blocking agents to interrupt or impede the various aspects of these complex and interacting pathways. A variety of these agents that appeared useful in experimental ARDS [51, 108, 120] have been tried in clinical settings without much success, including the nonsteroidal anti-inflammatory agent ibuprofen, which blocks the formation of thromboxane A_2, as well as steroids that reduce the propensity for the complement cascade induction [29]. More recently, specific blockers of PAF or of the leukotriene or cyclooxygenase pathways, as well as superoxide scavengers, have been attempted in experimentally induced ARDS [29, 51, 65]. At present, however, no specific pharmacotherapy for this disease exists. Although it is expected that a better understanding of the process of mediator activation may allow effective medical therapy to prevent or ameliorate this disease, the mainstay of contemporary therapy remains early and effective cardiovascular and ventilatory support of the respiratory function, until the initiating factors can be removed by excision of dead tissue and control of invading bacterial sepsis by surgical drainage and appropriate antibiotics [99].

Pathophysiologic Processes Leading to Abnormalities in Respiratory Gas Exchange

The consequence of the alveolar capillary injury induced by the sequence of mediator interactions in the ARDS process is a change in capillary permeability that induces an increased lymph flow, as well as an increase in the alveolar capillary interstitial fluid [110]. This alteration appears to follow the classic Starling's law of capillary action [64, 109], formulated as $\dot{Q}_f = K_f(P_{IV} - P_{EV}) - \sigma(II_{IV} - II_{EV})$, in which the flow of fluid from the alveolar capillary to the pulmonary interstitium ($\dot{Q}_f$) is a function of the permeability of the capillary membrane (K_f) times the intramicrovascular (P_{IV})-to–extramicrovascular (P_{EV}) pressure gradient, minus the reflection coefficient (σ) of the membrane to colloid, times the intramicrovascular (II_{IV})–to–extramicrovascular (II_{EV}) osmotic pressure gradient. Thus, the resuscitative process following a major injury that necessitates increasing intravascular volume by infusion, usually with crystalloids that lower intravascular colloid oncotic pressure, tends to increase the net lymph flow through the altered pulmonary alveolar capillary into the pulmonary interstitial space. This results in an impairment in the diffusion of oxygen from the alveolus across the capillary membrane into the blood, as well as a marked reduction in alveolar compliance, as it is harder to distend an alveolus surrounded by fluid. Consequently, the alveolar volume is reduced, as is the functional residual capacity (FRC) of the lung.

There also appear to be alterations in pulmonary airway resistance [106]. Staub [110] suggested that this was related to edema in the wall of small bronchi or bronchioles. This increased airway resistance appears to be the result of narrowing of the bronchial lumen, but the factors proposed as causative of this narrowing are not clearly defined. Speculation has included not only the presence of fluid in the airway, but also the decrease in FRC leading to a loss of the tethering effect. Direct bronchoconstriction, possibly endotoxin-mediated through the cyclooxygenase pathway by thromboxane A_2, has been implicated [27, 51, 108], as has reflex airway constriction (probably vagally mediated), compression of airways by adjacent congested arteries, and compression of small airways directly by the edema in their interstitium [110]. The latter two factors—compression of airways by interstitial fluid and congested arteries—have been shown by Michel et al. [71] probably not to have a role in the increased airway resistance. They found that interstitial edema did not compress small airways, or small-to-medium arteries. Fluid accumulation did not occur around the small airways; only around the larger bronchioles and bronchi did significant amounts of interstitial edema accumulate. The effect of the interstitial fluid accumulation on the larger airways may be counterbalanced by the interdependence between the parenchyma and the airways. These data support the contention that small airway compression is not an important mechanism for increased airway resistance but leave most of the other mechanisms as possibilities.

Increased airway responsiveness to nonantigenic aerosolized bronchoconstrictors has been reported in some survivors of ARDS [101] and in animal models of diffuse lung disease [54]. It is possible that the alterations in lung mechanics observed in some patients with ARDS involve acute bronchoconstriction secondary to increased airway responsiveness [107]. Although there is a relationship between pulmonary inflammation and altered airway responsiveness, a specific role for granulocytes or other inflammatory cells in the altered airway responsiveness observed following ARDS remains to be proven.

The ARDS process is not uniform in distribution. Although the presence of diffuse alveolar infiltration has, from the first descriptions of this entity [1, 74, 81, 83], been a part of the operational definition of this disease, and ARDS was initially considered a diffuse, homogeneous process, recent studies using computerized tomography (CT) have shown ARDS to be patchy and heterogeneous [39, 40, 70, 99]. Gattinoni et al. [39] consistently found the presence of normally aerated tissues in the nondependent regions of the lung, with a nonhomogeneous distribution of the lesions. Using CT scans performed at three levels of positive end-expiratory pressure (PEEP), they proposed a simple three-zone model of the ARDS lung: a healthy zone (zone H) with normal morphologic features and density, a recruitable zone (zone R), and a diseased zone (zone D) [40]. This nonuniformity of effect has been explained by a heterogeneity of the arteriolar vasoconstrictor and lung capillary endothelial permeability altering process in these different zones.

The magnitude of the lymph flow depends both on the degree of mediator insult to the alveolar capillary membrane, which appears to be flow-related with regard to the delivery of the mediators to the endothelial surface and to the relative position of the injured alveolus with regard to the left atrial pressure (LAP): i.e., the greater the level of pulmonary venous pressure for any given degree of membrane permeability, the higher the rate of interstitial fluid accumulation. The local abnormalities in lung mechanics, compliance, and resistance follow the local changes in capillary permeability and vasomotion. As a result, the superior, or dependent, position of the injured lung segment vis à vis the LAP sets the relative ventilation : perfusion ratio ($\dot{V}_A/\dot{Q}_T$) and thus influences both the rate of pulmonary capillary blood flow past the alveolus and the magnitude of respiratory gas exchange permitted into the alveolus. The more-dependent alveoli have higher blood flows, greater lymph flow into the interstitium, lower compliance, and higher airway resistance—and, consequently, a smaller ventilation. Thus the abnormalities in gas exchange that occur at the alveolar level and are reflected in the alveolar-arterial oxygen gradient are compounded by the tendency for an increased blood flow through those alveoli that are either reduced in volume or closed entirely. This produces a physiologic pulmonary shunt with a resulting pulmonary venoarterial admixture ($\dot{Q}_s/\dot{Q}_t$). At any specific inspired-oxygen concentration (FiO_2) and minute ventilation ($\dot{V}_E$), the net reduction in arterial oxygen tension (PaO_2) in ARDS is the direct result of both of these factors.

The Consequences of ARDS Pathophysiologic Alterations in Lung Mechanics

The progressive interstitial edema of ARDS alters the elastic properties of the lungs and is associated with decreased static and dynamic compliance of the lungs. In severely involved alveolar capillary segments the fluid accumulation progresses from filling of the interstitium to alveolar flooding, and localized pulmonary edema occurs. The earliest mechanical feature noted in the development of ARDS is an increase in the pressure required to distend the lung to a given volume: i.e., a reduction in lung compliance. The respiratory compliance is a good indicator of the amount of liquid in the lung interstitium and air spaces, as the loss of ventilating units accounts for the loss of compliance. Compliance is a measure of the elastic forces acting on the lung. At a given compliance (C), in order to increase lung volume (V), either the pleural pressure must be decreased or the alveolar pressure must be increased. The difference between these two pressures is the transpulmonary pressure (ΔP), or distending pressure.

$$\Delta V = \Delta P \times C$$

As ARDS develops, the decrease in compliance and in alveolar volume is manifested by a decrease in the FRC.

QUANTIFICATION OF THE MECHANICAL AND GAS EXCHANGE ABNORMALITIES IN ARDS

Assessment of Respiratory Mechanics in Ventilated ARDS Patients

Compliance is usually obtained by determining the slope of the pressure/volume curve, or the change in volume per unit change in pressure. Figure 12-1 shows the shift to the right in this relationship in acute ARDS and in the late fibrosis stage of chronic ARDS compared to normal. Bone [11] described a method of generating pressure-volume (P-V) curves by plotting volume against peak pressure and plateau pressure to obtain both a dynamic characteristics curve and a static compliance curve. Automated systems now available can generate P-V curves from each breath. We have developed a computer-based analytic system (Fig. 12-2) that allows us to evaluate respiratory flows (F), pressures (P), and volumes (V) in intubated and ventilated patients [97, 98] as a means of quantifying respiratory mechanics and adjusting the characteristics of ventilatory support therapy. The compliance of the normal human lung is about 0.2 liter/cm H_2O (200 ml/cm H_2O). To measure lung compliance, one needs a measure of both the intrapleural pressure and the intra-alveolar pressure. In humans it is difficult to measure the intrapleural pressure, and the esophageal pressure is usually substituted. The esophageal pressure, although not equal to pressure in the intrapleural space, does reflect the changes in pressure except in supine subjects (such as critically ill ICU patients), in whom the weight of the mediastinal structures interferes with the accuracy of measurement.

To obtain an assessment of the lung compliance of patients with ARDS, it has now become standard to measure total static respiratory compliance (C_{ST}), which is the sum of the lung compliance (C_L) and the compliance of the thoracic cage or chest wall (C_W) added in parallel:

$$\frac{1}{C_{ST}} = \frac{1}{C_L} + \frac{1}{C_W} \text{ and } C_{ST} = C_L \times \frac{C_W}{C_W + C_L}$$

Under equilibrium conditions, at FRC the chest wall is pulled inward while the lung is pulled outward, these two forces balancing each other. The normal total C_{ST} is approximately 0.1 liters/cm H_2O (100 ml/cm H_2O) and ranges from 0.040 (40 ml/cm H_2O) to 0.140 (140 ml/cm H_2O) liters/cm H_2O. It is affected by age, body size, and total lung capacity. C_{ST} can be decreased as a result of a decrease in the compliance of the lung or the thorax, or both.

The change in transpulmonary pressure—airway pressure (P_{AW}) minus

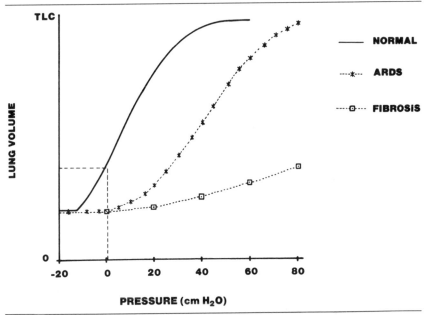

Fig. 12-1. Static compliance curve for lung and chest wall. Comparison of pressure-volume relationships under normal conditions in the early inflammatory phase of ARDS and in late fibrosis. (From J. H. Siegel, J. C. Stoklosa, and U. Borg, Cardiorespiratory Management of the Adult Respiratory Distress Syndrome. In J. H. Siegel (ed.), *Trauma: Emergency Surgery and Critical Care.* New York: Churchill Livingstone, 1987. Pp. 581–673.)

pleural pressure (P_{PL})—that produces a given tidal volume is similar whether it is generated by spontaneous breathing or by mechanical breathing. C_{ST} can be measured in patients with ARDS who are intubated and are on a ventilator, by measuring the tidal volume and the distending pressure required to deliver this volume. The distending pressure is determined by measuring the airway pressure at the points of zero airflow on both inspiration and expiration [the plateau pressure minus the end-expiratory pressure (PEEP)].

$$C_{ST} = \frac{\text{Tidal volume}}{\text{Plateau pressure} - \text{PEEP}}$$

It is possible to generate a total static respiratory compliance curve (P-V curve) by varying the tidal volume and measuring the plateau pressure at each new tidal volume level. This is demonstrated in Figure 12-1.

It is important to emphasize that in critically ill ventilated patients the conventional method of calculating C_{ST}—using the mechanically set PEEP as reflecting the end-expiratory pressure—may be in error. Jonson and co-workers [56], as well as Pepe and Marini [77], have shown that a positive alveolar pressure can be present throughout the breathing cycle when the

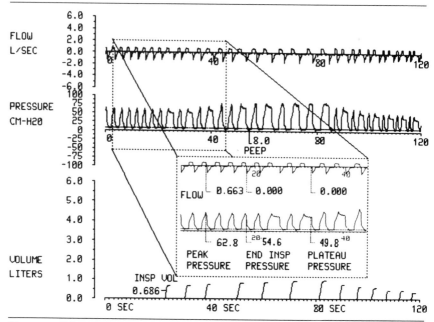

Fig. 12-2. Primary respiratory flow and pressure data showing methodology for the determination of total static compliance. Volume is obtained from integration of the area under the inspiratory and/or expiratory flow curve. When using the Servo Ventilator 900C in volume control mode and constant minute volume, by varying respiratory rate it is possible to produce a series of breaths at different tidal volumes. An inspiratory pause hold is used to obtain the plateau pressure. (From J. H. Siegel, J. C. Stoklosa, and U. Borg, Cardiorespiratory Management of the Adult Respiratory Distress Syndrome. In J. H. Siegel (ed.), *Trauma: Emergency Surgery and Critical Care.* New York: Churchill Livingstone, 1987. Pp. 581–673.)

patient is being mechanically ventilated, even though PEEP is not being applied. Pepe and Marini [77] demonstrated the presence of what they termed *auto-PEEP* by occluding the airway at end-expiration and delaying the onset of the next breath. Rossi et al. [86] showed the effect of what they termed *intrinsic positive end-expiratory pressure*, or $PEEP_i$, on the measurement of the C_{ST}. They studied mechanically ventilated patients with acute respiratory failure and measured airflow, airway pressure, and volume changes. The pressure at end-expiration ($PEEP_i$) was determined using the occlusion method of Pepe and Marini [77]. The C_{ST} was determined using the conventional method (using the mechanically set PEEP) and by using $PEEP_i$ determined by occluding the expiratory port at end-expiration. These findings were compared to a determination of effective PEEP from the flow and pressure tracings (using the airway pressure at which inspiratory airflow begins).

An example of this discrepancy between the set and measured PEEP level is shown in Figure 12-3. The difference (7.4 cm H_2O) between the *set*

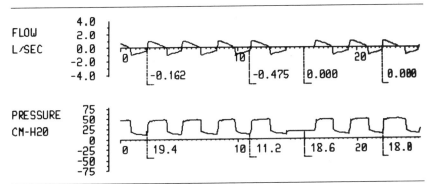

Fig. 12-3. Measurement of set versus intrinsic positive end-expiratory pressure (PEEP$_i$); by convention, inspiratory flows are shown as positive and expiratory flows as negative around the zero-flow point. (See text for details.)

PEEP of 11.2 cm H$_2$O and the pressure at the onset of inspiratory airflow (18.6 cm H$_2$O) represents the pressure the ventilator must generate to overcome the elastic recoil pressure producing expiratory airflow during passive exhalation. If expiration is not complete (as indicated in Fig. 12-3 by the expiratory flow rate of 0.475 liters/sec just prior to the beginning of the next positive-pressure breath and 0.162 liters/sec when the pressure had increased above the set PEEP level as the ventilator cycles to inspiration), then the pressure required for delivery of the volume is equal to the plateau pressure minus the pressure at the point at which inspiratory airflow actually begins (18.6 cm H$_2$O)—not the difference between the plateau pressure minus the mechanically set PEEP level (11.2 cm H$_2$O). The level of true PEEP will also vary with the time allowed for expiration. Using the set PEEP to calculate C$_{ST}$ has been shown to lead to an underestimation in calculated compliance of up to 48 percent [86].

It is very important to obtain an accurate measure of PEEP$_i$ in critically ill patients with altered compliance; otherwise, major impairments in venous filling of the right heart and consequent reductions in cardiac output can be induced while attempts are made to raise mean airway pressures to achieve an acceptable lung volume. When using the airway occlusion method to determine PEEP$_i$, care must be taken to see that occlusion of the expiratory port occurs precisely at end-expiration. Some ventilators, such as the Servo Ventilator 900C (which was used in Fig. 12-2), allow occlusion of the expiratory port at end-expiration and thus provide a true static measurement of PEEP$_i$.

When a measurement of C$_{ST}$ is done, the patient must be fully relaxed or paralyzed and in synchrony with the ventilator. Any respiratory efforts made at the time of measurement, whether inspiratory or expiratory, will change the compliance of the thoracic cage and thus affect the measurement of total compliance. C$_{ST}$ is used to track the elastic properties of the lungs, since it is generally assumed that the pressure-volume relationship of the chest wall is linear and unchanging. This may not be the case in the critically ill patient, whose chest wall distensibility may be disturbed by

Pt I.D. = 301

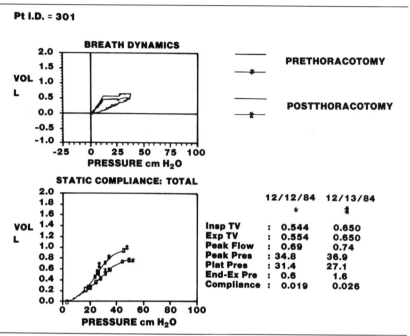

Fig. 12-4. The dynamic and static compliance relationships for total respiratory compliance, showing the effect of chest wall abnormalities in influencing CsT. Patient pre- and postthoracotomy for removal of chronic empyema with a pleural fibrotic peel. (From J. H. Siegel, J. C. Stoklosa, and U. Borg, Cardiorespiratory Management of the Adult Respiratory Distress Syndrome. In J. H. Siegel (ed.), *Trauma: Emergency Surgery and Critical Care.* New York: Churchill Livingstone, 1987. Pp. 581–673.)

abdominal distention, effusions, increased muscular tone, position, or recent surgery. In particular, the development of an acute empyema with a fibrin pleural peel may markedly reduce CsT by virtue of its reduction in chest wall compliance (Cw) (Fig. 12-4). Since this can be surgically corrected by decortication in the acute phase, its appearance under the appropriate clinical conditions may be first suggested by a deterioration in CsT with a compatible x-ray or CT scan picture.

When measuring the compliance of a patient who is on a ventilator, one needs to measure the tidal volume actually delivered to the patient (V_{T_a}), as well as the plateau pressure (PlatP), which is representative of the alveolar pressure at end-inspiration, and the pressure at end-expiration ($PEEP_i$) level. The plateau and end-expiratory pressures can be read from the manometer on the ventilator by utilizing a pause period at the end of inspiration and expiration to ensure a condition of *zero* airflow. When flow is stopped at end-inspiration, there is a fall in pause pressure from its peak until the true plateau level is reached (Fig. 12-2). This usually occurs within 2 seconds; however, it may take up to 4 seconds to achieve in some individuals with ARDS. If the patient has a nonuniform distribution of abnormalities in compliance and/or resistance—a situation now known to occur in patients with ARDS [24, 25, 39, 70, 79, 84, 97]—there are different time constants for alveolar expansion in the lung. (The time constant is the product of lung compliance and resistance and has the dimensions of seconds, with areas of ARDS lung having longer time constants than normal.) As a result, flow may still be occurring within the lung when it has ceased at the proximal airways, causing a continuing redistribution of volume from lung units with normal time constants to lung units with prolonged time constants, such as those located behind partially obstructed airways. These lung units may continue to fill when the rest of the lung has begun to empty, the so-called *pendelluft* effect. Sufficient pause time must be used to ensure equilibration of pressure between the alveoli and the point of measurement, whether this is at the proximal end of the endotracheal tube or within the ventilator. If adequate time is not allowed for equilibration, the lung will appear to be less compliant than it really is, with potentially disastrous consequences for therapeutic decision making, since this could lead to an inappropriate interpretation of the patient's response to a change in therapy.

It must be remembered that a continuing fall in the plateau pressure can be caused by air leaks within the system, whether at the site of the cuff of the endotracheal tube, in the ventilator, or because of the presence of a bronchopleural fistula. In this case, there will be a larger discrepancy between the set inspired tidal volume and the expired tidal volume measured at the expiration valve of the ventilator. If leaks are present, it is impossible to obtain an accurate assessment of compliance.

The tidal volume *actually delivered* to the patient (V_{T_a}) must be used to calculate compliance not the *set* tidal volume (V_{T_s}). There is always some compression of gas within the ventilator system, and this compressed, or "lost", volume (V_{T_c}) causes a lower volume of gas to be delivered to the patient than is set or measured by the ventilator ($V_{T_a} = V_{T_s} - V_{T_c}$) (Table 12-1). This compressibility factor (CF) is dependent upon the type of tubing, the humidification system and the ventilator used, the level to which heated humidifiers are filled, and the pressure required to deliver the set tidal volume. The compressibility factor can range from about 1 ml/cm H_2O, when small-bore tygon tubing (as for infant ventilation) and nose humidifiers are used, up to 5 ml/cm H_2O, when disposable tubing and partially filled heated humidifiers are used. An approximation of the compressed or "lost" volume (V_{T_c}) can be obtained by multiplying the distending pressure, which is the difference between the peak pressure at end-inspiration (PkP) and the set end-expiratory pressure ($PEEP_s$), by the compressibility factor (CF) determined for each ventilator setup.

The set end-expiratory pressure is equivalent to the PEEP level set on the ventilator ($PEEP_s$).

$$V_{T_c} = (PkP - PEEP_s) \times CF$$

This calculated volume is then subtracted from the tidal volume set on the ventilator to determine the actual delivered volume.

Table 12-1. Comparison between "set" tidal volume and delivered tidal volume

	800			800			800			800			800		
"Set" tidal volume (ml) [V_{T_3}]															
Distending pressure (cm H_2O)*	20			40			60			80			100		
Compression factor (ml/cm H_2O)#	1	3	5	1	3	5	1	3	5	1	3	5	1	3	5
"Lost" volume (ml) [V_{T_c}]	20	60	100	40	120	200	60	180	300	80	240	400	100	300	500
Actual tidal volume (ml) [V_{T_a}]	780	740	700	760	680	600	740	620	500	720	560	400	700	500	300
Exhaled tidal volume (ml)	800	800	800	800	800	800	800	800	800	800	800	800	800	800	800

*Peak pressure – PEEP; varies due to changes in compliance and/or resistance.
#Compression factor varies due to type of ventilator, tubing, humidification system used.

From the above equations, it is apparent that as the peak pressure increases, the magnitude of the "lost" volume also increases. Table 12-1 also shows a comparison between *set* and *actual* tidal volume using differing compressibility factors and peak pressures. The end-expiratory pressure is zero. If one fails to measure the actual tidal volume, then the derived compliance value will be higher than the true value.

Using the appropriately measured and calculated parameters total, static compliance (C_{ST}) can be assessed and followed.

$$C_{ST} = \frac{V_{T_S} - [(PkP - PEEP_s) \times CF]}{PlatP - PEEP_i}$$

Assessment of the Adequacy of Gas Exchange

The adequacy of ventilation is assessed by analysis of arterial blood for oxygen tension (PaO_2), carbon dioxide tension ($PaCO_2$), and pH. The alveolar CO_2 tension ($PACO_2$) is directly related to carbon dioxide production ($\dot{V}CO_2$) and inversely related to alveolar ventilation ($\dot{V}A$). For practical purposes, $PaCO_2$ can be substituted for $PACO_2$, and thus

$$PaCO_2 = \frac{\dot{V}CO_2 \times K}{\dot{V}A}$$

where K is a constant converting liters to mm Hg = 0.863. It is apparent that $PaCO_2$ can increase if alveolar ventilation decreases or if CO_2 production increases.

Alveolar ventilation can be decreased as a result of a decrease in total ventilation ($\dot{V}E$) or as a result of a ventilation-perfusion mismatching resulting in an increased dead space ventilation ($\dot{V}D$).

$$\dot{V}A = \dot{V}E - \dot{V}D$$

The volume of dead space can be measured by collecting mixed expired gas over a period of time and measuring minute ventilation ($\dot{V}E$) and the carbon dioxide tension of this mixed expired gas ($P\bar{E}CO_2$), as well as the $PaCO_2$:

$$\dot{V}D = \frac{PaCO_2 - P\bar{E}CO_2}{PaCO_2} \times \dot{V}E$$

This value represents the physiologic dead space, which includes the alveolar as well as the anatomic dead-space volume. The $\dot{V}D/\dot{V}T$ ratio, which represents the fraction of ventilation that is dead space ventilation, can be obtained by collecting a mixed expired gas sample as well as an arterial blood sample, and measuring the PCO_2 of both:

$$\dot{V}D/\dot{V}T = \frac{PaCO_2 - P\bar{E}CO_2}{PaCO_2}$$

A normal $\dot{V}D/\dot{V}T$ ratio is 0.20 to 0.40.

The end-tidal carbon dioxide tension ($P_{ET}CO_2$) is an approximation of the alveolar (P_ACO_2) and, in turn, of the arterial $PaCO_2$. It can be monitored using infrared sensors or a mass spectrometer. In normal individuals the $P_{ET}CO_2$ (or P_ACO_2) is only 1 to 4 mm Hg below the $PaCO_2$. However, when the distribution of ventilation becomes more uneven, as in obstructive lung disease or pulmonary emboli, or in ARDS where the pulmonary shunt ($\dot{Q}_s$/$\dot{Q}_t$) becomes very large, the $P_{ET}CO_2$ to $PaCO_2$ gradient widens. Correlation of the $P_{ET}CO_2$ with a simultaneously drawn arterial blood sample can be of value in alerting one to changes in the patient's status.

Skin sensors now available allow for the measurement of transcutaneous carbon dioxide tension ($P_{TC}CO_2$) and transcutaneous oxygen tension ($P_{TC}O_2$). Monitoring of the transcutaneous carbon dioxide tension is especially valuable when one is making changes in ventilator settings, since there is a close relationship between $PaCO_2$ and $P_{TC}CO_2$ when one is using heated sensors. Local heating is used to improve gaseous diffusion through the skin. This, however, leads to an increase in local CO_2 production, and as a result, transcutaneous CO_2 tension monitors usually report values higher than $PaCO_2$—a difference of 5 to 20 mm Hg. In patients with adequate cardiovascular function the linear correlation coefficient (r) approximates 0.8 to 0.9 [50, 118]. In a group of normodynamic or hyperdynamic posttrauma patients, we found the following relationship using a transcutaneous monitor incorporating an internal automatic correction for the temperature effect [112].

$$PaCO_2 = 0.76 \, (P_{TC}CO_2) + 0.06 \, (\% \text{ insp. } O_2) + 0.035 \, (P_{TC}O_2) + 4.1$$
$$N = 78, \, r^2 = 0.683, \, F_{2.76} = 53, \, P < 0.001$$

The arterial oxygen tension (PaO_2) is dependent upon the FIO_2, the alveolar ventilation, ventilation-perfusion inequality, the degree of shunting, and diffusion limitations for oxygen in the interstitial fluid separating the alveolus from the alveolar capillaries. However, abnormalities in diffusion are likely to be only a very minor component of the causes of hypoxemia in ARDS patients.

Alveolar hypoventilation as a cause for hypoxemia can be ascertained by calculating the alveolar-arterial oxygen tension gradient $P(A-a)DO_2$ utilizing the alveolar gas equation to calculate P_AO_2 and the measured PaO_2

$$P_AO_2 = FIO_2 \, (P_B - P_{H_2O}) - \frac{P_ACO_2}{R} + FIO_2 \times P_ACO_2 \frac{(1 - R)}{R}$$

where P_B is barometric pressure, P_{H_2O} is water vapor pressure (47 mm Hg at 37°C), FIO_2 is fractional concentration of inspired oxygen, R is the respiratory quotient (assumed to be 0.8), and P_ACO_2 is alveolar carbon dioxide (assumed to equal $PaCO_2$). For simplicity's sake, the last term, [$FIO_2 \times$

$PACO_2$ $[(1 - R)/R]$ is usually ignored and a value of 0.8 is used for R. Thus the alveolar-arterial O_2 gradient can be calculated as

$$PAO_2 = FIO_2 (PB - 47) - PaCO_2/0.8$$

and

$$P(A-a)DO_2 = PAO_2 - PaO_2$$

The normal gradient when breathing room air is 5 to 10 mm Hg but may be as high as 20 mm Hg in the aged individual. The gradient widens as the FIO_2 is increased, with a gradient of 100 mm Hg being considered normal on an $FIO_2 = 1.0$. If hypoxemia is present and the $P(A-a)DO_2$ is normal, then alveolar hypoventilation with its resultant increase in $PACO_2$ and $PaCO_2$ is the cause, since all other causes of hypoxemia result in a widened $P(A-a)DO_2$.

Oximetry is a means by which arterial oxygen saturation (SaO_2) can be continuously monitored noninvasively. This technique utilizes a probe that is attached to the earlobe or a digit. Oximetry is not markedly affected by skin pigmentation or jaundice and is accurate $(1 - 4\%)$ when the SaO_2 exceeds 75 to 80 percent. The tendency of most units to overestimate the true value becomes significant at lower saturations. Pulse oximeters are especially useful when changes are being made in ventilator settings, FIO_2, or PEEP levels, when weaning is occurring, and as an early warning of deterioration in a patient's oxygenation. The SaO_2 measured by the oximeter should be correlated periodically with a directly measured, *not calculated,* SaO_2, since taking instrument accuracy into account, an oximeter reading of 95 percent could be equivalent to a true saturation of 99 percent, or even 92 percent.

Transcutaneous gas monitoring also can be used to assess oxygen tension ($PTCO_2$). It measures the amount of oxygen in gas equilibrated above a warmed patch of skin using a membrane-covered polarographic electrode [88]. In adults, $PTCO_2$ underestimates the PaO_2 to a variable degree, although it does correlate well during hemodynamic stability (cardiac index ≥ 2.5 liters/m²) provided a regression-derived correction factor is used to adjust the TC value to that of the PaO_2 [112].

$$PaO_2 = 1.12 (PTCO_2) - 0.28 (\% \text{ insp. } O_2) + 45.5$$
$$N = 78, r^2 = 0.822, F_{2.76} = 173, P < 0.001$$

During periods of profound vasoconstriction or shock (cardiac index below 2.5 liters/m²) $PTCO_2$ appears to track the reduction in skin perfusion. This may provide an early indication of an impending perfusion crisis, if there is not a corroborating change in PaO_2 or SaO_2 indicating central arterial hypoxemia.

The PaO_2, SaO_2, and $P(A-a)DO_2$ are abnormal in ARDS patients. However, they are relatively insensitive indicators of the degree of abnormality in gas exchange, since they are altered not only by the level of overall ventilation but also by such nonpulmonary causes as changes in cardiac output, reductions in hemoglobin concentration, shifts in the oxygen dissociation curve, and changes in oxygen consumption that can affect the mixed venous oxygen content ($C\bar{v}O_2$). This can be seen by examining the Fick equation, which relates oxygen consumption ($\dot{V}O_2$), cardiac output ($\dot{Q}T$), arterial O_2 content (CaO_2), and mixed venous O_2 content ($C\bar{v}O_2$).

$$\dot{V}O_2 = \dot{Q}T(CaO_2 - C\bar{v}O_2)$$

$$C\bar{v}O_2 = CaO_2 - \frac{\dot{V}O_2}{\dot{Q}T}$$

Changes in CaO_2 may be due to changes in PaO_2, arterial O_2 saturation (SaO_2), or hemoglobin concentration (Hb).

$$CaO_2 = Hb \times 1.39 \times \frac{SaO_2}{100} + 0.0031\ PaO_2$$

therefore,

$$C\bar{v}O_2 = [Hb \times 1.39 \times \frac{SaO_2}{100} + 0.0031\ PaO_2] - \frac{\dot{V}O_2}{\dot{Q}T}$$

Under normal circumstances, any perturbations causing a decrease in $C\bar{v}O_2$ will be accompanied by compensatory changes in cardiac output or minute ventilation. In the critically ill individual, however, these compensatory mechanisms may not be fully operative, and a decrease in $C\bar{v}O_2$ will lead to a decrease in PaO_2 and widened $P(A-a)DO_2$.

The respiratory index (RI), which is the alveolar-arterial O_2 gradient divided by the PaO_2,

$$RI = \frac{[(P_B - P_{H_2O})\ FiO_2 - PaCO_2/0.8] - PaO_2}{PaO_2} = P(A-a)DO_2/PaO_2$$

helps to normalize for the effect of increasing FiO_2 in critically ill patients [89, 93]. This index provides a useful method of quantifying the severity of abnormalities in oxygen exchange and has been used to assess overall respiratory oxygen exchange in trauma [28, 62], sepsis or hepatic failure syndromes [89, 93, 94, 99], pneumonitis [53, 89, 159], and cardiogenic decompensation [89, 93]. When evaluated as a function of the simultaneously obtained total shunt ($\dot{Q}_s/\dot{Q}_t$), it can provide diagnostic information concerning the type of clinical process producing the oxygen exchange limitations [89].

The total cardiac output ($\dot{Q}T$) is made up of two major components: $\dot{Q}C$, which is the portion of the blood flow that exchanges perfectly with alveolar air; and $\dot{Q}s$, the shunt component, or that portion of blood flow that does not exchange at all with alveolar air.

$$\dot{Q}_T = \dot{Q}_C + \dot{Q}_S$$

Total shunt $(\dot{Q}_s/\dot{Q}_t)$ is largely determined by two factors: the fixed anatomic and pathologic anatomic shunt representing collapsed, consolidated, or absent alveoli; and the physiologic shunt representing flow through the alveoli of very low V_A/Q. A simple mixing equation is used to quantify the percent of blood flow being shunted and thus not undergoing gas exchange.

$$\dot{Q}_T(CaO_2) = \dot{Q}_S(C\bar{v}O_2) + (\dot{Q}_T - \dot{Q}_S)(CiO_2)$$

where CiO_2 is the O_2 content of fully saturated blood leaving the alveolar capillary unit. Arterial and mixed venous bloods are sampled directly, their pH, PCO_2, PO_2, Hb, and SO_2 are analyzed, and oxygen contents are calculated, utilizing the formula

$$CaO_2 = Hb \times 1.39 \times \frac{SaO_2}{100} + 0.0031\ PaO_2$$

$$C\bar{v}O_2 = Hb \times 1.39 \times \frac{S\bar{v}O_2}{100} + 0.0031\ P\bar{v}O_2$$

The oxygen content of the alveolar-capillary compartment must be calculated using the alveolar air equation to determine the correct alveolar PO_2 (PAO_2). When high FIO_2 mixtures are breathed, resulting in an alveolar $PAO_2 \geqslant 240$ mm Hg, one can assume that blood leaving the alveolar capillary unit is essentially completely saturated and CiO_2 can be calculated as

$$CiO_2 = (Hb \times 1.39) + 0.0031\ PAO_2$$

At levels below a PAO_2 of 240 mm Hg, the true end capillary O_2 saturation and content must be calculated using a mathematical algorithm [35, 58]. Shunt flow as a percentage of the total cardiac output is calculated as

$$\dot{Q}_s/\dot{Q}_t = \frac{CiO_2 - CaO_2}{CiO_2 - C\bar{v}O_2}$$

Factors other than true right-to-left shunt influence the calculated value of shunt when room air is being breathed. These include $\dot{V}_A/\dot{Q}$ inequality, diffusion, and the nonpulmonary factors that influence mixed venous oxygen content. As FIO_2 is increased, the contribution of these other factors diminishes, but the rate at which their influence is diminished varies and depends upon the underlying pathophysiology. At an FIO_2 of 1.0 (100 percent) breathed for a sufficient time to wash out nitrogen, the calculation will reflect the level of the true shunt [10]. Therefore, if factors other than true right-to-left shunt alone contribute to hypoxemia, there will be a linear fall in the calculated total shunt ($\dot{Q}_s/\dot{Q}_t$) as FIO_2 is increased [35]. In patients in whom true right-to-left shunt is the mechanism for the observed hypoxemia, the measured $\dot{Q}_s/\dot{Q}_t$ will be constant at any FIO_2, unless the actual shunt has changed.

Some studies have shown that shunt does indeed increase when FIO_2 is increased, and this phenomenon has been attributed to the reversal of compensatory hypoxic pulmonary vasoconstriction in areas with extremely low $\dot{V}A/\dot{Q}$ ratios and reabsorption microatelectasis as a result of denitrogenation of these lung units [30, 91]. Dantzker [24, 25] has claimed that this effect may only be theoretical—especially in patients with ARDS, in whom his anatomic and physiologic data suggested that lung units are either well-ventilated with normal or high $\dot{V}A/\dot{Q}$ ratios or totally collapsed. He believes that if there are areas with low $\dot{V}A/\dot{Q}$ ratios, their contribution is small and they are only intermittently ventilated at peak inspiration. However, other studies have suggested that a bimodal distribution of $\dot{V}A/\dot{Q}$ exists in ARDS, with some very low $\dot{V}A/\dot{Q}$ regions that may be collapsed if high FIO_2 levels are used [30, 68, 91]. In practice, most workers, including the authors, have utilized shunt calculations based on the patient receiving an $FIO_2 \geq 0.40$ ($\geq$40 percent), which should yield a PaO_2 in excess of 240 mm Hg, to avoid potential problems with a FIO_2 of 1.0.

When interpreting shunt, one must be aware that the level of the intrapulmonary shunt can be affected by the level of the cardiac output and that an increase or decrease can cause similar changes in $\dot{Q}_s/\dot{Q}_t$ (26, 94, 95, 108). The mechanism for this dependence may be related to the relative increase in perfusion of more-dependent low $\dot{V}A/\dot{Q}$ lung segments, so that physiologic shunt rises as flow increases [94]. One must always interpret changes in the level of the shunt in conjunction with concomitant changes in cardiac output [26, 94, 95, 105].

Recent observations by Sganga et al. [89] and by Laghi et al. [62] have demonstrated that the degree of severity in ARDS can be directly quantified by the difference in relationship between the respiratory index (RI), which reflects the alveolar-arterial oxygen gradient normalized by the arterial oxygen tension [P(A-a)DO$_2$/PaO$_2$)] and the percent of pulmonary shunt ($\dot{Q}_s/\dot{Q}_t$). This difference in relationship is shown in Figure 12-5. This figure demonstrates the difference in RI/($\dot{Q}_s/\dot{Q}_t$) relations for patients with ARDS who subsequently died compared with those for critically ill posttrauma patients without ARDS and those patients who had ARDS of a milder nature that was compatible with survival. As can be seen, the difference in the slopes of the RI shunt relationships in these two circumstances is highly significant. More recently, studies by De Gaetano et al. [28] have shown that a probability statistic can be constructed from the RI to $\dot{Q}_s/\dot{Q}_t$ relationship by which the probability (*P*) of death can be directly related to the distance along the RI/($\dot{Q}_s/\dot{Q}_t$) slope away from the origin.

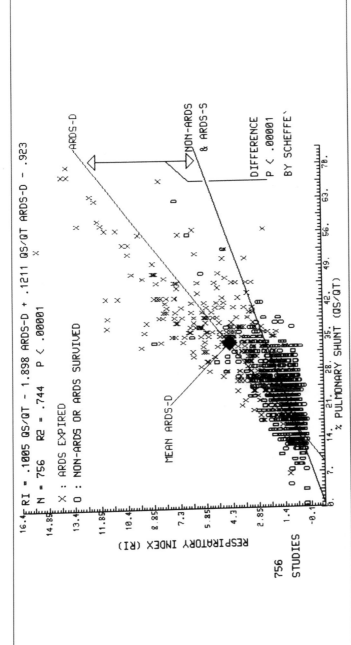

Fig. 12-5. Respiratory index–pulmonary shunt relationship in posttraumatic and septic ARDS. Note statistically different slope between nonsurviving ARDS patients (ARDS-D) and non-ARDS or ARDS survivors (ARDS-S). (From F. Laghi, et al. The respiratory index/pulmonary shunt relationship: Quantification of severity and prognosis in the posttraumatic adult respiratory distress syndrome. *Crit. Care Med.* 17:1121–1128, 1989.

This relationship can be expressed by a linear logistic equation:

$P \text{ death} = e^\lambda/1 + e^\lambda$

where

$\lambda = 0.628 \text{ RI} + 0.027 \, \dot{Q}_s/\dot{Q}_t - 1.991$

The statistical "goodness" of the prediction of outcome, using present modalities of therapy, from this probability-based equation is shown in Figure 12-6. Thus, a quantitative method of ascertaining the severity of the ARDS process can be developed *from blood gas measurements alone* and therefore easily obtained at the bedside of the critically ill ARDS patient. This measure of the adequacy of respiratory gas exchange can be used as a means of quantifying the net response to ventilatory, circulatory, or pharmacologic therapy used to address the abnormalities in this disease process [13, 99]. To facilitate its clinical use, a nomogram [28] for the estimation of the severity of respiratory insufficiency (i.e., *P* death), derived from the linear logistic equation for the respiratory index and the pulmonary shunt, is shown in Figure 12-7. The use of RI ($\dot{Q}_s/\dot{Q}_t$) in a number of clinical situations to assess the severity of ARDS and the response to therapy will be demonstrated later.

THERAPEUTIC CONSIDERATIONS IN ARDS

The Role of the Hyperdynamic Cardiovascular State in Compensation for Gas Exchange Abnormalities

The natural response to the development of respiratory insufficiency in the ARDS process is the development of a compensatory hyperdynamic state [21, 93, 94, 99]. This may also be induced by the same types of processes that are related to the evolution of the ARDS syndrome: namely, trauma and sepsis that in themselves result in a hyperdynamic process [21, 62, 94, 95, 99, 100]. This can be seen in Figure 12-8, which demonstrates the effective nonshunted pulmonary blood flow ($\dot{Q}_E/m^2$) as a function of the cardiac index (CI) in patients with nonseptic and septic hyperdynamic states, with or without a respiratory component. In the normal hyperdynamic response, an increase in cardiac index (such as occurs in cirrhosis or sepsis uncomplicated by pneumonitis or ARDS) is associated with an increased pulmonary shunt as the flow is increased [94, 95]. This reflects the increased perfusion of the more dependent lung segments that have a reduced ventilation-to-perfusion ratio (increased perfusion per unit ventilation). However, the development of pneumonitis (or ARDS, or a septic process with pulmonary involvement) produces a further shift to the right, so that for a given cardiac index there is a lower $\dot{Q}_E/m^2$. This difference is also reflected in the previously discussed RI($\dot{Q}_s/\dot{Q}_t$) relationship. As a result, in ARDS or pneumonitis, *a higher cardiac output is necessary to maintain any given level of effective pulmonary blood flow.*

Therefore, factors that deleteriously affect the cardiac function and prevent the maintenance of a high cardiac output will compound any given

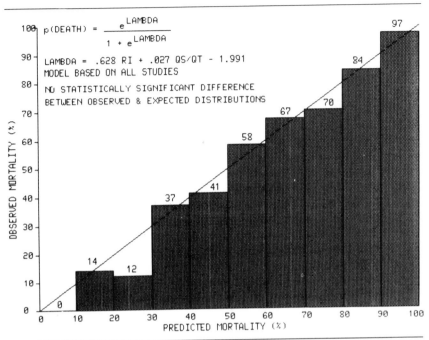

Fig. 12-6. Performance of linear logistic model for predicted mortality versus observed mortality in 849 studies from 227 trauma patients, 79 of whom developed ARDS. (A. De Gaetano, et al., Predicting the probability of death from ARDS after trauma. Submitted to *Surgery,* 1990.)

level of abnormality in net pulmonary gas exchange induced either by alveolar capillary dysfunction or by shunting. This can occur either with hypovolemia, which tends to reduce ventricular end-diastolic filling (*preload*), or with preexisting or shock-induced depressions in myocardial *contractility,* which reduce the cardiac ejection fraction at a given *afterload* (stroke volume times mean blood pressure). Also, marked increases in vasoconstriction, which increase the *afterload* and therefore reduce ejection fraction at a given level of contractility and blood volume, will have the same effect by reducing cardiac output and thus will reduce the effective pulmonary blood flow across an ARDS-limited pulmonary capillary gas exchange surface. Even a small reduction in myocardial contractility is extremely important in those hyperdynamic states in which there is a requirement for a high systemic oxygen consumption, since there is evidence that severe posttraumatic hypovolemic shock, the septic process per se, and the evolution to the multiple organ failure syndrome are all associated with a high incidence of biventricular myocardial depression on a metabolic basis [95, 100]. This is shown in Figure 12-9, which demonstrates the depression in left ventricular function in hyperdynamic patients in whom severe sepsis complicates the postsurgical or posttraumatic response [95].

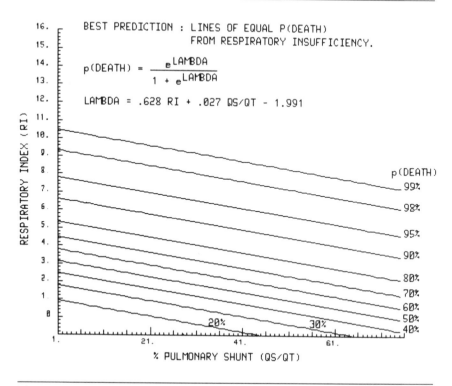

Fig. 12-7. ARDS severity nomogram based on linear logistic model for prediction of severity (*P* death). (A. De Gaetano, et al., Predicting the probability of death from ARDS after trauma. Submitted to *Surgery*, 1990.)

The Role of the Oxygen-Hemoglobin Dissociation Relation in ARDS Compensation

The reason for this phenomenon becomes clear on examination of the other major component of the physiologic response related to oxygen delivery and consumption: namely, the role of the oxygen-hemoglobin dissociation curve in mediating the effect of increased oxygen delivery on the level of arterial PO_2 and arterial oxygen content. As seen in this example (Fig. 12-10), at a given level of oxygen consumption (300 ml/min) and pulmonary shunt ($\dot{Q}_s/\dot{Q}_t = 30\%$), the relationship of flow to the obligatory level of oxygen consumption determines the position on the dissociation curve of the mixed venous oxygen tension ($P\bar{v}O_2$) point. In this example, it can be seen that at a cardiac output of 5 liters/min, the arterial-venous oxygen content difference [$C(a-\bar{v})DO_2$] is 6 ml/dl. The body's mandatory level of oxygen consumption (300 ml/min), which is generally increased over normal in postinjury and septic states, means with this level of flow (cardiac output) the total oxygen delivery (450 ml/min) is only sufficient to allow a reduced mixed venous O_2 tension ($P\bar{v}O_2 = 26$ torr), because the

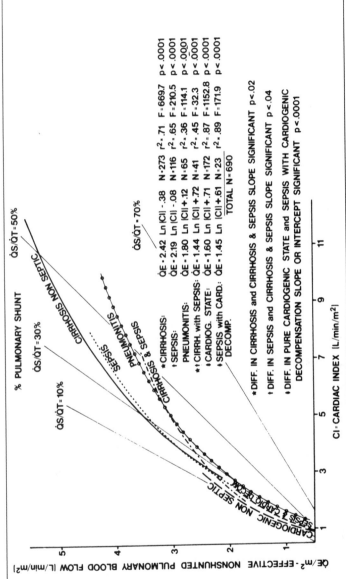

Fig. 12-8. Effect of cardiac index and percent pulmonary shunt on the maintenance of effective nonshunted pulmonary blood flow ($\dot{Q}_E/m^2$). Curved lines represent mean slope and intercept data for patients in various clinical conditions. Note that in patients with cirrhosis or sepsis, and especially in those with cirrhosis and sepsis or those with pneumonitis, an increased flow (CI) is necessary to maintain effective pulmonary blood flow ($\dot{Q}_E/m^2$), because of the high $\dot{Q}_S/\dot{Q}_T$. N = number of studies. (From J. H. Siegel, I. Giovannini, B. Coleman, et al., Pathologic synergy modulation of the cardiovascular, respiratory and metabolic response to injury by cirrhosis and/or sepsis: A manifestation of a common metabolic defect. *Arch. Surg.* 117:225–238, 1982.)

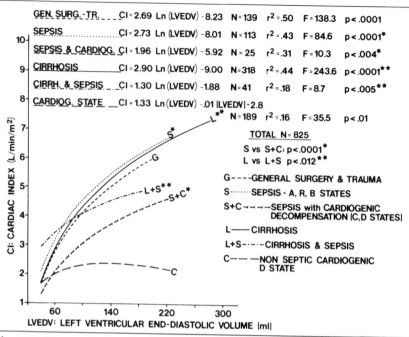

Fig. 12-9. Ventricular function mean slopes labeled by clinical condition in various states of critical illness. N = number of studies. From J. H. Siegel, I. Giovannini, B. Coleman, et al. Pathologic synergy modulation of the cardiovascular, respiratory and metabolic response to injury by cirrhosis and/or sepsis: A manifestation of a common metabolic defect. *Arch. Surg.* 117:225–238, 1982.

arterial desaturation produced by the 30 percent shunt is too great to be overcome. Thus, the highest level of arterial saturation that can be achieved will still be on the *steep* portion of the oxygen-hemoglobin dissociation curve, so that the arterial oxygen tension remains less than 60 torr. However, in this example when the cardiac output is doubled to 10 liters/min, thereby increasing the oxygen delivery from 450 ml/min to 1350 ml/min relative to the mandatory level of oxygen consumption (300 ml/min), the $C(a-\bar{v})DO_2$ narrows to 3 ml/dl. Thus, with a higher net O_2 content the mixed venous blood rises from a saturation of 50 percent to one of 76 percent as the O_2 delivery-to-consumption ratio increases from 1.5 to 4.5. Furthermore, with this O_2 delivery–mediated rise in the mixed venous oxygen saturation and tension level, the net result is to shift the arterial saturation versus PaO_2 point to the *horizontal* portion of the oxygen-hemoglobin dissociation curve. As a result, even though the shunt remains unchanged ($\dot{Q}_s/\dot{Q}_t = 30\%$), the small additional increase in arterial saturation from 89 to 94 percent causes the arterial oxygen tension to rise from 59 to 78 torr, producing a reasonable level of oxygen tension in the arterial blood and thus reducing the hypoxemia. Thus, the critical relationship that must be considered in achieving optimum cardiovascular thera-

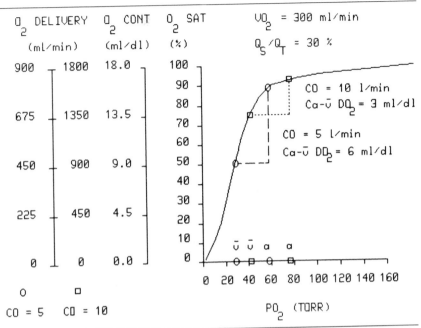

Fig. 12-10. The role of the oxygen-hemoglobin dissociation curve mediating the effect of an increased oxygen delivery on the level of arterial PO_2 and arterial oxygen content. (From J. H. Siegel, J. C. Stoklosa, and U. Borg, Cardiorespiratory Management of the Adult Respiratory Distress Syndrome. In J. H. Siegel (ed.), *Trauma: Emergency Surgery and Critical Care.* New York: Churchill Livingstone, 1987. Pp. 581–673.)

peutic compensation is that between the level of oxygen delivery and the oxygen consumption requirement at any given level of pulmonary dysfunction.

Cardiac Output Control of the Oxygen Delivery-to-Consumption Ratio

The application of this principle to improving PaO_2 by increasing cardiac output can be seen in Figure 12-11. This figure shows the level of arterial oxygen tension (PaO_2) as a function of the oxygen delivery-to-consumption ratio (O_2 DEL/O_2 CONS) and the percent of pulmonary venoarterial admixture ($\dot{Q}_s/\dot{Q}_t$). At low pulmonary venoarterial admixtures, very little effect on the maintenance of PaO_2 is to be gained by increasing the oxygen delivery-to-consumption ratio. However, at shunts greater than 30 percent the increase in the O_2 DEL/O_2 CONS ratio has a major effect in raising the PaO_2. In general, *patients with shunts of greater than 30 percent require a O_2 delivery-to-consumption ratio in excess of 5 to 1,* whereas under normal circumstances a 2 or 3 to 1 ratio would suffice for an adequate PaO_2. It is important to emphasize that since oxygen delivery is the arterial oxygen content (CaO_2) *times* the cardiac output and that oxygen consumption is the arterial-venous oxygen content difference ($Ca-\bar{v}O_2$) *times* the cardiac

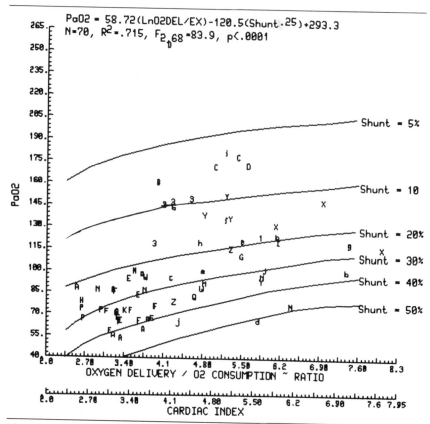

Fig. 12-11. Relation of oxygen delivery-to-consumption ratio and percent pulmonary shunt ($\dot{Q}_s/\dot{Q}_t$) on the maintenance of arterial oxygen tension (PaO_2).

output, in this relationship the cardiac output drops out and therefore the oxygen delivery-to-consumption ratio can be accurately described as the ratio $CaO_2/C(a-\bar{v})DO_2$. These three measurements [PaO_2, CaO_2, $C(a-\bar{v})DO_2$] can be easily and repeatedly obtained at the bedside to evaluate the success of therapeutic cardiovascular manipulation, *if both arterial and mixed venous blood samples are obtained simultaneously.*

In summary, *maintenance of effective pulmonary gas exchange requires as its foundation the maintenance of adequate pulmonary perfusion. When the net surface for pulmonary gas exchange is reduced or is impaired in terms of oxygen diffusion it is critical to optimize the cardiac output at the highest possible level. This means that the net flow must be considerably higher than the level of oxygen delivery that would be required to meet the body's oxygen consumption requirements. This can be achieved by increasing blood volume and by increasing the hemoglobin concentration so as to raise the oxygen-carrying capacity in the blood to the maximum degree possible. This will allow the oxygen delivery to be maximized at any given flow, especially if myocardial function is limited by shock- or sepsis-induced contractile abnormalities, age, or preexisting cardiovascular disease [96, 100]. This, combined with appropriate use of cardiac inotropic support to increase ejection fraction, as well as vasodilator agents to reduce afterload, facilitates a greater cardiac ejection fraction to increase stroke volume and net body flow.*

Also, since pulmonary perfusion is highly dependent on right heart function, it is critical to strengthen right heart contractility in ARDS, in which pulmonary vascular resistance is increased [21, 27, 51, 62, 75, 79, 99, 107, 110]. In this setting, a nonvasoconstricting inotropic agent such as dobutamine (5–10 µg/kg/min) is a valuable therapeutic modality [96, 99]. It is often important to reduce the afterload to the right heart, which is less able to handle high-pressure loads. This may mean that specific vasodilator therapy directed at the pulmonary circulation may be helpful. In our experience the use of low-dose isoproterenol (0.25–1.0 µg/min, *total dose*), which has inotropic but little chronotropic effect [96], has been useful in producing pulmonary arterial vasodilatation whose net effect is to increase total pulmonary perfusion even though there may be some tendency for an increase in pulmonary shunt. However, for the reasons noted above, the net effect of a major increase in pulmonary blood flow usually more than compensates for the small increases in pulmonary shunt that may be caused by any additional ventilation-perfusion abnormalities induced by the dobutamine or isoproterenol. Other vasodilator agents delivered into the pulmonary artery—such as nitroprusside, which also increases shunt—may also be useful in these circumstances, if combined with cardiac inotropic support; but in all instances the relative increase in PaO_2 due to the rise in O_2 DEL/O_2 CONS ratio must be quantitatively evaluated against the proportionate increase in shunt (Fig. 12-11).

Ventilation in ARDS

The goal of mechanical ventilation in this syndrome must be to increase alveolar gas exchange, either by increasing alveolar volume and functional residual capacity or by increasing the rate of exchange of inspired respiratory gas across the remaining reduced alveolar to pulmonary capillary gas exchange surface. To carry out this goal, it is essential to modify the characteristics of mechanical ventilation to compensate for the abnormalities in pulmonary pressure-volume relationships. These can be quantified by the alterations in pulmonary compliance. The characteristics of ventilation must also be used to overcome the ARDS-associated abnormalities in pulmonary airway resistance that impair gas exchange into partially occluded alveoli. *The ventilatory modality chosen must be one that does not further exaggerate the already extent ventilation-perfusion maldistribution characteristic of the ARDS syndrome.*

It is also imperative that any mode of mechanical ventilation provide the maximum exchange for respiratory gas *at the lowest possible airway pressures*, so as to reduce the effects of barotrauma and its potential complications of pneumothorax, pneumomediastinum, or pneumoperitoneum. Excessively high peak, mean, and end-expiratory pressures can cause impairment of right atrial filling due to increased intrathoracic pressure or because a high-pressure bronchial leak has produced a sudden pneumopericardium. These complications can reduce the effective cardiac output by limitations in inflow volume (preload). In the case of pneumopericardium, *immediate subxiphoid pericardial decompression is mandatory,* even if an associated pneumothorax has been treated by thoracostomy tube. The techniques for achieving optimization of ventilatory function at any given level of cardiovascular adequacy in compensation for ARDS respiratory exchange limitations are discussed in the remaining portions of this chapter.

Position

The interrelationship between the nonuniform alterations in capillary permeability and the maldistribution of the pulmonary blood flow in the hyperdynamic state produces some of the unique features of ARDS. The nonuniform ARDS pathology is often concealed by the apparent uniformity of the radiographic findings. As noted earlier, in many cases the interstitial and alveolar infiltrates appear to be distributed fairly uniformly throughout the upper and lower lung fields on an anteroposterior (AP) x-ray. However, on computed tomographic (CT) scan or at autopsy, it can be clearly seen that the most involved segments of the lung are in the dependent portions, which in the case of the severely ill supine patient are the posterior aspects of both upper and lower lobes. Since the AP film does not distinguish anterior from posterior lung segments, but rather projects them, one on the other, what is really a gravitationally influenced progress appears to a large extent to be pathologic change uniformly distributed throughout the lung fields. *The implications of this observation are that no segment of the lung should be allowed to be dependent for any great length of time, and that frequent change in position represents an important modality of therapy.*

The influence of changes in position on improving blood gases by altering the relative $\dot{V}A/\dot{Q}$ distribution is seen in Figure 12-12, which shows data from a patient who sustained a closed head injury and bilateral pulmonary contusion as a result of a motor vehicle accident. He developed pneumonia and ARDS, and his chest radiographs revealed greater involvement of the left lung than the right lung. The use of the noninvasive transcutaneous monitor allowed identification of a significant deterioration in the patient's respiratory status with a change in position from sitting at 60 degrees to left-side-down and with suctioning. Note the improvement when he was placed in the right lateral position (right-side-down). The transcutaneous data generally correlated well with the measured arterial carbon dioxide tension and was within 10 percent of the PaO_2 when the $PTcO_2$ was adjusted by the regression-derived constants described earlier [112].

This case also makes the point that the transcutaneous monitor is useful as a trend monitor and is especially valuable when making changes in ventilator settings in normodynamic or hyperdynamic posttrauma patients.

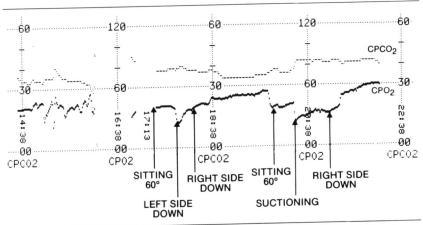

Fig. 12-12. Effect of changing position on the maintenance of arterial blood gases as determined from transcutaneous O_2 and PCO_2 measures. (From J. H. Siegel, J. C. Stoklosa, and U. Borg, Cardiorespiratory Management of the Adult Respiratory Distress Syndrome. In J. H. Siegel (ed.), *Trauma: Emergency Surgery and Critical Care.* New York: Churchill Livingstone, 1987. Pp. 581–673.)

An improvement or a decrease in oxygenation noted on the transcutaneous or pulse oximeter when a patient is moved from the supine to the right or left lateral decubitus position may be an indication for use of independent lung ventilation.

PEEP

Positive end-expiratory pressure (PEEP) can be defined as an above-atmospheric pressure applied to the airway at the end of expiration. The clinical use of PEEP in cardiogenic pulmonary edema was first described in the 1930s by Poulton and Oxon [83], who used a continuous-flow system utilizing a spring-loaded PEEP valve to maintain continuous positive airway pressure (CPAP), and by Barach et al. [7], who used an underwater seal to create PEEP. As a means of supporting oxygenation in patients who developed ARDS, PEEP became part of routine medical management as a result of the work of Ashbaugh, Petty, and coworkers in the late 1960s [2, 81].

Despite the ubiquitous use of PEEP, there is no direct evidence of any therapeutic benefit to the lungs from PEEP, nor has any study demonstrated a significant increase in survival from ARDS since the "state of the art" first included the use of PEEP. Pepe and colleagues [76] demonstrated that the early application of PEEP at 8 cm H_2O did not influence the incidence of ARDS, even though there was improvement in the PaO_2/FiO_2 ratio during PEEP in patients who developed ARDS. This is unsurprising, since the time course of the initiating humoral response would not be expected to be influenced by a strictly mechanical therapy, which although not useful in preventing ARDS alterations, may help to compensate for the altered permeability and ventilation-perfusion ratio induced by this disease process.

Petty [80] expressed doubt that a prospective, randomized, controlled study will ever be performed to show a survival effect from PEEP, since more good than harm apparently comes from the use of PEEP in the range of 5 to 15 cm H_2O. PEEP, therefore, is a supportive adjunct used to improve oxygenation and allow for a decrease in supplementary oxygen. It allows critical gas-exchange processes to occur at nontoxic levels of inspired oxygen, thereby buying time for natural processes to heal injured tissue [80, 90, 119].

The postulated mechanisms for the improvement in oxygenation by PEEP, as manifested by an increase in PaO_2, include the holding open of respiratory bronchioles with the prevention of alveolar collapse. In addition, direct measurement [57, 84, 119] has demonstrated that PEEP leads to an increase in FRC. This is accomplished by an increase in both alveolar size and alveolar recruitment, the latter occurring when ARDS-induced alveolar atelectatic pathology is present [76, 84, 87, 90]. Figure 12-13 illustrates the effect of increasing the PEEP from 0.5 to 25.3 cm H_2O. Displayed are the inspiratory and expiratory flows, the airway pressures, and from integration of the flow, the inspiratory and expiratory volumes. The pressure level was increased on the third breath. Note that whereas inspired volume remained constant for the subsequent breaths, expiratory volume was less than inspired until the seventh breath, when the inspired and expired volume again became equal. This difference in volume amounted to 0.817 liters and *is equivalent to the increase in the FRC level* achieved by PEEP of 25.3 cm H_2O above that at 0.5 cm PEEP.

The increase in volume (ΔV) that occurs in already open lung units in response to a change in the end-expiratory pressure level (ΔP) is dictated by the elastic behavior of the lung (C_L) and chest wall (C_w),

$$\Delta V = \Delta P \times C_L \times \frac{C_w}{C_L + C_w}$$

and usually occurs within the first breath or two. The recruitment phase may take longer. In most patients, four to five breaths suffice to complete more than 90 percent of the eventual volume change [57]. In some patients, however, it may require minutes to hours for the full effect of PEEP to occur [63]. But to recruit fluid-filled or atelectactic areas it appears to be necessary to overdistend those more-normal alveoli operating on the favorable portion of their pressure-volume curve—the point at which compliance is greatest. Below a certain critical volume, alveoli tend to collapse and expand only at a much higher pressure than that originally needed to maintain expansion. The volume of each alveolus, and of the lung as a unit, is determined by the distending pressure multiplied by the compliance. As a result, the markedly compliant alveoli have more volume.

What level of PEEP is "best," or "optimal"? What level results in a balance between the pressure needed to prevent airway and alveolar collapse

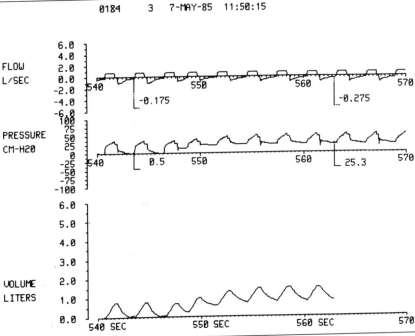

0184   3   7-MAY-85   11:50:15

Fig. 12-13. Effect of increasing positive end-expiratory pressure (PEEP) from 0.5 cm H$_2$O to 25.3 cm H$_2$O on level of functional residual capacity (FRC). (From J. H. Siegel, J. C. Stoklosa, and U. Borg, Cardiorespiratory Management of the Adult Respiratory Distress Syndrome. In J. H. Siegel (ed.), *Trauma: Emergency Surgery and Critical Care*. New York: Churchill Livingstone, 1987. Pp. 581–673.)

and promote alveolar recruitment and that which causes overexpansion of the more compliant areas of the lung? Such overdistention can result in hemodynamic compromise and worsening of $\dot{V}A/\dot{Q}$ relationships, due to the transmission of high airway pressures to the alveolar capillary vasculature, which acts as a Starling resistor to blood flow, with diversion of blood flow away from the well-ventilated areas. The fraction of the end-expiratory airway pressure (PAW ex) transmitted depends on the relative compliances of the lung and chest wall.

$$\Delta V_L = C_L \times \Delta(PAW\ ex - P_{PL})$$
$$\Delta V_W = C_W \times \Delta P_{PL}$$

since $\Delta V_L = \Delta V_W$,

$$\Delta P_{PL} = \Delta PAW\ ex \frac{C_L}{C_L + C_W}$$

Normally, C_L equals approximately C_W over the tidal volume range, so that

$$\frac{\Delta P_{PL}}{C_L + C_W} \text{ equals approximately } \tfrac{1}{2}\Delta P_{AW} \text{ ex } C_L$$

Therefore, about one-half of the PEEP increment is reflected in the pleural pressure. With stiff lungs a lesser fraction of the PEEP is transmitted, whereas with a stiff chest wall a greater fraction will be transmitted. This increase in transmission must be kept in mind when dealing with patients who have essentially normal lung compliances but who may have a decreased chest wall compliance and thus a reduced total static compliance, due to abdominal distention or the presence of a pleural effusion or fibrin peel (Fig. 12-4). The harmful effects of using excessive PEEP in this situation are related to an overdistention of the more compliant alveoli with diversion of alveolar capillary blood flow to the less compliant, poorly exchanging alveoli. This will convert the overdistended alveoli to dead space and will result in an increase in blood flow to low $\dot{V}_A/\dot{Q}$ areas with a rise in physiologic shunting. Thus, there will be a further fall in PaO_2 and often a rise in $PaCO_2$.

Depending on the degree of distention of the lung and chest wall prior to the initiation of PEEP, compliance may be either increased or decreased by PEEP and ventilation-perfusion relationships in the lung, and PaO_2 and $PaCO_2$ can be improved, can be unchanged, or can deteriorate when PEEP is used. There are also varying effects on the volume of dead space. Dead space can be decreased if the application of PEEP leads to a more even distribution of a constant tidal volume as a result of reexpansion of previously collapsed alveoli. Dead space can increase if the size of conducting airways is increased, if normal alveoli are overexpanded, or if there is a reduction in the amount of perfusion to normal alveoli due to increased intra-alveolar pressure that exceeds that in the alveolar capillary bed.

Tissue oxygen delivery is the ultimate goal of treatment of a patient with refractory hypoxemia. No one formula can predict the level of PEEP that will maximally benefit the patient, but Suter et al. [114, 115] showed that systemic oxygen transport (arterial oxygen content times cardiac output) was maximal when total compliance was highest in a series of 15 clinically normovolemic patients with acute pulmonary failure. They demonstrated that PaO_2 varied with end-expiratory pressure. Cardiac output, and therefore oxygen transport, decreased when PEEP was increased beyond the level that produced the maximum compliance. Among the factors thought to cause this change in compliance is the curvilinear form of the lung–chest wall pressure-volume relationship, at the lower end of which is superimposed the effect of recruitment of atelectatic alveoli and stress relaxation of the lung and chest wall. Katz et al. [57] found that about 60 percent of the improvement in compliance seen with addition of increments of PEEP was due to the lung and the remainder to the chest wall, suggesting that stress relaxation of the chest wall is an important component.

To the extent that changes in total static compliance do reflect changes in lung compliance, with increases reflecting recruitment and decreases

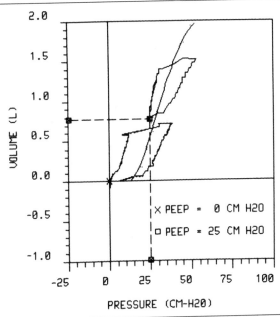

Fig. 12-14. Total static compliance curve (CST) obtained by increasing inspired volume from 0 to 2.0 liters at a PEEP of 0 cm H_2O. Superimposed are the dynamic curves of two breaths, one starting at a PEEP level of 0 cm H_2O and the other at a PEEP level of 25 cm H_2O. Note increase in functional residual capacity (FRC) by 0.78 liters and the change in the dynamic characteristics of the breath as the FRC level is raised as a new starting point for the tidal volume at a PEEP of 25 cm H_2O. (From J. H. Siegel, J. C. Stoklosa, and U. Borg, Cardiorespiratory Management of the Adult Respiratory Distress Syndrome. In J. H. Siegel (ed.), *Trauma: Emergency Surgery and Critical Care.* New York: Churchill Livingstone, 1987. Pp. 581–673.)

overdistention, this is a relatively simple way to assess what level of PEEP provides optimal gas exchange. As a general rule, Suter [114, 115] feels that those levels of PEEP or tidal volume that lower the compliance value should not be used unless objective evidence of improved O_2 delivery is obtained. Other investigators have established the importance of blood volume and other hemodynamic factors in determining the mean airway pressure above which cardiac output decreases. It is dangerous simply to assume that gas exchange will be most favorable when compliance is greatest. *Therefore, it is imperative that all parameters affecting oxygen delivery, including arterial and mixed venous blood gases and oxygen saturation, hemoglobin level, and cardiac output, be assessed when PEEP levels are being adjusted.* However, when the lung is grossly abnormal and high inflation pressures are required during mechanical ventilation, the use of the total static compliance (CST) relationship and the generation of the dynamic pressure-volume curve may be very useful in determining the best combination of PEEP, tidal volume, and ventilatory dynamics to raise FRC, minimize barotrauma, and maximize respiratory gas exchange (Fig. 12-14). This optimization will be discussed at the conclusion of the chapter.

As previously described, the level of end-expiratory pressure in the alveolus may be different from the set PEEP—the so-called auto-PEEP, or intrinsic PEEP (PEEP$_i$), effect seen when mechanical ventilation is used. PEEP$_i$ is usually considered a complication of mechanical ventilation due to pulmonary gas trapping caused by insufficient expiratory time. A significant level of PEEP$_i$ above set PEEP has been noted in patients with chronic obstructive pulmonary disease, when high minute ventilation or respiratory rates are used and with the use of small endotracheal tubes [9]. Among the adverse effects of PEEP$_i$ are hemodynamic compromise, misinterpretation of pulmonary capillary wedge pressure, increased work of breathing, barotrauma, and miscalculation of compliance [9]. It is therefore imperative that PEEP$_i$ be measured directly, using the methodology previously described. Clinical techniques that can be utilized to minimize pulmonary gas trapping are aggressive bronchodilitation, secretion removal, increases in the size of the endotracheal tube, and modification of the ventilatory pattern.

Increasing the level of the set PEEP can at times ameliorate gas trapping by splinting the airways, as in pursed-lips breathing. This technique should be used cautiously, since increasing external PEEP could contribute further to the increase in PEEP$_i$. If PEEP$_i$ decreases or remains the same when this technique is used, the increased set PEEP can be considered advantageous. Two newer techniques of mechanical ventilation, combined high-frequency ventilation (CHFV) and inverse-ratio ventilation (IRV), deliberately employ auto-PEEP to improve oxygenation. These techniques will be discussed in the section on mechanical ventilation. Under appropriate circumstances, auto-PEEP can be therapeutic when an oxygenation deficit requires the use of PEEP and the measured PEEP$_i$ is considered as part of the management. *In this situation it must be understood that manipulation of respiratory rate, minute ventilation, inspiratory flow rate, inspiratory : expiratory (I : E) ratio, and/or set PEEP can all impact on the level of auto-PEEP, and careful and routine monitoring of PEEP$_i$ is mandatory.*

Continuous Positive Airway Pressure in the Spontaneously Breathing Patient

Continuous positive airway pressure (CPAP) is a means of maintaining positive end-expiratory pressure in the spontaneously breathing patient. It was developed by Gregory and coworkers [47] for the treatment of infants with the idiopathic respiratory distress syndrome and has become an accepted method of treatment in adults who develop ARDS. It is delivered utilizing a breathing circuit with a threshold resistance underwater seal on the expiratory limb to maintain the selected PEEP and a source of gas to provide continuous inspiratory flow.

The cardiopulmonary effects of PEEP and CPAP in the spontaneously breathing patient were assessed by Sturgeon and associates [113], who found no differences in expiratory transpulmonary pressures but an increase in inspiratory effort with PEEP. There was a decrease in effective cardiac filling pressures without a change in stroke volume with CPAP, whereas with PEEP effective cardiac filling pressures were not modified but stroke volume was increased.

The use of PEEP in the spontaneously breathing patient significantly increases the work of breathing, since the patient must generate greater negative pressure to initiate inspiration. The use of a CPAP system should require less work, since a positive inspiratory pressure is maintained utilizing a source of continuous gas flow. However, work may still be greater than it would be without the use of PEEP, unless there is a significant improvement in compliance as a result of the use of PEEP.

Mechanical Ventilation Techniques

The successful ventilation of the patient with ARDS must accommodate to a number of pathophysiologic mechanisms, ranging from decreased compliance and reduced FRC (due to alveolar collapse) to major bronchopleural or parenchymal air leaks. The types and functions of the various modes of mechanical ventilation now available must be fully understood and their characteristics matched to the patient [59, 99].

Types of Ventilators

There are three basic types of ventilators:

Time-cycled: inspiration terminated after a preset time.
Volume-cycled: inspiration terminated after delivery of a preset volume.
Pressure-cycled: inspiration terminated after a preset pressure is attained at the mouth or elsewhere in the apparatus.

More than one method of cycling can be included in one apparatus.

Characteristics of Ventilator Operation

TIME-CYCLED VENTILATION. In time-cycled ventilators, a pressure generator will deliver a smaller volume in the face of an increased resistance and a true flow generator will deliver almost the correct volume, provided the raised pressure does not exceed a set safety value.

If compliance is diminished, the flow generator should again deliver the correct tidal volume and the pressure generator would deliver a reduced tidal volume in proportion to the reduction in compliance.

VOLUME-CYCLED VENTILATION. A flow generator should deliver the correct tidal volume in the normal time. The minute volume should, therefore, be independent of moderate changes in compliance and resistance.

PRESSURE-CYCLED VENTILATION. Only flow generators can be pressure-cycled, and a constant-pressure generator must be cycled by either time or volume.

Cycling by pressure has the disadvantage that if the resistance increases or the compliance decreases, the mouth pressure will reach the set or critical level at a smaller tidal volume than it would with normal respiratory function.

Controlled Ventilation

There are two types of controlled ventilation: volume-controlled (VC) and pressure-controlled (PC). In the control mode the patient is unable to initiate a breath and, unless paralyzed or anesthetized, will "fight" the ventilator if the settings are inadequate to provide for optimal gas exchange. The usual practice when choosing the appropriate ventilator setting at which to begin therapy is to use a tidal volume of 12 to 15 ml/kg and a rate sufficient to maintain $PaCO_2$ between 36 and 44 mm Hg. If the control mode of ventilation is utilized initially, the respiratory rate is usually set between 10 and 16 breaths/min and all ventilation is provided by the ventilator.

VOLUME-CONTROLLED VENTILATION. In VC ventilation (Fig. 12-15), a set volume is delivered to the patient. The volume to be delivered is determined by selecting the respiratory rate (RR) and tidal volume, or the RR and minute ventilation. The pressure required to deliver each tidal volume is dependent on the patient's compliance and resistance. A pressure limit is set on the ventilator to guard against excessively high airway pressures. If this pressure limit is exceeded, the volume actually delivered will be less than the set tidal volume. As noted earlier (Table 12-1), the volume delivered to the patient is also dependent upon the amount of gas compressed within the ventilator itself and on its tubing and humidification system.

Volume-controlled ventilators are either time-cycled or volume-cycled. Time-cycled ventilators terminate inspiratory gas flow at a predetermined time, thus allowing for adjustments of inspiratory and expiratory time. The inspiratory : expiratory (I : E) ratio is set. Volume-cycled ventilators stop gas flow when a predetermined volume (as signaled by a measuring device such as a flow sensor, potentiometer, or bellows) has been delivered. The I : E ratio is variable, since it is dependent upon the inspiratory flow rate. With some ventilators, the operator can set a period of inflation-hold (inspiratory pause) at the end of the inspiratory period; this phase is usually considered a part of inspiration. Inflation-hold is used to improve gas distribution when lung areas have differing time constants. Varying inspiratory flow patterns are also available on many ventilators now used in critical care. Flow is usually constant (as shown in Fig. 12-15) but can be set for a given time related pattern in some ventilator systems (i.e., sine wave, accelerating, or decelerating). The availability of these different patterns of flow is especially useful in ventilating patients who have markedly dissimilar time constants in differing lung areas because of the asymmetric distribution of their disease process.

PRESSURE-CONTROLLED VENTILATION. In PC ventilation, gas is delivered at a constant pressure and for a set period of time. The flow rate is a decelerating pattern—that is, flow is initially high and decreases throughout the

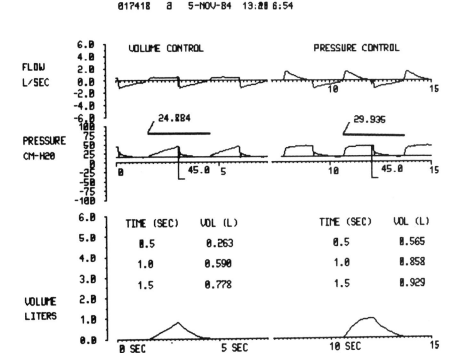

Fig. **12-15.** Comparison of volume control and pressure control ventilation at the same respiratory rate and controlled peak pressure limit (45.0 cm H_2O). Note the constant flow in volume control mode versus decelerating flow in pressure control mode and the increase in rate of inspiratory volume, as well as absolute inspiratory volume, under PC mode, at the cost of a somewhat higher mean airway pressure—24.9 cm H_2O (VC) versus 29.9 cm H_2O (PC). (From J. H. Siegel, J. C. Stoklosa, and U. Borg, Cardiorespiratory Management of the Adult Respiratory Distress Syndrome. In J. H. Siegel (ed.), *Trauma: Emergency Surgery and Critical Care.* New York: Churchill Livingstone, 1987. Pp. 581–673.)

inspiratory cycle (Fig. 12-15). The volume delivered is determined by the set inspiratory pressure, the rate, and the time for inspiration. In the example shown in Figure 12-15, comparing constant flow in the VC mode to constant pressure in the PC mode, the PC mode results in a larger tidal volume delivered earlier in inspiration, but at the cost of a somewhat higher mean airway pressure.

However, in the PC mode the volume delivered will vary depending on the patient's compliance and airway resistance, as well as on the actual or "intrinsic" PEEP level, and close monitoring of the actual volume delivered is essential. Any increase in airway resistance caused by bronchospasm, or a decreased lumen of the endotracheal tube due to secretions, will result in a decrease in the tidal volume actually delivered, since there will be a decrease in the flow rate delivered by the ventilator.

Patient-Assisted Ventilation

In the *assist-control* mode the patient initiates the machine breath by generating a pressure that is negative in relation to the baseline or end-expiratory pressure. The patient controls the rate and minute volume delivered. In this mode of ventilation the tidal volume remains constant, and if the patient's ventilatory rate falls below a set level, the ventilator will automatically deliver the number of breaths set as the "backup" rate.

Two modes of ventilation that can be used not only for control mode but also for spontaneous breathing are *intermittent mandatory ventilation (IMV)* and *synchronized intermittent mandatory ventilation (SIMV)*. The IMV mode utilizes a control mode ventilator with attached circuitry that allows the patient to spontaneously breathe gas of the same temperature, humidity, and FIO_2 as provided by the ventilator. At preset intervals, a VC breath is delivered by the ventilator. To ensure unimpeded spontaneous ventilation, a continuous gas flow with a flow rate at least four times the patient's minute ventilation must be provided, and care must also be taken that the circuitry does not cause any increase in resistance to breathing.

The SIMV mode utilizes a ventilator in the assist-control mode with circuitry that also allows the patient to breathe spontaneously. Unlike with the IMV mode, however, the ventilator breath is initiated by the patient's inspiratory effort. As in the assist-control mode, if the patient does not initiate the breath, the ventilator will automatically deliver it. A demand-flow system for the spontaneous breath is used in SIMV, since a continuous-flow system does not allow for generation of the subbaseline pressure necessary for this means of synchronizing volume delivery by the ventilator to the patient's inspiratory effort.

The SIMV mode was developed due to concerns that using the IMV mode would result in "stacking" of a ventilator breath on top of a machine-initiated breath, with production of excessively high airway pressures and their subsequent effect on cardiorespiratory function. In actuality, "stacking" does not have any significant effect on function, and SIMV has no demonstrable physiologic advantage over IMV. One practical advantage, however, is that one can easily monitor the minute ventilation of the patient, as well as his or her spontaneous tidal volume, using the SIMV mode.

When rates of greater than 8 per minute are used in the IMV or SIMV mode, the ventilator is essentially providing controlled ventilatory support. At rates below this, the patient is providing a significant portion of his or her ventilatory requirement.

There is much controversy concerning the reputed advantages of the IMV or SIMV modes of mechanical ventilation over the controlled, or assist-controlled, mode of ventilation. Weisman et al. [122] discussed the advantages and disadvantages of intermittent mandatory ventilation, and readers may wish to consult this article to come to their own conclusions regarding the value of these techniques for ARDS-patient management. Assist-control modalities are of some value in weaning the patient from ventilatory support, especially if the patient has been on some form of controlled ventilation for a prolonged period and may have wasting of the accessory muscles of respiration, so that he or she tires easily after a brief period of spontaneous breathing.

A new mode of assisted ventilation, *pressure support,* used either with SIMV or alone, has been utilized to augment the weaning patient's spontaneous tidal volume [15, 67]. Gradually decreasing levels of pressure support (PC) are used to wean this type of patient from ventilator dependence. In our experience, this appears to be a more reliable method of weaning, affording less chance of allowing muscle weakness to induce respiratory failure due to hypoventilation, with the weaning complications of CO_2 retention and respiratory acidosis.

Ventilatory Patterns of Respiratory Gas Delivery

The distribution of inspired gas is normally inhomogeneous, due to the presence of varying time constants within the lung. During controlled mechanical ventilation, there is an accentuation of this maldistribution, with the inspirate going preferentially to the dead space. Studies on the effect of varying inspiratory flow patterns on this maldistribution have yielded conflicting results: some authors have found sinusoidal flow better than constant flow [23, 92] in patients or lung models with disparate airway resistances, whereas others have found the opposite [66]. However, in a comparison of the decelerating flow pattern to constant or accelerating flow patterns in patients with acute respiratory failure, decelerating flow was found to be superior [1, 55, 72].

A tidal volume delivered using a decelerating flow pattern, as in PC ventilation [15], theoretically should accentuate any maldistribution of gas in lungs with inhomogeneous ventilation, since gas distribution is presumably most sensitive to flow rate early in inspiration. With decelerating flow, however, the mean lung volume during the inspiratory phase is *larger* than with constant, sinusoidal, or accelerating flow patterns, since a greater portion of the tidal volume is given earlier in the inspiratory time (Fig. 12-15) and the duration of fresh gas dilution of the FRC will be increased for a given inspiratory time. Therefore, distribution uniformity may be more dependent on time than inspiratory waveform. The use of an inspiratory pause hold may also improve gas distribution [23]. When mechanical ventilation is instituted, the ratio of inspiration to expiration (I : E) is routinely 1 : 3. When an inspiratory pause is added, the I : E ratio will change, since the time for expiration will decrease. Ratios of 1 : 2 and even 1 : 1 can be used in patients with ARDS if there is no evidence of obstructive lung disease. These ratios can result in lower peak and plateau airway pressures but produce a higher mean airway pressure with improved gas exchange, as discussed below.

Mean Airway Pressure

The mean airway pressure ($\overline{PAW}$) is a reflection of all pressures transmitted to the airways. Factors that affect the $\overline{PAW}$ include peak inspiratory pressure (PIP); PEEP; inspiratory time, including inflation hold or end-inspiratory pause (EIP); rate of ventilation; and the type of pressure waveform created by the ventilator. Recent studies [14, 20, 38, 78] have shown that improvement in oxygenation is directly correlated with changes in mean airway pressure irrespective of how the increase in $\overline{PAW}$ was achieved—whether by increasing PEEP, changing the inspiratory pressure waveform, increasing inspiratory time by decreasing inspiratory flow rate, or using an inflation-hold. However, changes in cardiac output must be considered when using increases in mean airway pressure to improve oxygenation, since the increase in $\overline{P_{AW}}$ may also reduce cardiac output, thus producing an undesirable decrease in peripheral oxygen delivery.

The increase in mean airway pressure with PC (Fig. 12-15) can be significant especially when the inspiratory time is prolonged, as with an inspiratory pause hold or a reverse I : E ratio; also, in hypovolemic conditions it may adversely affect cardiac output and thus oxygen delivery, as well as result in an increased risk of barotrauma, and these must be monitored when it is used.

New Techniques of Mechanical Ventilation in ARDS

Conventional methods of ventilatory support, which apply their volume and pressure characteristics indiscriminately to all lung regions, may lead to a worsening of ventilation-perfusion ($\dot{V}_A/\dot{Q}$) relationships in the normally aerated regions now shown to be present in ARDS [39, 40, 70]. There is a therapeutic paradox imposed by this pathophysiologic problem: conventional mechanical ventilation (CMV) with generalized PEEP may increase flow through low-$\dot{V}_A/\dot{Q}$, low-compliance lung while reducing that through high-compliance, high-$\dot{V}_A/\dot{Q}$ lung. This occurs even though the PEEP effect assists in opening underventilated alveoli by raising mean airway pressures above the now-increased critical opening pressures in the injured lung. This pathophysiologic sequence has led to the modification of conventional modes of ventilation.

Inverse I : E Ratio Ventilation

Recently, a ventilatory technique of supplying conventional mechanical ventilation with the I : E ratio greater than 1 : 1, *inverse ratio ventilation (IRV)*, has been used in infants and adults with severe pulmonary dysfunction. Ratios of up to 4 : 1, where inspiration time is prolonged to 80 percent of the respiratory cycle with a concomitant drop of expiratory time to 20 percent, have been used [48, 61, 116]. Proponents of this mode of therapy have postulated that the improvement in gas exchange seen (Fig. 12-16) could be due to improved gas diffusion and recruitment and stabilization of alveolar units [48]. When IRV is used, care must be taken in choosing the correct means of increasing inspiratory time. In the VC mode, decreasing the inspiratory flow rate will increase the time required to deliver a given volume and result in a lower mean lung volume during the entire inspiratory phase, with a potential deleterious effect on gas exchange. If the VC mode is to be used, adding an inspiratory pause hold, rather than extending the time to full tidal volume, should be the method utilized to increase the I : E ratio. Currently, the pressure-controlled, time-cycled mode is used to deliver IRV (PC-IRV) (Fig. 12-16). Lachmann compared the VC to the PC mode and documented the superiority of PC ventilation [61].

When IRV is used, the "auto"- or "intrinsic"-PEEP level (PEEP$_i$) must be measured [32] at each setting, since if it is correctly applied, expiratory flow will still be occurring when the next breath is delivered to the patient

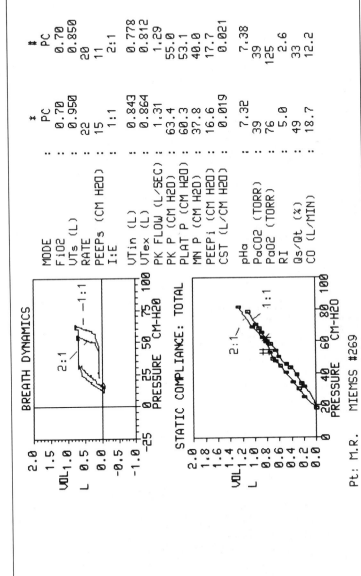

	*	#
MODE	PC	PC
FiO2	0.70	0.70
VTs (L)	0.950	0.850
RATE	22	20
PEEPs (CM H2O)	15	11
I:E	1:1	2:1
VTin (L)	0.843	0.778
VTex (L)	0.864	0.812
PK FLOW (L/SEC)	1.31	1.29
PK P (CM H2O)	63.4	55.0
PLAT P (CM H2O)	60.3	53.1
MN P (CM H2O)	37.8	40.0
PEEPi (CM H2O)	16.6	17.7
CST (L/CM H2O)	0.019	0.021
pHa	7.32	7.38
PaCO2 (TORR)	39	39
PaO2 (TORR)	76	125
RI	5.0	2.6
Qs/Qt (%)	49	33
CO (L/MIN)	18.7	12.2

Pt: M.R.   MIEMSS #269

Fig. 12-16. Static compliance and breath dynamics in ARDS patient in pressure control mode. Effect of increasing I : E ratio from 1 : 1 to 2 : 1 on lung mechanics and gas exchange.

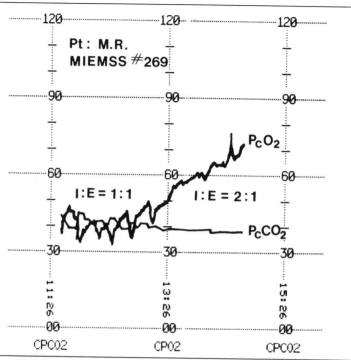

Fig. 12-17. Effect of increasing I : E ratio on arterial blood gases as measured from transcutaneous O_2 and CO_2. Note the increase in P$\text{TC}O_2$ with a slight decrease in P$\text{TC}CO_2$ following the increase in the I : E ratio. At an I : E ratio equal to 1 : 1, the regression-corrected PaO_2 = 76 torr and the regression-corrected $PaCO_2$ = 40 torr. Two hours after institution of an increase in I : E ratio equal to 2 : 1, the regression-corrected PaO_2 = 108 torr and that for $PaCO_2$ = 36 torr. Patient CST data previously shown in Figure 12–16.

(Fig. 12-3). As previously mentioned, this will result in the generation of a higher PEEP level than that mechanically set on the ventilator (Fig. 12-16). Figure 12-16 also shows the reduction in peak airway pressure (PKP), plateau pressure (PLAT P), PaO_2, RI, and shunt ($\dot{Q}_s/\dot{Q}_t$) in spite of a fall in cardiac output (CO) when the I : E ratio was increased from 1 : 1 to 2 : 1. The time course of the regression [112] uncorrected transcutaneous O_2 (P$\text{TC}O_2$) and P$\text{TC}CO_2$ for this patient is shown in Figure 12-17, demonstrating the brisk rise in oxygen tension with little change in carbon dioxide tension as the I : E ratio was increased. In addition to routine monitoring of hemodynamics, tidal volume, minute ventilation, and peak and mean airway pressures, graphical display of flow and pressure curves (Fig. 12-3) should be considered when using IRV. At present, IRV should be considered an experimental technique and should only be undertaken by those cognizant of its potentially adverse effects. It should not be used in patients with low cardiac output syndromes.

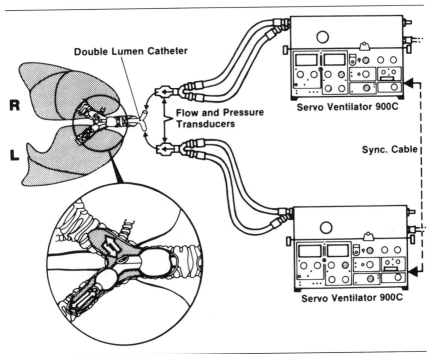

Fig. 12-18. Therapeutic system for simultaneous independent lung ventilation (SILV). (From J. H. Siegel, J. C. Stoklosa, U. Borg, et al., Quantification of asymmetric lung pathophysiology as a guide to the use of simultaneous independent lung ventilation in posttraumatic and septic ARDS. *Ann. Surg.* 202:425–439, 1985.)

Simultaneous Independent Lung Ventilation

Respiratory failure in patients with asymmetric lung disease cannot be treated effectively with conventional methods of ventilatory support, which apply their volume and pressure characteristics indiscriminately to all lung regions. In *simultaneous independent lung ventilation (SILV)*, the use of two ventilators (Fig. 12-18) allows the ventilatory pressures and time patterns of the volume delivery to be tailored for each lung, so as to alter perfusion to obtain better $\dot{V}A/\dot{Q}$ distribution and to interfere less with cardiac filling and cardiac output levels. Synchronization of the ventilators allows for simultaneous inspirations, and tidal volume, inspiratory time, pause time, PEEP, and FiO_2 can be adjusted separately for each lung. The SILV technique has been applied with some success to unilateral lung contusion [43, 97], ARDS [5, 97], lobar pneumonia [18, 85], and refractory unilateral atelectasis [87, 97]. It is particularly useful for treating massive bronchial repair leaks such as may occur after unilateral pneumonectomy with disruption of the bronchial suture link [19] and is also of great value in maintaining ventilation of the dependent lung during thoracotomy in the lateral position [99]. More recently, it has been suggested that even acute asymmetric bilateral lung pathology may be treated by independent lung ventilation in the lateral position [4, 5, 6, 97, 99], thus artificially creating a situation in which one lung (the dependent) has increased perfusion and the other (nondependent) has increased ventilation. Then, by using selective PEEP and pressure- or volume-controlled ventilation, it may be possible to shift perfusion upward to the hyperventilated nondependent lung while simultaneously increasing ventilation to the hyperperfused dependent lung, thereby effecting a more even $\dot{V}A/\dot{Q}$ matching [4, 5, 6].

Difficulties in achieving an optimal ventilatory solution to this set of clinical problems have been encountered in three areas: (1) the need for an easily insertable double-lumen bronchial catheter for separation of the two lungs; (2) the need for a suitable dual-ventilator system with sufficient flexibility to accommodate all of the variations in PEEP, volume, flow, I : E ratio, and modalities of pressure- and volume-controlled support required to meet all possible clinical situations; (3) the need for a simple, clinically applicable bedside technique of ventilatory assessment whereby the magnitude of the asymmetric pathologic lung condition can be rapidly assessed, criteria for the initiation of SILV established, and management of this therapy effected.

The method of carrying out SILV is shown in Figure 12-18 [97]. In this therapeutic system, two advanced Servo ventilators are synchronized to start of inspiration. Each complete system is connected to one lumen of a dual-lumen Broncho-cath* catheter. Regardless of the side of greatest pathologic change, the long arm of a left-angled Broncho-cath is placed in the left mainstem bronchus, to avoid obstruction to the right upper lobe segmental bronchus. The proximal balloon occludes the trachea, providing a closed system, and when the distal balloon is inflated the right and left lungs can be independently ventilated by the two Servo ventilators using different tidal volumes, PEEPs, I : E ratios, and pause times—and in some instances, totally different ventilatory modes (i.e., volume-controlled in one lung and pressure-controlled in the other). To start the SILV process, the total tidal volume is divided in half, the pressures monitored, and a compliance curve created for each lung. Then, adjustment to an appropriate pressure-volume point for each lung is carried out. The value of this approach can be seen in Figure 12-19, in which the different static total compliance curves of the right and left lungs mandate two different volume optimization points at different PEEPs [97].

In using this technique, the cardiac output (CO) should be measured by thermodilution or cardiogreen dye dilution at frequent intervals and after all major ventilatory changes. Arterial and mixed venous oxygen saturations and the blood partial pressures of respiratory gases (PO_2, PCO_2) and pH should also be measured at the same time, and the oxygen content difference [$C(a-\bar{v})DO_2$], percent pulmonary venoarterial admixture ($\dot{Q}_s/\dot{Q}_t$), and respiratory index (alveolar-arterial O_2 gradient/PaO_2 ratio) should be

*National Catheter Corp., Argyle, N.Y.

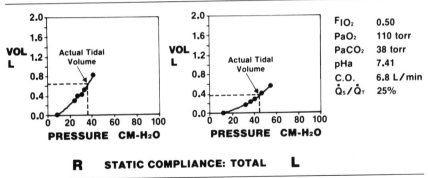

Fig. 12-19. Total static compliance curves for right (R) and left (L) lungs under simultaneous independent lung ventilation, showing optimization points at different tidal volumes and PEEP levels. (From J. H. Siegel, J. C. Stoklosa, U. Borg, et al., Quantification of asymmetric lung pathophysiology as a guide to the use of simultaneous independent lung ventilation in posttraumatic and septic ARDS. *Ann. Surg.* 202:425–, 1985.)

computed to permit accurate quantification of physiologic changes in response to SILV therapy [10, 89, 93].

High-Frequency Ventilation

Since the introduction of high-frequency ventilation (HFV), three types of systems have been used clinically: high-frequency positive-pressure ventilation (HFPPV) [102, 103], high-frequency jet ventilation (HFJV) [17, 19, 60], and high-frequency oscillation (HFO) [16, 46]. The rationale for the use of HFV is that delivery of a small tidal volume (less than the volume of the physiologic dead space) at a high ventilatory rate could result in lower peak and mean airway pressures than those seen with conventional tidal volumes and rates, thus decreasing the risk of barotrauma, cardiocirculatory embarrassment, and compounding of the existing ventilation-to-perfusion mismatch [12, 103]. Early experimental studies suggested that HFV maintained lower peak and mean airway pressures and produced less cardiocirculatory impairment; however, these experimental advantages could not be convincingly repeated in clinical investigations in patients with ARDS. Positive effects were noted in terms of improved intrapulmonary gas distribution, and in some cases, lower peak airway pressures were achieved.

HFJV and HFO are the most commonly used HFV techniques, but both are limited by a lack of sufficient control of volume delivery and by the need for continuous monitoring to protect against very high airway pressures that can compromise patient safety. Combined high-frequency ventilation (CHFV), a mode of HFV introduced in 1983, utilizes two different breathing rates—a high-frequency rate superimposed on a base rate [33]. The superimposed HFV pulses are thought to improve gas distribution

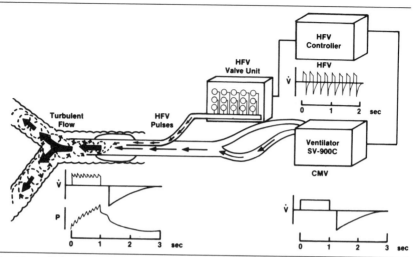

Fig. 12-20. Schematic diagrams for combined high-frequency ventilation system (CHFV). The HFV controller is electronically connected to the Servo ventilator (SV 900C), which generates trigger pulses regulating the start and stop of the superimposed high-frequency pulses from the HFV valve unit. Also shown are the flow patterns for the SV 900C and HFV controller. (From J. H. Siegel, J. C. Stoklosa, and U. Borg, Cardiorespiratory Management of the Adult Respiratory Distress Syndrome. In J. H. Siegel (ed.), *Trauma: Emergency Surgery and Critical Care.* New York: Churchill Livingstone, 1987. Pp. 581–673.)

through enhanced convection and use of frequency-dependent *pendelluft* effects [34], and the basal breath provides sufficient pressure above the critical opening pressure to open and stabilize the airways. As originally described, CHFV was associated with an increase in the effective end-expiratory and mean airway pressures, at times to unacceptable levels, in patients with noncompliant lung parenchyma. This increase in intrathoracic pressures, which is also seen in HFPPV, HFJV, and HFO, is attributable to inadvertent gas trapping that can occur in patients with relatively compliant respiratory systems ventilated at high I : E ratios. Gas trapping can be assessed by measuring airway pressure under static conditions after airway occlusion using the methodology previously described for measuring plateau pressure and intrinsic PEEP.

Using a modification of CHFV, in which a flexible-purpose, multicomponent system consisting of a conventional ventilator and a high-frequency ventilator was used to superimpose HFV on conventional volume- or pressure-controlled ventilation (Fig. 12-20) at clinically acceptable basal respiratory rates (8–32/min), researchers evaluated 35 patients suffering from posttraumatic and/or septic ARDS [13]. These patients were refractory to conventional modes of ventilatory support and had a probability-of-death index (*P* death) greater than 85 percent. Figure 12-21 demon-

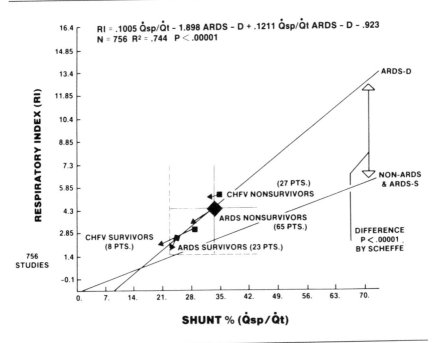

RI = .1005 $\dot{Q}sp/\dot{Q}t$ - 1.898 ARDS - D + .1211 $\dot{Q}sp/\dot{Q}t$ ARDS - D - .923
N = 756 R² = .744 P < .00001

ARDS-D

NON-ARDS & ARDS-S

(27 PTS.) CHFV NONSURVIVORS

ARDS NONSURVIVORS (65 PTS.)

DIFFERENCE P < .00001 , BY SCHEFFE

CHFV SURVIVORS (8 PTS.)

ARDS SURVIVORS (23 PTS.)

756 STUDIES

RESPIRATORY INDEX (RI)

SHUNT % ($\dot{Q}sp/\dot{Q}t$)

Fig. 12-21. Effect of combined high-frequency ventilation (CHFV) in posttrauma ARDS. Pre- and poststudy period mean values for ARDS survivors and nonsurvivors treated by controlled mechanical ventilation (CMV) and pre- and post-CMV mean values for CHFV nonsurvivors and CHFV survivors. Data superimposed on slopes of respiratory index/($\dot{Q}_s/\dot{Q}_t$) relationship described by Laghi [62]. Note mean and −1 standard deviation lines for ARDS nonsurvivors treated by CMV. Prior to CHFV, there were no significant differences between the means of any of the groups. However, CHFV allowed treated survivors to move into a region of RI and shunt compatible with successful outcome. (From U. Borg, J. C. Stoklosa, J. H. Siegel, et al., Prospective evaluation of combined high frequency ventilation in posttrauma patients with ARDS refractory to optimized conventional ventilatory management. *Crit. Care Med.* 17:1129–1142, 1989.)

strates the mean RI/($\dot{Q}_s/\dot{Q}_t$) ratio of 8 patients who had failed conventional controlled mechanical ventilation (CMV) and were then successfully ventilated by CHFV. Prolonged support by CHFV—in some cases, as long as 25 days—stabilized the potentially salvageable patients by increasing total minute ventilation, by increasing the low-pressure HFV volume component while decreasing the higher peak pressure volume component. Because of this, CHFV lowered the mean airway pressure from that on CMV and reduced the ventilatory barotrauma until the acute inflammatory phase of the disease subsided. As can be seen in Figure 12-21, the RI/($\dot{Q}_s/\dot{Q}_t$) ratio was returned to the non-ARDS range by CHFV therapy in a group of ARDS patients whose mean severity level was not significantly different from that of CMV-treated nonsurviving patients. In addition, CHFV is also useful in managing ARDS patients with a large air leak through a bronchopleural fistula, since by lowering peak airway pressure, ventilation is improved while the air leak is reduced. This study [13] indicates that CHFV appears to be an effective and safe modality for the ventilatory management of critically ill ARDS patients. It can produce a favorable outcome in selected ARDS patients who on CMV have severe impairment of gas exchange parameters and respiratory mechanics at levels that cannot be distinguished from those found in nonsurviving ARDS patients. However, this study, although prospective, was not randomized. A prospective, randomized study using the CHFV technique earlier in the patient's course as compared with CMV is planned to test the efficacy of CHFV and to categorize those ARDS patients most likely to benefit from early use of CHFV.

Nonconventional Methods of Ventilation
Conventional mechanical ventilators are designed using the underlying principle that for adequate gas exchange to occur the tidal volume must exceed the dead space volume. However, because of the relatively large tidal volumes traditionally required for the effective ventilation of patients with ARDS, there is an increased risk for the development of complications, including hemodynamic compromise and pulmonary barotrauma. To obviate these problems, new techniques of ventilation and oxygenation have been developed based on a large number of studies indicating that gas exchange can occur under conditions in which the traditional concepts of gas transport no longer hold [104]. Included in these techniques are *apneic oxygenation, low-frequency positive-pressure ventilation with extracorporeal removal of CO_2 (LFPPV-ECCO$_2$R), and constant-flow ventilation (CFV)*. Apneic ventilation and CFV at present are not applicable to the patient with ARDS. Gattinoni and colleagues [41, 42] in an uncontrolled clinical study on humans with severe respiratory failure and a predicted mortality rate greater than 90 percent, found that use of their technique of LFPPV-ECCO$_2$R was associated with a mortality rate of 48.8 percent, but previous prospective randomized studies of extracorporeal oxygenation (ECMO) showed no statistically significant difference in outcome between ECMO and conventional mechanical ventilation [124]. A prospective, controlled study is required before LFPPV-ECCO$_2$R can be recommended for use in the treatment of ARDS.

Practical Considerations in the Assessment and Optimization of Mechanical Ventilation in ARDS
Assessment of the appropriateness of a particular ventilator setting can be accomplished not only by the routine monitoring of gas exchange and hemodynamic parameters, but also by the measurement of airway pressure, airflow characteristics, and the volume delivered. Construction of a total static compliance curve can aid in the selection of the tidal volume and PEEP levels that not only can result in optimum gas exchange, but also can assist in the prevention of needless barotrauma [11, 56, 98, 99]. Studies show that patients with high peak airway pressures and patients who are treated with high levels of PEEP have an increased incidence of alveolar

rupture or barotrauma, but no study has looked prospectively at the factors usually listed as causative, to assess their relative importance in patients with ARDS. Among these factors are peak airway pressure, mean airway pressure, inspiratory pressure and flow pattern, and peak distending volume, as well as underlying the disease process. At present, no published data implicates any particular mode of mechanical ventilation as more likely to cause barotrauma.

Pierson [82], in discussing the relative importance of peak airway pressure and tidal volume in the production of barotrauma, pointed out that it is high alveolar pressure that causes the alveolar rupture. Although the peak airway pressure measured on the ventilator may be quite high—especially when the increase in peak airway pressure is due to a high inspiratory flow rate or to increased resistance within the ventilator circuitry, endotracheal tube, or conducting airways—the alveolar pressure is not necessarily increased. Rather, it appears that the maximum distending volume is most important in the production of alveolar rupture. Consequently, tidal volumes greater than 12 ml/kg should be avoided if possible in ARDS, especially when PEEP is used. The plateau, or static inflation-hold pressure more accurately reflects alveolar conditions and should be used as the primary monitor of the risk for alveolar rupture. The use of pressure-volume curves at varying tidal volumes can assist in avoiding excessively dangerous settings. The generation of a family of compliance curves at varying PEEP levels can aid in determining the "best" or "optimal" PEEP and tidal volume settings to be used when ventilating ARDS patients [57, 69, 97, 99, 114, 115]. Selection of the "best" settings results in a balance between the pressure needed to prevent airway and alveolar collapse and to promote alveolar recruitment and the pressure level that causes dangerous overexpansion of the more compliant areas in the lung. Such overdistention can result in hemodynamic compromise and worsening of $\dot{V}A/\dot{Q}$ relationships, due to the transmission of high airway pressures to the alveolar capillary vasculature, which then acts as a Starling resistor to blood flow, with diversion of blood flow away from the well-ventilated areas.

As an example of this approach, three representative P-V curves from a patient with ARDS are shown in Figure 12-22. The PEEP level was varied from 0 to 23 cm H_2O in 3–cm H_2O increments and maintained at the new level for 15 to 30 minutes, and the data for the construction of the P-V curve obtained. The three curves shown in Figure 12-21 were obtained at PEEP values of 0, 12, and 23 cm H_2O, respectively. Inspection of the zero-PEEP curve shows that the pressure rose to 6 cm H_2O before there was any increase in volume; that there was an early inflection point, or area where there was a change in slope, at a pressure of 12 cm H_2O; and that above 17 cm H_2O the P-V curve became grossly linear. The presence of an early inflection point has been demonstrated in the presence of pulmonary edema and in ARDS related to high opening pressures due to increased alveolar capillary permeability [22]. It has been correlated with the stage of ARDS and the pattern of the chest radiograph [69]. Glaister et al. [45] explained this inflection in the inflation P-V curve as resulting from the reopening of lung units that had closed during the period of deflation. If this is indeed the explanation, then the level of PEEP should be set above

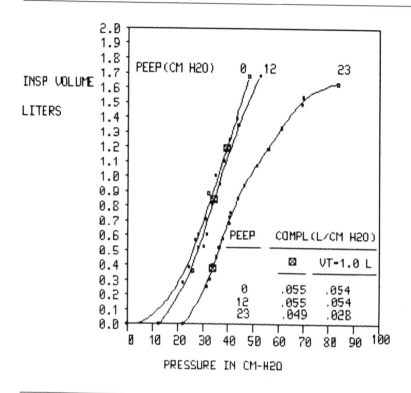

Fig. 12-22. Determination of "best" PEEP from total static compliance curves. Shown are curves obtained at 0, 12, and 23 cm H_2O. The point of equivalent lung volume is indicated by the marker box on each of the compliance curves. (From J. H. Siegel, J. C. Stoklosa, U. Borg, Cardiorespiratory Management of the Adult Respiratory Distress Syndrome. In J. H. Siegel (ed.), *Trauma: Emergency Surgery and Critical Care.* New York: Churchill Livingstone, 1987. Pp. 581–673.)

the pressure level at the point of early inflection, to prevent distal airway collapse at the end of expiration (Fig. 12-22).

When comparing the P-V curves from an ARDS patient shown in Figure 12-22, it can be seen that the curve obtained at *zero* PEEP had an early inflection point at about 20 cm H_2O and then was essentially linear above an inspired volume of 0.3 liters. In contrast, at a PEEP of 12 cm H_2O the P-V curve was linear up to a volume of 1.4 liters, but at a PEEP of 23 cm H_2O the linear portion extended only to an inspired volume of 0.8 liters and then the pressure rose rapidly as V_T was increased toward the ARDS-reduced total lung capacity (TLC). It should be recalled that when the end-expiratory pressure level is increased, there is an associated increase in the volume of the FRC (Figs. 12-13 and 12-14). In the patient shown in Figure 12-22, when the PEEP level was increased from zero to 12 cm H_2O, the

FRC increased by 0.38 liters, and at a PEEP level of 23 cm H_2O, it was further increased by an additional 0.82 liters above the FRC volume at zero PEEP.

A frequent concern is overdistention of lung units as PEEP, and thus FRC, is increased. With the institution of PEEP, there is a movement of the end-expiratory point from the lower flatter portion of the P-V curve to the steeper portion. As the FRC level approaches TLC, tidal ventilation (VT) now occurs on the upper, flatter portion of the curve (Fig. 12-22). If the compliance, which is a measurement of the slope of the P-V curve at a given point, is increasing or remains the same, it is assumed that overdistention is not occurring. This movement up the P-V curve is demonstrated in Figure 12-22, in which equivalent lung volumes are indicated by the square markers placed at an inspired volume of 1.2 liters on the zero-PEEP curve, 0.85 liters on the curve at a PEEP level of 12 cm H_2O, and at 0.38 liters on the curve at 23 cm H_2O. The slopes of the P-V curves at these points, as represented by the compliance values, are 0.055, 0.055, and 0.049 liters/cm H_2O, respectively. If one were to use an equivalent inspired tidal volume (VT) of 1.0 liters to ventilate the patient at each of these PEEP levels, one would see that at the PEEP levels of 0 and 12 cm H_2O, ventilation is still occurring on the steep linear portion of the curve and the compliance is essentially unchanged: 0.054 liters/cm H_2O. In contrast, at a PEEP level of 23 cm H_2O, the end-inspiratory point has moved from the steep portion toward the flatter upper portion of the P-V curve, and the compliance has fallen to 0.028 liters/cm H_2O, indicating that some alveoli have reached their distensible limits. Reduction of the tidal volume to 0.7 liters at the PEEP level of 23 cm H_2O would again return ventilation to the steeper portion of the curve. *Pressure-volume curves should be monitored daily, since the same PEEP level in a patient whose compliance is improving will result in the patient becoming more and more hyperinflated on the same level of PEEP.*

Even once a given PEEP level has been chosen, the complete total static compliance curve should be defined by a variety of trial tidal volume breaths that are greater or smaller than the actual ventilator setting. This technique will define the optimum point on the specific CST curve at which ventilation should take place. Figure 12-23 depicts the standard graphic report generated when a patient is evaluated to determine optimum ventilator settings. The report shows the pressure-volume dynamics of four breaths of varying tidal volumes using PC mode with an I : E ratio of 1 : 1, the total static compliance curve, the blood gas data at the actual settings, and the lung-mechanics data for the actual and trial settings. The compliance value at each tidal volume is plotted on the compliance curve.

No early inflection point was noted on the total static compliance curve shown, nor was any increase in the compliance values as the tidal volume is increased, suggesting that the actual PEEP level (PEEP$_i$) was adequate to prevent collapse at end-expiration. Despite this, the patient had a decreased PaO_2 (68 torr) at an FIO_2 % 60 with an increased shunt ($\dot{Q}_s/\dot{Q}_t$ = 29%) and an RI of 4.3. At the set tidal volume of 0.9 liters, the compliance was 0.050 liters/cm H_2O, the peak pressure was 35.3 cm H_2O, and the pla-

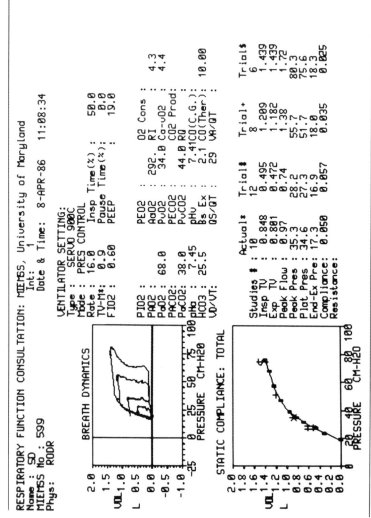

Fig. 12-23. Respiratory function consultation in ARDS patient, showing actual pulmonary mechanics and blood gases (*) at I : E ratio of 1 : 1 positioned on the static compliance curve and compared with three trial runs at different inspired tidal volumes (#, +, $), demonstrating the effect of higher and lower volumes on peak, plateau, and PEEP pressures in compliance. The study demonstrates how the optimum point on the pressure-volume curve for that particular patient is chosen to maximize tidal volume at best acceptable compliance and PEEP pressure.

teau pressure was 34.6 cm H_2O. Note that this actual breath (study No. 10) and trial breath No. 12 fall on the steep portion of the total static compliance curve, whereas trial breaths Nos. 8 and 6 fall on the flat portion that occurs above a volume of 1.1 liters. On the flat portion of the P-V curve, relatively small changes in volume lead to large changes in pressure. As shown by trial breaths Nos. 8 and 6, the use of the conventionally recommended tidal volumes of 0.012 to 0.015 liters/kg (12–15 ml/kg)—a volume equivalent 1.1 to 1.4 liters in this 95-kg man—would have resulted in a decrease in compliance to 0.035 liters/cm H_2O at 1.2 liters and 0.025 liters/cm H_2O at 1.4 liters.

Increasing the tidal volume by 0.46 liters (study breaths Nos. 10 and 8) led to a 20.4–cm H_2O increase in peak pressure and a 17.1–cm H_2O increase in plateau pressure. Contrast this to the changes seen when using tidal volumes in the steep range of the total static compliance curve (study breaths Nos. 12 and 10), where increasing the volume by 0.35 liters, from 0.50 to 0.85, only resulted in an increase in peak and plateau pressure of 7.1 and 7.3 cm H_2O. In the flat range (breaths Nos. 6 and 8), above a tidal volume of 1.1 liters, a change in tidal volume of 0.23 liters resulted in an increase in peak and plateau pressure of 24.6 and 23.9 cm H_2O, respectively.

Based on the results of this study, it was decided to try a period of inverse ratio ventilation (IRV). The pause time was increased to 10 percent of the total breath cycle, resulting in an I : E ratio of 1.5 : 1. Three hours later, at the same FIO_2 (0.6), the PaO_2 had increased from 68 to 110 torr and the RI had decreased from 4.3 to 1.7. The patient remained on the same I : E ratio and PEEP, and the next day, on an FIO_2 of 0.45, the PaO_2 was 107 torr, the RI was 1.3, and the shunt had decreased from 29 percent to 17 percent with essentially no change in cardiac output.

SUMMARY

Thus, it is possible to see how one can progress from an understanding of the pathophysiologic abnormalities that produce the ARDS syndrome, through a knowledge of the cardiovascular and ventilatory responses in ARDS, to a mechanism for taking practical, physiologically sound measures to improve ventilation, perfusion, and gas exchange in this disease entity. In conclusion, it is critical to emphasize that there is *no* substitute for precise analytic quantification of the ARDS patient's specific set of cardiorespiratory abnormalities as a means of developing a physiologically correct therapeutic prescription for effective treatment of this highly lethal process.

REFERENCES

1. Al-Saady, N., and Bennett, E. D. Decelerating inspiratory flow waveform improves lung mechanics and gas exchange in patients on intermittent positive-pressure ventilation. *Intensive Care Med.* 11:68, 1985.
2. Ashbaugh, D. G., Petty. T. L., Bigelow, D. B., and Harris, T. M. Continuous positive pressure breathing (CPPB) in adult respiratory distress syndrome. *J. Thorac. Cardiovasc. Surg.* 57:31, 1969.

3. Bachofen, M., and Weibel, E. R. Structural alterations of lung parenchyma in the adult respiratory distress syndrome. *Clin. Chest Med.* 3:35, 1982.

4. Baehrendtz, S., Bindslev, L., Hedenstierna, G., and Santesson, J. Selective PEEP in acute bilateral lung disease: Effect on patients in the lateral posture. *Acta Anaesthesiol. Scand.* 27:311, 1983.

5. Baehrendtz, S., and Hedenstierna, G. Differential ventilation and selective positive end-expiratory pressure: Effects on patients with acute bilateral lung disease. Anesthesiology 61:511, 1984.

6. Baehrendtz, S., Santesson, J., Bindslev, L., et al. Differential ventilation in acute bilateral lung disease: Influence on gas exchange and central hemodynamics. *Acta Anaesthiol. Scand.* 27:270, 1983.

7. Barach, A. L., Marin, J., and Eckman, M. Positive pressure respiration and its application to the treatment of acute pulmonary edema. *Ann. Intern. Med.* 12:754, 1938.

8. Bell, R. C., Coalson, J. J., et al. Multiple organ system failure and infection in adult respiratory distress. *Ann. Intern. Med.* 99:293, 1983.

9. Benson, M. S., and Pierson, D. J. Auto-PEEP during mechanical ventilation of adults. *Respiratory Care* 33:557, 1988.

10. Berggren, S. M. The oxygen deficit of arterial blood caused by nonventilating parts of the lung. *Acta Physiol. Scand.* Suppl. II, 1942.

11. Bone, R. C. Diagnosis of causes for acute respiratory distress by pressure-volume curves. *Chest* 70:740, 1976.

12. Borg, U., Eriksson, I., Sjostrand, U., and Wattwil, M. Experimental studies of continuous positive pressure ventilation and high frequency positive pressure ventilation. *Resuscitation* 9:1, 1981.

13. Borg, U., Stoklosa, J. C., Siegel, J. H., Wiles, C. E., Belzberg, H., Blevins, S., Cotter, K., Laghi, F., and Rivkind, A. Prospective evaluation of combined high frequency ventilation in posttrauma patients with ARDS refractory to optimized conventional ventilatory management. *Crit. Care Med.* 17: 1129, 1989.

14. Boros, S. J. Variations in inspiratory : expiratory ratio and airway pressure wave form during mechanical ventilation: The significance of mean airway pressure. *J. Pediatr.* 94:114, 1979.

15. Boysen, P. G., and McGough, E. Pressure-control and pressure-support ventilation: Flow patterns, inspiratory time and gas distribution. *Respiratory Care* 33:126, 1988.

16. Butler, W. J., Bohn, D. J., Bryan, A. C., and Froese, A. B. Ventilation by high frequency oscillations in humans. *Anesth. Analg.* 59:577, 1980.

17. Carlon, G. C., and Groeger, J. S. High Frequency Jet Ventilation Compared to Volume-Cycled Ventilation: A Prospective Randomized Evaluation. In P. A. E. Scheck, U. H. Sjostrand, and R. B. Smith (eds.), *Perspectives in High Frequency Ventilation.* The Hague: Martinus Nijhoff, 1983.

18. Carlon, G. C., Kahn, R., Howland, W. S., et al. Acute life-threatening ventilation-perfusion inequality: An indication for independent lung ventilation. *Crit. Care Med.* 6:380, 1978.

19. Carlon, G. C., Ray, C., Jr., Klain, M., and McCormack, P. M. High frequency positive-pressure ventilation in management of a patient with bronchopleural fistula. *Anesthesiology* 52:160, 1980.

20. Ciszek, T. A., Modanlou, H. D., Owings, D., and Nelson, P. Mean airway pressure-significance during mechanical ventilation in neonates. *J. Pediatr.* 99:121, 1981.

21. Clowes, G. H. A., Jr., Zuschneid, W., Dragacevic, S., et al. The nonspecific pulmonary inflammatory reactions leading to respiratory failure after shock, gangrene and sepsis. *J. Trauma* 8:899, 1968.

22. Cook, C. P., Mead, J., Schreiner, G. L., et al. Pulmonary mechanics during induced pulmonary edema in anesthetized dogs. *J. Appl. Physiol.* 14:177, 1959.
23. Dammann, J. F., McAslan, T. C., and Maffeo, C. J. Optimal flow pattern for mechanical ventilation of the lungs. II. The effect of a sine versus square wave flow pattern with and without an end-inspiratory pause on patients. *Crit. Care Med.* 6:293, 1978.
24. Dantzker, D. R. Gas exchange in the adult respiratory distress syndrome. *Clin. Chest Med.* 3:57, 1982.
25. Dantzker, D. R., Brook, C. J., Dehart, P., et al. Ventilation-perfusion distributions in the adult respiratory distress syndrome. *Am. Rev. Respir. Dis.* 120:1039, 1979.
26. Dantzker, D. R., Lynch, J. P., and Weg, J. G. Depression of cardiac output is a mechanism of shunt reduction in the therapy of acute respiratory failure. *Chest* 77:636, 1980.
27. Deby-Dupont, G., Braun, M., Lamy, M., et al. Thromboxane and prostacyclin release in adult respiratory distress syndrome. *Intensive Care Med.* 13:167, 1987.
28. De Gaetano, A., Siegel, J. H., Stoklosa, J. C., et al. Predicting the probability of death from ARDS after trauma. Submitted to *Surgery,* 1990.
29. Demling, R. H. The role of mediators in human ARDS. *J. Crit. Care* 3:56, 1988.
30. Douglas, M. E., Downs, J. B., Dannemiller, F. J., et al. Change in pulmonary venous admixture with varying inspired oxygen. *Anesth. Analg.* 55:688, 1976.
31. Drazen, J. M., Austen, K. F., Lewis, R. A., et al. Comparative airway and vascular activities of leukotrienes C-1 and D in-vivo and in-vitro. *Proc. Natl. Acad. Sci.* 77:4354, 1980.
32. Duncan, S. R., Rizk, N. W., and Raffin, T. A. Inverse ratio ventilation, PEEP in disguise? *Chest* 92:390, 1987.
33. El-Baz, N., El-Ganzouri, A., and Invahovich, A. Combined High Frequency Ventilation for Treatment of Severe Respiratory Failure. In P. A. E. Scheck, U. H. Sjostrand, and R. B. Smith (eds.), *Perspectives in High Frequency Ventilation.* The Hague: Martinus Nijhoff, 1983.
34. Eriksson, I. The role of conducting airways in gas exchange during high frequency ventilation—A clinical and theoretical analysis. *Anesth. Analg.* 61:483, 1982.
35. Farrell, E. J., and Siegel, J. H. Investigation of cardiorespiratory abnormalities through computer simulation. *Comput. Biomed. Res.* 5:161, 1973.
36. Fowler, A. A., Hamman, R. F., Good, J. T., Benson, K. N., Baird, M., Eberle, D. J., Petty, T. L., and Hyers, T. M. Adult respiratory distress syndrome: Risk with common predispositions. *Ann. Intern. Med.* 98:593, 1983.
37. Fowler, A. A., et al. Adult respiratory distress syndrome: Prognosis after onset. *Am. Rev. Respir. Dis.* 132:472, 1985.
38. Gallagher, T. J., and Banner, M. J. Mean airway pressure as a determinant of oxygenation. *Crit. Care Med.* 8:244, 1980.
39. Gattinoni, L., Mascheroni, D., Torresin, A., et al. Morphological response to positive end-expiratory pressure in acute respiratory failure. Computerized tomography study. *Intensive Care Med.* 12:137, 1986.
40. Gattinoni, L., Pesenti, A., Avalli, T., Rossi, F., and Bombino, M. Pressure-volume curve of total respiratory system in acute respiratory failure. *Am. Rev. Respir. Dis.* 136:730, 1987.
41. Gattinoni, L., Pesenti, A., Marcolin, R., and Damia, G. Extra-corporeal support in acute respiratory failure. *Intensive Careworld* 5:42, 1988.

42. Gattinoni, L., Pesenti, A., Mascheroni, D., et al. Low frequency positive-pressure ventilation with extracorporeal CO_2 removal in severe acute respiratory failure. *J.A.M.A.* 256:881, 1986.
43. Geiger, K. Differential lung ventilation. *Int. Anesthesiol. Clin.* 21:83, 1983.
44. Gens, D., Rivkind, A., and Siegel, J. H. Adult respiratory distress syndrome in the trauma patient: A prospective clinical study of incidence, predisposing factors and outcome. Submitted to *J. Trauma,* 1989.
45. Glaister, D. H., Schroter, R. C., Sudlow, M. F., and Milic-Emili, J. Transpulmonary pressure gradient and ventilation in excised lungs. *Resp. Physiol.* 17:365, 1973.
46. Goldstein, D., Slutsky, A. S., Ingram, R. H., Jr., et al. CO_2 elimination by high frequency oscillatory ventilation (4–10 Hz) in normal subjects. *Am. Rev. Respir. Dis.* 123:251, 1981.
47. Gregory, G. A., Kitterman, J. A., Phibbs, R. H., et al. Treatment of the idiopathic respiratory distress syndrome with continuous positive airway pressure. *N. Engl. J. Med.* 284:1333, 1971.
48. Gurevitch, M. J., VanDyke, J., Young, E. S., and Jackson, K. Improved oxygenation and lower peak airway pressure in severe adult respiratory distress syndrome. Treatment with inverse ratio ventilation. *Chest* 89:211, 1986.
49. Hammerschmidt, D. E., Weaver, L. J., Hudson, L. D., et al. Association of complement activation and elevated C_5a with adult respiratory distress syndrome. *Lancet* 1:947, 1980.
50. Harris, K. Noninvasive monitoring of gas exchange. *Respiratory Care* 32:544, 1987.
51. Hechtman, H. B., Lelcuk, S., Alexander, F., and Shepro, D. Humoral Mediators in Adult Respiratory Distress Syndrome. In J. H. Siegel (ed.), *Trauma: Emergency Surgery and Critical Care.* New York: Churchill Livingstone, 1987. Pp. 565–580.
52. Heffner, J. E., Sahn, S. A., and Repine, J. E. The role of platelets in the adult respiratory distress syndrome: Culprits or bystanders? *Am. Rev. Respir. Dis.* 135:482, 1987.
53. Hegi, T., and Hiatt, I. M. Respiratory index: a simple evaluation of severity of idiopathic respiratory distress syndrome. *Crit. Care Med.* 7:500, 1979.
54. Hutchinson, A. A., Hinson, J. M., Jr., Brigham, K. L., et al. Effect of endotoxin on airway responsiveness to aerosol histamine in sheep. *J. Appl. Physiol.* 54:1463, 1983.
55. Johansson, H. Effects of different inspiratory gas flow patterns on thoracic compliance during respirator treatment. *Acta Anaesthiol. Scand.* 19:89, 1975.
56. Jonson, B., Nordstrom, L., Olsson, S. G., and Akerback, D. Monitoring of ventilation and lung mechanics during automatic ventilation. A new device. *Bull. Eur. Physiopathol. Respir.* 11:729, 1975.
57. Katz, J. A., Ozanne, G. M., Zinn, S. E., Fairley, H. B. Time course and mechanics of lung-volume increase with PEEP in acute pulmonary failure. *Anesthesiology* 54:9, 1981.
58. Kelman, G. B. Digital computer subroutine for conversion of oxygen tension into saturation. *J. Appl. Physiol.* 21:1375, 1966.
59. Kirby, R. R., Smith, R. A., and Desautels, D. A. (eds.). *Mechanical Ventilation.* New York: Churchill Livingstone, 1985.
60. Klain, M., and Smith, R. B. High frequency percutaneous transtracheal jet ventilation. *Crit. Care Med.* 5:280, 1977.
61. Lachmann, B., Danzmann, E., Haendly, B., and Jonson, B. Ventilator Settings and Gas Exchange in Respiratory Distress Syndrome. In

O. Prakash (ed.), *Applied Physiology in Clinical Respiratory Care*. The Hague: Martinus Nijhoff, 1982.

62. Laghi, F., Siegel, J. H., Rivkind, A. I., Chiarla, C., De Gaetano, A., Blevins, S., Stoklosa, J. C., Borg, U. R., and Belzberg, H. The respiratory index/pulmonary shunt relationship: Quantification of severity and prognosis in the posttraumatic adult respiratory distress syndrome. *Crit. Care Med.* 17:1121, 1989.

63. Lamy, M., Fallat, R. J., Koeniger, E., et al. Pathologic features and mechanisms of hypoxemia in adult respiratory distress syndrome. *Am. Rev. Respir. Dis.* 114:267, 1976.

64. Levine, O. R., et al. The application of Starling's law of capillary exchange to the lungs. *J. Clin. Invest.* 46:934, 1967.

65. Lewis, R. A., and Austen, K. F. The biologically active leukotrienes: Biosynthesis, metabolism and pharmacology. *J. Clin. Invest.* 73:889, 1984.

66. Lyager, S. Influence of flow pattern on the distribution of respiratory air during intermittent positive pressure ventilation. *Acta Anaesthiol. Scand.* 12:191, 1968.

67. MacIntyre, N. R. Weaning from mechanical ventilatory support: Volume-assisting intermittent breaths versus pressure-assisting every breath. *Respiratory Care* 33:121, 1988.

68. Markello, P., Winter, P., and Olszowka, A. Assessment of ventilation-perfusion inequalities by arterial-venous nitrogen differences in intensive care patients. *Anesthesiology* 37:4, 1972.

69. Matamis, D., Lemaire, F., Harf, A. et al. Total respiratory pressure-volume curves in the adult respiratory distress syndrome. *Chest* 88:58, 1984.

70. Maunder, R. J., Shuman, W. P., McHugh, J. W., Marglin, S. I., and Butter, J. Preservation of normal lung region in the adult respiratory distress syndrome. Analysis by computed tomography. *J.A.M.A.* 255:2463, 1986.

71. Michel, R. P., Zorchi, L., Rossi, A., Cardinal, G. A., Ploy-Song-Sang, Y., Poulsen, R. S., Milic-Emili, J., and Staub, N. C. Does interstitial lung edema compress airways and arteries? Amorphometric study. *J. Appl. Physiol.* 62:108, 1987.

72. Modell, H. I., and Cheney, F. W. Effects of inspiratory flow pattern on gas exchange in normal and abnormal lungs. *J. Appl. Physiol.* 46:1103, 1979.

73. Montgomery, A. B., Stager, M. A., Carrico, C. J., and Hudson, L. P. Causes of mortality in patients with the adult respiratory distress syndrome. *Am. Rev. Respir. Dis.* 132:485, 1985.

74. Moore, F. D., Lyons, J. H., Pierce, E. C. et al. *Post-Traumatic Pulmonary Insufficiency*. Philadelphia: Saunders, 1969.

75. Murray, J. F., Matthay, M. A., Luce, J. M., and Flick, M. R. An expanded definition of the adult respiratory distress syndrome. *Am. Rev. Respir. Dis.* 138:720, 1988.

76. Pepe, P. E., Hudson, L. D., and Carrico, C. J. Early application of positive end-expiratory pressure in patients at risk for the adult respiratory distress syndrome. *N. Engl. J. Med.* 311:281, 1984.

77. Pepe, P. E. and Marini, J. J. Occult positive end-expiratory pressure in mechanically ventilated patients with airflow obstruction: The auto-PEEP effect. *Am. Rev. Respir. Dis.* 126:166, 1982.

78. Pesenti, A., Marcolin, R., Prato, P., et al. Mean airway pressure vs. positive end-expiratory pressure during mechanical ventilation. *Crit. Care Med.* 13:34, 1985.

79. Petty, T. L. ARDS: Refinement of concept and redefinition. *Am. Rev. Respir. Dis.* 138:724, 1988.

80. Petty, T. L. The use, abuse and mystique of positive end-expiratory pressure. *Am. Rev. Respir. Dis.* 138:475, 1988.

81. Petty, T. L., and Ashbaugh, D. G. The adult respiratory distress syndrome: Clinical features, factors influencing prognosis and principles of management. *Chest* 60:233, 1971.

82. Pierson, P. J. Alveolar rupture during mechanical ventilation: Role of PEEP, peak airway pressure, and distending volume. *Respiratory Care* 33:472, 1988.

83. Poulton, E. P., and Oxon, D. M. Left-sided heart failure with pulmonary edema. *Lancet* 2:981, 1936.

84. Powers, S. R., Mannel, R., Neclerio, M., Monaco, V., and Leather, R. Physiologic consequences of positive end-expiratory pressure (PEEP) ventilation. *Ann. Surg.* 178:265, 1973.

85. Powner, D. J., Eross, B., and Grenvik, A. Differential lung ventilation with PEEP in the treatment of unilateral pneumonia. *Crit. Care Med.* 5:170, 1977.

86. Rossi, A., Gottfried, S. B., and Zocchi, L. Measurements of static compliance of the total respiratory system in patients with acute respiratory failure during mechanical ventilation. The effect of intrinsic positive end-expiratory pressure. *Am. Rev. Respir. Dis.* 131:672, 1985.

87. Sachdeva, S. P. Treatment of post-operative pulmonary atelectases by active inflation of the atelectatic lobe(s) through an endobronchial tube. *Acta Anaesthiol. Scand.* 19:65, 1974.

88. Severinghaus, J. W. Transcutaneous blood gas analysis. *Respiratory Care* 27:152, 1982.

89. Sganga, G., Siegel, J. H., Coleman, B., Giovannini, I., Boldrini, G., and Pittiruti, M. The physiologic meaning of the respiratory index in various types of critical illness. *Circ. Shock* 17:179, 1985.

90. Shapiro, B. A., Cane, R. D., and Harrison, R. A. Positive end-expiratory pressure therapy in adults with special reference to acute lung injury: A review of the literature and suggested clinical correlations. *Crit. Care Med.* 12:127, 1984.

91. Shapiro, B. A., Cane, R. D., Harrison, R. A., and Steiner, M. C. Changes in intrapulmonary shunting with administration of 100 percent oxygen. *Chest* 77:138, 1980.

92. Shykoff, B. E., Grondelle, A. V., and Chang, H. K. Effects of unequal pressure swings and different waveforms on distribution of ventilation: A non-linear model simulation. *Respir. Physiol.* 48:157, 1982.

93. Siegel, J. H., Farrel, E. J., Miller, M., et al. Cardiorespiratory interactions as determinants of survival and the need for respiratory support in human shock states. *J. Trauma* 13:602, 1973.

94. Siegel, J. H., Giovannini, I., and Coleman, B. Ventilation : perfusion maldistribution secondary to the hyperdynamic cardiovascular state as the major cause of increased pulmonary shunting in human sepsis. *J. Trauma* 19:432, 1979.

95. Siegel, J. H., Giovannini, I., Coleman, B., Cerra, F. B., and Nespoli, A. Pathologic synergy modulation of the cardiovascular, respiratory and metabolic response to injury by cirrhosis and/or sepsis: A manifestation of a common metabolic defect? *Arch. Surg.* 117:225, 1982.

96. Siegel, J. H., Linberg, S. E., and Wiles, S. E. III. Therapy of Low-Flow Shock States. In J. H. Siegel (ed.), *Trauma: Emergency Surgery and Critical Care.* New York: Churchill Livingstone, 1987. Pp. 201–284.

97. Siegel, J. H., Stoklosa, J., Borg, U., Wiles, C. E., Sganga, G., Geisler, F. H., Belzberg, H., Wedel, S., and Goh, K. Quantification of asymmetric lung

pathophysiology as a guide to the use of simultaneous independent lung ventilation in posttraumatic and septic ARDS. *Ann. Surg.* 202:425, 1985.

98. Siegel, J. H., Stoklosa, J., Geisler, F. H., et al. Computer-based evaluation of cardiopulmonary function for the optimization of ventilatory therapy in the adult respiratory distress syndrome. *Int. J. Clin. Monit. Comput.* 1:107, 1984.

99. Siegel, J. H., Stoklosa, J. C., and Borg, U. Cardiorespiratory management of the adult respiratory distress syndrome. In J. H. Siegel (ed.), *Trauma: Emergency Surgery and Critical Care.* New York: Churchill Livingstone, 1987. Pp. 581–673.

100. Siegel, J. H., and Vary, T. C. Sepsis, abnormal metabolic control and the multiple organ failure syndrome. In J. H. Siegel (ed.), *Trauma: Emergency Surgery and Critical Care.* New York: Churchill Livingstone, 1987. Pp. 411–501.

101. Simpson, D. L., Goodman, M., Spector, S.L., et al. Long-term follow-up and bronchial reactivity testing in survivors of the adult respiratory distress syndrome. *Am. Rev. Respir. Dis.* 117:449, 1978.

102. Sjostrand, U. Pneumatic systems facilitating treatment of respiratory insufficiency with alternative use of IPPV/PEEP, HFPPV/PEEP, and CPPB or CPAP. *Acta Anaesthiol. Scand.* 64(Suppl.):123, 1977.

103. Sjostrand, U. Review of the physiological rationale for and development of high frequency positive pressure ventilation-HFPPV. *Acta Anaesthiol. Scand.* 64(Suppl.):7, 1977.

104. Slutsky, A. S. Nonconventional methods of ventilation. *Am. Rev. Respir. Dis.* 138:175, 1988.

105. Smith, G., Cheney, F. V., Jr., and Winter, P. M. The effect of change in cardiac output on intrapulmonary shunting. *Br. J. Anaesthesiol.* 46:337, 1974.

106. Snapper, J. R. Lung mechanics in pulmonary edema. *Clin. Chest Med.* 6:393, 1985.

107. Snapper, J. R., and Brigham, K. L. Inflammation and airway reactivity. *Exp. Lung Res.* 6:83, 1984.

108. Snapper, J. R., Hutchinson, A. A., Ogletree, M. L., et al. Effects of cyclooxygenase inhibitors on the alterations in lung mechanics caused by endotoxemia in the unanesthetized sheep. *J. Clin. Invest.* 72:63, 1983.

109. Starling, E. H. On the absorption of fluids from the connective spaces. *J. Physiol.* (Lond) 19:312, 1896.

110. Staub, N. C. State of the art review. Pathogenesis of pulmonary edema. *Am. Rev. Respir. Dis.* 109:358, 1974.

111. Stephens, K. E., Ishizaka, A., Larrick, J. W., and Raffin, T. A. Tumor necrosis factor causes increased pulmonary permeability and edema: Comparison to septic acute lung injury. *Am. Rev. Respir. Dis.* 137:1364, 1988.

112. Stokes, C., Blevins, S., Stoklosa, J. C., Cotter, K., Goh, K. C., Belzberg, H., and Siegel, J. H. Prediction of arterial blood gas by transcutaneous O_2 and CO_2 in critically ill hyperdynamic trauma patients. *J. Trauma* 27:1240, 1987.

113. Sturgeon, C. L., Jr., et al. PEEP and CPAP: Cardiopulmonary effects during spontaneous ventilation. *Anesth. Analg.* 56:633, 1977.

114. Suter, P. M., Fairley, B., and Isenberg, M. D. Optimum end-expiratory airway pressure in patients with acute pulmonary failure. *N. Engl. J. Med.* 292:284, 1975.

115. Suter, P. M., Fairley, H. B., and Isenberg, M. D. Effect of tidal volume and positive end-expiratory pressure on compliance during mechanical ventilation. *Chest* 73:158, 1978.

116. Tharratt, R. S., Allen, R. P., and Albertson, T. E. Pressure controlled inverse ratio ventilation in severe adult respiratory failure. *Chest* 94:755, 1988.

117. Till, G. O., Johnson, K. J., Kunkel, R., and Ward, P. A. Intravascular activation of complement after acute lung injury dependency on neutrophils and toxic oxygen metabolites. *J. Clin. Invest.* 69:1126, 1982.
118. Tremper, K. K., Shoemaker, W. C., and Shippy, C. R. Transcutaneous PCO_2 monitoring on adult patients in the ICU and operating room. *Crit. Care Med.* 9:752, 1981.
119. Tyler, D. C. Positive end-expiratory pressure: A review. *Crit. Care Med.* 11:300, 1983.
120. Utsunomiya, T., Krausz, M. M., Shepro, D., and Hechtman, H. B. Treatment of aspiration pneumonia with ibuprofen and prostacyclin (PGI_2). *Surgery* 90:170, 1981.
121. Weiland, J. E., Davis, W. B., Holter, J. F., et al. Lung neutrophils in the adult respiratory distress syndrome: Clinical and pathophysiologic significance. *Am. Rev. Respir. Dis.* 133:218, 1986.
122. Weisman, I. M., Rinaldo, J. E., Rogers, R. M., and Sanders, M. H. Intermittent mandatory ventilation. *Am. Rev. Respir. Dis.* 127:641, 1983.
123. Wright, D. G. The Neutrophil as a Secretory Organ of Host Defense. In J. Gallin and A. S. Farice (eds.), *Advances in Host Defense Mechanisms,* vol. 1. New York: Raven Press, 1982. Pp. 75–110.
124. Zapol, W. M. Extracorporeal membrane oxygenation in severe acute respiratory failure. *J.A.M.A.* 242:2193, 1979.
125. Zapol, W. M., Trelstad, R. L., Coffey, W., et al. Pulmonary fibrosis in severe acute respiratory failure. *Am. Rev. Respir. Dis.* 119:547, 1979.

Pulmonary Embolism

Franz-Peter Lenhart
Lorenz Frey
Klaus Peter

INCIDENCE AND MORTALITY

In the United States, pulmonary embolism is the third most-frequent cause of death, with 200,000 cases per year [4, 12, 17]. Pulmonary embolism is the most common disease connected to the lungs, even if it is not a disease that is due to the organ "lung" itself. Pulmonary emboli are detected by autopsy in about 25 percent of all deaths [3]. However, only 20 to 30 percent of these are diagnosed antemortem [18]. Pulmonary embolism is thus one of the most frequently overlooked acute diseases with a potentially fatal outcome [9]. Owing to the nonspecificity of the clinical signs, false-positive results are to be reckoned within 70 to 80 percent of cases after checking with objective methods. Today, the putative diagnosis can be confirmed in about 30 percent of cases, owing to the introduction of new methods and the improvement of such well-proved procedures as perfusion scintigraphy, ventilation scintigraphy, angiography, and more recently, computed tomography (CT) and nuclear magnetic resonance imaging (MRI). This rate was only 15 percent as recently as 30 years ago [25, 27]. Figures obtained in the studies on the incidence and mortality of pulmonary embolism must be regarded as estimates, however. The real figures might thus be even higher [53]. A consistent strategy of diagnosis and recognition of risk groups may contribute to a lowering of mortality from pulmonary embolism.

Although the clinical signs of pulmonary embolism are highly nonspecific, they should nevertheless always give rise to the suspicion of pulmonary embolism.

ETIOLOGY AND RISK FACTORS

Most emboli that pass into the pulmonary circulation derive from deep venous thrombosis of the pelvis or the deep veins of the lower limbs. At especially high risk for development of pulmonary embolism are patients with already-existing thrombophlebitis, patients over 50 years old, bedrid-

Table 13-1. Risk factors

Thrombophlebitis
Immobilization
Age (50–65)
Postoperative
Preexisting cardiac disease (atrial fibrillation, congestive heart failure)
Major trauma (fractures, burning)
Obesity (>20% ideal body weight)
Malignancy
Pregnancy (especially postpartum period)
Women receiving oral contraceptives (especially in combination with cigarette
    smoking and hypertension)
Polycythemia
Abnormalities in blood clotting mechanisms (e.g., antithrombin III deficiency)
Diabetes mellitus
Chronic respiratory disease

den and immobilized patients, patients after operations, women in pregnancy and postpartum, patients after trauma (especially after femoral neck
fractures), excessively obese patients, patients with malignancies, and
women who take contraceptives—above all, when they smoke or have
high blood pressure. In addition, patients with disorders of blood clotting
are affected to a greater extent (Table 13-1).

PATHOPHYSIOLOGY
There are very few clinical measurements of and data on the effects of
acute pulmonary embolism on hemodynamics and gas exchange. Information obtained with noninvasive methods of investigation, such as echocardiography, Doppler sonography, and scintigraphy, only allow an ori-
entative impression of cardiac function after acute pulmonary embolism
[6, 30]. Our understanding of the pathophysiology in acute pulmonary embolism therefore has been obtained almost exclusively in the animal experimental model of pulmonary embolism. Statements on the efficacy of
pharmacotherapeutic measures also derive from such animal experiments
[31, 48, 63].

Pulmonary embolism causes an acute restriction in the transverse section of the pulmonary vascular bed, with a simultaneous increase in resistance of the still-perfused residual pulmonary vascular bed, so that the
pressure in the right ventricle rises [50]. Owing to the low wall thickness
of the right ventricle, this can produce pressures rarely higher than 50 to
60 mm Hg systolic or 30 to 40 mm Hg mean pressure in the pulmonary
artery in acute pressure load. Higher pressures regularly lead to acute right
ventricular failure. Patients with preexistent pulmonary hypertension may
also develop higher pressures, owing to the adaptation of the right ventric-

ular wall [37, 62]. In acute pressure loading, the right ventricle dilates and assumes an increasingly spherical form, so that the intraventricular septum can shift into the left ventricle. Consequently, there is a loss of left ventricular filling volume and thus a decrease in left ventricular stroke volume [56].

Cardiac function is affected by three mechanisms in acute pulmonary embolism. On the one hand, there is an increase of the afterload of the right ventricle [36]. Belonging to the lowered cardiac output is a reduction of myocardial perfusion. An impairment of the oxygen supply results from hypoxemia occurring in parallel to this. These three factors result in a deterioration in myocardial contractility that can give rise to terminal right ventricular heart failure [57].

The mechanisms that contribute to disturbance of gas exchange have not yet been completely clarified. Disorders of ventilation and perfusion, as well as the development of an intrapulmonary right-to-left shunt, are partially responsible for the disturbance of gas exchange [13, 14, 33, 61, 62]. In unclosed foramen ovale, which is to be found in about 50 percent of patients, a cardiac right-to-left shunt may occur under the pressure conditions after an acute increase in resistance in the pulmonary circulation. A reduced cardiac output gives rise to a high oxygen extraction in the periphery and thus a reduced mixed venous oxygen saturation. Under these conditions, V_T/Q_T disorders accentuate an existing or developing hypoxemia. After embolization of a pulmonary arterial branch, the surfactant production stops in the distally located areas of the lung and, consequently, development of atelectasis occurs [33]. In addition, the release of mediators that have an effect on the microcirculation in the lungs and originate from thrombocytes of the embolus and the endothelial structures concerned is discussed [22, 23, 39, 44].

CLINICAL SIGNS

The clinical appearance of pulmonary embolism is characterized by nonspecific symptoms and a diversity of clinical signs, the occurrence and severity of which depend not only on the size and localization of the affected pulmonary arteries or the vessel cross-section involved, but also on prodromal conditions or the current clinical state of the patient. Pulmonary emboli in which less than 50 percent of the pulmonary vessel cross-sections are involved frequently have a clinically occult course. The following clinical signs may be manifested: dyspnea, tachypnea, pleuritic thorax pain, coughing, hemoptysis, congestion of the jugular vein, hypotension, and syncopes. Various authors have investigated the frequency of occurrence of different clinical signs (Table 13-2) [7, 25, 41, 48, 53]. States of confusion, fever and arrhythmias, rhonchi, and pleural and pericardial friction are observed more rarely. The second heart sound may be emphasized, but a split second heart sound may sometimes also occur. When acute hypotension is manifested in combination with tachycardia and chest pain and signs of right ventricular failure, a massive, potentially fatal pulmonary embolism must be assumed.

Table 13-2. Incidence of signs and symptoms (%)

	Valenzuela [53]	Rubin [41]	Stein [48]	Greenfield [20]
SYMPTOMS				
Dyspnea	81	81	84	80
Pleuritic pain		72	74	60
Pleurisy	73			
Cough	60	54	50	50
Apprehension	59	59	63	60
Hemoptysis	34	34	28	27
Syncope		14	13	22
SIGNS				
Tachypnea	46		85	88
Tachycardia	43		58	63
Temperature >37.5°C	41		50	
Accentuated P_2		53	57	
Rales		53	56	51
Pleural rub		23	18	17
Thrombophlebitis		33	41	

DIAGNOSTIC TESTS

Since the clinical signs of pulmonary embolism are so diverse, and thus do not permit definitive diagnosis, the probability of a suspected diagnosis must be rendered objective by technical methods. The basic investigatory techniques in cases of suspected pulmonary embolism include electrocardiogram (ECG), chest x-ray, and analysis of blood gases. These techniques allow the differential diagnosis of pulmonary embolism to a certain extent. The ECG will show a right axis shift, disorders of impulse propagation and repolarization, and cardiac arrhythmias owing to the acute strain on the right ventricle. Intermittent atrial flutter or fibrillations are frequently observed. Alterations of the ST segment occur most frequently (about 40% of cases). The S_IQ_{III} pattern (McGinn-White syndrome) "typical" for embolism is observed in only 10 to 15 percent of cases with acute pulmonary embolism [41, 49]. Massive pulmonary embolism frequently leads to right bundle branch block phenomena in the ECG. With dissolution of the thrombus, the ECG alterations are reversible in most cases. The ECG alterations may be indications of both the severity of the pulmonary embolism and its course. The main function of the ECG is to exclude myocardial infarction. The arterial *blood gases* deteriorate depending on the degree of pulmonary embolism. On average, partial pressures of oxygen of 50 to 75 mm Hg are measured. However, normal PaO_2 values in excess of 80 mm Hg do not rule out pulmonary embolism. Blood gas measurements do provide an indication of the severity of the disorder of gas exchange and of the course of this disorder at follow-up.

The alterations in the *chest x-ray* depend on the degree of pulmonary embolism, and x-rays should always be compared with previous films. Besides elevation of the diaphragm and pleural effusion on the affected side, foci of radioopacity in the region of the embolus, vascular discontinuations, hilus amputation (Westermark sign), hyperemia of the contralateral lung, and broadening of the heart silhouette to the right may occur. All these signs are non-specific and also occur in many other pulmonary diseases [21]. In this constellation the x-ray is indicated on one hand to exclude other causes (e.g., pneumothorax), and on the other to increase the rate of correct diagnosis in pulmonary embolism, in combination with a perfusion lung scan.

Perfusion scintigraphy of the lung is the routine noninvasive method in diagnosis of pulmonary emboli. The frequency of pulmonary embolism detected antemortem has risen from about 10 percent in the 1950s to about 30 percent since the introduction of pulmonary scintigraphy methods [19]. Perfusion scintigraphy documents the blood flow in the lungs by measurement of radioactively labeled albumin microspheres or microaggregates. With this method, perfusion defects up to a size of about 2 cm can be detected in views at several levels. An appraisal of the cause of the perfusion defect is not possible. The low specifity of this method of investigation has been demonstrated in several studies [10, 27, 28]. Depending on the extent of the defect demonstrated, it fluctuates between 21 and 71 percent [28]. But when used in combination with a chest x-ray and, in particular, with ventilation scintigraphy, the specificity of this test is markedly improved. A normal perfusion scintigraphy rules out pulmonary embolism.

Ventilation scintigraphy is carried out with radioactive gases or radioactive aerosols. Assuming that lung areas with loss of perfusion due to emboli continue to be ventilated, perfusion defects of other genesis may be differentiated by the combination of perfusion and ventilation scintigraphy. However, the specifity of perfusion scintigraphy cannot be appreciably raised by combination with ventilation scintigraphy, as has been shown by both animal experiments and clinical studies [5, 27, 28, 40]. The probable relevance of the data provided by this method could be markedly raised by the introduction of a classification scheme. This schedule takes into account the size and number of perfusion defects, as well as the incidence of corresponding ventilation defects [10, 27, 28, 38]. Analysis of the two scintigraphic methods led to the specification of "high," "moderate," and "low" probabilities of pulmonary embolism. In control studies, this method was validated with pulmonary angiography, and it was shown that among patients in whom a "high" probability of pulmonary embolism was reported after analysis of the combined ventilation/perfusion scintigraphy, this diagnosis was confirmed in 86 percent [11, 27, 28]. However, a pulmonary embolism was also demonstrated angiographically in 25 to 40 percent of the patients with a "low" probability. The appraisal of a "low" probability is thus relatively nonspecific, and further diagnostic measures must be carried out to rule out or to verify the diagnosis [59].

Pulmonary angiography must still be regarded as the "gold standard" in the diagnosis of pulmonary embolism. Imaging of a filling defect or a reduction in perfusion in the pulmonary vascular tree renders the diagnosis definitive. The occurrence of cut-off vessels is typical. These signs must be demonstrable on several images in sequence. The technique of pulmonary angiography has been improved in recent years [16], and selective pulmonary angiography with repeated administration of small-contrast medium boli has reduced the rate of side effects. Nevertheless, side effects must be reckoned with in 3 to 4 percent of patients—mainly tachyarrhythmias, injuries to the endocardium and myocardium, perforations, allergic reactions, and cardiac arrests [50].

Phlebography provides the most reliable proof of venous thrombosis of the lower limbs or the pelvis, but it is an invasive and expensive procedure. In only 20 to 30 percent of patients with pulmonary embolism can deep venous thrombosis of the lower limbs and pelvis be detected [27]. In these cases, phlebography can confirm the diagnosis of pulmonary embolism, and anticoagulatory therapy can be established. If phlebography is negative, further diagnostic evaluations (e.g., ventilation lung scan or pulmonary angiography) are necessary. Allergy to radiographic agents is a contraindication for phlebography. Other side effects are pain, swelling, and erythema (postphlebography syndrome), as well as tissue necrosis in case of extravasation of contrast material.

Magnetic resonance imaging (MRI) may be of assistance in diagnosing pulmonary emboli. Difficulties in differential diagnosis occur with regard to pulmonary hypertension, however, and peripheral pulmonary emboli cannot be diagnosed. MRI may constitute an alternative method for hemodynamically unstable patients, since it is noninvasive [60].

TREATMENT

The treatment of acute pulmonary embolism generally consists of symptomatic and specific causally related measures. One of the first *general measures* is administration of *oxygen,* since hypoxia of various extents is encountered. The degree of hypoxia or the result of oxygen administration must be checked by repeated analyses of blood gases. Because spontaneous breathing can be restricted by chest pain, *analgesics* are indicated. However, analgesics may intensify or elicit hypotension; for this reason, a dose of, for example, 1 mg morphine sulfate is initially administered intravenously, and this dose can be raised to 5 to 10 mg as required. If hypotension occurs as a result of pulmonary embolism, a *volume substitution* with crystalloids is necessary. By improvement of the preload of the right ventricle, the contractility is increased (Frank-Starling). If the hypotension cannot be improved by volume substitution, positive *inotropic substances,* such as dobutamine or dopamine, must be administered. When an adequate perfusion pressure cannot be attained with these measures, administration of vasopressors (e.g., phenylephrine or noradrenaline) is indicated [57].

The objective of the *specific pharmacotherapy* of pulmonary embolism is dissolution of the thrombus and thus elimination of the pathologic effects of the obstruction on the right ventricle and the pulmonary vascular bed.

Systemic *anticoagulation* with heparin is the basic therapy of acute pulmonary embolism. A current coagulation profile of the patient must be taken before the beginning of therapy. This includes activated partial thromboplastin time (PTT), thrombin time (TT), antithrombin III (AT III) levels, and thrombocyte count [26]. Heparin does not bring about dissolution of the embolus but prevents its enlargement and recurrent emboli. The dissolution or reduction in size of the embolus takes place on the subsequent days owing to autologous spontaneous fibrinolysis [46]. Animal experiments show that a 50 percent reduction of the embolus size is possible within 1 week as a result of spontaneous fibrinolysis [49].

Heparin therapy begins with a bolus injection of 5000 to 10,000 units, followed by continuous infusion of 1000 units per hour. The subsequent dosage depends on the results of the laboratory tests of PTT and TT. A PTT and TT of about 1.5 to 2 times the control value is aimed for. Uncontrolled studies have ascribed a better effectiveness to heparin therapy at a higher dosage when the rate of hemorrhage is not raised [29]. Under heparin therapy, the PTT and TT must be checked every 4 to 6 hours [58]. The thrombocyte count is checked daily. If an AT III deficiency is present, adequate anticoagulation cannot be achieved with the specified dosage, and AT III must then be substituted. The patient must receive long-term anticoagulant medication for prophylaxis of recurrences. After the acute phase, long-term anticoagulation with coumarin derivatives is indicated. A heparin-induced thrombocytopenia occurs in 3 to 5 percent of patients [8]. Since this side effect is more frequent with bovine heparin, switching to porcine heparin or continuation of therapy with coumarin derivatives is recommended. In the course of anticoagulation, large hemorrhages are reported in 1 percent of patients [42]. Particularly at risk are patients after surgical operations, trauma, and gastrointestinal diseases.

With *thrombolytics,* the embolus can be effectively dissolved. Streptokinase and urokinase are the main representatives of this group of drugs. Streptokinase is a product of streptococci; urokinase is isolated from human urine or nephrogenic cell cultures. Compared to streptokinase, urokinase has the advantage of not eliciting any allergic reactions. Newly developed second-generation thrombolytics, such as the tissue plasminogen activator (tPA), prourokinase, or acetylated streptokinase specifically lyse the thrombus or embolus [32], so that a systemic fibrinolysis is avoided and the fibrinolysis remains largely restricted to the embolus. Streptokinase and urokinase activate plasminogen to plasmin, which inhibits the clotting factors V, VII, and XII and thus leads to a general inhibition of blood coagulation. On the other hand, plasmin actively cleaves fibrinogen and fibrin proteolytically [52]. The half-life of streptokinase is about 80 minutes, and that of urokinase is about 16 minutes.

Hemorrhage is the most frequent complication of thrombolytic therapy, with a reported incidence of up to 50 percent [19, 34, 35]. The risk of an intracranial hemorrhage in patients under thrombolytic therapy is reported to be 1 to 2 percent—twice the frequency found in patients on heparin therapy [2, 46]. The second-generation thrombolytics are reported to give rise to fewer bleeding problems, because of their more-specific fibrinolytic activity [1].

The allergic side effects of streptokinase can be largely avoided by prophylactic intravenous administration of 100 mg hydrocortisone. With a raised antistreptolysin titer, such as may occur after infections with streptococci or after previous treatment with streptokinase, there is loss of activity or even absence of an effect. The antistreptolysin titers are correspondingly raised for about 6 months after streptococcal infections or after streptokinase treatment. Patients with raised antistreptolysin titers should receive urokinase as thrombolytic therapy.

Before therapy with thrombolytics, the basic test parameters of coagulation must be measured on principle. Determination of activated PTT, TT, the thrombocyte count, and fibrinogen and the fibrinogen degradation products is necessary. Streptokinase therapy consists of a bolus administration of 250,000 units intravenously over 30 minutes followed by continuous long-term infusion of 100,000 units per hour. Patients receiving urokinase are given a bolus of 4400 units intravenously per kilogram of body weight over 10 minutes and afterward a continuous infusion of 4400 units/kg/hr. The fibrinogen and the degradation products of fibrinogen and fibrin, as well as the TT, are checked with clinical tests in the subsequent period. The fibrinogen level falls to about one-half to one-third of its initial value, the fibrinogen degradation products are markedly raised and the TT is doubled or tripled under this therapy. The duration of therapy depends on the size of the embolus. Therapy is continued until there is a therapeutic result—as a rule, for 24 to 72 hours.

A chronic heparinization is administered subsequent to the thrombolytic treatment, to prevent recurrent emboli. The beginning of heparin therapy after thrombolysis depends on the PTT value, which should not be more than twice as high as the control value at the beginning of thrombolytic therapy. As a rule, 2 to 4 hours elapse between the end of thrombolytic therapy and the beginning of heparin therapy.

As yet no controlled study has documented the superiority of the thrombolytic therapy over heparin therapy with regard to long-term mortality [47, 51]. However, there are indications that the functional long-term results are better with regard to pulmonary restitution and the physiologic data in the pulmonary circulation in patients who have had thrombolytic therapy. The capillary blood volume of the lungs and the diffusion capacity in pulmonary embolism patients show better results 1 year after the event in patients who received thrombolytics compared with patients who were treated with heparin alone [45]. On the other hand, it has been demonstrated that treatment with thrombolytics leads to a more rapid improvement of the clinical symptoms. Taking these results and clinical observations into account, indications for thrombolytic therapy in confirmed pulmonary embolism are as follows: (1) patients who have suffered massive pulmonary embolism and in whom more than 50 percent of the vessel cross-section is obstructed (in these patients, a further embolus may result in exitus); (2) patients who are hemodynamically unstable and do not respond to corresponding symptomatic measures under heparin therapy; and (3) patients with preexisting severe cardiopulmonary disorders to which the effects of pulmonary embolism are additive. In the last-named group of patients, the chronic long-term damage resulting from pulmonary

Table 13-3. Contraindications to thrombolytic therapy

ABSOLUTE
Active bleeding
Cerebral hemorrhage ($<$2 months)
Surgical procedures ($<$10 days), including biopsies and punctures
Recent trauma
CPR
Recent bleeding from peptic ulcer
Postpartum ($<$10 days)
Heparin-associated severe thrombocytopenia
RELATIVE
Hypertension
Coagulation defects
Arterial lines
Central venous lines

embolism is especially manifest—a finding that provides an additional argument for the administration of thrombolytics. The precise indications and the advantages of the new second-generation thrombolytics are still to be established in controlled studies. So far, a higher effectiveness or a lower rate of hemorrhagic complications has only been described episodically or in small groups of cases for this class of agent [34, 54, 55].

Active hemorrhages, along with cerebrovascular conditions or neurosurgical operations within the last 2 months [45], are regarded as absolute contraindications for lytic therapy. Relative contraindications are surgical procedures within the last 14 days and pregnancy. Vascular puncture and, in particular, arterial punctures require a correspondingly substantiated indication, in view of the risk of hemorrhage (Table 13-3).

If the clinical symptoms do not improve within the first 1 to 2 hours after exhaustion of all conservative measures, *surgical embolectomy* must be considered. The mortality rate of embolectomy is about 50 to 60 percent. With the use of a bypass, the mortality rate could be lowered by 10 percent [15, 43]. Verification of the diagnosis and localization of the embolus by pulmonary angiography is absolutely necessary. The mortality rate associated with overlooked myocardial infarction is 100 percent.

If recurrent pulmonary embolism occurs despite long-term anticoagulation, *ligature* of the inferior vena cava or insertion of a *cava filter* may be considered. The mortality of untreated pulmonary emboli is about 30 percent. This group of patients is still subject to a mortality risk of 8 percent even under adequate long-term anticoagulation. With a cava filter, this risk can be further reduced to 1 to 4 percent. However, the surgical mortality resulting from this operation varies between 0.5 and 10 percent [24], depending on the filter type in various studies.

An algorithm to diagnostic steps and therapeutic decisions in suspected pulmonary embolism is shown in Figure 13-1. This flow chart does not show the whole picture, but it should provide a helpful guide to decision making in pulmonary embolism.

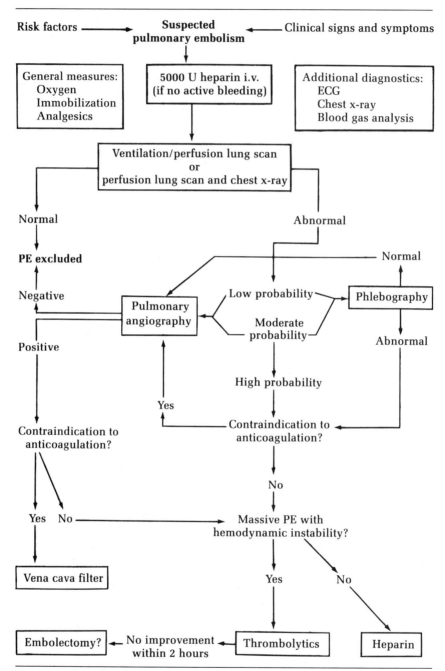

Fig. 13-1. Algorithm for diagnosis and therapy of pulmonary embolism (PE).

REFERENCES

1. Agnelli, G., et al. Sustained thrombolysis with DNA-recombinant tissue type plasminogen activator in rabbits. *Blood* 66:399, 1985.
2. Aldrich, M. S., Sherman, S. A., and Greenberg, H. S. Cerebrovascular complications of streptokinase infusion. *J.A.M.A.* 253:1777, 1985.
3. Alpert, J. S., et al. Mortality in patients treated for pulmonary embolism. *J.A.M.A.* 236:1477, 1976.
4. Alpert, J. S., et al. Left ventricular function in massive pulmonary embolism. *Chest* 71:108, 1977.
5. Austin, J. H. M., and Sagel, S. S. Alterations of airway caliber after pulmonary embolization in the lung. *Invest. Radiol.* 7:135, 1972.
6. Bell, W. R., and Simon, T. L. A comparative analysis of pulmonary perfusion scans with pulmonary angiograms. *Am. Heart J.* 92:700, 1976.
7. Bell, W. R., Simon, T. L., and DeMets, D. L. The clinical features of submassive and massive pulmonary emboli. *Am. J. Med.* 62:355, 1977.
8. Bell, W. R., and Royall, R. M. Heparin-associated thrombocytopenia. A comparison of three heparin preparations. *N. Engl. J. Med.* 303:902, 1980.
9. Bell, W. R., and Simon, T. L. Current status of pulmonary thromboembolic disease: Pathophysiology, diagnosis, prevention and treatment. *Am. Heart J.* 103:239, 1982.
10. Biello, D. R., et al. Ventilation-perfusion studies in suspected pulmonary embolism. *A.J.R.* 133:1033, 1979.
11. Braun, S. D., et al. Ventilation-perfusion scanning and pulmonary angiography: Correlation in clinical high-probability embolism. *A.J.R.* 143:977, 1984.
12. Dalen, J. E., et al. Pulmonary embolism, pulmonary hemorrhage and pulmonary infarction. *N. Engl. J. Med.* 296:1431, 1977.
13. D'Alonzo, G. E., et al. The mechanisms of abnormal gas exchange in acute massive pulmonary embolism. *Am. Rev. Respir. Dis.* 128:170, 1983.
14. Dantzker, D. R., and Bower, J. J. Alterations in gas exchange following pulmonary thrombo-embolism. *Chest* 81:495, 1982.
15. DelCampo, C. Pulmonary embolectomy. A review. *Can. J. Surg.* 28:111, 1984.
16. Fedullo, P. F., and Shure, D. Pulmonary vascular imaging. *Clin. Chest. Med.* 8:53, 1987.
17. Gillum, R. F. Pulmonary embolism and thrombophlebitis in the United States, 1970–1985. *Am. Heart J.* 114:1262, 1987.
18. Goldhaber, S. Z., et al. Factors associated with correct antemortem diagnosis of major pulmonary embolism. *Am. J. Med.* 73:822, 1982.
19. Goldhaber, S. Z., et al. Acute pulmonary embolism treated with tissue plasminogen activator. *Lancet* 2:886, 1986.
20. Greenfield, L. J. Acute venous thrombosis and pulmonary embolism. In J. D. Hardy et al. (eds.), *Textbook of Surgery* (2nd ed.). Philadelphia: Lippincott, 1988. Pp. 1002–1015.
21. Greenspan, R. H., et al. Accuracy of the chest radiograph in the diagnosis of pulmonary embolism. *Invest. Radiol.* 17:539, 1982.
22. Gurewich, V., Cohen, M., and Thomas, D. P. Humoral factors in massive pulmonary embolism. *Am. Heart J.* 76:784, 1968.
23. Halmagyi, D., Starzecki, B., and Norner, G. Humoral transmission of cardio respiratory changes in experimental lung embolism. *Circ. Res.* 14:546, 1964.
24. Hirsh, J., Genton, E., and Hull, R. Treatment of Venous Thromboembolism. In: J. Hirsh, et al. (eds.) *Venous Thromboembolism.* New York: Grune & Stratton, 1981. Pp. 122–144.
25. Hirsh, J., Hull, R. D., and Raskob, G. E. Diagnosis of pulmonary embolism. *J. Am. Coll. Cardiol.* 8:128B, 1986.
26. Hirsh, J. Treatment of pulmonary embolism. *Ann. Rev. Med.* 38:91, 1987.

27. Hull, R. D., et al. Pulmonary angiography, ventilation lung scanning, and venography for clinically suspected pulmonary embolism with abnormal perfusion scan. *Ann. Intern. Med.* 98:891, 1983.

28. Hull, R. D., et al. Diagnostic value of ventilation-perfusion in patients with suspected pulmonary embolism and abnormal perfusion lung scans. *Chest* 88:819, 1985.

29. Hyers, T. M. Antithrombotic therapy for venous thromboembolism. *Clin. Chest. Med.* 5:479, 1984.

30. Jardin, F., et al. Hemodynamic factors influencing arterial hypoxemia in massive pulmonary embolism with circulatory failure. *Circulation* 59:909, 1972.

31. Johnson, W. C., et al. Effect of streptokinase on canine pulmonary emboli: Local vs. peripheral infusion. *J. Surg. Res.* 24:366, 1978.

32. Loscalzo, J., and Braunwald, E. Tissue plasminogen activator. *N. Engl. J. Med.* 319:925, 1988.

33. Manier, G., Castaing, Y., and Guenard, H. Determinants of hypoxemia during the acute phase of pulmonary embolism in humans. *Am. Rev. Respir. Dis.* 132:332, 1985.

34. Marder, V. J. The use of thrombolytic agents: Choice of patient, drug administration, laboratory monitoring. *Ann. Intern. Med.* 90:802, 1979.

35. Marder, V. J., and Sherry, S. Thrombolytic therapy: Current status. *N. Engl. J. Med.* 318:1512, 1988.

36. McIntyre, K. M., and Sasahara, A. A. Hemodynamic and ventricular response to pulmonary embolism. *Progr. Vasc. Dis.* 17:175, 1974.

37. McIntyre, K. M., Sasahara, A. A., and Littmann, D. Relation of the electrocardiogram to hemodynamic alterations in pulmonary embolism. *Am. J. Cardiol.* 30:205, 1972.

38. McNeil, B. J. Ventilation-perfusion studies and the diagnosis of pulmonary embolism. *J. Nucl. Med.* 21:319, 1980.

39. Moser, K. M. Pulmonary Thromboembolism. In Petersdorf, R. G., et al. (eds.), *Harrison's Principles of Internal Medicine* (11th ed.). New York: McGraw-Hill, 1987. Pp. 1105–1111.

40. Robinson, A. E., et al. In vivo demonstration of small-airway bronchoconstriction following pulmonary embolism. *Radiology* 109:283, 1973.

41. Rubin, L. J. Southwestern Internal Medicine Conference: Pulmonary thromboembolic disease—Diagnosis, management and prevention. *Am. J. Med. Sci.* 290:167, 1985.

42. Salzman, E. W., et al. Management of heparin therapy: Controlled prospective trial. *N. Engl. J. Med.* 292:1046, 1975.

43. Sautter, R. D., et al. Pulmonary embolectomy: A review and current status. *Prog. Cardiovasc. Dis.* 17:371, 1975.

44. Seeger, W., and Neuhof, H. Pathophysiologie der Lungenembolie. *Hämostaseologie* 3:72, 1984.

45. Sharma, G. V. R. K., et al. Thrombolytic therapy. *N. Engl. J. Med.* 306:1268, 1982.

46. Sherry, S., et al. Thrombolytic therapy in thrombosis: A National Institutes of Health consensus development conference. *Ann. Intern. Med.* 93:141, 1980.

47. Stehle, G., and Schettler, G. Review and current status of thrombolytic therapy with streptokinase. *Tokai J. Exp. Clin. Med.* 11:51, 1986.

48. Stein, P. D., Willis, P. W., and DeMets, D. L. History and physical examination in acute pulmonary embolism in patients without preexisting cardiac or pulmonary disease. *Am. J. Cardiol.* 47:218, 1981.

49. Strauer, B. E., Motz, W., and Cade, R. Pathophysiologie und Klinik der Lungenembolie. *Dtsch Ges. Herz- u. Kreislaufforsch* 49:41, 1983.

50. Strauer, B. E. Pathophysiologie und Klinik der Lungenembolie. *Internist* 25:108, 1984.
51. Tibbutt, D. A., et al. Comparison by controlled clinical trial of streptokinase and heparin in treatment of life-threatening pulmonary embolism. *Br. Med. J.* 1:343, 1974.
52. Tsapogas, M. J. Pulmonary embolism. Part II: Management. *Ala. J. Med. Sci.* 25,1:59, 1988.
53. Valenzuela, T. D. Pulmonary embolism. *Emerg. Med. Clin. North. Am.* 6:253, 1988.
54. Verstraete, M., et al. Intravenous and intrapulmonary recombinant tissue-type plasminogen activator in the treatment of acute massive pulmonary embolism. *Circulation* 77:353, 1988.
55. Verstraete, M. Treatment of acute massive pulmonary embolism with recombinant tissue-type plasminogen activator. In K. Peter, et al. (eds.), *Intensivmedizin 1988 Band 67* (S. 61–63). Stuttgart, New York: Georg Thieme, 1988.
56. Visner, M. S., et al. Alterations in left ventricular three dimensional dynamic geometry and systolic function during acute right ventricular hypertension in the conscious dog. *Circulation* 67:353, 1983.
57. Vlahakes, G. J., Turley, K., and Hoffmann, J. I. E. The pathophysiology of failure in acute right ventricular hypertension. Hemodynamic and biochemical correlation. *Circulation* 63,1:87, 1981.
58. Walker, A. M., and Jick, H. Predictors of bleeding during heparin therapy. *J.A.M.A.* 244:1209, 1980.
59. Wellman, H. N. Pulmonary thromboembolism: Current status report on the role of nuclear medicine. *Semin. Nucl. Med.* 16:236, 1986.
60. White, R. D., Winkler, M. L., and Higgins, Ch. B. MR imaging of pulmonary arterial hypertension and pulmonary emboli. *A.J.R.* 149:15, 1987.
61. Wichert, v. P. Auswirkungen der akuten pulmonalen Hypertension auf Lungendurchblutung und kleinen Kreislauf. In K. Peter, et al. (eds.), *Intensivmedizin 1988 Band 67* (S. 31–35). Stuttgart, New York: Georg Thieme, 1988.
62. Wilson, J. E., et al. Hypoxemia in pulmonary embolism, a clinical study. *J. Clin. Invest.* 50:481, 1971.
63. Young, T. E., et al. Comparative effects of nifedipine, verapamil, and diltiazem on experimental pulmonary hypertension. *Am. J. Cardiol.* 51:195, 1983.

Cardiac Arrhythmias

William J. Mandel

The management of arrhythmias plays a major role in the care of the critically ill patient, since the presence of even minor arrhythmias in this clinical setting may have profound negative hemodynamic effects. It is therefore essential to have accurate electrocardiographic (ECG) evaluation of all patients who are critically ill, preferably by continuous monitoring techniques. Adequate therapy for the arrhythmias encountered can be accomplished only by careful analysis of the ECG waveform. In many instances atrial activity cannot readily be recognized, necessitating the use of special surface lead positions (i.e., Lewis lead), esophageal leads, and/or intracardiac electrogram recordings.

A key part of the management of patients with arrhythmias is to recognize that extracardiac problems may be largely responsible for the basic arrhythmia encountered. Therefore, it is essential to recognize and correct alterations in acid-base balance, gas exchange, electrolyte disorders, hypotension, catecholamine excess, and hypermetabolic states such as hyperthyroidism.

ANTIARRHYTHMIC DRUG THERAPY

Multiple attempts have been made to classify antiarrhythmic drugs. The most widely used classification is that of Vaughan-Williams (Table 14-1). Although not universally accepted, this classification has provided the clinician with some understanding of the relationship between the electrophysiologic and the clinical effects of antiarrhythmic drugs.

Type I_A Agents

Quinidine

ELECTROPHYSIOLOGIC EFFECTS. Quinidine has a variety of electrophysiologic effects that are dependent on the particular cardiac tissue studied. Quinidine prolongs atrial refractoriness and depresses intraventricular conduction. In general, it shortens atrioventricular (AV) nodal conduction; the latter effect may be due to a direct or a vagolytic action of the drug.

303

Table 14-1. Antiarrhythmic drug types

Type	Repolarization	ECG	Examples
I			
A. Block of Na$^+$ channels; ↓ in rate of membrane depolarization; depression of conduction velocity MOD ↓ in CV ↑ APD; ↑ ERP	↑↑	↑ QT ±↑ QRS	Quinidine, procainimide, Disopyramide (?Cibenzoline) (?Pirmenol)
B. Minimal ↓ in CV ↓ APD; rel. ↑ ERP	↓→	QRS – QT± →	Lidocaine, Tocainide, Mexiletine Phenytoin (?Ethmozine)
C. Significant ↓ in CV ± APD; ± ERP	±	↑ PR ↑ QRS ±↑ QT	Flecainide, Encainide, (Lorcainide) (?Propafenone)
II			
Beta-blocking agents (sympatholytic/antiadrenergic)	– – –	↓ HR ↑ PR	Propranolol Acebutolol
III			
Significant prolongation of repolarization; no Δ in velocity	↑↑↑	↑ QT ↓ HR ↑ PR ↑ QT	Amiodarone Bretylium (Sotalol)
IV			
Slow channel blocking agents	– – – –	↓ HR ±↑ PR	Verapamil Diltiazem

↓ = decrease; ↓↓ = significant decrease; ↑ = increase; ↑↑ = significant increase
Δ = change

HEMODYNAMIC EFFECTS. Quinidine is a negative inotropic agent and also causes peripheral vasodilation, possibly by adrenergic blocking action.

ABSORPTION AND METABOLIC FATE. Quinidine, the dextro-isomer of quinine, is almost completely absorbed by the gastrointestinal tract; the extent and rate are dependent on gastric acidity, gastrointestinal tract motility, and the amount of food in the gastrointestinal tract. The molecule is unchanged during absorption. Quinidine is highly protein-bound (approximately 80%), with a peak serum concentration being achieved between 1 and 2 hours. The heart has a high affinity for quinidine, and rapid binding occurs (less than 1 min). Skeletal muscle concentration appears to be only one-tenth that of ventricular muscle concentration, and the concentration in the ventricle is greater than that in the atrium. Quinidine's half-life is between 2 and 3 hours; 95 percent of the administered dose can be recovered in the urine as either quinidine or one of its metabolites. As yet, no significant data are available concerning the antiarrhythmic properties of the metabolites of quinidine.

DOSAGE, ROUTE, AND SERUM LEVELS. In general, quinidine is administered by the oral route every 6 hours. However, occasional patients may require administration every 3 or 4 hours. The total daily dose required is usually 1.2 to 3.4 gm, with a therapeutic serum level range of 2 to 6 mg/liter. The method of quinidine serum level determination may be important in evaluating the dosage. The protein precipitate method measures quinidine plus all metabolites, including water-soluble metabolites. The double-extraction technique measures only quinidine and its dihydroxyquinidine derivative. Stable serum levels during oral quinidine therapy are not observed for 2 to 3 days. In moderate to severe renal failure (with or without dialysis), no significant change in dose is needed.

TOXICITY. The most common side effect of quinidine therapy is gastrointestinal tract toxicity, usually manifested by nausea, vomiting, and diarrhea. These symptoms are occasionally severe enough to warrant discontinuance of the drug. Another significant side effect is the development of cinchonism, which is characterized by tinnitus, visual difficulty, vertigo, and headache. Rarely, one may see thrombocytopenic purpura, exfoliative dermatitis, fever, and respiratory paralysis. In addition, quinidine syncope has been described, which appears to be related to the development of ventricular arrhythmias (i.e., torsade de pointes). This event is not clearly dose-related, but it may be related to rapidly increasing QT_c. Hypotension and diminished cardiac output may also occur because of quinidine's negative inotropic effects and may prove a significant problem in patients with borderline hemodynamic function. Acceleration of the ventricular rate during atrial fibrillation or atrial flutter may occur because of potential vagolytic effects on AV nodal transmission. Quinidine administration in digitalized patients may result in significant elevation of the serum digitalis level and possible precipitation of digitalis intoxication. Rarely, decrease in sinus node function may occur.

SPECIFIC INDICATIONS. Oral quinidine therapy is useful for the treatment of both atrial and ventricular arrhythmias of all types. Furthermore, it may be used prophylactically following conversion to sinus rhythm from atrial fibrillation, as well as in the early stages of myocardial infarction. Also, it has been shown to have prophylactic benefits in the long-term management of patients with paroxysmal atrial tachycardia, with or without Wolff-Parkinson-White syndrome.

AVAILABLE PREPARATIONS. Quinidine for oral administration is available as the sulfate in tablets of 200 or 300 mg, as the polygalacturonate (Cardioquin) in 275-mg tablets, as sustained-release quinidine gluconate (Quinaglute) in 330-mg tablets, or as sustained-release quinidine sulfate (Quinidex) in 300-mg tablets. The sustained-release or long-acting quinidine preparations have been stated to be effective over periods of 8 to 12 hours. The peak level of quinidine achieved with quinidine gluconate generally is lower for equal amounts of quinidine sulfate, but the half-life is longer. The usual dose for quinidine gluconate in an average-sized patient with normal renal function is 660 mg every 8 hours. Intravenous administration should be utilized only by physicians experienced with its use. Continuous ECG and frequent blood pressure monitoring is essential.

Procainamide

ELECTROPHYSIOLOGIC EFFECTS. The electrophysiologic effects of procainamide are essentially identical to those of quinidine. Specifically, this drug prolongs the effective refractory period of the atrium and His-Purkinje system and abbreviates the effective refractory period of the AV node.

HEMODYNAMIC EFFECTS. Procainamide may significantly lower cardiac output and peripheral vascular resistance. Intravenous administration may also significantly depress glomerular filtration rate and effective renal plasma flow.

ABSORPTION AND METABOLIC FATE. The absorption of procainamide from the gastrointestinal tract is rapid, with the peak effect being seen in 1 to 1½ hours. This drug is sparingly protein-bound and is highly concentrated in cardiac muscle. Approximately 90 percent of the unchanged drug or its metabolites are excreted via the renal route. The half-life for procainamide is approximately 2 to 3 hours. Acetylation is a major method of pronestyl metabolism/excretion. Slow or fast acetylators are frequently encountered in clinical practice, accounting for unanticipated high (slow acetylators) or low (fast acetylators) serum pronestyl levels. The corresponding metabolite [N-acetyl procainamide (NAPA)] will be altered in a way opposite to the parent compound, pronestyl. NAPA appears to have some (but less) antiarrhythmic action. Elevated NAPA levels are frequently seen in patients with moderate or severe renal failure.

DOSAGE, ROUTE, AND SERUM LEVELS. Therapy with oral procainamide usually requires a total daily dose of 50 mg/kg given in divided doses every 3 hours. For a more rapid onset of action with oral therapy, it is suggested that a loading dose of 1 gm be given intramuscularly, eliminating the long equilibration that may be necessary by the oral route. Procainamide requires 1 to 2 days to establish a stable serum level when administered orally. Sustained-release pronestyl preparations are available with a dosage schedule of every 6 hours.

In contrast with quinidine, procainamide is frequently administered by intravenous injection and by chronic infusion. Intravenous administration may be carried out using a dose of 30 to 50 mg/min until a total dose of 10 to 15 mg/kg is given or the arrhythmia is terminated. The dose necessary for satisfactory results with constant infusion is 20 to 80 μg/kg/min, with an expected plateau time of approximately 12 hours. Therapeutic serum levels are 4 to 8 μg/ml. In some instances levels of 10 to 20 μg/ml are needed.

TOXICITY. Procainamide may produce clinically significant ventricular arrhythmias that apparently are the result of excessive blood levels. Syncopal episodes, as reported with quinidine, may occur, presumably due to ventricular arrhythmias. Rarely, a decrease in sinus node function has been observed.

In addition, significant depression of blood pressure and cardiac output may be seen. Agranulocytosis and transient psychoses may develop. Other side effects include anorexia, fever, drug rash, nausea, and vomiting. A lupus-like syndrome occurs in a relatively small percentage of patients, usually after at least 2 weeks of oral therapy. However, elevated antinuclear antibody titers will develop in nearly all patients after 12 months of oral therapy. Moderate to severe renal failure will produce a significant increase in the pronestyl levels, as well as prolong the half-life (see above).

SPECIFIC INDICATIONS. Indications of procainamide are identical to those for quinidine therapy; these drugs have been found to be effective in a variety of atrial and ventricular arrhythmias.

AVAILABLE PREPARATIONS. Procainamide is available in capsules of 250, 375, and 500 mg for oral administration. It is available as the hydrochloride for parenteral administration in 10-ml ampules containing 100 mg/ml. Procan SR is an oral preparation of procainamide that enables the clinician to administer the drug every 6 hours. This preparation is available in 250-, 500-, 750-, and 1000-mg tablets.

Disopyramide

Since this agent (Norpace) was introduced in the United States in 1977, significant experience has been gained in its use for the treatment of supraventricular and ventricular arrhythmias.

ELECTROPHYSIOLOGIC EFFECTS. Disopyramide is similar but not identical with quinidine with regard to electrophysiologic effects. It decreases action potential amplitude and upstroke velocity, resulting in decreased conduction and prolongation of refractoriness in the intraventricular conduction system.

This drug has potent anticholinergic properties that balance the direct depressant effects on the sinus node.

HEMODYNAMIC EFFECTS. Disopyramide has been found to have minor negative inotropic effects. However, in the setting of acute myocardial infarction, the negative inotropic effects seem to be accentuated.

ABSORPTION AND METABOLIC FATE. The drug is well (83%) absorbed from the gastrointestinal tract. The reported half-life has been variable, ranging from 8 to 18 hours.

A significant portion of the unchanged drug and its major metabolite is excreted by the kidneys. The protein binding is concentration-dependent, and the free form increases as the total drug concentration increases—i.e., nonlinear pharmacokinetics. The major metabolite is formed in the liver. Renal insufficiency necessitates significant reduction in the frequency of administration and the total dose administered per day.

DOSAGE, ROUTE, SERUM LEVELS. Disopyramide is clinically available only as an oral agent. Doses range from 300 to 1600 mg/day administered in divided doses every 6 hours. The therapeutic serum levels are 2 to 5 μg/ml. A controlled-release (CR) preparation is available allowing a dosage regimen of every 12 hours.

TOXICITY. Side effects are generally related to the drug's potent anticholinergic effects—i.e., dry mouth, blurred vision, constipation, urinary retention, and psychosis. Intraventricular conduction disturbances may occur, especially in patients with preexisting conduction abnormalities.

SPECIFIC INDICATIONS. Disopyramide is particularly useful in the treatment of ventricular arrhythmias. Its usefulness in the treatment of supraventricular arrhythmias has been less clearly elucidated.

AVAILABLE PREPARATIONS. Capsules are available in 100- and 150-mg sizes.

Type I_B Agents

Lidocaine

ELECTROPHYSIOLOGIC EFFECTS. Lidocaine's electrophysiologic effects differ significantly from those of procainamide and quinidine. The drug has little effect on the sinus node, atrial muscle, or AV node but has a profound effect on the ventricular conduction system and ventricular muscle. It has been shown to shorten markedly the refractory period and action potential duration of both Purkinje fibers and ventricular muscle.

HEMODYNAMIC EFFECTS. No significant changes in cardiac output, left ventricular end-diastolic pressure, dp/dt, or stroke work are observed. Peripheral vascular resistance is variably affected.

ABSORPTION AND METABOLIC FATE. Lidocaine is available only for parenteral administration. Its half-life is short (108 min), requiring repeated administration of intravenous boluses or chronic constant infusion. Nevertheless, 6 to 10 hours are required before stable plateau levels are achieved with chronic infusion. The serum blood levels of lidocaine are influenced substantially by decrease in hepatic blood flow with resultant increases in expected serum levels; this is a particular problem in the setting of congestive heart failure or liver insufficiency. If it is deemed essential to increase the infusion rate of lidocaine in response to increasing ventricular arrhythmias, it would appear most prudent to administer sequential small (i.e., 25-mg) boluses at repeated 15-min intervals, in addition to increasing the infusion rate, until a new stable state is achieved. Lidocaine is metabolized by the liver, without any significant renal excretion; it is less than 10 percent bound to plasma proteins. In the setting of acute myocardial infarction, an increase in the level of carrier protein (AAG) results in a "spurious" increase in the total serum lidocaine level but *not* in the free (unbound) lidocaine level.

DOSAGE, ROUTE, AND SERUM LEVELS. In general, the drug is administered by an intravenous bolus of 1 mg/kg followed by continuous infusion. Lidocaine's effective plasma levels are 2 to 6 mg/liter, necessitating an infusion rate of 20 to 50 μg/kg/min. Lidocaine may also be given by intramuscular (deltoid) injection. Doses of 300 mg will result in prompt therapeutic serum levels that will be maintained for more than 1 hour.

TOXICITY. The toxic effects of lidocaine are usually restricted to central nervous system dysfunction. These effects in turn are usually related to the serum level of the drug, with toxic manifestations being seen at serum levels above 7.5 mg/liter. These toxic manifestations range from drowsiness and confusion to respiratory arrest and convulsions.

SPECIFIC INDICATIONS. Lidocaine has been found most useful for the treatment of serious ventricular arrhythmias. The drug appears to have no significant effectiveness in the treatment of atrial arrhythmias or AV block. However, in the setting of digitalis intoxication with prolonged AV conduction and ventricular arrhythmias, lidocaine appears to be of great clinical utility.

AVAILABLE PREPARATIONS. Lidocaine as the hydrochloride (without epinephrine) comes in single-dose and multidose ampules in concentrations of 1%, 2%, 4%, and 20%.

Mexiletine
Mexiletine is a structural analog of lidocaine that shows many clinical and electrophysiologic effects similar to those of its sister compound. In contrast to lidocaine, it is available for oral administration.

ELECTROPHYSIOLOGIC EFFECTS. Studies in isolated cardiac tissue have demonstrated that mexiletine has effects similar to lidocaine. It decreases the maximum rate of depolarization and shortens the refractory period more than it shortens action potential duration. Its effect on depolarization is, however, minor. It has been shown to suppress normal and abnormal automatic mechanisms at concentrations that have a limited effect on sinus node function. It also has some minimal effect on slow-channel–dependent events in Purkinje fibers.

In patients, it appears to have limited, if any, effects on sinus or AV node, with effects limited to the His-Purkinje system.

HEMODYNAMIC EFFECTS. Data suggest that mexiletine has a limited effect on hemodynamic performance in both patients with normal and patients with abnormal ventricular function.

ABSORPTION AND METABOLIC FATE. Mexiletine is rapidly and nearly completely absorbed with oral administration. There is some abnormality of absorption in patients with myocardial infarction and in patients who have received narcotics. Mexiletine is generally eliminated by hepatic metabolism, with only 10 percent of the drug excreted unchanged in the urine. The elimination half-life is approximately 12 hours. Approximately 70 percent of the drug is protein-bound.

DOSAGE, ROUTE, AND SERUM LEVELS. Mexiletine is administered as an oral agent, although experimentally it can be given intravenously. Dosage ranges from 150 mg every 12 hours to 300 mg every 8 hours. Therapeutic serum levels range from 0.5 to 2 μg/ml.

TOXICITY. The major side effects of mexiletine therapy appear to be related to gastrointestinal upset and neurologic problems. Gastrointestinal complaints include nausea, vomiting, and dyspepsia. These side effects can be modified by administration of the drug with food. Neurologic effects include tremor, nystagmus, dizziness, ataxia, confusion, etc. Rare hematologic side effects have been described, including thrombocytopenia and a positive ANA.

SPECIFIC INDICATIONS. Mexiletine is indicated for the treatment of ventricular arrhythmias of all sorts, including isolated ventricular premature complexes, complex ventricular arrhythmias, and sustained recurrent ventricular tachycardia. Its effectiveness in the latter group of patients is relatively limited, however. It has no specific indication for the treatment of supraventricular arrhythmias.

AVAILABLE PREPARATIONS. Capsules of 150, 200, and 250 mg are available.

Tocainide

Tocainide is another lidocaine analog, and its spectrum of action and clinical effectiveness are similar to those of mexiletine. It is only available clinically for oral administration.

ELECTROPHYSIOLOGIC EFFECTS. Isolated cardiac tissue studies have demonstrated that tocainide has similar electrophysiologic effects to lidocaine and mexiletine.

HEMODYNAMIC EFFECTS. Little or no negative effects on cardiac hemodynamics or peripheral vascular hemodynamics have been identified with the use of tocainide in clinically appropriate concentrations.

ABSORPTION AND METABOLIC FATE. Tocainide is rapidly absorbed by oral administration and has a high bioavailability. A significant portion of the drug is metabolized by the liver, but at least 40 percent may be eliminated by the kidney in unchanged form. The elimination half-life of the drug is approximately 12 hours (10–17 hours); 50 percent of the drug is bound to plasma protein.

DOSAGE, ROUTE, AND SERUM LEVELS. Tocainide is available only for oral administration with dosages from 400 mg every 12 hours to as much as 1200 mg every 8 hours. Titration of dose should be done infrequently—i.e., a minimum of 4 days between each dosage change. Total dosage utilized will clearly be dependent upon clinical toxicity (see below). Effective serum concentrations are 4 to 10 μg/ml.

TOXICITY. Tocainide's major toxicity is similar to that of mexiletine—i.e., gastrointestinal and neurologic side effects. Unusual side effects reported include agranulocytosis and pulmonary toxicity with fibrosis.

SPECIFIC INDICATIONS. Tocainide, like mexiletine, is specifically indicated for ventricular arrhythmias of all types. Its effectiveness for recurrent/sustained ventricular tachycardia, like mexiletine, is relatively low. It has no specific indication for the treatment of supraventricular arrhythmias.

AVAILABLE PREPARATIONS. Tablets are available in 400- and 600-mg sizes.

Diphenylhydantoin Sodium

ELECTROPHYSIOLOGIC EFFECTS. Diphenylhydantoin appears to be identical to lidocaine in its electrophysiologic effects. Specifically, it has limited effect on the sinus node or atrial musculature, abbreviates AV conduction, and markedly shortens the effective refractory period and action potential duration in Purkinje fibers and ventricular muscle.

HEMODYNAMIC EFFECTS. Diphenylhydantoin decreases myocardial contractility, increases coronary flow, increases coronary vascular resistance, and has a variable effect on peripheral resistance and left ventricular end-diastolic pressure.

ABSORPTION AND METABOLIC FATE. Diphenylhydantoin is absorbed slowly from the gastrointestinal tract and has a long half-life. The peak plasma level is achieved 6 to 12 hours after oral administration. Oral administration requires 6 to 7 days before a plateau is reached. The drug is approximately 50 percent bound by plasma protein and is excreted to a very limited extent by the renal route; its main metabolic pathway is that of the liver. Therefore, in patients with decreased hepatic perfusion, liver insufficiency, or both, elevated blood levels of this agent may be anticipated.

DOSAGE, ROUTE, AND SERUM LEVELS. Diphenylhydantoin may be administered orally, intramuscularly, or intravenously. Oral administration requires 300 to 600 mg/day administered once or in divided doses every 6 or 8 hours. A decreasing loading dose over the first 3 days of therapy may be clinically useful. Intravenous administration can be carried out by giving 100 mg every 3 to 5 minutes until a total dose of 600 mg is achieved or the arrhythmia is terminated. Effective serum levels are 10 to 18 mg/liter.

TOXICITY. Diphenylhydantoin produces central nervous system toxic manifestations, generally in direct relation to the amount of drug administered. These symptoms include tremors, ataxia, nystagmus, drowsiness, and confusion. In addition, with parenteral administration, asystole has been observed, but rarely. Further toxic manifestations include gum hypertrophy, megaloblastic anemia, pseudolymphoma, and drug interaction.

SPECIFIC INDICATIONS. Diphenylhydantoin appears to be useful in the treatment of ventricular arrhythmias with or without AV block in the setting of digitalis intoxication and may also be effective in the treatment of other types of ventricular arrhythmias. Parenteral administration is more successful than oral administration.

AVAILABLE PREPARATIONS. Capsules are available in 30- and 100-mg sizes. A suspension of 30 or 125 mg per 5 ml is also available. Parenteral preparations consist of 2- or 5-ml ampules (50 mg/ml) to be mixed just before use.

Type I$_C$ Agents

Flecainide
Flecainide was first released for treatment of ventricular arrhythmias in 1985. Subsequently, it was found to have a broad spectrum of action.

ELECTROPHYSIOLOGIC EFFECTS. Microelectrode studies have shown that this agent markedly decreases the upstroke velocity in all cardiac tissue; in addition, significant depression of AV nodal conduction and His-Purkinje conduction have been observed. In humans, it also has been noted to depress sinus node function.

Electrophysiologic studies in humans have demonstrated a significant prolongation of the A–H and H–V intervals, as well as prolongation of the QRS duration. Refractoriness in the ventricle was not increased.

Electrocardiographic findings include the fact that the P–R interval and QRS duration are generally increased with substantial increase in the Q–T interval.

HEMODYNAMIC EFFECTS. Myocardial performance is depressed by all parameters measured. Caution is warranted in patients with significant depression of left ventricular function.

ABSORPTION AND METABOLIC FATE. Oral administration of flecainide demonstrates an excellent bioavailability. The maximum plasma concentration is achieved 2 to 4 hours after oral dose. Elimination half-life is 14 to 20 hours. The drug is approximately 33 percent bound to plasma protein. The drug is metabolized by the liver, but about 25 percent of the parent compound is excreted unchanged in the urine. It is advisable to reduce the dose in the setting of renal failure, and probably in the setting of congestive heart failure as well.

DOSAGE, ROUTE, AND PLASMA ADMINISTRATION. Plasma concentrations from 200 to 1000 ng/ml are considered to be in the therapeutic range. Dosage for the oral preparation begins at 100 mg every 12 hours and increases 50 mg every 4 to 7 days until a maximum of 200 mg every 12 hours is reached.

The drug is available as an intravenous compound only for investigational use. Previous studies have demonstrated that it is effective at a dose of approximately 2 mg/kg.

TOXICITY. The predominant side effects are neurologic and cardiac problems. The most common side effects are blurred vision, headache and nausea, worsening congestive heart failure, and proarrhythmia. This drug should be used with caution in patients with significant left ventricular dysfunction or recurrent sustained ventricular tachycardia.

No significant drug interactions have been noted.

SPECIFIC INDICATIONS. Currently, flecainide has been approved for the treatment of ventricular arrhythmias. In more than 95 percent of patients it reduces ventricular ectopy by greater than 75 percent. In comparative studies, it has been found to be more effective than quinidine or disopyramide.

Preliminary clinical studies have demonstrated that this drug is quite effective in the prevention of a variety of supraventricular arrhythmias.

Encainide

Because this agent (Enkaid) has only recently been introduced for clinical use, extensive experience has not yet been gained with this drug in the management of a variety of arrhythmias. Nevertheless, it appears to have utility for the treatment of both ventricular and supraventricular arrhythmias.

ELECTROPHYSIOLOGIC EFFECTS. Studies in isolated cardiac tissue have shown that encainide significantly decreases depolarization from isolated Purkinje fibers in a rate-dependent manner, as well as shortening action-potential duration. Apparently, it does not shorten action-potential duration in ventricular muscle. It appears to have no effect on calcium channel events. Only relatively limited data are available in isolated tissue electrophysiologic studies.

Clinical studies have demonstrated that encainide causes a significant increase in the AV nodal refractory period, as well as prolongation of the H–V interval and QRS duration. It also prolongs the refractory period of atrial and ventricular muscle. Q–T prolongation apparently has not been observed.

HEMODYNAMIC EFFECTS. This drug appears to have significant negative inotropic effects, and large doses should be used with significant caution in patients with depressed left ventricular function.

ABSORPTION AND METABOLIC FATE. The absorption of this drug is highly variable; bioavailability ranging between 7 and 80 percent. This may be due, in large part, to a first-pass effect. The major route of elimination is hepatic metabolism, and the drug should be used with caution in patients with liver disease. The elimination half-life varies fairly widely between 1.5 and 4 hours.

Encainide has at least two active metabolites: O-demethyl encainide and N,O-demethyl encainide (ODE, MODE). The half-lives of ODE and MODE are longer than that of the parent compound. These metabolites are clinically active and may, in fact, be the major mechanism of the antiarrhythmic effect of this drug.

DOSAGE, ROUTE, AND SERUM LEVELS. Encainide is available only as an oral agent. Dosage ranges from 25 mg every 12 hours to 50 mg every 6 hours. Higher doses—i.e., greater than 150 mg—should be used with caution and followed carefully with serial electrocardiograms. Therapeutic serum levels have not been clearly defined, because of the drug's active metabolites.

TOXICITY. Major side effects of encainide relate to an incidence of proarrhythmic effect, with potentially life-threatening ventricular arrhythmias being precipitated in patients at high risk who are treated with higher doses. The proarrhythmic effect has been reported to be approximately 10 percent. Additional side effects include headache, increase in blood pressure, and gastrointestinal side effects.

SPECIFIC INDICATIONS. Encainide has been found to be very effective for suppression of ventricular ectopy in most clinical situations.

Type II Agents

β-Blocking Agents

There are now at least nine beta blockers clinically available for use in the United States. Only three (propranolol, acebutolol, and esmolol) are approved for use as antiarrhythmic agents. These drugs are competitive β-adrenergic blocking agents, which will inhibit myocardial response to catecholamines. Cardioselective β-blocking agents have been released for use as antihypertensive agents. These drugs may have special use in patients with asthma who have need for a β-blocker.

Propranolol

ELECTROPHYSIOLOGIC EFFECTS. Propranolol, in Purkinje fibers, decreases the rate of rise of the action potential upstroke and prolongs the refractory period and conduction time. It also shortens action potential duration. Studies in both experimental animals and humans have determined that propranolol significantly prolongs the AV nodal conduction time without altering intraventricular conduction times.

A pronounced electrophysiologic alteration seen following propranolol administration is the decrease in spontaneous sinus node activity.

HEMODYNAMIC EFFECTS. Propranolol is a potent negative inotropic agent and so decreases the force of contraction. In addition, there is a decrease in both the velocity and the extent of fiber shortening following propranolol administration, as well as a drop in dp/dt and an elevation of left ventricular end-diastolic pressure. It also may decrease coronary flow and cause arteriolar constriction and venodilatation. Propranolol produces a decrease in adenyl cyclase activity in the myocardium.

In spite of its effect on the peripheral arterial system, propranolol, especially in hypertensive patients, may produce a significant hypotensive effect.

ABSORPTION AND METABOLIC FATE. Highly variable plasma levels of propranolol are obtained from different patients, suggesting marked variation in the rate of absorption from the gastrointestinal tract from patient to patient, or alterations in metabolism, or both. Peak absorption is 1½ to 2 hours after the oral dose in the fasting state and 2 to 4 hours if taken with a meal. The plasma half-life is 3.2 hours after oral administration; up to 90 percent of the drug is protein-bound. The drug is extensively metabolized, with only minimal amounts excreted unchanged by the kidneys. The major site of metabolism appears to be the liver.

DOSAGE, ROUTE, AND SERUM LEVELS. For the treatment of recurrent arrhythmias, oral administration of propranolol is usually begun with 10 mg every 6 hours. The dosage can be increased in a stepwise fashion to as much as 480 mg/day in recalcitrant cases. During oral administration a stable serum level is achieved in 1 to 2 days.

Propranolol can also be administered intravenously for the urgent treatment of arrhythmias. A dosage schedule should be at the rate of 1 mg intravenously every 1 to 3 minutes, for a total dose of up to 20 mg.

TOXICITY. The major toxic effect of propranolol is the development of sinus arrest or marked sinus bradycardia. Complete AV block may also be observed. These findings have generally been seen during intravenous administration at too rapid a rate and in too large a dose.

Hemodynamic side effects include a significant decrease in cardiac output and peripheral blood pressure. In addition, patients may manifest bronchospasm, gastrointestinal distress, or masked hypoglycemia.

SPECIFIC INDICATIONS. Propranolol's most potent clinical effect is the production of delay in AV nodal conduction. It is very effective for the rapid induction of partial AV nodal delay. It is most appropriately used clinically to slow the ventricular rate in atrial tachyarrhythmias, such as atrial fibrillation and atrial flutter and/or atrial tachycardia. Furthermore, it has been suggested to be of significant benefit for the elimination of arrhythmias due to reentry involving the AV nodal conducting system, such as those seen during episodes of paroxysmal atrial tachycardia. Oral administration has been helpful in the treatment of significant ventricular arrhythmias, especially those that are related to catecholamines, digitalis intoxication, or both.

AVAILABLE PREPARATIONS. Propranolol is supplied in 10-, 20-, 40-, 60-, 80-, and 90-mg tablets; long-acting 80-, 120-, and 160-mg capsules; and 1-mg vials for intravenous administration.

ADDITIONAL β-BLOCKING AGENTS. There are a variety of β-blocking agents available, having slightly different effects in terms of cardiac and extracardiac manifestations of β blockade as compared with propranolol. Advantages over propranolol in the treatment of arrhythmias may reflect duration of action or the spectrum of side effects.

Esmolol

This drug is an ultra–short-acting "cardioselective" β_1-adrenergic blocking agent available for intravenous use only. It has apparently no intrinsic sympathomaimetic activity. Its half-life is 9 minutes! It has no obvious membrane stabilizing activity. Its short duration of action is related to its metabolism via red blood cell esterases. It is 55 percent bound to protein.

As an intravenous infusion, the steady state is achieved in approximately 3 to 5 minutes. Dose-hemodynamic response curves identify a linear response within an infusion range of 25 to 300 µg/kg/min. Initial therapy is to give a loading dose of 500 µg/kg/min for 30 to 60 seconds followed by an initial dose of 25 µg/kg/min as an infusion. Every 4 to 5 minutes, the dose can be increased, if necessary, to a maximum of 300 µg/kg/min.

Studies comparing intravenous verapamil with esmolol indicate a similar rate of conversion of supraventricular tachyarrhythmias to sinus rhythm. In addition, esmolol is equally effective in slowing the ventricular rate of atrial arrhythmias. Side effects, however, appear less profound and of shorter duration.

Clinically, this drug appears to be extremely useful for the acute management of a variety of supraventricular tachycardias, either in terms of conversion (i.e., paroxysmal supraventricular tachycardia) or a slowing of the ventricular response (i.e., atrial fibrillation or flutter).

Type III Agents

Bretylium

Bretylium was recognized as a potent antiarrhythmic drug in 1965. Previously, the drug was used as an antihypertensive agent with modest clinical success.

ELECTROPHYSIOLOGIC EFFECTS. Bretylium has complex electrophysiologic effects based on its ability to cause, initially, catecholamine release. In Purkinje fibers, the drug prolongs action potential duration and refractory period, but it does not do this in atrial muscle. It also has been shown to have differential effects in infarcted myocardium. On rare occasions, this agent has been found to convert ventricular fibrillation. More commonly, it has been effective in preventing ventricular fibrillation.

HEMODYNAMIC EFFECTS. The hemodynamic effects of bretylium are, in part, related to initial release and subsequent blockade of norepinephrine from adrenergic nerve endings.

In clinical use, bretylium produces an initial mild increase and subsequent modest decrease in systemic pressure. No significant effects have been noted with regard to other parameters of ventricular function—i.e., wedge pressure, cardiac index, and stroke work index.

ABSORPTION AND METABOLIC FATE. Pharmacologic data are limited, but in studies with intramuscular dosage the plasma half-life was between 3 and 10 hours. Approximately 80 percent of the drug was excreted in the urine. Suppression of the arrhythmia was not related to the plasma levels of the drug.

DOSAGE, ROUTE, AND SERUM LEVELS. Acute intravenous administration with bretylium is in a 5- to 10-mg/kg dose given over at least 10 minutes. Maintenance dosage may be given by constant infusion at a dosage of 1 to 7 mg/min, with mandatory monitoring of blood pressure.

Intramuscular administration may also be utilized with a dosage of 5 to 10 mg/kg given every 6 hours. It has been recommended that the total 24-hour dosage not exceed 30 mg/kg.

Blood level determinations are not clinically available at this time. However, dosage should be reduced in significant renal insufficiency.

TOXICITY. Hypotension is a frequently observed effect. Nausea and vomiting are also commonly observed, especially if the dose is administered too rapidly. Ventricular arrhythmias may be enhanced in the early stages of administration. Bradycardia has been noted. Rarely, episodes of parotitis have been clinically recognized.

SPECIFIC INDICATIONS. Bretylium is specifically indicated for the treatment of intractable ventricular arrhythmias, especially recurrent ventricular fibrillation. Clinically, the drug has been used only in patients refractory to routine antiarrhythmic agents.

AVAILABLE PREPARATIONS. The drug is available presently only for parenteral use. A 10-ml ampule containing 500 mg is available. The drug should be diluted to a minimum of 50 ml of 5% D/W or saline.

Amiodarone

Amiodarone is an agent with complex pharmacologic effects and very broad spectrum of antiarrhythmic drug efficacy. This drug was intensively and extensively studied prior to its recent introduction in the United States.

ELECTROPHYSIOLOGIC EFFECTS. It has been very difficult to evaluate the electrophysiologic effects of amiodarone on isolated cardiac tissue because of its unusual pharmacokinetics—i.e., its extremely long half-life and the availability of a major metabolite. Nevertheless, studies have shown that it significantly depresses sinus node automaticity and prolongs action potential duration. It also has some effects on abnormal automatic mechanisms dependent on slow-channel events. Studies on Purkinje fibers have suggested that it markedly prolongs action potential duration without significant influence on upstroke velocity.

HEMODYNAMIC EFFECTS. In patients with depressed left ventricular dysfunction, large oral doses in the loading phase of therapy may significantly depress hemodynamic performance. Generally, however, in the maintenance phase of therapy the drug is well tolerated, with limited negative inotropic effects being clinically recognized.

ABSORPTION AND METABOLIC FATE. Amiodarone demonstrates unique pharmacologic properties, in that its distribution and accumulation in the body are extremely slow, presumably secondary to extensive uptake by adipose tissue. The proposed elimination half-life for oral administration of amiodarone has been reported to be from 1 week to several months!

Oral absorption of amiodarone is relatively slow, with peak serum concentration being achieved approximately 5 hours after a single oral dose. Oral bioavailability is approximately 35 percent. Amiodarone appears to be metabolized via the hepatic route. Its major metabolite, desethyl-amiodarone, may possess significant antiarrhythmic effects. Investigators have suggested that amiodarone fits into a three-compartment pharmacokinetic distribution model, with the third, or "deep," compartment being adipose tissue. This may account for its very prolonged half-life.

Dosage of amiodarone does not appear to be significantly influenced by renal insufficiency.

DOSAGE, ROUTE, AND SERUM LEVELS. Amiodarone is available for oral administration. Dosage schemes are dependent on the type of arrhythmia and the need for "rapid" accumulation of the drug. In patients with life-threatening ventricular arrhythmias, a variety of oral loading dose schemes have been utilized, ranging from 1000 mg per day to as high as 5000 mg per day, for periods of 1 to 14 days. This loading phase has been followed by tapering oral administration with daily doses ranging initially from 400 to 800 mg per day, reducing to maintenance dosages from 800 mg per day to as low as 100 mg three times per week. The drug can be administered daily as a single oral dose or in divided dosages that may produce fewer gastrointestinal side effects if administered with meals.

Amiodarone therapeutic serum levels are between 1 and 2.5 μg/ml. Similar serum level values appear to apply to the major metabolite desethylamiodarone. Serum levels should not be ordered for chronic therapy unless steady state has been achieved—i.e., approximately 3 months of stable dose.

TOXICITY. Amiodarone has manifested a wide spectrum of side effects, with multiple systems being involved in its toxicity profile. Recognized side effects include: (1) corneal microdeposits associated with blurring of vision, halo vision, and decreased visual acuity; (2) sun sensitivity with marked increase in "sun burning"; (3) abnormalities in liver function studies; (4) neurotoxicity with tremor, ataxia, and proximal muscle weakness; (5) thyroid function test abnormalities. Hypothyroidism, and occasionally hyperthyroidism, have been noted clinically; (6) slate gray/blue discoloration to the skin, especially of the face; and (7) pulmonary toxicity manifested by a wide spectrum of chest x-ray abnormalities and clinical symptoms of breathlessness, cough, etc.

It is essential that serial laboratory studies be done and periodic chest x-rays performed for evaluation of side effects when amiodarone is administered chronically.

Amiodarone causes significant slowing of ventricular rate, and on rare occasions, permanent pacemaking therapy may be needed. It also causes significant prolongation of AV conduction and marked prolongation of the Q–T interval. Electrocardiographic follow-up is mandatory.

Interaction with a variety of agents has been determined, including (1) potentiating coumadin effect; (2) elevating serum levels of quinidine and pronestyl with conjoint administration; (3) elevating digoxin levels with conjoint administration; (4) slowing of the heart rate when administered with beta blockers or calcium-channel blockers; (5) rarely, a proarrhythmic effect has been noted (i.e., torsade de pointes), especially when amiodarone is administered with agents with a propensity to develop torsade de pointes (i.e., quinidine).

SPECIFIC INDICATIONS. Amiodarone is indicated for a wide spectrum of atrial and ventricular arrhythmias. Atrial arrhythmias appear to require much smaller chronic doses. With serious ventricular arrhythmias, large loading-dose therapy may be necessary to produce a more rapid onset of action.

Amiodarone is also useful in slowing the ventricular rate in patients who have chronic atrial fibrillation or atrial flutter with rapid ventricular rates.

Although not available clinically, intravenous amiodarone has been utilized for urgent therapy for both supraventricular and ventricular arrhythmias.

AVAILABLE PREPARATIONS. Amiodarone is available in tablets of 200 mg.

Type IV Agents

Verapamil

Verapamil became available for use in the United States in 1982. Its use has been generally restricted to the treatment of supraventricular tachyarrhythmias.

ELECTROPHYSIOLOGIC EFFECTS. Microelectrode studies have demonstrated that this agent differs from other previous antiarrhythmic agents in that in therapeutic concentrations it has little or no effect on normal Purkinje fibers. However, when Purkinje fibers are depressed—i.e., resting potentials less negative than -60 mV—verapamil depresses depolarization. This effect appears to be due to blocking of the channel that carries predominantly calcium ions (the slow channel). Verapamil also suppresses depolarization in depressed atrial and ventricular muscle fibers, which demonstrate spontaneous electrical activity or abnormal after-depolarization currents. This latter effect of verapamil terminates "ectopic" automatic arrhythmias, some of which may be due to a triggered automaticity.

HEMODYNAMIC EFFECTS. Verapamil does depress myocardial contractility, but it also has peripheral vasodilatation effects. Therefore, it may be difficult to predict whether cardiac output may be increased or decreased in patients. In patients with overt congestive heart failure, verapamil should be used with caution. Intravenous administration of verapamil has been rarely associated with severe hypotension, severe bradycardia, and in some instances, asystole. Therefore, continuous electrocardiographic and hemodynamic monitoring is essential when this drug is being used intravenously.

ABSORPTION AND METABOLIC FATE. Verapamil is eliminated largely by liver metabolism, with only 5 percent of the drug being found in the urine in unchanged form. A major metabolite with pharmacologic activity has been identified (indemethyl verapamil). Verapamil has low bioavailability, which appears in large part to be due to first-pass hepatic elimination. The half-life of the drug is dose-related, with a single oral dose having a half-life of approximately 6 hours (2–15 hours). However, this half-life increases to 12 hours (9–25 hours) after 10 or more weeks of daily oral therapy. Effective serum levels have been reported to be 100 to 300 ng/ml.

A reduction in the elimination of verapamil occurs in patients with liver disease or compromised left ventricular function, necessitating possible reduction in dosage amounts or reduction in the frequency of administration. Approximately 90 percent of verapamil is bound to plasma protein.

DOSAGE, ROUTE, AND SERUM LEVELS. Verapamil is given intravenously in urgent situations in doses ranging from 2.5 to 10 mg. It is advisable to give this drug slowly—i.e., over 1 to 2 minutes. Repeat doses can be given. At present, it appears to be the drug of choice for the treatment of sustained supraventricular tachycardia. Its onset of action is very rapid (less than 3 minutes), with reversion to sinus rhythm occurring in greater than 80 percent of patients with supraventricular tachycardia (PAT) following intravenous administration. It is also useful in treatment of atrial fibrillation/atrial flutter to slow the rapid ventricular response.

Although not officially approved, constant intravenous infusion of verapamil at doses ranging from 5 to 40 mg/hr has been utilized. The dose must be carefully titrated.

Intravenous verapamil has been utilized in patients with the Wolff-Parkinson-White syndrome. However, it is hazardous to do so in patients with atrial fibrillation, the Wolff-Parkinson-White syndrome, and a rapid ventricular response. In these patients, verapamil may cause acceleration of ventricular rates, with rare instances of precipitation of ventricular fibrillation. It is therefore recommended that verapamil *not* be used in patients with atrial fibrillation or flutter and the Wolff-Parkinson-White syndrome.

Verapamil has been administered intravenously for the treatment of unusual forms of ventricular tachycardia. To date, patients with this form of ventricular tachycardia responsive to verapamil are infrequently identified, and therefore verapamil generally should not be used under these circumstances.

Intravenous verapamil has been associated with conversion of atrial fibrillation and flutter to sinus rhythm, but this conversion rate is low (i.e., less than 15%).

Oral verapamil may be administered in doses of 80 mg 3 times a day to 120 mg 4 times a day. Rarely, higher doses may be needed, if tolerated.

Serum levels have been reported to be from 100 to 400 ng/ml.

TOXICITY. Verapamil is generally well tolerated. With intravenous administration, bradyarrhythmias, hypotension, asystole, or in rare instances, acceleration of ventricular response with precipitation of life-threatening ventricular arrhythmias have been reported. With oral administration, depression of left ventricular contractility, sinus bradycardia, and/or depression of AV nodal conduction may be observed. Constipation, headache, gastrointestinal upset, and dizziness have been reported, with constipation being the most common side effect. It is important to note that verapamil, in contrast to beta blockers, will not increase airway resistance and can therefore be administered to patients with asthma.

SPECIFIC INDICATIONS. Verapamil is useful for the treatment of a variety of supraventricular arrhythmias, either to terminate (acute/intravenous administration) or to slow supraventricular tachycardias with rapid ventricular rates (acute/intravenous administration). It is useful as an adjunct to slow the ventricular rate in chronic atrial arrhythmia such as atrial fibrillation or flutter. It is also useful in preventing recurrent supraventricular tachycardias when given orally. It has a limited role, if any, in the treatment of ventricular arrhythmias.

AVAILABLE PREPARATION. Verapamil is available in ampules of 5 mg and in tablets of 40, 80, and 120 mg. It is also available in sustained release tablets of 240 mg to be given every 12 hours.

Miscellaneous Antiarrhythmic Drugs

Various additional agents have been found helpful for the treatment of arrhythmias in man. Of particular interest is ancillary therapy, such as the use of tranquilizing agents in the setting of recurrent tachyarrhythmias. It has been suggested that central nervous system alterations may be partly responsible for the development or perpetuation of arrhythmias seen in humans. In this regard, drugs such as hydroxyzine, chlordiazepoxide, and pentazocine have been found to have some antiarrhythmic effects.

In addition, there are agents available outside the continental United States or only for experimental trial in the United States that are reported to have significant antiarrhythmic action, such as propafenone, sotalol, ethmozine, cibenzoline, ATP, adenosine, and lorcainide. To date, only limited data are available concerning the clinical efficacy of these drugs.

Drug Interactions

The introduction of an assay for digoxin serum levels resulted in the discovery of alterations in digoxin levels associated with concomitant drug administration. The first such drug interaction was the observed increase in digoxin levels when quinidine therapy was added. Digoxin levels at least doubled in many patients so treated. The mechanism of this increase is related to (1) a decrease in the digoxin volume of distribution, (2) a decrease in the systemic clearance of digoxin, and (3) an increase in the bioavailability of digoxin.

Other agents that have demonstrated clear, but less profound, increases in digoxin serum levels include amiodarone, flecainide, and verapamil.

Also, amiodarone administration increases the serum levels of pronestyl, procainamide, and quinidine; propranolol administration has been shown to increase the lidocaine levels; and finally, cimetidine administration has been shown to increase serum levels of lidocaine, quinidine, procainamide, propranolol, and verapamil.

ARRHYTHMIAS IN DIGITALIS INTOXICATION

A significant percentage of arrhythmias seen in the clinical setting are due to digitalis overdosage. The gamut of arrhythmias produced by digitalis intoxication covers such arrhythmias as paroxysmal atrial tachycardia with block, multiform ventricular premature complexes, and second- and higher-degree AV block. The treatment of these arrhythmias is dependent on the type observed clinically. For the treatment of significant ventricular arrhythmias, diphenylhydantoin, lidocaine, and procainamide appear to be highly efficacious. For various types of AV block, diphenylhydantoin appears to be particularly effective because it shortens AV nodal conduction time. In addition, potassium administration is usually of value in all these patients, including those with various forms of AV block. The use of oral or intravenous potassium in the setting of digitalis-induced AV block can be considered appropriate if the serum potassium level is less than 4.5 mEq/liter. Digoxin-specific antibody has recently been released for clinical use. This agent (purified fragments of digoxin-specific antibody FAB), has

been administered intravenously in patients with life-threatening arrhythmias secondary to digoxin. Clinical trials have indicated that this agent is of great use in the management of these critically ill patients.

CARDIOVERSION

The use of electrical conversion of tachyarrhythmias has become commonplace since the introduction of the first capacitor-discharged defibrillator by Lown and his coworkers. Cardioversion requires the use of a synchronizer circuit that will result in discharge of the waveform at the time of the QRS. This timed discharge will therefore eliminate the possibility of induction of ventricular fibrillation by delivering the electrical discharge outside the vulnerable period of ventricular repolarization.

Indications for Use

Cardioversion is considered appropriate for attempted conversion of atrial fibrillation to sinus rhythm, especially if the atrial fibrillation is of short duration. Anticoagulation for approximately 3 weeks should be used if the patient has a history of mitral valve disease, systemic embolization, or both. Cardioversion is also of great value for the treatment of ventricular tachyarrhythmias and supraventricular tachyarrhythmias that are recalcitrant to medical management. Cardioversion would not be considered beneficial for the treatment of paroxysmal arrhythmias that are self-terminating, short-lived, or both.

Cardioversion can be performed in patients who have been receiving digitalis if initial power settings are of very low magnitude. Initial cardioversion in these instances should be attempted with a power setting of 5 to 10 watt-seconds, then increased in a graded fashion with constant ECG monitoring. A bolus of lidocaine (1 mg/kg) should be administered just prior to the cardioversion. If ventricular extrasystoles are seen, cardioversion should be discontinued. However, if no ventricular extrasystoles are observed, increasing power settings should be used until cardioversion is successful.

Adverse Effects

The complications resulting from cardioversion vary. The development of pulmonary edema following successful cardioversion of atrial fibrillation has been reported; the mechanism responsible appears to be possible electromechanical dissociation with mechanical paralysis of the left atrium. In addition, ventricular tachyarrhythmias may be precipitated in the digitalized patient. Other problems include the development of asystole following cardioversion in patients with sinoatrial node disease or in patients treated with β-blocking agents. Cerebrovascular accidents presumed secondary to embolism are also a potential, serious problem. A variety of enzymes will be released from skeletal muscle following closed chest cardioversion, resulting in elevation of serum enzymes. Finally, chest burns may occur if electrode solution or paste is not appropriately applied to the chest.

Ancillary Cardioversion Procedures

Various analgesic agents have been used to medicate patients before the use of cardioversion, but the most popular agent at present appears to be diazepam in doses from 2.5 to 30 mg given by slow intravenous infusion. This drug should not be administered into intravenous tubing, but directly into the vein. It appears most prudent to consider the ancillary use of premedication such as intravenous meperidine before the use of diazepam, so that lower doses of the latter drug may be given and more rapid "anesthesia" induced.

Medazolam given intravenously in doses of 0.5 to 1 mg may offer an alternative to diazepam administration. This drug has a more rapid onset of action and a shorter half-life than diazepam. Repeat doses can be given as clinically indicated.

Oxygen should be available for inhalation at the time of cardioversion. Atropine (0.5–1.0 mg) and lidocaine (50–100 mg) should also be at the bedside for intravenous administration if needed. Intubation equipment is also essential.

VASOPRESSOR THERAPY

Many of the serious tachyarrhythmias are associated with significant peripheral hypotension. Nevertheless, restoration of systemic pressure with the use of vasopressors does not usually convert ventricular tachyarrhythmias to normal sinus rhythm; sympathetic stimulation in these patients may in fact enhance the frequency or result in further rhythm deterioration. Therefore, in the setting of serious ventricular arrhythmias with hypotension, immediate attention should be given to restoration of normal sinus rhythm by other means.

However, in the setting of paroxysmal atrial tachycardia, elevation of the peripheral arterial pressure frequently activates parasympathetic input to the heart through carotid sinus and arch reflexes. This intense parasympathetic stimulation frequently converts these arrhythmias if they are due to reentrant activity. It is essential to recognize that relatively modest elevations in blood pressure usually are satisfactory in conversion of these tachycardias—i.e., a systolic pressure rise to 160 mm Hg maximum. Extreme care must be used in monitoring the peripheral arterial pressure during the vasopressor administration to prevent an overshoot of systemic pressure; marked elevations in systemic pressure might result in cerebrovascular accidents due to intracranial hemorrhage. Phenylephrine hydrochloride (Neo-Synephrine) and metaraminol (Aramine) are the drugs generally used, but any vasoconstrictor with α-stimulating characteristics would be appropriate.

ADDITIONAL MEASURES USEFUL FOR THE TREATMENT OF ARRHYTHMIAS

Carotid Sinus Massage

Carotid sinus massage is extremely useful for the diagnosis and treatment of certain paroxysmal arrhythmias. It is especially useful for the produc-

tion of AV nodal conduction delay to enable full identification of underlying atrial arrhythmias. Furthermore, certain paroxysmal arrhythmias, such as paroxysmal atrial tachycardia, can be converted with the use of carotid sinus massage. It is interesting to note that the right carotid sinus has been suggested to have dominant innervation of the sinus node area, whereas the left carotid sinus appears to innervate predominantly the AV nodal area.

It is essential to recognize that carotid sinus massage in the elderly patient may produce cardiac asystole, significant cerebrovascular insufficiency, or even central blindness from emboli from the carotid artery. One should not consider the use of carotid sinus massage in patients with bruits in the neck.

Edrophonium Administration

Edrophonium administration has been found useful for the treatment of paroxysmal supraventricular tachyarrhythmias because of its anticholinesterase activity, which resembles that of acetylcholine and therefore results in intense parasympathetic stimulation. This drug may be administered either in an acute intravenous dose (10 mg) or by continuous infusion at a rate of 0.25 to 2.0 mg/min. Its use has been generally supplanted by the use of intravenous verapamil or esmolol (as well as by adenosine and ATP, when they become clinically available).

Atropine Administration

Frequently, clinical situations are encountered of moderate bradycardia or second-degree AV block that appears to be due to enhancement of parasympathetic tone. In these cases, intravenous administration of atropine in doses from 0.5 to 2.0 mg as a bolus will restore normal sinus rate and AV conduction. Under other circumstances, bradycardia may result in more serious arrhythmias, such as those observed during myocardial infarction with the development of idioventricular tachycardia. The latter rhythm can frequently be treated by increasing the sinus rate with atropine administration. However, the resultant sinus rate cannot be predicted from the dose of atropine administered; therefore, episodes of sinus tachycardia may result in patients who are highly responsive to atropine. This overshoot in cardiac rate may be a potential problem because of diminished coronary flow.

TREATMENT OF SPECIFIC ARRHYTHMIAS

Atrial Premature Complexes

Atrial premature complexes are usually considered to be benign. However, frequent premature atrial complexes with very short coupling intervals (less than 450 msec) may be precursors of atrial fibrillation. Therefore, in the latter case, antiarrhythmic drug therapy should be considered, with the major drug being quinidine, digitalis, or procainamide. On rare occasions, atrial premature complexes may initiate ventricular tachycardia.

Occasional instances occur when frequent, blocked premature atrial complexes will impair the functional ventricular rate. Antiarrhythmic drug therapy will be required to reestablish an effective ventricular rate.

Premature Ventricular Complexes (PVCs)

Premature ventricular complexes may be observed in patients without evidence of cardiovascular disease. In general, these patients should not be treated unless they are symptomatic or have frequent PVCs. On occasion, patients respond to the withdrawal of stimulants, caffeine, tobacco, and/or alcohol. If encountered in the setting of organic heart disease, PVCs should be treated if any of the following criteria are met: (1) there are more than 6 ventricular complexes per minute; (2) the ventricular prematures interrupt the T wave; and (3) the ventricular prematures occur in salvos.

The antiarrhythmic drugs that have been found to be successful in the treatment of PVCs include, with varying success, all agents discussed. If significant congestive heart failure is associated with PVCs, the arrhythmias may respond to digitalis therapy.

Paroxysmal Supraventricular Tachycardia

Paroxysmal supraventricular tachycardia (PSVT) is usually seen in young patients without obvious organic heart disease. Atrial activity is only occasionally discernible, with ventricular rates between 150 and 250 per minute. The rhythm is generally perfectly regular, and the QRS duration is usually normal. However, during these episodes, occasional patients manifest rate-related bundle branch block that may simulate ventricular tachyarrhythmias.

Treatment of an acute episode should be initiated with performance of a Valsalva maneuver. In the young patient, carotid sinus massage should be used after careful auscultation of both carotid arteries to ensure that bruits are not present. If the tachycardia is not terminated, intravenous administration of verapamil or esmolol should be utilized. Other agents to be considered are rapid intravenous digitalization or edrophonium administration. If clinically necessary, emergent cardioversion should be employed. The patient with recurrent episodes of paroxysmal tachycardia should be treated with a combination of (1) digoxin and beta-blocking agent, or (2) digoxin and verapamil, or (3) digoxin and flecainide, or (4) digoxin and quinidine. However, patients with recurrent episodes of PSVT should be considered for evaluation by electrophysiologic studies.

Paroxysmal Atrial Tachycardia with Block

Paroxysmal atrial tachycardia with block, a dysrhythmia characterized by an atrial rate of 150 to 250 per minute and a variable ventricular rate, is considered to be due to digitalis toxicity in approximately two-thirds of cases. In general, the P-wave configuration resembles sinus rhythm; in contrast, the atrial rate in atrial flutter is 250 to 350 per minute and has a sawtooth configuration to the P waves.

When this rhythm is related exclusively to digitalis intoxication, digitalis administration should be discontinued immediately. If the clinical situation is stable, observation of the rhythm disturbance may be all that is needed. However, if the serum potassium is in the lower range of normal, potassium may be administered by mouth or intravenously to elevate the serum potassium to the upper range of normal. In addition, cautious administration of intravenous verapamil or esmolol may be used to increase the degree of AV block if clinically indicated.

Atrial Fibrillation

Atrial fibrillation is a common arrhythmia characterized in the untreated state by chaotic atrial activity and a rapid ventricular response, usually 140 to 200 per minute. P waves are not discernible on the ECG; atrial fibrillation characterized by coarse electrical activity may be observed with a bizarre baseline or with a fine baseline not demonstrating any significant fibrillatory waves. On occasion, with rapid ventricular rates, bizarre QRS configurations may be identified, which may be due to aberrant conduction within the ventricular conducting system.

Extremely rapid ventricular rates due to atrial fibrillation may be seen on rare occasions. Patients with ventricular rates in excess of 250 per minute should be presumed to have Wolff-Parkinson-White syndrome.

In general, this rhythm disturbance is due most frequently to atrial fibrosis and occurs secondary to mitral valve disease or to atherosclerotic or hypertensive cardiovascular disease. Furthermore, atrial fibrillation can develop in patients with significant hyperthyroidism and is usually accompanied by a rapid ventricular rate in such patients. Finally, occasional patients are observed who have paroxysmal atrial fibrillation without a discernible cause ("lone" fibrillators). Rarely, atrial fibrillation may be due to pericarditis, and in older patients, carcinomatous pericardial implantation may be responsible.

Hemodynamically, the loss of the atrial contribution to ventricular filling may result in a diminished cardiac output, with decreases of up to 25 percent. An additional complication is the presence of systemic embolization in patients who have paroxysmal episodes of atrial fibrillation.

The hemodynamic advantage of restoration of sinus rhythm varies from patient to patient. In a younger patient without evidence of atrial disease, restoration of sinus rhythm may result in an increase in cardiac output of up to 25 percent. However, in the older patients with advanced atrial disease, restoration of sinus rhythm may produce little or no increase in cardiac output.

Medical Treatment

The method of choice for the control of the ventricular rate in the untreated patient is the administration of digitalis, usually intravenously. The end point for digitalization would be the presence of a resting heart rate of 60 to 90 per minute, with only a minimal increase observed during mild exercise. Maintenance digitalis should be administered according to the patient's weight and renal function status.

In an occasional patient in whom immediate control of rapid ventricular rates is necessary, the intravenous use of propranolol, verapamil, or esmolol may be considered.

On occasion, patients will present with atrial fibrillation with a controlled rate (i.e., 60–80/min). In these circumstances no therapeutic intervention should be considered unless the patients require the use of inotropic drugs as part of their medical management.

Methods of Conversion to Sinus Rhythm

In all patients, an attempt should be made to convert atrial fibrillation to sinus rhythm when the patient first presents with arrhythmia. The success rate for conversion to sinus rhythm is dependent largely on the duration of the atrial fibrillation and the size of the left atrium. The success rate diminishes significantly when the duration exceeds 1 month. Furthermore, maintenance of sinus rhythm following successful conversion is highly variable and appears to be related to the underlying pathologic condition.

Anticoagulation should be considered mandatory in all patients who have a history of systemic embolization and in patients who have mitral valve disease. Anticoagulation should be administered for a total of 3 weeks before attempting conversion.

CARDIOVERSION. Patients who are on maintenance digitalis can be electively cardioverted using the graded cardioversion technique. It is generally suggested that the morning dose of digitalis be deleted on the day of cardioversion.

PHARMACOLOGIC CONVERSION. All patients should be adequately digitalized to obtain controlled ventricular rates prior to the attempt at pharmacologic conversion.

In general, the most effective agent for the conversion to sinus rhythm is quinidine sulfate. A variety of regimens have been developed for the administration of quinidine for the conversion of atrial fibrillation to sinus rhythm, including the Sokolow method and the Levine method. The Sokolow regimen consists of 5 doses of quinidine sulfate administered at 2-hour intervals, the initial dose being 200 mg. If conversion does not occur, the dose is increased the next day by 100 mg and repeated over the 5 daily doses. The end point is either conversion to sinus rhythm or a daily dosage of up to 4 gm. In contrast, the Levine regimen consists of three daily doses at 4-hour intervals. Each dose is increased by 200 mg until a total daily dose of 3 gm is given.

Utilizing present pharmacologic concepts, one may devise any number of different regimens for quinidine administration. At our institution, we administer 200 to 400 mg of quinidine sulfate every 4 hours, depending on body size. If conversion does not occur after four doses, the dosage is increased by 100 mg and 4 additional doses are given. Serial ECG and blood pressure data should be obtained. If the blood pressure significantly decreases, QRS significantly increases or the peak (i.e., 2 hours after dose) serum levels are above 6.5 μg/ml, then the drug should be discontinued.

It is essential that the electrocardiogram be continuously recorded during these medical cardioversion procedures, so that early signs of toxicity may be detected.

Intravenous pronestyl administration has proved to be effective as a means of converting atrial fibrillation, if the left atrial size is less than 4.6 cm. Intravenous administration of 15 to 20 mg/kg at a rate of 30 to 50 mg/min is utilized. This regimen requires serial blood pressure and ECG monitoring. A serum sample for a pronestyl level should be obtained at the end of the infusion. Conversion to sinus rhythm generally requires a serum level of 12 µg/ml.

POSTCONVERSION AND MAINTENANCE THERAPY. *At the time of cardioversion.* No definitive information is available to date on the efficacy of prophylactic antiarrhythmic therapy prior to electrical cardioversion. Nevertheless, it appears prudent to consider the use of intramuscular quinidine a half-hour prior to the attempted cardioversion in doses of 200 mg for a 70-kg patient or oral therapy with any agent considered appropriate for long-term treatment—i.e., pronestyl, quinidine, flecainide, norpace, etc.

Maintenance antiarrhythmic drug therapy. The long-term prognosis for maintenance of sinus rhythm is dependent on the nature of the underlying disease. Nevertheless, it appears prudent to consider long-term antiarrhythmic therapy for most patients. Doses should be administered so that effective blood levels will be obtained around the clock. The dosage regimen should be tailored to the patient's body weight and renal function. To date, however, no definitive studies are available on the long-term effects of antiarrhythmic prophylactic drug therapy in these patients.

Atrial Flutter

Atrial flutter is characterized by regular atrial rates between 250 and 350 beats per minute. The etiology of this rhythm disturbance is generally considered to be identical with that of atrial fibrillation, except that it is seen more often in patients with pulmonary disease. Morphologically, the P wave has a biphasic or sawtooth configuration, which is most clearly seen in leads II, III, and a VF. In the untreated patient there is usually 2 : 1 conduction to the ventricles, with a ventricular rate of 150 per minute. On occasion, it may be difficult to identify atrial flutter waves clearly. In the latter instance, gentle coronary sinus massage may be utilized to increase the degree of AV block and further delineate flutter waves. Furthermore, prominent *a* waves may be noted in the jugular veins.

This rhythm is usually treated by digitalis administration. In patients with rapid ventricular rates, intravenous digitalis administration should be considered. However, patients with atrial flutter generally need much more digitalis than usual to produce significant AV block. Digitalis administration may result in either increased degrees of AV block, conversion to atrial fibrillation, or conversion to sinus rhythm. In addition, for immediate control of a rapid ventricular rate, the use of intravenous propranolol, verapamil, or esmolol (see Atrial Fibrillation) may be considered. However, atrial flutter, in contrast with atrial fibrillation, is very sensitive to electrical conversion, and cardioversion is therefore the therapy of choice. Power settings of less than 100 watt-seconds are frequently successful for the conversion of this rhythm disturbance.

Ventricular Tachycardia

Ventricular tachycardia is characterized by ventricular rates of 100 to 250 per minute. Independent atrial activity can occasionally be observed on the ECG. The QRS configuration is bizarre, but the ventricular rate is generally regular. Patients who have ventricular tachycardia usually have significant hemodynamic depression, with dizziness, syncope, and evidence of acute left-sided failure or angina pectoris, or both. The treatment of sustained ventricular tachycardia should be immediate cardioversion if the patient is hemodynamically compromised. Otherwise, medical management may be considered. In the setting of recurrent bouts of ventricular tachycardia, medical management is essential. Medical therapy includes: (1) lidocaine, (2) oral or intravenous procainamide, or (3) any of the previously noted oral agents.

In the setting of recurrent ventricular tachycardia, intravenous lidocaine and pronestyl may be used in combination. The pronestyl level needed may be as high as 15 to 20 mg/ml to maintain sinus rhythm. Intravenous bretylium may be needed, with an initial loading dose of 5 to 10 mg/kg over 30 minutes followed by an infusion of 1 to 4 mg/min.

Recurrent overdrive termination of ventricular tachycardia can be done with a temporary pacing catheter. This overdrive termination should be done only by an experienced electrophysiologist.

Overdrive suppression—i.e., atrial or ventricular pacing at rates of approximately 100/min—has occasionally been of help. In patients with significant coronary artery disease, the insertion of an intraaortic balloon may be crucial in patient management.

Surgical therapy may be considered in the patient whose arrhythmia is recalcitrant to medical therapy and in whom there is evidence suggestive of ischemic heart disease with or without ventricular aneurysm formation. Such a patient may be found to be a suitable candidate for revascularization procedures, ventricular aneurysm resection, or both.

Electrophysiologically oriented surgery is routinely used in centers with special expertise in intraoperative endocardial mapping. This may be performed in association with implantation of an automatic defibrillator device.

An additional form of ventricular tachycardia has been observed that can be characterized as an escape ventricular rhythm, generally with rates of 50 to 120 per minute. This is seen most frequently in patients with acute myocardial infarction, usually with an inferior infarct. The patients do not appear to have significant hemodynamic abnormalities during this rhythm disturbance. At present, the prognosis of the rhythm disturbance has not been fully delineated, and the need for antiarrhythmic drug therapy is thus uncertain. Attempted medical management should consist of agents that would elevate the basic sinus rate, such as atropine or its derivatives, and possibly the use of antiarrhythmic agents, such as lidocaine.

WOLFF-PARKINSON-WHITE SYNDROME

The Wolff-Parkinson-White syndrome is characterized by alterations in electrical activity secondary to ventricular preexcitation and is frequently associated with a history of paroxysmal arrhythmias. In the majority of patients who have a history of such arrhythmias, paroxysmal supraventricular tachycardia without a Δ wave is observed during this tachyarrhythmia. Medical management for these patients is highly dependent on the electrophysiologic characteristics of the bypass tract(s) and AV conducting system. Therapy should be tailored to the individual patient and should be based on studies directed at defining the electrical characteristics of these conducting networks.

Atrial fibrillation develops in a small percentage of patients with the Wolff-Parkinson-White syndrome. This group appears to be in jeopardy because of the potential development of extremely rapid ventricular rates due to anterograde conduction through the bypass tract or tracts. This bypass conduction leads to ventricular rates that on occasion may exceed 300 per minute. These rapid ventricular rates may result in syncopal episodes or in the development of ventricular fibrillation.

In the setting of atrial fibrillation with the Wolff-Parkinson-White syndrome, digitalis administration should be considered contraindicated because digitalis can shorten refractoriness in the bypass tract or tracts and may result in a more rapid ventricular rate. The therapy of choice would be immediate cardioversion or the intravenous administration of drugs that preferentially block the bypass tract, such as lidocaine and procainamide.

CARDIAC ARREST

Cardiac arrest may be due to the development of either ventricular fibrillation or cardiac asystole. In the setting of a witnessed cardiac arrest, it is suggested that a sharp blow with a clenched fist be administered to the midsternum. However, in an unwitnessed arrest, immediate cardiopulmonary resuscitation should be instituted.

Resuscitation

Single-Person Resuscitation Technique

In the single-person resuscitation technique, the airway should be checked, foreign bodies removed, and mouth-to-mouth resuscitation begun with four superimposed respirations to hyperinflate the lungs. The carotids should then be immediately checked for restoration of cardiac activity, and if no pulse is discernible, closed-chest massage should be instituted immediately at a cadence of 80 compressions per minute. After 15 chest compressions, the resuscitator should ventilate the patient twice and then resume closed-chest compression for an additional 15 compressions. This should be continued, alternating 15 compressions and 2 respirations, until cardiac action is restored. Every attempt should be made to obtain additional help.

Two-Person Cardiopulmonary Resuscitation

In the two-person technique, chest compression is performed by one member at a rate of 60 compressions per minute, and the other member performs one respiration after every fifth chest compression; the team alternates when necessary.

Medical Management at the Time of Cardiopulmonary Arrest

If ancillary help is available and an arrest cart is nearby, an intravenous line must be inserted immediately and the patient defibrillated at once. If monitoring is available and the patient was noted to be asystolic, intracardiac administration of epinephrine, 1 ml of 1 : 1000, is required. If fibrillation ensues, the patient should then be defibrillated.

If the patient is found on the floor, resuscitative procedures should continue in this position. If the patient is in bed, a board must be slid under the patient's back to allow for adequate chest compression.

Under no circumstances should any significant delay be allowed to occur before the institution of closed-chest massage. Furthermore, no significant interruptions should be allowed in the sequence of closed-chest massage and ventilation.

In the setting of poor myocardial contractility, consideration should be given to the administration of 10 ml of intracardiac calcium chloride.

If possible, arterial blood gases and serum potassium should be obtained for analysis. All attempts should be made to correct acid-base balance through the use of intravenous bicarbonate. In addition, at the earliest possible point, the patient should be intubated either by the nasotracheal or orotracheal route, so that artificially assisted ventilation may be instituted.

If the patient's arrest occurs outside the hospital, every attempt should be made to ensure rapid transport to the nearest hospital facility that has adequate resources to handle the patient's emergency care.

Atrioventricular Block

The use of intracardiac recording techniques has substantially increased the information available to the clinician relative to the etiology of heart block in man. Utilizing these techniques, investigators have observed that first- and second-degree AV block may occur because of abnormalities throughout the entire AV conduction system—i.e., within the atrium, the AV node, the bundle of His, and the bundle branches. Therefore, therapy should be guided by knowledge of the underlying site of AV block.

In general, it has been observed that the width of the QRS on the standard ECG may serve as an indicator of the area of block that will be encountered by electrophysiologic studies: a narrow QRS generally identifies a supraventricular site of AV block, and a wide QRS identifies a distal conducting system site. Although this relation usually holds regardless of the degree of AV block encountered, there are significant exceptions. Thus, the decision to insert a permanent pacemaker should not be made unless electrophysiologic studies are performed to define clearly the site of block within the AV conducting system.

First-Degree Atrioventricular Block

First-degree AV block is characterized by the presence of a P-R interval in excess of 210 milliseconds. In the majority of patients with first-degree AV block, the delay is due to an abnormality of conduction in the AV node. Nevertheless, block may occur because of delay within the atrium, bundle of His, or bundle branches. In the latter circumstance, first-degree AV block due to delay in the distal conducting system may be of grave prognostic significance if the patient has any evidence suggestive of additional intraventricular conduction delay—i.e., bundle branch block, fascicular block, or both.

Second-Degree Atrioventricular Block

Second-degree AV block is usually divided into two subgroups.

TYPE I. Type I second-degree AV block is characterized by the presence of gradual prolongation of the P-R interval with associated gradual shortening of the R-R interval, until a P wave is not conducted to the ventricles. As observed with first-degree AV block, this rhythm disturbance may be due to delay in conduction within the atrium, the AV node, or the bundle of His. In general, this rhythm disturbance is considered benign and should not warrant medical or pacemaker therapy if the ventricular rate is adequate and the patient suffers no adverse hemodynamic consequences. Nevertheless, in patients who have distal conduction delay accounting for Wenckebach periods, a less optimistic prognosis has been suggested, and these patients should be followed extremely carefully.

TYPE II. Type II second-degree AV block is characterized by stable P-R and stable R-R intervals until suddenly a P wave or waves are found not to conduct to the ventricle. This rhythm disturbance is generally considered to have a poor prognosis, in that more advanced degrees of AV block, syncope, or both frequently develop. Therefore, in a large percentage of patients, permanent pacemaker therapy should be considered. A peculiar situation exists for patients who have second-degree AV block with 2 : 1 conduction to the ventricles. Regardless of the site of AV block, these patients may have significant alterations in hemodynamics because of the extremely slow ventricular rate sometimes observed. Furthermore, these patients may not respond appropriately to exercise in that it may increase the degree of AV block. Therefore, regardless of the site of AV block, many of these patients require pacemaker therapy.

Chronic Advanced AV Block

CONGENITAL TYPE. Congenital AV block is characterized generally by the presence of a narrow escape pacemaker configuration with ventricular rates of 35 to 60. In addition, the ventricular rate in these patients frequently increases slightly with exercise. The site of block in these patients is generally within the AV node. Their long-term prognosis appears to be reasonably good, although there is evidence to suggest that Adams-Stokes syndrome develops in such patients on occasion. Pacemaker therapy is not indicated in the majority of these patients, but careful long-term follow-up is essential.

ACQUIRED TYPE. The majority of the patients with acquired AV block appear to have distal conducting system disease with escape ventricular pacemakers with rates of 15 to 50 per minute and a wide QRS duration.

Some patients manifest this rhythm disturbance on a chronic basis and appear to have a reasonably good hemodynamic function. However, in the majority this rhythm disturbance is acute and there are associated seizure episodes (Adams-Stokes syndrome). The latter group is universally treated by permanent pacing. If chronic advanced AV block is seen in the adult patient without symptoms, permanent pacemaker insertion is not mandatory, but extremely careful follow-up should be instituted.

MANAGEMENT OF ADAMS-STOKES SYNDROME. The immediate management of Adams-Stokes syndrome should be the insertion of a transvenous pacemaker on an emergency basis. If this cannot be done, pharmacologic measures should be taken immediately to enhance the ventricular rate until a pacemaker may be inserted. Isoproterenol appears to be the drug of choice, given by the intravenous route. Immediate intravenous infusion should be begun at a rate of at least 3 μg/min. The patient's ECG should be followed continuously and the dose of isoproterenol altered in response to the rate of the ventricular escape pacemaker. If medical management is not successful, cardiopulmonary resuscitation should be instituted at once until it is possible to insert an emergency transvenous pacemaker. Recently, external cardiac pacing has been reintroduced with an updated device. This unit may prove a lifesaving measure until more suitable forms of pacing can be established.

SELECTED READINGS

Anderson, J. L. Current clinical perspectives on anti-arrhythmic drug therapy. *Fed. Proc.* 45:2213, 1986.

Fenster, P. E. Clinical pharmacology—Clinical use of pharmacokinetic principles in prescribing cardiac drugs. *Med. Clin. North Am.* 68:1281, 1984.

Mandel, W. J. (ed.). *Cardiac Arrhythmias—Their Mechanisms, Diagnosis and Management* (2nd ed.). Philadelphia: Lippincott, 1987.

Michelson, E. L., and Dreifus, L. S. Newer anti-arrhythmic drugs. *Med. Clin. North Am.* 72:275, 1988.

Nestico, P. F., Morganroth, J., and Horowitz, L. N. New anti-arrhythmic agents. *Drug* 35:286, 1988.

Reiser, H. J., and Sullivan, M. E. Anti-arrhythmic drug therapy: New drugs and changing concepts. *Fed. Proc.* 45:2206, 1986.

Rosen, M. R., and Spinelli, W. Some recent concepts concerning the mechanism of action of anti-arrhythmic drugs. *PACE* 11:1485, 1988.

Rotmensch, A. H., and Belhassen, B. Amiodarone in the management of cardiac arrhythmias—Current concepts. *Med. Clin. North Am.* 72:321, 1988.

Standards and guidelines of cardiopulmonary resuscitation and emergency cardiac care. *J.A.M.A.* 255:2905, 1986.

Acute Heart Failure

Kanu Chatterjee

Heart failure may manifest rapidly, and sometimes precipitously, with unstable clinical, hemodynamic, and pathophysiologic consequences. Acute heart failure may be caused by myocardial, pericardial, or valvular heart disease. Occasionally, arrhythmias may precipitate acute or subacute heart failure in the absence of myocardial or valvular disease. The clinically important etiologies of acute and subacute heart failure are summarized in Table 15-1.

ACUTE MYOCARDIAL INFARCTION

Heart failure of varying severity is a relatively common complication of acute myocardial infarction. Left ventricular infarction is by far the most frequent underlying pathophysiologic mechanism. The extent of recent myocardial injury and ischemia, coupled with the extent of prior myocardial infarction, determines the magnitude of overall left ventricular dysfunction and the severity of heart failure. Limiting the "infarct size" therefore is one of the major objectives of treatment of acute myocardial infarction, to minimize the degree of left ventricular dysfunction and, consequently, the severity of heart failure. Total thrombotic occlusion of the infarct-related coronary artery and interruption of blood flow to the myocardium at risk is the principal mechanism of myocardial necrosis in the vast majority of patients (over 90%) with acute myocardial infarction. Presently, recanalization of the occluded infarct-related artery and establishment of reperfusion to the ischemic myocardium is the most promising and effective method for limiting infarct size. Recanalization of the infarct-related artery can be achieved by mechanical means, such as coronary artery angioplasty, by coronary artery bypass surgery, or by intracoronary and intravenous thrombolytic therapy. The principal determinant for the salvage of ischemic myocardium by reperfusion therapy is the elapsed time for recanalization after the onset of symptoms. Most studies have reported that recanalization of the infarct-related artery 6 hours after the onset of ischemic pain is not associated with any significant improvement in

Table 15-1. Etiology of acute and subacute heart failure

A. Acute myocardial infarction
   1. Left ventricular failure without mechanical defects
   2. Left ventricular failure with mechanical defects: left ventricular
      aneurysm, papillary muscle infarction, ventricular septal rupture
   3. Right ventricular infarction
   4. Ventricular free wall rupture—cardiac tamponade
B. Myocarditis and cardiomyopathies
   1. Acute viral myocarditis
   2. Septic myocarditis
   3. Heart failure with septic shock
   4. Peripartum cardiomyopathy
   5. Alcoholic cardiomyopathy
C. Valvular heart disease
   1. Acute mitral regurgitation
   2. Acute aortic regurgitation
   3. Acute tricuspid regurgitation
   4. Sudden deterioration of chronic valvular heart disease
D. Pericardial disease—cardiac tamponade
E. Postoperative heart failure
F. Tachycardic-cardiomyopathy

---

survival and left ventricular function. Usually, a considerable amount of time is required to perform angioplasty or coronary artery bypass surgery, and thus intravenous thrombolytic therapy has become the therapy of choice for recanalization of the infarct-related artery. Except in patients with cardiogenic shock, angioplasty is not usually attempted following thrombolytic therapy. Currently, streptokinase (1.5 million units in 90 minutes) and recombinant tissue plasminogen activator (rtPA, 100 mg in 3 hours) are the two most commonly used thrombolytic agents in this country. However, newer thrombolytic agents, such as urokinase and anysolited plasminogen activator complex, are undergoing clinical trials. Patients with anterior myocardial infarction, inferior infarction with previous infarction, and right ventricular infarction are the appropriate candidates for thrombolytic therapy.

Despite thrombolytic therapy, many patients develop heart failure. Patients who do not receive thrombolytic therapy also may develop heart failure due to complications of acute myocardial infarction. The management of left ventricular failure is better approached by determining the clinical and hemodynamic subsets. The clinical subsets are recognized by the presence of signs of hypoperfusion or of pulmonary congestion, or of both. Hypoperfusion usually indicates low cardiac output, and pulmonary congestion is associated with an elevated pulmonary capillary wedge pressure. The hemodynamic correlates of the clinical subsets are summarized in Table 15-2.

In patients in clinical subset I, hemodynamic monitoring is not required. In patients who present with pulmonary congestion, hemodynamic monitoring is also not required if there is prompt clinical improvement follow-

Table 15-2. Hemodynamic correlates of
clinical subsets of acute myocardial infarction

Subset	Clinical signs	Cardiac index (liters/min/m₂)	Pulmonary artery wedge pressure (mm Hg)
I	No pulmonary congestion No hypoperfusion	> 2.2	< 18
II	Pulmonary congestion No hypoperfusion	> 2.2	> 18
III	No pulmonary congestion Hypoperfusion	< 2.2	< 18
IV	Pulmonary congestion Hypoperfusion	< 2.2	> 18

K. Chatterjee, Bedside Hemodynamic Monitoring. In W. W. Parmley and K. Chatterjee (eds.), *Cardiology*. Philadelphia: Lippincott, 1988. Reproduced with permission.

ing administration of diuretics, analgesics, nitroglycerin, nitrates, and supplemental oxygen. If the signs and symptoms of pulmonary congestion persist, hemodynamic monitoring is indicated. In patients in subsets III and IV, hemodynamic monitoring is required for prompt assessment of the results of therapy.

MANAGEMENT OF COMPLICATIONS OF ACUTE MYOCARDIAL INFARCTION
Pulmonary Congestion Without Hypoperfusion
(Refer to subset II, Table 15-2.) Mild pulmonary congestion is common, particularly at the onset of myocardial infarction. Symptoms of pulmonary congestion are frequently rapidly relieved following the adminstration of diuretics and/or venodilators (nitroglycerin and nitrates). Supplemental oxygen should be administered to ensure adequate arterial oxygenation. Intravenous furosemide (20–40 mg) may cause prompt reduction of pulmonary capillary wedge pressure even before diuresis starts. Nitroglycerin and nitrates are also effective in reducing pulmonary venous pressure. Initially, sublingual nitroglycerin followed by topical nitroglycerin or oral isosorbide dinitrate frequently relieves pulmonary congestion, and usually no further therapy is required. Repeated and aggressive diuretic therapy, however, should be avoided, since hypotension and low output state may result from excessive reduction of left ventricular preload.

Acute Pulmonary Edema Without Hypoperfusion requires prompt, aggressive therapy to maintain adequate gas exchange and to decrease pulmonary capillary wedge pressure. High concentrations of oxygen (60–100%) should be administered by face mask. Endotracheal intubation is required in patients who are unable to maintain an arterial PO_2 of at least 60 mmHg with a face mask and who develop a progressive rise in PCO_2 or a declining arterial PH.

Nitroglycerin and nitrates, which are predominantly venodilators, cause a significant reduction of pulmonary capillary wedge pressure by venous pooling and reduction of venous return to the heart. Initially, nitroglycerin or isosorbide dinitrate should be administered sublingually. Intravenous diuretics and morphine sulfate are also administered concurrently. After initial therapy, hemodynamics should be determined and subsequent treatment should be adjusted according to the hemodynamic abnormalities. If cardiac output is adequate, there is no evidence of metabolic acidosis, and pulmonary capillary wedge pressure remains elevated, nitroglycerin therapy, preferably intravenously, 20 to 300 μg/min, should be continued. In hypertensive patients (e.g., arterial pressure exceeding 160/90 mmHg), sodium nitroprusside, 15 to 300 μg/min may be more effective than nitroglycerin. Nitroprusside is also preferable in patients who develop pulmonary edema due to mitral regurgitation. Digitalis and aminophylline are generally not effective for the treatment of acute pulmonary edema complicating myocardial infarction. After recovery from pulmonary edema and stabilization of hemodynamics, evaluation of cardiac function, the severity of coronary artery disease, and the extent of myocardial ischemia should be undertaken.

Hypoperfusion without Pulmonary Congestion

(Refer to subset III, Table 15-2.) Hemodynamic monitoring is useful in establishing the pathophysiologic mechanism of hypoperfusion and the absence of pulmonary congestion. Both right ventricular infarction and hypovolemic shock are associated with this similar clinical profile. Right ventricular infarction, however, results in elevated right atrial pressure, whereas the hemodynamics of hypovolemic shock are characterized by both lower right atrial and pulmonary artery wedge pressures, in addition to hypotension and decreased cardiac output. Initial therapy for hypovolemic shock consists of rapid administration of intravenous fluids, 100 to 200 cc in 10 to 15 minutes each time, while monitoring changes in right atrial and pulmonary capillary wedge pressures and in cardiac output. Fluid therapy is continued and the rate of fluid administration is adjusted to maintain pulmonary capillary wedge pressure between 10 and 18 mmHg. If, during initial intravenous fluid therapy, pulmonary capillary wedge pressure increases rapidly and exceeds 20 to 25 mmHg, fluid administration should be discontinued, because of the potential risk of precipitating pulmonary edema. In some patients there is little or no increase in cardiac output, despite maintenance of optimal filling pressures during intravenous fluid therapy. In these patients, appropriate therapy for pump failure should be instituted and adequate filling pressures maintained with intravenous fluids.

Hypoperfusion and Pulmonary Congestion

(Refer to subset IV, Table 15-2.) A marked reduction in cardiac output and an elevated pulmonary capillary wedge pressure cause hypoperfusion and pulmonary congestion and result from marked depression of cardiac function. The major objectives of therapy of severe pump failure, with or without the clinical syndrome of cardiogenic shock, are (1) to improve cardiac performance, (2) to normalize hemodynamic abnormalities, and (3) to limit the infarct size.

General supportive therapy, which includes maintenance of adequate oxygenation, correction of acid-base abnormalities, and relief of pain, is similar to that employed for other subsets of patients with acute myocardial infarction. Control of dysrhythmias is also essential.

Improvement in cardiac performance and correction of hemodynamic abnormalities with pharmacologic agents require the use of vasodilator drugs, which decrease left ventricular ejection impedance, or positive inotropic drugs, which enhance contractility. In many patients, a combination of vasodilator and inotropic therapy is required to optimize hemodynamic improvement. Hemodynamic monitoring is indicated to assess the response to therapy.

Inotropic Agents

The inotropic agents digitalis, isoproterenol, norepinephrine, dopamine, and glucagon are potentially capable of increasing cardiac output by increasing contractility. An increase in contractility, however, increases myocardial oxygen demand, which may exceed oxygen supply in the presence of severe obstructive coronary artery lesions, thereby enhancing existing myocardial ischemia. Paradoxically, an increase in contractility may cause deterioration of cardiac performance. The chronotropic effect of some of the inotropic drugs (e.g., isoproterenol, norepinephrine) may also contribute to an increase in myocardial oxygen demand by inducing tachycardia. Most inotropic agents are essentially arrhythmogenic.

Furthermore, improvement in cardiac performance in patients with recent myocardial infarction depends on the degree of responsiveness of the noninfarcted myocardium to inotropic stimulation. Recent studies indicate that the level of circulating endogenous catecholamines is already high in these patients and is higher in patients with pump failure and cardiogenic shock. It is possible that noninfarcted myocardial segments are already maximally or near maximally inotropically stimulated, and administration of inotropes may therefore not produce adequate and expected responses.

Digitalis Preparations

When pump failure is not precipitated by atrial arrhythmias in patients with recent myocardial infarction, digitalis usually does not improve cardiac output significantly (<10% of output), and the decrease in pulmonary venous pressure is also minimal. Digitalis may also increase infarct size. Furthermore, in the presence of recent infarction, ventricular irritability is enhanced by digitalis. Therefore, digitalis should be avoided for the management of pump failure complicating myocardial infarction. Digitalis, however, is indicated for the treatment of atrial fibrillation or flutter with rapid ventricular response. Digoxin, when given intravenously, should be administered by infusion, not by bolus. With infusion of digoxin (0.5–1 mg), given in 15 to 20 minutes, adverse peripheral vascular effects can be minimized. Once the ventricular rate has been controlled, digoxin should be continued with 0.125 to 0.25 mg, once a day, as a maintenance dose. At this stage, quinidine or procainamide will frequently convert atrial fibrillation or flutter into sinus rhythm, and these type IA antiarrhythmic drugs may be helpful in maintaining sinus rhythm. (See Chapter 14.)

Norepinephrine

Like digitalis, norepinephrine is of little use in the management of pump failure complicating recent myocardial infarction. With higher doses of norepinephrine (>10 µg/min), systemic vascular resistance increases, which might further decrease stroke volume. Left ventricular end-diastolic pressure, and therefore pulmonary venous pressure, may also concomitantly increase. Furthermore, like any other inotropic agent, norepinephrine has the disadvantage of enhancing myocardial ischemia. It is used to maintain arterial pressure only in severely hypotensive patients.

Isoproterenol

Despite some improvement in cardiac output that might occur in a dose range of 1 to 8 µg/min, isoproterenol increases myocardial ischemia by its marked inotropic and chronotropic effects. It is also a potent arrhythmogenic. Therefore, it is not recommended for the treatment of pump failure complicating myocardial infarction.

Glucagon

With an initial intravenous loading dose of 5 mg, followed by a maintenance dose of 1 mg/min, glucagon may improve cardiac performance, but only in patients with mild-to-moderate left ventricular failure. In patients with severe pump failure or cardiogenic shock, it has little beneficial effect. Nausea, vomiting, and marked hyperglycemia limit its use. Furthermore, it is weaker than other inotropic drugs, and thus it is now seldom used.

Dopamine

A relatively low dose of dopamine (1–4 µg/kg/min) activates predominantly dopamine one and two receptors and produces renal and mesenteric vasodilatation. Low-dose dopamine may also activate β_1 receptors and increase contractility, although this usually occurs with higher doses of dopamine (4–10 µg/kg/min). With a further increase in the dose, peripheral α receptors are activated, and systemic vascular resistance and arterial pressures increase. To increase cardiac output, a lower dose should be used, and to increase arterial pressures, higher doses should be used. A renal dose of dopamine (1–4 µg/kg/min) is used primarily to improve renal plasma flow and urine output. With dopamine, pulmonary capillary wedge pressure and total pulmonary resistance either remain unchanged or increase. Tachycardia generally develops, particularly with larger doses. Augmented contractility and tachycardia increase myocardial oxygen demand and may enhance myocardial ischemia in patients with acute myocardial infarction. The principal indications for the use of dopamine are for the treatment of hypotension accompanying pump failure and for the improvement of renal function when the cardiac output is maintained with the use of vasodilators or other inotropic agents.

Dobutamine
Dobutamine is a new synthetic catecholamine that predominantly activates β-adrenergic receptors. It is predominantly a β_1 receptor agonist, but it also activates β_2 and α receptors to a smaller extent; with larger doses, systemic vascular resistance may decrease markedly, and hypotension may result despite a significant increase in cardiac output.

In patients with heart failure, dobutamine at infusion rates of 2.5 to 15 μg/kg/min increases cardiac output and decreases left ventricular filling pressure significantly. Some increase in heart rate and systolic arterial pressure usually accompanies an increase in cardiac output. Enhanced contractile state and tachycardia increase myocardial oxygen demand, coronary blood flow, and myocardial oxygen consumption. The principal indication for the use of dobutamine is to increase cardiac output in the absence of significant hypotension.

Amrinone
Amrinone is a bipyridine derivative and a nonglycosidic, nonadrenergic inotropic agent. In patients with severe left ventricular failure, it increases cardiac output and stroke volume and decreases left ventricular filling pressure, indicating improved cardiac performance. It does not cause any significant change in heart rate or arterial pressure, but it decreases systemic vascular resistance. Since its mode of action is different from that of digitalis or catecholamines, it can be combined with these inotropic agents to produce synergistic effects on left ventricular function. Because amrinone does not appear to cause significant tachycardia or hypertension, an excessive increase in myocardial oxygen demand and, therefore, adverse effects on myocardial metabolism are less likely to occur in patients with ischemic heart disease. After a single intravenous dose (0.75–2.5 mg/kg), the onset of action has been noted within 2 minutes, reaching a maximum in 10 minutes, with the hemodynamic effects lasting 60 to 90 minutes. With a continuous infusion (6–10 μg/kg/min) sustained hemodynamic effects are expected.

Vasodilator (Afterload-Reducing) Agents
Changes in resistance to left ventricular ejection alter left ventricular pump function. Decreased resistance enhances left ventricular stroke volume and cardiac output. Vasodilator agents such as nitroprusside or phentolamine have been shown to reduce peripheral resistance and thereby to improve cardiac performance. Furthermore, because of the venous pooling effect, left ventricular end-diastolic volume and pressure (preload) and pulmonary venous pressure usually decrease. There is some decrease in arterial pressure without any change in heart rate and contractile state. Overall myocardial oxygen demand tends to decrease.

Vasodilator therapy may improve the immediate prognosis in patients with recent infarction complicated by severe pump failure with or without clinical features of cardiogenic shock. The major disadvantage of vasodilator therapy, however, is the decrease in arterial pressure, which, if pronounced, might restrict coronary blood flow and enhance ischemia. Arterial pressure, left ventricular filling pressure (LVFP)—pulmonary wedge capillary pressure (PCWP) or pulmonary artery end-diastolic pressure (PADP)—and, if possible, cardiac output should therefore be monitored during vasodilator therapy.

For the treatment of pump failure complicating myocardial infarction, vasodilator agents with quickly reversible hemodynamic effects have been advocated. Sodium nitroprusside and phentolamine are examples; the hemodynamic effects are usually reversed within 5 to 10 minutes after discontinuation of these drugs. Both drugs are used intravenously, and the initial dosage should not exceed 16 μg/min. If there is no significant decrease in PCWP and arterial pressure or increase in cardiac output, the dose is increased by 10 to 15 μg every 5 to 10 minutes until the hemodynamic response is adequate. At any dose level, if arterial pressure decreases markedly without significant decrease in PCWP or increase in cardiac output, the therapy should be discontinued. If phentolamine is used (this use of phentolamine is not stated in the manufacturer's official directive), the initial dose should not exceed 0.1 mg/min. Every 5 to 10 minutes, the dose may be increased by 0.1 mg/min, up to 2 mg/min.

Nitroglycerin and nitrates are predominantly venodilators, although when given intravenously, they appear to exert some arteriolar-dilating effects. Whether given intravenously or nonparenterally, nitroglycerin and nitrates cause a substantial reduction in pulmonary capillary wedge and right atrial pressures with only a modest or no increase in cardiac output. Mean arterial pressure may decrease, but the heart usually remains unchanged. In patients with persistent left ventricular failure, nitroglycerin is usually administered intravenously (usual dose, 20–200 μg/min), and the usual indication for its use is to decrease pulmonary capillary wedge and right atrial pressures. If cardiac output is significantly decreased, along with an increased systemic vascular resistance and pulmonary capillary wedge pressure, sodium nitroprusside is preferable to nitroglycerin. However, if myocardial ischemia is suspected, and when cardiac output is only slightly reduced, nitroglycerin is the vasodilator of choice.

Complications of Vasodilator Therapy
Several complications may be associated with vasodilator therapy. (1) Unexpected, sudden, significant hypotension may occur; in such circumstances, therapy should be discontinued temporarily, and the legs should be elevated. (2) When nitroprusside is used for more than 2 weeks, hypothyroidism may be induced. (3) Involuntary muscular twitching and even frank convulsions may occur. (4) Hiccups, the mechanism of which remains unexplained, may occur in some patients. (5) Cardiac output may not increase; indeed, it may decrease if there is a marked decrease in LVFP. In such patients, the dose of the vasodilator should be adjusted to maintain the PCWP or PADP between 14 and 18 mmHg. (6) Cyanide poisoning, thiocyanate toxicity, and methemoglobinemia are rare complications of nitro-

prusside therapy. During prolonged nitroprusside therapy, particularly in patients with renal failure, serum levels of thiocyanate should be monitored. The lethal concentration of thiocyanate is approximately 12 mg/100 ml.

Role of Diuretics in the Management of Pump Failure

Potent diuretics such as furosemide are helpful in reducing pulmonary venous congestion. Intravenous furosemide decreases pulmonary venous pressure in 5 to 10 minutes, even before there is any significant increase in urinary output. This early reduction is related to increased peripheral venous capacitance. Potent diuretics should be used cautiously, because they may induce marked and rapid diuresis, with precipitation of hypovolemic shock. Furthermore, associated urinary potassium loss may enhance ventricular irritability. A single intravenous dose of 20 mg of furosemide should be tried initially. Although they decrease pulmonary congestion, diuretics do not increase cardiac output. Therefore, in the presence of low cardiac output, diuretics alone are not effective.

Combination Inotropic and Vasodilator Therapy

If a vasodilator agent such as sodium nitroprusside or phentolamine does not improve left ventricular failure appreciably, an inotropic agent such as dopamine or dobutamine may be added. This combination therapy may prove particularly beneficial in patients with severe pump failure associated with hypotension. In such patients, dopamine or dobutamine infusion should be started and then a vasodilator drug (nitroprusside) added when arterial pressure is adequate. If there is a substantial increase in cardiac output with an inotropic agent, without a significant decrease in pulmonary capillary wedge pressure, nitroglycerin can be added instead of sodium nitroprusside.

Intra-aortic Balloon Counterpulsation

As is illustrated in Figure 15-1, the two major objectives of intra-aortic balloon counterpulsation are (1) to increase arterial pressure during diastole (diastolic augmentation) to maintain or enhance coronary artery perfusion pressure, and (2) to decrease left ventricular and arterial pressures (systolic unloading) to reduce myocardial work and oxygen demand and to increase stroke volume and cardiac output. With effective systolic unloading, the left ventricular diastolic and pulmonary capillary wedge pressures decrease along with the left ventricular diastolic volume.

Although an improvement in hemodynamics and a reversal of shock syndrome have been demonstrated in some patients with severe pump failure and cardiogenic shock, the prognosis has not significantly improved with intra-aortic balloon counterpulsation alone. Surgical therapy, when feasible, following stabilization with the use of intra-aortic balloon counterpulsation may improve the prognosis. The indications for the use of intra-aortic balloon counterpulsation in patients with acute myocardial infarction are (1) cardiogenic shock, for stabilization prior to surgery; (2)

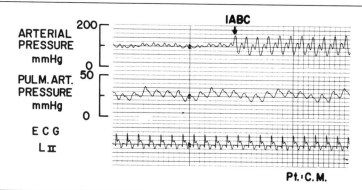

Fig. 15-1. Intra-aortic balloon counterpulsation.

severe mitral regurgitation with hypotension; (3) postinfarction ventricular septal rupture; (4) selected patients with postinfarction angina.

Surgery and Pump Failure

The role of surgical therapy in the management of pump failure and cardiogenic shock in the absence of mechanical defects is controversial. Aortocoronary artery bypass surgery provides supplementary channels of blood supply to the ischemic myocardium. Coronary artery bypass surgery with or without infarctectomy has been attempted to revascularize the ischemic myocardium in the peri-infarction zone. It has been hoped that by such revascularization, the function of the ischemic myocardium can be significantly restored and pump failure can be reversed. Although some success has been reported, the surgical mortality rate remains extremely high.

Percutaneous Coronary Artery Angioplasty

Rapid recanalization of the infarct-related artery following the intravenous administration of thrombolytic agents—streptokinase or rtPA—has been reported to decrease mortality of patients with cardiogenic shock in uncontrolled studies. As the mortality rate for patients with conventional therapy—i.e., vasodilators, inotropic agents, intra-aortic balloon counterpulsation with or without coronary artery bypass surgery—remains very high (exceeding 50%), recanalization treatment is worth considering in these patients, although no controlled studies have been performed to demonstrate efficacy of such therapy. It needs to be emphasized, however, that in addition to recanalization therapy, aggressive supportive pharmacotherapy and intra-aortic balloon counterpulsation are still required to maintain adequate cardiac performance in these patients. The therapeutic approach for the treatment of left ventricular failure complicating acute myocardial infarction is outlined in Table 15-3 and Figure 15-2.

Table 15-3. Therapeutic approach to the treatment of left
ventricular failure complicating acute myocardial infarction

1. *Subset I* (no pulmonary congestion or hypoperfusion). No specific treatment
   indicated until a complication supervenes.
2. *Subset II* (pulmonary congestion, no hypoperfusion). Nitroglycerin or
   nitrates, supplemental oxygen, morphine or diuretics. (a) Improvement:
   observe. (b) No improvement: hemodynamic monitoring, subsequent
   treatment as in subset IV.
3. *Subset III* (hypoperfusion, no pulmonary congestion). Hemodynamic
   monitoring preferable. Low cardiac output with low right atrial and
   pulmonary capillary wedge pressure: intravenous fluid therapy to maintain
   pulmonary capillary wedge pressure between 14 and 18 mmHg. (a)
   Improvement: continued intravenous fluid therapy. (b) No improvement:
   subsequent treatment as in subset IV.
4. *Subset IV* (hypoperfusion and pulmonary congestion). Hemodynamic
   monitoring usually required. (a) Elevated pulmonary capillary wedge
   pressure, slight reduction in cardiac output, adequate arterial pressure:
   intravenous nitroglycerin and diuretics. (b) Elevated pulmonary capillary
   wedge pressure, low cardiac output, adequate arterial pressure, and elevated
   systemic vascular resistance: nitroprusside. (a) Improvement: continue
   nitroprusside. (b) Increased cardiac output but persistent elevation of
   pulmonary capillary wedge pressure, adequate arterial pressure: add
   intravenous nitroglycerin. (c) Decreased pulmonary capillary wedge pressure
   but inadequate increase in cardiac output: add inotropic drugs and consider
   intra-aortic balloon counterpulsation. (c) Elevated pulmonary capillary
   wedge pressure, low cardiac output, and hypotension: vasopressor and intra-
   aortic balloon counterpulsation. (a) Adequate arterial pressure, little or no
   increase in cardiac output, and lower pulmonary capillary wedge pressure:
   add vasodilator such as nitroprusside. (b) Adequate arterial pressure,
   adequate increase in cardiac output with elevated pulmonary capillary
   wedge pressure: add nitroglycerin and diuretics. (c) Modest increase in
   arterial pressure, low cardiac output, and elevated pulmonary capillary
   wedge pressure: add inotropic drugs such as dobutamine or amrinone. All
   patients should be evaluated for potentially surgically correctable lesions.
5. Early cardiogenic shock: consider thrombolytic therapy and immediate
   percutaneous angioplasty of the infarct-related artery in addition to treatment
   outlined for patients in subset IV.

Correction of Contributing Factors in Pump Failure

Acid-Base Imbalance

Hypoxia, acidosis, and electrolyte imbalance, such as hyperkalemia, not
only precipitate but also perpetuate pump failure. Frequent determinations
of arterial blood gases and serum electrolytes are mandatory for the proper
management of pump failure. Intubation and arterial ventilation should
not be delayed if the usual methods of oxygen administration fail to correct
hypoxia.

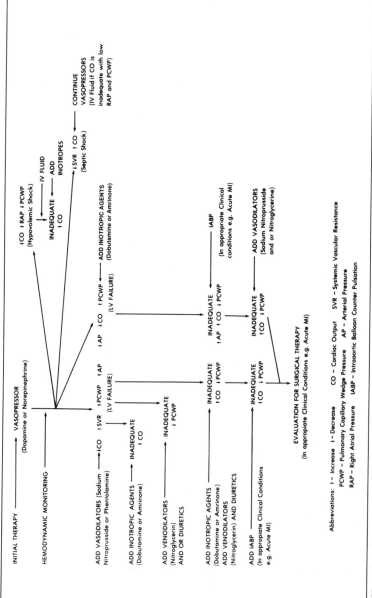

Fig. 15-2. Hypotension in critically ill patients: stepwise therapeutic approach based on hemodynamics.

Arrhythmias

In some patients, persistent sinus bradycardia and atrioventricular (AV) block or dissociation with relatively slow ventricular response may precipitate severe pump failure. It is desirable in such cases to increase the heart rate to an optimal level. Sinus bradycardia can usually be corrected by intravenous atropine sulfate (0.6 mg initial dose; this can be repeated until 1–2 mg have been given), but it should be administered cautiously, because a sudden and rapid ventricular response may enhance ventricular irritability by increasing myocardial oxygen demand. Similarly, isoproterenol may enhance ischemia and ventricular arrhythmias and therefore should be avoided. In such circumstances, atrial pacing may be a safer method of elevating the heart rate. In the presence of AV block, however, ventricular pacing is needed. For management of severe pump failure associated with AV block, ventricular pacing alone may not adequately improve cardiac output. Atrioventricular sequential pacing may in some instances significantly improve cardiac output and should be attempted.

Mechanical Defects and Pump Failure

Severe mitral regurgitation due to papillary muscle infarction and ventricular septal rupture, although uncommon complications of acute myocardial infarction (occurring in approximately 1% of cases), may precipitate severe pump failure and cardiogenic shock despite the presence of a relatively small infarct. Prompt diagnosis and immediate therapeutic intervention are essential. Clinical differentiation between mitral regurgitation and ventricular septal rupture is often difficult. Bedside hemodynamic monitoring with the use of a balloon floatation (Swan-Ganz) catheter resolves the difficulty in diagnosis. The presence of giant *v* waves in the PCWP tracing indicates mitral regurgitation (Fig. 15-3); significantly higher oxygen saturation in the pulmonary artery blood as compared with right atrial blood confirms the diagnosis of ventricular septal rupture (Fig. 15-4).

The prognosis of patients with severe mitral regurgitation resulting from papillary muscle infarction or rupture is extremely poor: approximately 50 percent mortality within 24 hours and 94 percent mortality within 8 weeks. Although some patients appear to improve with medical therapy, such improvement is usually transient and, usually, multiple organ failure occurs with expectant medical treatment. Early surgical correction of mitral regurgitation by mitral valve replacement or repair can salvage 60 to 70 percent of patients.

However, in preparation for cardiac catheterization and surgery, aggressive supportive therapy should be instituted without delay for stabilization. Hemodynamic monitoring is required to employ appropriate therapy and to assess the response to therapy. If arterial pressure is adequate and systemic vascular resistance is elevated in the presence of low cardiac output and elevated pulmonary capillary wedge pressure, intravenous sodium nitroprusside is effective in increasing forward cardiac output and in decreasing the regurgitant volume and the pulmonary capillary wedge pressure. With intravenous nitroglycerin, although pulmonary capillary wedge pressure and regurgitant volume decrease, forward stroke volume

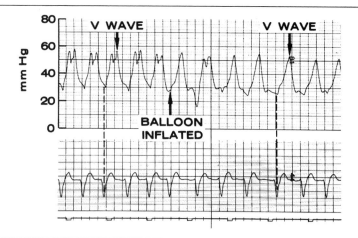

Fig. 15-3. PCWP tracing; giant *v* waves indicate mitral regurgitation.

or cardiac output usually remains unchanged. Thus, sodium nitroprusside is preferable to nitroglycerin in these circumstances. In the presence of hypotension, vasodilators cannot be used initially, because of the risk of inducing further hypotension. In the presence of hypotension, a vasopressor or inotropic agent is used initially and then a vasodilator agent can be added, depending on the hemodynamic response. The systolic unloading effect of intra-aortic balloon counterpulsation increases forward cardiac output and decreases regurgitant volume, and diastolic augmentation helps to maintain coronary artery perfusion pressures. Thus, intra-aortic balloon counterpulsation is particularly useful in patients with hypotension. After the institution of intra-aortic balloon counterpulsation, vasodilators, inotropic agents, and diuretics are added as required to stabilize these patients prior to cardiac catheterization and corrective surgery.

Rupture of the interventricular septum, another catastrophic complication of acute myocardial infarction, occurs in 0.5 to 2 percent of cases. Rupture of the interventricular septum causes left-to-right shunt and produces right ventricular volume overload, increased pulmonary blood flow, and decreased systemic blood flow. Low-output state, along with elevated pulmonary and systemic venous pressure and varying degrees of hypotension, is precipitated. Until these hemodynamic abnormalities are promptly corrected, the prognosis remains grave. The mortality is approximately 24 percent within 24 hours, 46 percent within 1 week, and 67 to 82 percent within 2 months. Early repair of the ventricular septal defect with or without coronary artery bypass surgery may be associated with 48 to 75 percent short-term survival. Cardiogenic shock, right ventricular infarction, and severe right heart failure and evidence for end-organ (pulmonary, renal) failure are associated with a higher perioperative mortality.

Patients with ventricular septal rupture also require aggressive supportive therapy for stabilization prior to surgery. Although vasodilators can

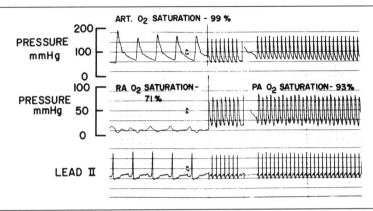

Fig. 15-4. Significantly higher oxygen saturation in the pulmonary artery blood compared to that in the right atrial blood confirms the diagnosis of ventricular septal rupture.

decrease the magnitude of left-to-right shunt and increase systemic flow in some patients, vasodilators—particularly those that can also decrease pulmonary vascular resistance in addition to systemic vascular resistance (nitroprusside, nitroglycerin)—should be used cautiously. If the relative reduction in pulmonary vascular resistance is greater than that in systemic vascular resistance, the magnitude of left-to-right shunt may increase and systemic flow may decrease. For a reduction of left-to-right shunt, a predominantly arteriolar dilator such as hydralazine is preferable to nitroprusside or nitroglycerin. Intra-aortic balloon counterpulsation is particularly useful in patients with ventricular septal defect, as it causes a selective "unloading" of the left ventricle, with a concomitant increase in systemic flow and reduction in the magnitude of left-to-right shunt. Thus, intraaortic balloon counterpulsation treatment should be started whenever feasible, and vasodilators and/or inotropic agents should be added depending on the hemodynamic response. As in patients with papillary muscle infarction, however, the objective of aggressive supportive therapy is to stabilize these patients before an early corrective surgery is performed.

Right Ventricular Infarction
Right ventricular infarction occurs almost always in association with left ventricular inferior or inferoposterior wall infarction. The incidence of right ventricular infarction in patients with inferior myocardial infarction is between 28 and 44 percent. Diagnosis of right ventricular infarction is suspected clinically when there is evidence for right heart failure (elevated jugular venous pressure, right ventricular S3 gallop) in the absence of pulmonary congestion or pulmonary edema. Kussmaul's sign, when present, is a very helpful diagnostic clue. S–T segment elevations in leads V_1 and V_4R and a greater Q wave in lead III compared to lead AVF, in the presence of electrocardiographic evidence of inferior-wall myocardial infarction, al-

most always indicate right ventricular infarction. Radionuclide ventriculography and echocardiography usually demonstrate a dilated, poorly contracting right ventricle, reduced right ventricular ejection fraction, and right ventricular segmental wall motion abnormalities. Technetium-99m pyrophosphate scintigraphy that reveals its uptake by the infarcted right ventricular free wall provides definitive diagnosis of right ventricular infarction. Hemodynamic monitoring is not required to establish the diagnosis of right ventricular infarction; however, determination of hemodynamics is useful during management of low-output state. The two major complications of right ventricular infarction are bradyarrhythmias and low-output state with hypotension. The incidence of complete atrioventricular block is approximately 20 percent, which is higher than its overall incidence in patients with acute myocardial infarction. Ventricular pacing in patients with right ventricular infarction is usually ineffective in correcting low-output state. Atrioventricular sequential pacing causes a greater increase in cardiac output and is the pacing mode of choice in these patients.

Decreased systemic output in patients with right ventricular infarction results from decreased left ventricular preload. Reduction of left ventricular preload (end-diastolic volume, transmural pressure) is caused by decreased right ventricular stroke volume and the constraining effects of pericardium, which also restrict left ventricular filling. The interventricular septum also shifts toward the left ventricle during diastole, and this also reduces left ventricular preload. The mechanisms for reduced right ventricular stroke volume are decreased right ventricular contractility due to infarction and a secondary increase in right ventricular afterload.

To improve systemic output and correct hypotension, it is necessary to increase right ventricular stroke volume, which, in turn, increases left ventricular preload. When right and left ventricular filling pressures are relatively low (right atrial pressure <10–12 mmHg, pulmonary capillary wedge pressure <15 mmHg), intravenous fluid therapy may increase right ventricular stroke volume by the Frank-Starling mechanism, and systemic output may also increase. However, when the right ventricle is already markedly dilated with a higher right atrial pressure, volume expansion is usually ineffective in increasing systemic output. The vasodilators, such as sodium nitroprusside and nitroglycerin, can potentially decrease pulmonary vascular resistance (i.e., right ventricular afterload) and increase right ventricular stroke volume. Thus, these vasodilators are useful in increasing systemic output; however, concomitant intravenous fluid therapy is also required to maintain adequate right and left ventricular preload.

The inotropic drugs dobutamine and dopamine are also effective in improving systemic output in patients with right ventricular infarction. With relatively larger doses of dopamine, total pulmonary resistance and pulmonary capillary wedge pressure may increase, enhancing right ventricular afterload. In contrast, dobutamine does not cause any change or may even decrease total pulmonary resistance and pulmonary capillary wedge pressure. Amrinone also decreases pulmonary vascular resistance, right atrial and pulmonary capillary wedge pressures. Thus, for the treatment of

Table 15-4. Therapeutic approach to treatment of
"low output" in patients with right ventricular infarction

1. Right ventricular infarction compensated without hypotension or
   manifestations of low cardiac output: no specific therapy required. Avoid
   diuretics, nitroglycerin, and nitrates, which may precipitate hypotension.
2. Low cardiac output and lower pulmonary capillary wedge pressure (< 15
   mm Hg): initially, intravenous fluids to maintain pulmonary capillary wedge
   pressure between 15 and 18 mm Hg.
   a. Improvement with intravenous fluids: continue intravenous fluid
      therapy.
   b. No improvement with intravenous fluids: add vasodilators.
   c. No improvement: add inotropic agents.
3. Low cardiac output, elevated pulmonary capillary wedge and right atrial
   pressures, or elevated arterial pressure: initial therapy, vasodilators.
   a. Improvement with fall in right atrial and pulmonary capillary wedge
      pressures: add intravenous fluids.
   b. Improvement without fall in right atrial and pulmonary capillary wedge
      pressures: continue vasodilators.
   c. No improvement: add inotropic drugs.
4. Low cardiac output, elevated pulmonary wedge and right atrial pressures,
   and hypotension: inotropic drugs such as dobutamine or dopamine,
   depending on the level of blood pressure.
   a. Improvement: continue inotropic drugs.
   b. No improvement: add vasodilators.

primary right heart failure, as in patients with right ventricular infarction,
dobutamine or amrinone is preferable to dopamine. However, in hypotensive patients, dopamine should be considered initially and once hypotension is corrected, vasodilators (dobutamine or amrinone) can be added to
optimize hemodynamic improvement. In patients with severe right heart
failure, unresponsive to pharmacotherapy, pulmonary artery balloon
counterpulsation and right ventricular assist pneumatic pump have been
used with occasional success. The therapeutic approach for the correction
of low output state in patients with right ventricular infarction is outlined
in Table 15-4.

CARDIAC TAMPONADE

Diagnosis

Cardiac tamponade is another form of acute heart failure caused by markedly increased intrapericardial pressure. Increased intrapericardial pressure restricts diastolic filling of the heart and causes a marked decrease in
cardiac output. Cardiac tamponade may occur with a small or a large pericardial effusion. Rising jugular venous pressure, tachycardia, and falling
blood pressure with pulsus paradoxus (inspiratory decrease in systolic
blood pressure of more than 10 mm Hg) strongly suggest tamponade in a
patient with suspected or known pericardial effusion. Echocardiography
is the investigatory method of choice for the diagnosis of pericardial effu-

sion and tamponade. Determination of hemodynamics that demonstrate equalization of right atrial and pulmonary capillary wedge pressure is not required for the diagnosis of tamponade except in rare instances.

Pericardiocentesis

Treatment of cardiac tamponade is specific: removal of the pericardial fluid or the pericardium, or both. Intravenous fluids, vasodilators, and inotropic agents have been shown to improve hemodynamics in the presence of tamponade. However, such therapy should never be entertained as substitutes for pericardiocentesis.

Procedure

For closed pericardiocentesis, the following equipment should be available: 5- and 50-ml syringes; 14-, 18-, and 20-gauge needles (3 in. in length with short bevels); three-way sterile stopcock; rubber connecting tubing; sterile alligator clamps; and an ECG machine and defibrillation equipment. Premedication is usually not required. Pericardiocentesis should be performed with the patient elevated at 60 degrees with proper aseptic technique.

After administering local anesthesia to the skin and subcutaneous tissue of the selected area, a 20-gauge needle is connected to a 50-ml syringe through a three-way stopcock. The V lead to the electrocardiography (ECG) machine is then connected to the shank of the needle through the alligator clamp (the ECG machine must be properly grounded). The ECG is monitored continuously. The needle is slowly advanced, without sudden movement and with intermittent gentle suction. Fluid is usually encountered at a depth of 3 to 4 cm with these approaches. Epicardial contact is marked by premature beats or by S–T or P–R segment elevation, and the needle is then drawn back. After the presence and depth of fluid has been ascertained, a larger needle may be substituted, and polyethylene catheters may be placed in the pericardial cavity. Pericardiocentesis can also be performed with echocardiographic and/or fluoroscopic guidance.

Potential Sites for Closed Pericardiocentesis

The potential sites for closed pericardiocentesis are as follows.

1. Subxiphoid. The needle is inserted directly inward at the left xiphocostal angle to the level of the inner rib cage and directed at about 30-degree angle superiorly, posteriorly, and toward the left shoulder.
2. Apical. The needle is inserted in the fifth intercostal space about 2 to 3 cm lateral to the apex beat, or just inside the left border of cardiac dullness.
3. Left sternal border. The potential site is the fifth or sixth intercostal space, and the needle is directed medially.
4. Right-sided approach. If the effusion appears to be mainly on the right, one can insert the needle in the fourth intercostal space just inside the right border of cardiac dullness, directing the needle slightly medially.

Possible Complications of Closed Pericardiocentesis

The possible complications of closed pericardiocentesis include entry into a cardiac chamber; arrhythmia; damage to the coronary artery, liver, stomach, or lungs; subepicardial hematoma; and infections from contamination. When bloody fluid is aspirated, hematocrit determinations should be done to identify the source of the fluid. It should also be observed whether or not the fluid clots easily; pericardial fluid usually does not clot. The location of the catheter can also be determined by monitoring the pressure. If ventricular pressure is recorded, the catheter should be withdrawn.

THERAPY OF ACUTE HEART FAILURE OWING TO SEVERE SYSTEMIC HYPERTENSION

A sudden severe increase in arterial blood pressure may precipitate left ventricular failure and acute pulmonary edema by increasing the resistance to left ventricular ejection and thereby decreasing stroke volume and increasing end-diastolic volume and pressure. The treatment of hypertensive heart failure and pulmonary edema is no different from the usual treatment of heart failure and pulmonary edema from any cause—namely, administration of oxygen, morphine, diuretics, and nitroglycerin. It is also important in the management of such patients to attempt to decrease arterial pressure. The diastolic arterial pressure may occasionally exceed 140 mmHg in some of these patients. Blood pressure can be reduced rapidly with the use of diazoxide, trimethaphan, nitroprusside, intravenous nitroglycerin, sublingual nifedipine, and the intravenous angiotensin-converting enzyme inhibitor enalaprilats (see Chap. 16).

ACUTE HEART FAILURE DUE TO VALVULAR REGURGITATION

Acute severe mitral regurgitation may precipitate pulmonary edema and low-output state precipitously and requires aggressive supportive therapy for clinical and hemodynamic stabilization. Besides acute myocardial infarction and papillary muscle ischemia, bacterial endocarditis and spontaneous rupture of the chordae tendineae are important etiologies for acute severe mitral regurgitation. Diagnosis can usually be confirmed by echo Doppler studies, which may also reveal the underlying mechanism, such as vegetations due to bacterial endocarditis, flail mitral leaflets, or ruptured chordeae. Supportive therapy is similar to that in patients with postinfarction mitral regurgitation. In some patients, intra-aortic balloon counterpulsation therapy is required to improve systemic hemodynamics. All patients with acute severe mitral regurgitation with hemodynamic compromise are potential candidates for surgical correction of mitral regurgitation. Even in patients with bacterial endocarditis, who of course require the appropriate antibiotics, surgical treatment should not be withheld if the clinical status and hemodynamic abnormalities do not improve promptly with aggressive medical therapy.

Acute aortic valvular regurgitation can also induce severe left ventricular failure, pulmonary edema, and low cardiac output. Bacterial endocarditis and aortic dissection are the two important causes of acute aortic regurgitation. Echo Doppler, magnetic resonance imaging, and computed tomography are useful noninvasive ways to establish the etiology. Contrast angiographic studies are also required in some patients for the diagnosis of the cause of aortic regurgitation.

Vasodilators, inotropic agents, and diuretics, in addition to appropriate antibiotics, are the initial therapies for aortic regurgitation resulting from bacterial endocarditis. Intra-aortic balloon counterpulsation, however, is contraindicated in the presence of significant aortic regurgitation. Aortic valve replacement should be considered even during the acute phase of bacterial endocarditis, if heart failure does not improve with supportive therapy.

Aortic regurgitation in patients with thoracic aortic dissection always indicates type A dissection (involvement of ascending aorta) and is an indication for urgent surgery. Type A thoracic aortic dissection is associated with an ominous prognosis (70–80% mortality within first 3 days). Immediate therapy is directed to lower arterial pressure with intravenous nitroprusside or trimethaphan and to lower aortic dp/dt with β-adrenergic blocking drugs. Diuretics and nitroglycerin are also helpful in decreasing pulmonary venous pressures. However, surgical therapy should not be delayed in these patients.

MYOCARDIAL, PERIPARTUM, ALCOHOLIC CARDIOMYOPATHY

Supportive treatment for heart failure resulting from infectious myocarditis or toxic and peripartum myocardiopathies is similar to the treatment of heart failure resulting from other causes. Diuretics, vasodilators, and angiotensin-converting enzyme inhibitors are the initial therapies of choice. Digitalis is sometimes poorly tolerated by patients with infectious or toxic myocarditis. Digitalis is primarily used for the control of ventricular response in patients with atrial fibrillation or flutter. Patients unresponsive to vasodilators and/or angiotensin-converting enzyme inhibitors, intravenous inotropic therapy (dobutamine, amrinone) with or without additional vasodilators, and angiotensin-converting enzyme inhibitors frequently require hemodynamic monitoring for stabilization. Patients who have a rapidly deteriorating clinical status and who are unresponsive to aggressive vasodilator and inotropic therapy should be considered for cardiac transplantation.

In some forms of infectious myocarditis (rheumatic, diphtheritic), corticosteroid therapy is sometimes useful. In viral myocarditis, however, early intervention with steroids (within 6 weeks) may cause deterioration. Presently, endomyocardial biopsy is recommended and steroids and/or cytotoxic drug therapy are recommended only in those patients in whom myocardial biopsy is positive for inflammatory changes. Even in these patients the benefits of such therapy have not been firmly established.

In patients with alcoholic cardiomyopathy, thiaminic treatment may occasionally be associated with clinical improvement, but abstinence from alcohol use is mandatory. During the end-stages of alcoholic cardiomyopathy, however, abstaining from alcohol use does not cause any reversal of the cardiomyopasthic process.

A substantial number of patients with peripartum cardiomyopathy improve with conservative medical therapy, and cardiac function becomes normal. In these patients, subsequent pregnancies may not cause recurrence of heart failure. Patients with persistent heart failure and residual left ventricular dysfunction should be advised against further pregnancies.

SELECTED READINGS

Chatterjee, K., et al. Hemodynamic and metabolic responses to vasodilator therapy in acute myocardial infarction. *Circulation* 48:1183, 1973.

Chatterjee, K., and Parmley, W. W. Vasodilator therapy in heart failure. *Prog. Cardiovasc. Dis.* 19:301, 1977.

Chatterjee, K. Digitalis, catecholamines and other positive inotropic agents. In W. W. Parmley and K. Chatterjee, (eds.), *Cardiology.* Philadelphia: Lippincott, 1988. Pp. 1(17):1–46.

Chatterjee, K. Bedside hemodynamic monitoring. In W. W. Parmley and K. Chatterjee (eds.), *Cardiology.* Philadelphia: Lippincott, 1988. Pp. 1(55):1–19.

Cohn, J. N., et al. Right ventricular infarction. Clinical and hemodynamic features. *Am. J. Cardiol.* 33:209, 1974.

Goldberg, L. L., et al. Newer catecholamines for treatment of heart failure and shock: An update on dopamine and first look at dobutamine. *Prog. Cardiovasc. Dis.* 19:327, 1977.

Lejemtel, T. H., et al. Amrinone: A new non-glycoside, non-adrenergenic cardiotonic agent effective in the treatment of intractable myocardial failure in man. *Circulation* 59:1098, 1979.

Matthay, M., and Chatterjee, K. Respiratory and hemodynamic management after cardiac surgery. In W. W. Parmley and K. Chatterjee (eds.), *Cardiology.* Philadelphia: Lippincott, 1988. Pp. 2(74):1–20.

Mueller, H. S., et al. Effect of dopamine on hemodynamics and myocardial metabolism in shock following acute myocardial infarction in man. *Circulation* 57:361, 1978.

Sanders, C. A., et al. Mechanical circulatory assist: Current status and experience with combining circulatory assistance, emergency coronary angiography, and acute myocardial revascularization. *Circulation* 45:1292, 1972.

Hypertension

Dwight L. Makoff

Hypertension has traditionally been defined as an elevation of arterial pressure above 140 to 150/90 mm Hg. There is evidence, however, that no true cutoff point exists at which normal blood pressure proceeds to hypertension. Rather, there is a continuum of increasing systolic, diastolic, and thus mean blood pressures, which appears to represent ever-increasing risk factors in the development of target-organ damage. Hypertension is a proven risk factor for the development of atherosclerotic disease of the brain, kidney, and heart. Additionally, hypertension increases the workload on the heart and may lead to left ventricular hypertrophy and heart failure. Intracranial hemorrhage and aortic aneurysm are more prone to develop in the setting of elevated blood pressure.

In approaching the critically ill hypertensive patient, it is important to consider the cause of the blood pressure elevation. Often, however, treatment must be instituted before a specific etiologic diagnosis can be made. Therapy should be selected based on the target organs most prominently affected and the rapidity with which blood pressure control is required.

PATIENT EVALUATION

Diagnosis

The diagnosis of a hypertensive disorder rests on the objective finding of an elevated systolic or diastolic blood pressure, or both. A single blood pressure recording may be misleading, because emotional factors may have a profound effect on the blood pressure of some people. Care must be taken to evaluate the blood pressure in both arms; proximal arterial stenosis may produce a spuriously lowered reading. A sphygmomanometer cuff with a bladder too short to encircle the arm may lead to erroneously elevated blood pressure readings.

Isolated systolic hypertension occurs most frequently in elderly patients and reflects in part the lack of distensibility of vessels associated with the aging process. However, evidence indicates that systolic hypertension correlates independently from diastolic pressure with risks of stroke, ischemic heart disease, and congestive heart failure [14]. To what degree the risks associated with systolic hypertension can be lessened by antihypertensive therapy is uncertain. Any treatment offered to a patient with isolated systolic hypertension must be carefully monitored to avoid postural hypotension and cerebrovascular insufficiency.

Clinical Status

History
An attempt should be made in taking the history to establish the duration of hypertension, any family history of hypertension, and the presence of symptoms of disorders that cause hypertension. A statement should be included in the history noting when the pressure had last been normal, or whether or not the blood pressure had ever been measured previously. Age of onset of hypertension before 30 or after 55, as well as the absence of a family history of hypertension, increases the possibility of a secondary cause of blood pressure elevation.

Essential hypertension is best considered a disease with variable or no symptoms. Specifically, a history of headaches, epistaxis, lightheadedness, or tinnitus has shown a variable relation to either systolic or diastolic blood pressure [15].

Vascular Examination
Assessment of vascular damage caused by hypertension is a critical part of the patient examination. Funduscopic examination allows direct visualization of damage to small vessels. Narrowing of the arteriolar lumen correlates with the severity of hypertension. Hemorrhages, exudates, and papilledema reflect consequences of severe hypertension.

Larger vessels should be evaluated by careful palpation and auscultation of pulses, with particular emphasis on lower-extremity vessels and carotid arteries. Patients with significant cerebrovascular disease may not tolerate the postural drop in blood pressure that may be induced by certain medications. A bruit may be heard over the abdomen of patients with renovascular hypertension.

Cardiac Status
Careful history and physical examination, electrocardiogram (ECG), and chest x-ray are crucial to evaluate heart disease in every hypertensive patient. Both coronary artery disease and left ventricular hypertrophy or failure are complications related to hypertension that may be detected by these means. Prominent left ventricular impulse, loud aortic component of the second heart sound, and S4 gallop are cardiac findings that should be expected in severe hypertension. A two-dimensional echocardiogram is an excellent modality for assessing left ventricular wall thickness.

Renal Assessment
Hypertension can produce renal disease if it is sustained or severe. Conversely, intrinsic renal disease often produces hypertension. It is important to establish by history if the patient had hypertension prior to the devel-

opment of renal disease. A patient who has had proteinuria, abnormal urine sediment, or azotemia before the onset of elevated blood pressure has intrinsic renal disease with secondary hypertension. Urinalysis and serum creatinine are the two most useful screening tests for renal disease.

BLOOD PRESSURE CONTROL

Determinants of Arterial Pressure and Organ Perfusion

Blood pressure is the product of the cardiac output times the mean arterial resistance. Cardiac output is determined by diastolic filling and intrinsic myocardial factors. Certain hypertensive states are associated with an increased cardiac output. Peripheral resistance is a function of arteriolar tone, which is influenced by neural, humoral, and intrinsic blood vessel factors. Stroke volume and arterial compliance affect mainly systolic blood pressure, whereas the state of arteriolar tone determines mainly diastolic blood pressure. Blood flow to an organ will be determined not only by the perfusion pressure, but also by the vascular resistance in that organ. In states in which there is a high peripheral vascular resistance in an organ due to increased vascular tone or pathologic fixed blood vessel narrowing, the arterial pressure must be high to perfuse the organ adequately.

Renal Factors

The kidneys play a key role in blood pressure control by virtue of the release of certain humoral factors, as well as through intrarenal mechanisms that are important in the regulation of body fluid volume. Normally, sodium reabsorption in the proximal and distal renal tubules is regulated to maintain an optimal total extracellular fluid volume. Proximal tubular sodium reabsorption varies with the state of the effective arterial volume and is controlled by the distribution of blood flow within the kidneys, renal interstitial pressure, plasma protein concentration, and possibly a humoral factor or factors. Distal tubular sodium handling is controlled through the renin-angiotensin-aldosterone system, which itself is also intricately involved in the regulation of blood pressure.

In normal persons, a fall in pressure at the afferent glomerular arteriole will ultimately lead to release from the juxtaglomerular apparatus of renin, which activates two mechanisms that will serve to help restore blood pressure: (1) generation of angiotensin II, a potent vasoconstrictor; and (2) secretion of aldosterone, a mineralocorticoid that promotes sodium retention. Disturbances in sodium balance or alterations in the renin-angiotensin-aldosterone system may have a profound effect on blood pressure. Other, less-well-understood renal mechanisms involved in blood pressure regulation are control of the level of extrarenal pressor substances and renal production of a vasodilator substance, possibly a prostaglandin, present in high concentrations in the renal medulla.

Atrial natriuretic hormone (ANF) is secreted by granules in the atria of the heart. This secretion of ANF occurs with increased intra-atrial pressure and leads to an unloading effect on the heart by causing an increase in glomerular filtration rate, natriuresis, and vasodilation. ANF reduces renin secretion, blocks aldosterone secretion, opposes the vasoconstrictive effects of angiotensin II, and opposes the salt-retaining effect of aldosterone. ANF antagonizes vasoconstriction caused by vasopressin, angiotensin II, and catecholamines. Understanding of the role ANF may play in the pathogenesis of hypertension remains incomplete [10].

Neurogenic Factors

The autonomic nervous system is intimately involved with blood pressure regulation. Baroreceptors in the carotid sinus and aorta, as well as stretch receptors in the cardiac atria and great veins, provide information to the medulla in the brain about circulatory dynamics. Efferent sympathetic discharge controls constriction of resistance and capacitance vessels, cardiac output, and even the release of hormones such as catecholamines from the adrenal gland and renin from the kidney.

Despite the clear role of the autonomic nervous system in normal blood pressure regulation, a precise role for disordered nervous system regulation in most hypertensive states has not been found. It has been argued, however, that some patients labeled as having essential hypertension in fact have neurogenic hypertension [6]. These patients are characterized by adrenergic cardiovascular excitement with increased heart rate, cardiac index, total peripheral resistance, and shortened pre-ejection index. Plasma norepinephrine concentration in this group is high, although not so high as characteristically seen in association with pheochromocytoma.

Primary Vascular Factors

Intrinsic characteristics of the blood vessels themselves are important in blood pressure control, because of their influence on peripheral vascular resistance. The capacitance of the vascular tree is reduced as a consequence of aging, and this reduced distensibility of vessels will tend to cause an elevation of blood pressure. Although pressor substances tend to increase vasomotor tone, the responsiveness of the vessels to these substances is variable and not completely understood. It is now thought that the potent vasoconstrictor angiotensin II is produced locally in vessel walls and is important in local organ perfusion as well as overall blood pressure control. Catecholamines, vasopressin, prostaglandins, and bradykinins are among the various modulators of vascular tone. Factors that seem to alter the reactivity of vessel walls are the sodium and water content and the calcium content of the vessel wall itself [8].

Miscellaneous Humoral Factors

Glucocorticoid is necessary for normal function of the neurocirculatory homeostatic mechanisms. Hypotension occurs in instances in which there is primary glucocorticoid deficiency. Glucocorticoid excess, such as in Cushing's syndrome and adrenocorticotropic hormone (ACTH)–secreting tumors, is often associated with hypertension. Adrenal mineralocorticoids, primarily aldosterone, are needed for the maintenance of normal sodium balance. Hypertension secondary to mineralocorticoid excess occurs in primary aldosteronism due to an adrenal adenoma or hyperplasia or to 11-hydroxylase or 17-alpha-hydroxylase deficiency.

Androgens, estrogens, and progesterone-like compounds may affect

Table 16-1. Causes of hypertension

Essential hypertension

Renal hypertension
  Intrinsic renal disease
  Renovascular disease
  Renin-producing tumor

Adrenocorticoid hypertension
  Primary hyperaldosteronism
    Adrenal adenoma
    Bilateral adrenal cortical hyperplasia
  Cushing's syndrome
  Mineralocorticoid excess due to enzyme defects
    11-hydroxylase deficiency
    17-α-hydroxylase deficiency

Pheochromocytoma

Coarctation of the aorta

Toxemia of pregnancy

Oral contraceptives

Hypercalcemia

blood pressure through changes in sodium balance. Furthermore, estrogens may increase renin substrate and cause hypertension.

Although acromegaly may be associated with some increase in blood pressure, the role of growth hormone in blood pressure control has not been well studied. Parathyroid hormone has not been implicated as a regulator of blood pressure; however, ionized plasma calcium is of importance. Hypercalcemia is often associated with an increase in blood pressure. This is thought to represent either a direct effect of calcium on vascular smooth muscle or possibly a result of renin release stimulated by hypercalcemia.

CAUSES OF HYPERTENSION

Table 16-1 lists the causes of hypertension. Although the majority of patients with hypertension have what has been termed *essential hypertension,* secondary causes of hypertension must be considered in each patient. A decision regarding what studies to perform in a particular patient will be dependent on the patient's age, the presence of target-organ damage, the severity of hypertension, at times the response to medical therapy, and clues from the history and physical examination regarding the possibility of a secondary cause of hypertension. It is beyond the scope of this chapter to discuss the tests to be performed to exclude all such causes.

THERAPEUTIC CONSIDERATIONS IN HYPERTENSION

Goals of Therapy

The treatment of the patient with hypertension who does not have immediate complications is aimed at maintaining a sustained lowering of blood pressure to prevent the long-term cardiovascular consequences of uncontrolled hypertension. Because of limitations in the medical therapy of hypertension, often it is not possible to normalize blood pressure in all positions and under all circumstances. One should attempt, however, to maintain a diastolic blood pressure less than 90 to 100 mm Hg in the standing position. Therapy can generally be initiated on an ambulatory basis unless a hypertensive emergency exists. The latter requires hospitalization and often initiation of therapy with parenterally administered agents.

Renin Profile

Plasma renin activity (PRA) can be stimulated in normal individuals by a low-salt diet, upright posture, or diuretic drug administration. When patients with essential hypertension are compared with normal individuals after a standardized protocol of PRA stimulation, it is possible to identify low-, normal-, and high-renin essential hypertensives [9]. The mechanism accounting for hypertension may be different among these groups, although there may well be heterogeneity within the various groups.

There is no convincing evidence at present that renin has prognostic value or is a risk factor for end-organ complications independently of the degree of hypertension. Furthermore, renin profiling appears to be of limited value in guiding therapy by predicting response to various antihypertensive drugs [18]. For these reasons, empiric antihypertensive therapy in essential hypertension remains an acceptable standard of care.

Practical Therapeutic Principles

The patient with routine essential hypertension should be treated with the smallest dose of the fewest drugs possible to control blood pressure. The use of drug combinations in which small doses of each drug are used has a rationale if side effects are minimized by limiting the drug dose. In addition, one drug may enhance the action of another by blocking compensatory mechanisms that would otherwise come into play to limit blood pressure control. Consideration should be given to drug cost and convenience of administration, which are important factors in compliance with a long-term drug therapy program.

At times a patient may have a medical problem in addition to hypertension that might be treatable with an antihypertensive medication. The choice of treatment might be influenced by the possibility of treating two conditions with a single agent. Examples of this would be the use of a calcium blocker and/or β-blocker in a patient with migraine headaches or angina, or a diuretic in a patient who retains sodium.

HYPERTENSIVE CRISES

Definition

Marked elevation of blood pressure to levels greater than 200/120 mm Hg requires immediate attention. The urgency of the situation will be determined by a combination of the absolute level of blood pressure elevation and the clinical state of the patient [5]. An emergency exists if the severely hypertensive patient is encephalopathic, pregnant with toxemia, having acute myocardial ischemia and/or congestive heart failure, having an aortic dissection, or evolving a hemorrhagic or nonhemorrhagic stroke.

The choice of therapy will be dictated by the clinician's view of whether the situation is semi-emergent or represents a true emergency. Monitoring capabilities may play a role in the medication utilized, since intravenous infusion therapy will require an intensive care unit and, optimally, an arterial line for continuous blood pressure monitoring. Bolus intravenous drug therapy, sublingual medications, or oral medications are alternatives depending upon the clinical state of the patient. Newer medications have offered more alternatives in treatment of hypertension (Tables 16-2 and 16-3).

Encephalopathy

Hypertensive encephalopathy is a syndrome of diffuse cerebral dysfunction characterized by headache, somnolence, and sometimes coma and convulsions. Localizing sensory or motor defects may occur, but by definition they will be fleeting rather than fixed. Ultimately the diagnosis is confirmed by return to normal neurologic status after blood pressure is controlled.

Cerebral vessels normally are able to autoregulate by constriction to maintain blood flow constant; when blood pressure rises, cerebrovascular resistance rises. At some point, however, autoregulation fails as blood pressure rises and vasoconstriction cannot be maintained. Hyperperfusion occurs and results in cerebral edema. Initially this occurs in localized areas, but later it becomes diffuse and produces global cerebral dysfunction.

Chronically hypertensive individuals develop hypertrophy of arteriolar walls and are better able to autoregulate cerebrovascular resistance as blood pressure rises [13]. For this reason, hypertensive encephalopathy is more likely to develop in acutely hypertensive individuals and may appear at levels of blood pressure well tolerated by chronic hypertensives. Acute glomerulonephritis, toxemia of pregnancy, and ingestion of tyramine-containing foods by individuals taking monoamine oxidase inhibitors are three hypertensive disorders arising acutely in previously normotensive individuals that are frequently associated with encephalopathy.

Malignant Hypertension

Malignant hypertension is a clinical diagnosis made when severely elevated blood pressure, virtually always in excess of 125 to 135 mm Hg diastolic, has caused acute hypertensive retinopathy manifested by hemorrhages, exudates, and papilledema. Renal end-organ involvement with azotemia, proteinuria, and hematuria or central nervous system involvement with hypertensive encephalopathy may coexist [12]. A semantic distinction may be made and the disorder termed *accelerated hypertension* when papilledema is absent but other features are present. The pathologic and clinical features are perhaps best considered as a continuum.

Hypertension of any etiology, either essential or secondary, may enter into an accelerated or malignant phase. Essential hypertension is the most common underlying disorder. Once a malignant phase is entered, the hypertension is self-perpetuating and will be fatal if not treated.

The pathologic hallmark of malignant hypertension is fibrinoid necrosis

Table 16-2. Preferred pharmacologic agents in hypertensive crises

	Nitroprusside	Labetalol	Nifedipine	Clonidine	Hydralazine	Diuretics	Trimethaphan	β-blockers	Diazoxide	Nitroglycerin	Phentolamine
Malignant ↑ BP and encephalopathy	++++ with β-blockers	+++	+++	++	+	++	++	++++ with nitroprusside or hydralazine	++	No	No
Dissecting aneurysm	++++	?	No	No	No	No	++++	++++ with nitroprusside	No	No	No
↑ BP and cerebral ischemia	++	++	++	No	++	No	No	++	No	No	No
Toxemia of pregnancy	No	++	?	No	++++	No	No	+ with hydralazine	++	No	No
↑ BP and acute heart failure	++++	No	++	?	No	+++++	No	No	No	++	No
↑ BP and myocardial ischemia	++	?	+	No	No	+	+	++	No	++++	No
Catecholamine-related ↑ BP	++++	No	?	+	No	No	No	+++ with nitroprusside	No	No	++++
Autonomic hyperreflexia and ↑ BP	++++	?	?	?	No	No	No	++++ with nitroprusside	No	No	++++

++++ → + most to least desirable agents

Table 16-3. Pharmacologic agents for intravenous therapy for hypertensive crises

Drug	Intravenous dosage		Comments
	Bolus	Continuous	
Sodium nitroprusside		0.5–10.0 µg/kg/min	Parenteral agent of choice when careful titration of BP needed
Labetalol	20 mg/2 min followed by 40–80 mg q 10 min prn; maximum dose 300 mg	2 mg/min until maximum of 300 mg, then oral maintenance	Continuous monitoring not needed; contraindicated when β-blockade not desired
Hydralazine	5–10 mg q 20–30 min	50–150 µg/min	Mostly used for hypertensive crises of pregnancy
Diazoxide	50–100 mg miniboluses q 5–10 min; maximum 150–600 mg		Profound decrease in BP can occur limiting use in patients with cerebral or myocardial ischemia
Nitroglycerin		5 µg/min initial, increase by 5 µg/min increments as needed	Most used in myocardial ischemia
Phentolamine	1–5 mg over 5 min		Most used in catecholamine-related crises, although nitroprusside equally effective in this setting
Methyldopa	250–500 mg q 6–8 hours		Slow onset of action (2–4 hr) and sedation limit its use
Diuretics Furosemide Ethacrynic acid Butethamide	20–200 mg q 4–6 hours 50–100 mg q 4–6 hours 0.5–5 mg q 4 hours		Rapid onset of action useful; may induce electrolyte imbalance and hypovolemia; larger doses may be needed in renal failure; large doses may cause hearing disturbances

of arterioles. In addition, proliferative endarteritis may be seen. This characteristically affects afferent arterioles in the kidney and leads to glomerular obsolescence. Plasma renin activity is commonly elevated in malignant hypertension, sometimes to very high levels. The renin-angiotensin system may perpetuate the hypertension; however, activation of this system does not appear to be necessary to initiate malignant hypertension. Aldosterone levels are high, and hypokalemia often results.

Clinically, patients with malignant hypertension are likely to have pulmonary edema from high cardiac afterload. Neurologic manifestations may be prominent. In some patients, oliguric renal failure with uremia may be present when the patient is seen initially. Microangiopathic hemolytic anemia related to microvascular disease is often present and may contribute to the renal failure.

Therapy of hypertensive encephalopathy and malignant hypertension is urgent blood pressure reduction to prevent life-threatening complications. Blood pressure need not be reduced to normal levels initially to control end-organ involvement. Anecdotal reports of stroke and myocardial infarction associated with blood pressure reduction below systolic pressures of 130 mm Hg suggest that reduction in blood pressure to the range of 150 to 160/100 mm Hg may be an appropriate goal for the first several days.

The definition of a hypertensive emergency relates not only to the blood pressure itself, but to evidence of new or progressive end-organ damage. Elevated blood pressure alone rarely requires urgent therapy. Parenteral and oral agents used for therapy of hypertensive emergencies are listed in Tables 16-2 and 16-3.

Because hypertensive patients retain sodium when blood pressure is reduced, diuretics are often necessary adjuncts in drug therapy. With the advent of angiotensin-converting enzyme inhibitors and calcium-channel blockers, the need for diuretics has become less necessary in some patients. In patients with malignant hypertension who have edema from heart or renal failure at the time of presentation, diuresis with a rapid-acting potent diuretic such as furosemide may be essential to normalize expanded plasma volume so that blood pressure can be controlled. There appears to be, however, a subset of patients with malignant hypertension who are characterized by intravascular volume depletion, probably related to augmented renal sodium excretion induced by severe systemic hypertension. These patients may have high plasma renin activity and may have tachycardia, postural hypotension, and signs of enhanced sympathetic tone (diaphoresis, tremor). Diuretic administration may actually make hypertension more difficult to control in these patients, presumably because further renin release and sympathetic stimulation are produced.

Renal function must be evaluated at the onset of therapy and followed very carefully. As blood pressure is lowered, there may be a decrease in renal function. At times the impairment will be transient and improvement in renal function will occur as blood pressure is maintained under control. Dialysis may be needed transiently or permanently after blood pressure reduction, but overall patient survival is promoted by maintenance of controlled blood pressure.

Acute Dissecting Aneurysm of the Aorta

Emergency medical treatment of dissecting aneurysm of the aorta is based on the objective of reducing blood pressure to diminish pulsatile forces within the aorta while maintaining perfusion to vital organs [16]. When clinical features suggest acute aortic dissection, radiographic studies are required to confirm the diagnosis. However, blood pressure should be controlled while diagnostic studies are in progress.

Dissecting aneurysms carry a major risk of causing aortic rupture, occlusion of arteries arising from the aorta, and aortic insufficiency. As blood pressure is controlled, with a systolic blood pressure of 100 to 120 mm Hg or lower as tolerated, disappearance of the tearing pain that follows the course of the aorta correlates with limitation of dissection.

Medical control of blood pressure should be attempted only with agents that decrease the pulsatile forces within the aorta while maintaining perfusion of vital organs. Agents meeting these criteria include trimethaphan, which is an adrenergic blocker; a combination of propranolol and nitroprusside; and labetalol. If nitroprusside is used, the patient should initially have a beta blocker to block reflex adrenergic effects on the heart. Labetalol may be a suitable alternative because of its blockade of α_1- and β-receptors. However, its prolonged duration of action and limited experience with this agent in this condition should be considered.

When the diagnosis is established, the decision regarding medical versus surgical management must take into account the success rate of surgical intervention in the institution in which the operation is to be done. In many centers, surgical therapy is carried out for acute dissection when there are no medical contraindications and when the origin of the dissection can be identified. Surgical therapy must, of course, be undertaken when there is acute aortic insufficiency, rupture of the aneurysm, or occlusion of a vital artery. Furthermore, surgical management appears to be more satisfactory than medical treatment when the dissection is in the proximal aorta just distal to the aortic valve. In distal dissection beyond the origin of the left subclavian artery, the results of medical and surgical therapy appear to be about the same.

Medical therapy is indicated for patients who are not suitable candidates for surgery because of advanced age or superimposed medical illness, particularly chronic obstructive pulmonary disease. Furthermore, if the dissection began more than 2 weeks before the patient is first seen, the therapy will often be pharmacologic lowering of blood pressure.

Drug therapy is initiated with continuous infusion of an agent that will lower systolic blood pressure to 90 to 130 mm Hg and diastolic blood pressure to 60 to 80 mm Hg. An excellent combination therapy for acute aortic dissection is intravenous propranolol and a nitroprusside drip. Propranolol reduces the rate of increase of left ventricular pressure during systole ("shearing" force) and reduces cardiac output. Propranolol can be given intravenously in a dose of 1 mg every 5 minutes until the heart rate is reduced to 60 to 80 beats per minute. With monitoring of heart rate subsequent therapy can be given orally in doses of 40 to 80 mg every 6 hours unless bradycardia requires a lower dose. Nitroprusside infusion can be titrated to lower arterial pressure by vasodilation. An alternative means of therapy would include infusion of the ganglionic blocking agent trimethaphan in a dose of 1 mg/min, which as a single agent reduces the rate of rise of left ventricular pressures and reduces afterload by neuronal blockade. A third alternative for therapy would include labetalol infusion at a rate of 1 to 3 mg/min or intravenous boluses of 20 to 80 mg as needed. The latter agent provides a combination of α- and β-blockade.

Stroke

Patients with severe hypertension who have markedly lateralizing fixed neurologic signs usually have cerebrovascular thrombosis or intracranial hemorrhage rather than hypertensive encephalopathy. In both circumstances blood pressure reduction must be undertaken carefully [4].

Cerebrovascular thrombosis appears to impair cerebral blood flow autoregulation. Thus, hypertension may lead to hyperperfusion and cerebral edema, whereas systemic hypotension could enhance ischemic damage. Reduction of systolic pressure to no lower than 160 mm Hg is a reasonable goal in thrombotic stroke. Agents used to treat excessive hypertension in this setting should not lead to reduced cerebral perfusion. Labetalol infusions of 2 mg/min or less do not reduce cerebral perfusion and may be useful in this setting. Nifedipine appears to maintain normal cerebral flow. However, there are potential risks involved in using an oral or sublingual medication that might cause an unpredictably excessive fall in blood pressure in a patient in an unstable state of cerebral circulation. Hydralazine has been used for many years and has the advantage of not reducing cardiac output or cerebral perfusion. Clonidine and trimethaphan lead to reduced cerebral perfusion. There is concern that nitroprusside may shunt blood away from ischemic tissue.

Both intracerebral hemorrhage and ruptured intracranial aneurysm are more likely to occur in the setting of hypertension. However, raised intracranial pressure from hemorrhage may lead to reflex hypertension. It is possible that to some extent this is a protective mechanism to restore blood flow. The optimal blood pressure in such clinical circumstances has not been defined.

A 20 to 30 percent reduction in systolic blood pressure in the setting of intracranial hemorrhage in patients with a systolic blood pressure greater than 200 mm Hg is generally recommended. Patients with less severe hypertension should have blood pressure reduced toward a goal of 160/100 mm Hg.

Toxemia of Pregnancy

Hypertension may complicate pregnancy and increase perinatal mortality. Women with underlying hypertension, as well as those with chronic renal disease, are susceptible to marked worsening of hypertension associated with pregnancy. Some women, particularly primigravidas, may develop toxemia of pregnancy in the last trimester, characterized by hypertension and proteinuria. This disorder may progress to oliguria, neuromuscular irritability, and convulsions (eclampsia). The precise pathogenesis is unknown, although relative uteroplacental hypoperfusion is believed to be involved. The pregnant individual may be more susceptible to end-organ damage from hypertension.

Toxemia is treated in the hospital with bed rest. Magnesium sulfate may be useful in reducing neuromuscular irritability. Drug therapy is needed to counter the intense vasoconstriction if blood pressure does not fall steadily with bed rest alone. The main concern with lowering blood pressure is a possible decrease in uteroplacental perfusion [11].

Hydralazine has been used extensively in treating hypertensive pregnant patients. It should be used in small doses by intravenous bolus or continuous infusion. Although it generally enhances uteroplacental flow, in some instances reduced perfusion may occur, with fetal distress being induced. Furthermore, as in other instances, tachycardia may limit its use as monotherapy. Intravenous labetalol has also proven to be useful and relatively safe, and it may enhance uteroplacental circulation. The resistant patient may be managed with intravenous miniboluses of diazoxide. Nifedipine is effective in lowering blood pressure, but its safety at the time of this writing is not firmly established. Nitroprusside is generally not recommended in this setting, because of concerns about increased uteroplacental perfusion and cyanide toxicity in mother and fetus.

Ganglionic blockers may reduce uterine blood flow, as well as produce meconium ileus in the fetus, and thus are contraindicated. Because of depletion of effective intravascular volume in toxemia, as well as evidence of adverse effects on placental circulation, diuretics are generally not recommended in modern obstetric practice. Hypertension in toxemia resolves when the uterus is evacuated. Patients ill with toxemia with diastolic pressures greater than 100 mm Hg who fail to improve with drug therapy after 24 hours should have pregnancy terminated. If blood pressure and proteinuria improve with drug therapy in the hospital, it may be possible to allow gestation to continue to term.

Acute Pulmonary Edema

Although the initial therapy of pulmonary edema in the patient with an elevated blood pressure should continue to be the use of tourniquets, morphine, intermittent positive-pressure breathing, diuretics, and at times digitalization, there is a place for reduction in arterial pressure. Frequently, improvement in pulmonary edema following the onset of diuresis will be accompanied by a prompt reduction in blood pressure. However, when blood pressure remains elevated, reducing the afterload by reducing diastolic blood pressure may be effective in improving the acute left heart failure. The drug of choice for prompt reduction in blood pressure in these instances is intravenous sodium nitroprusside. This drug has the additional advantage of reducing cardiac preload because of its effect on venous capacitance vessels.

In patients with myocardial ischemia, there is concern that coronary artery vasodilation with nitroprusside may lead to shunting of blood from ischemic areas. If ischemia is evident, the patient can be treated with intravenous nitroglycerin, which causes potent venodilation with reduction in preload. In contrast to nitroprusside, this agent increases blood flow to ischemic tissues.

Reduction of preload and afterload is of key importance in the emergency and long-term therapy of the patient with impaired myocardial reserve. Angiotensin-converting enzyme inhibitors are the most effective unloading agents for chronic therapy. Therapy can be started with small doses of captopril orally (usually 6.25 mg) or with intravenous or oral doses of enalaprilat or enalapril in doses of 1.25 or 2.5 mg, respectively. Excessive hypotensive responses to angiotensin-converting enzyme inhibitors and adverse effects on glomerular filtration rate may occur. The latter tends to occur in patients with renal artery occlusive disease. In patients who cannot tolerate angiotensin-converting enzyme inhibitors, hydralazine or prazocin may be useful as unloading agents to prevent pulmonary vascular congestion.

CATECHOLAMINE-INDUCED HYPERTENSIVE CRISES
Pheochromocytoma
Paroxysms of hypertension in pheochromocytoma can be treated by specific therapy in the form of a potent α-blocker such as phentolamine. Alternatively, sodium nitroprusside works equally well. Long-term management requires excision of the hormone-producing tumor or use of a long-term α- and possibly β-blocker, such as phenoxybenzamine (Dibenzyline) and propranolol, respectively.

Drug Withdrawal Syndromes
Sympathetic overactivity can occur as a consequence of sudden cessation of clonidine, methyldopa, and guanabenz. Catecholamines that are stored in nerve endings are suddenly released if the medication is suddenly stopped.

Mild symptoms can be treated by simply restarting the prior medication. In extreme cases, nitroprusside and phentolamine can be used.

Monoamine Oxidase Inhibitors and Tyramines
Intracellular norepinephrine, epinephrine, and dopamine accumulate in storage granules in nerve endings when patients are treated with monoamine oxidase (MAO) inhibitors. Ingestion of tyramine-rich foods in patients taking MAO inhibitors can lead to an outpouring of norepinephrine that can cause a severe hypertensive crisis with symptoms that mimic a pheochromocytoma. Foods capable of inducing such a state are certain natural or aged cheeses, chocolate, coffee, soy sauce, pickled herring, certain beers, Chianti wine, yeast, chicken liver, avocados, broad bean pods, bananas, fermented sausage, and canned figs [2].

Symptoms occur within 2 hours of consumption of the offending agent and may last from minutes to as long as 6 hours.

Therapy is directed at vasodilation to reduce the blood pressure and to block cardiac arrhythmias that may occur. Infusions of sodium nitroprusside or phentolamine are effective in controlling blood pressure, and β-blockers are effective in blocking cardiac effects. β-blockers should not be used alone, since this may cause further increases in blood pressure.

AUTONOMIC HYPERREFLEXIA

An unusual type of hypertensive crisis can be seen in quadriplegic patients with spinal cord lesions above T6. Paroxysmal attacks of hypertension associated with headaches, facial flushing, sweating, and bradycardia are seen. Episodes can be triggered by bowel or bladder distention, or by certain cutaneous stimuli. The pathophysiology of the disorder relates to sympathetic discharge that is not modulated sufficiently by higher centers in the nervous system. Favorable results have been achieved treating this condition with sodium nitroprusside, trimethaphan, or phentolamine.

ANTIHYPERTENSIVE DRUGS

Following is a discussion of the main antihypertensive drugs (see Tables 16-2 and 16-3).

Sodium Nitroprusside

Sodium nitroprusside has many characteristics that make it an ideal drug for hypertensive emergencies. The drug acts specifically to relax vascular smooth muscle in arterial resistance, as well as venous capacitance beds. It is direct-acting and not mediated by the nervous system, so neither sedation nor ganglionic blockade occurs. Its onset of action is within 1 to 2 minutes, and the effect of the drug disappears rapidly when infusion is discontinued. For this reason careful dosage titration—ideally, guided by direct intra-arterial pressure monitoring—is essential. With remarkable predictability, blood pressure of any magnitude can be titrated to an optimal level at the desired rate.

Nitroprusside has been used with success in the treatment of malignant hypertension and hypertensive encephalopathy. Since both cardiac preload and afterload are reduced, the drug is useful in acute pulmonary edema when hypertension is present. Since it does not result in reflex cardiac stimulation, nitroprusside has an advantage over other direct-acting vasodilators in this setting. As noted previously, combined with propranolol to achieve myocardial depression, nitroprusside has been used successfully in the medical management of acute aortic dissection.

Dosage

The drug is available as a powder that can be diluted with sterile dextrose in water. The usual rate of infusion varies from 0.5 to 8.0 μg/kg/min. Patients on other antihypertensive agents may be very sensitive to the antihypertensive action of nitroprusside.

Side Effects

Prolonged administration of sodium nitroprusside can result in the accumulation of thiocyanate formed in the liver from cyanide liberated by the interaction of nitroprusside with sulfhydryl groups in red cells and tissue proteins. Nausea, fatigue, muscle twitching, and disorientation have occurred in association with elevated thiocyanate levels. If the drug is to be continued beyond 3 days, or if renal function is impaired, serum thiocyanate levels should be monitored. The drug should be discontinued if levels exceed 10 to 12 mg per 100 ml. A case of hypothyroidism associated with long-term nitroprusside administration has been reported.

Diazoxide

Diazoxide is a nondiuretic thiazide derivative that is a potent, rapid-acting vasodilator. Almost instantly after intravenous injection arterial pressure falls rapidly to normal. Hypotensive overshoot is rare. Blood pressure may remain depressed for as long as 5 hours after a single dose. The subsequent rise in blood pressure is gradual and predictable.

Diazoxide acts directly on arteriolar smooth muscle to reduce vascular resistance. The drug has little effect on venous capacitance vessels and does not impair cardiovascular autonomic reflexes. Thus, the barorecep-tors are activated as pressure falls, and a reflex increase occurs in heart rate, cardiac output, and left ventricular ejection velocity.

Hypertensive emergencies, including hypertensive encephalopathy, have been treated with diazoxide. The advantage of rapid action without the requirement for constant patient monitoring after treatment may be a tac-tical consideration in some situations. The drug should not be used in the treatment of aortic dissection or intracranial hemorrhage, because of the danger of augmented mechanical shearing forces induced by the reflex cardiac response. Since the drug does not reduce cardiac preload, it is less useful than nitroprusside for the treatment of pulmonary edema associated with severe hypertension. Angina and myocardial infarction have been precipitated with diazoxide, presumably related either to increased myo-cardial oxygen demands resulting from reflex cardiac stimulation or to de-creased coronary perfusion from abrupt blood pressure reduction. The drug should not be used in the setting of ischemic heart disease.

Dosage

The drug is given with the patient supine, with doses of 50 to 150 mg intravenous boluses every 10 minutes until the desired effect is achieved. The usual cumulative dose is 200 to 300 mg. Because diazoxide binds read-ily to plasma proteins, rapid injection produces higher levels of free drug to reach and activate arteriolar receptors.

Side Effects

Diazoxide will cause severe pain and cellulitis if extravasated during rapid injection. In addition to potential adverse effects related to rapid blood pressure lowering and cardiac stimulation, the drug commonly produces hyperglycemia and hyperuricemia. Renal sodium retention occurs with the drug; loop-acting diuretics such as furosemide are indicated when the drug is used.

Nitroglycerin

Intravenous nitroglycerin acts as a vasodilator, with venodilation being more prominent at lower doses and accompanying arterial dilation at higher doses. Regional blood flow in the myocardium is improved with nitroglycerin, which thus is thought to be more beneficial than nitroprus-side in patients having acute myocardial ischemia and hypertension [3].

Dosage

Intravenous nitroglycerin has an onset of action within minutes and a half-life of 1 to 4 minutes. The dosage ranges from 25 to 300 μg per minute using polyvinyl chloride (PVC) tubing, which absorbs 40 to 80 percent of the drug. Special infusion sets that absorb only small amounts of drug have been developed that require decreasing to an initial infusion rate of 5 μg per minute and increasing by 5-μg-per-minute increments. If adequate blood pressure control cannot be achieved, a change to nitroprusside may be indicated.

Side Effects

Hypotension is the most important side effect and will be most problematic if the patient is volume-depleted. Other side effects include nausea, restlessness, palpitations, abdominal pain, muscle twitching, and headaches.

Hydralazine

Hydralazine is a direct vasodilator that acts on smooth muscle in arterial resistance vessels. To a much lesser extent, it affects venous capacitance vessels. As peripheral resistance falls, reflex sympathetic stimulation occurs through activation of baroreceptor mechanisms. The resultant increase in cardiac output to some extent diminishes the antihypertensive action of the drug. When combined with a β-adrenergic blocking agent to control cardiac stimulation, the usefulness of hydralazine increases.

Blood flow to vital organs is not decreased by hydralazine. This makes the drug useful in the treatment of hypertension complicated by renal failure or vascular insufficiency—e.g., mesenteric insufficiency. It is particularly useful in toxemia of pregnancy, which, as discussed above, is thought to be related to uteroplacental ischemia. The tachycardia and increased velocity of cardiac contraction that occur with hydralazine prevent the drug's use as sole therapy in patients with ischemic heart disease or acute aortic aneurysm dissection.

Dosage

The blood pressure response to intramuscular or intravenous hydralazine is variable and occasionally results in sustained hypotension after a 10-mg dose. The intravenous route is preferable, because absorption from intramuscular sites is too variable. The onset of action is 10 to 30 minutes, and the duration is 3 to 9 hours. In hypertensive crises of pregnancy, various centers have treated the patients with intermittent intravenous bolus therapy or infusion. Initially an intravenous bolus of 5 mg may be used, followed by boluses of 5 to 10 mg every 20 to 30 minutes until the desired blood pressure is achieved. Others have used a slow infusion of 15 to 40 mg over 60 to 90 minutes until the desired blood pressure is achieved. Since patients with toxemia tend to be hypovolemic, it is necessary to monitor blood pressure closely to avoid excessive hypotension. An infusion can be mixed with 100 mg in 250 ml of one-half normal saline to yield 400 μg/ml. After initial loading, a maintenance infusion of 50 to 150 μg/min. is generally satisfactory to control the blood pressure in most instances, although lower doses may be desirable in preeclamptic patients.

Side Effects
Hydralazine used alone is limited by adverse effects. Throbbing headache, palpitations, and nausea may occur. These effects can be reduced by gradual upward titration of drug dosage and by concomitant administration of β-adrenergic blocking drugs.

Long-term oral use of hydralazine has been associated with drug fever, skin rash, and peripheral neuropathy. These appear more frequently with higher doses or in patients who are slow acetylators of the drug. Doses in excess of 300 to 400 mg per day sustained for several months have been associated with a lupuslike syndrome. Lupus erythematosus (LE) cells may appear in the blood, and an elevated antinuclear antibody titer may persist for several years. The syndrome is generally reversible when the drug is withdrawn, although resolution may be slow or may require corticosteroid therapy.

Methyldopa
The antihypertensive action of methyldopa was originally attributed to dopa decarboxylase inhibition, resulting in decreased norepinephrine stores at nerve terminals. This explanation has proved inadequate. Methyldopa appears to act by conversion in the central nervous system to α-methylnorepinephrine, which exerts a direct α-sympathomimetic inhibitory action upon a brain stem vasomotor center. Blood pressure falls because of a decrease in peripheral vascular resistance. Renal perfusion is maintained. Cardiac output is not substantially affected. Plasma renin activity falls.

Use of methyldopa for hypertensive emergencies is limited by its sedative properties, delayed onset of action, and variable effectiveness. It is of use in settings in which blood pressure control can safely be delayed for 4 or more hours and in which drug-induced somnolence will not be confused with progression of an underlying neurologic condition. Relative freedom from adverse cardiac effects offers an advantage in the use of methyldopa in situations such as myocardial infarction. It is useful in patients who by necessity have abruptly been withdrawn from clonidine.

Dosage
Gastrointestinal absorption of methyldopa varies. Maximal effects are seen 4 to 8 hours after intravenous administration. The daily dose ranges from 500 to 3000 mg given in divided doses. Patients with impaired renal function should be started on smaller doses—i.e., 250 to 500 mg daily—because of reduced clearance of the drug. Because of the fluid retention, refractoriness to methyldopa will often occur with continued use. For this reason, the drug should be administered with a diuretic agent.

Side Effects
Common side effects are drowsiness, nasal congestion, and dry mouth. Less frequent reactions are Coombs' positive anemia, fever, hepatitis, and impotence.

β-*Adrenergic Blocking Agents*

Propranolol in low doses has a modest antihypertensive effect that can be correlated with the degree of renin suppression produced. At higher doses, blood pressure is lowered independently of changes in plasma renin activity by what is theorized to be a central nervous system effect. In addition, β-adrenergic blockers allow utilization of vasodilators such as hydralazine and minoxidil at doses that might otherwise lead to intolerable symptoms related to reflex cardiac stimulation. By preventing a secondary rise in cardiac output, β-adrenergic blockers potentiate the antihypertensive effects of vasodilators.

Dosage

Propranolol, or its equivalent, can be initiated at doses of 40 mg per day and titrated upward to 480 mg per day in 2 or 3 divided doses if required, or administered as the sustained release formulation.

Side Effects

Adverse effects of β-adrenergic blocking agents include symptomatic bradycardia. Congestive heart failure may be precipitated. Patients with decreased cardiac function in whom cardiac output is maintained by intense sympathetic tone are at the greatest risk for precipitation of congestive heart failure. Bronchospasm may occur even in those not previously diagnosed as asthmatic. Intermittent claudication may worsen in patients with peripheral vascular disease, presumably because of unopposed α-adrenergic vasoconstriction.

Mental depression, gastrointestinal disturbances, and Peyronie's disease have been reported with propranolol. The drug should be withdrawn gradually, since sudden withdrawal of propranolol has been reported to provoke angina pectoris in patients with ischemic heart disease.

A variety of newer cardioselective β-blockers are available which cause less blockade of the β_2-receptors of the bronchi and blood vessels. Some of the newer β-blockers have less central nervous system penetration with lower brain lipid solubility, thus causing fewer central nervous system side effects.

Ganglioplegic Agents

Ganglioplegic drugs are potent antihypertensive agents, but their use is limited by side effects. They reduce transmission of nerve impulses through the ganglia of the autonomic nervous system by interfering with the action of acetylcholine on the ganglionic cells. The major antihypertensive action of these drugs is to inhibit venous capacitance vessels from constricting and thus to reduce venous return. Cardiac output falls because sympathetic reflexes are blocked.

Unpleasant side effects related to parasympathetic and sympathetic blockade have caused these drugs virtually to disappear from use in the treatment of chronic hypertension. The most rapidly acting ganglionic blocking agent, trimethaphan camsylate, has some use in certain acute settings. Because it reduces cardiac output, blood pressure, and cardiac contractility, it is useful as a single agent in the treatment of acute aortic dissection. Its use should never continue beyond several days.

Dosage
Trimethaphan camsylate is supplied in a 10-ml multidose vial containing 50 mg/ml. One vial should be diluted to 500 ml with 5% D/W to yield a concentration of 1 mg trimethaphan per milliliter. The solution should be administered intravenously at a rate of 0.5 to 5.0 mg/min and titrated to achieve the desired drop in blood pressure. The onset of action is immediate, and the hypotensive effect of the drug disappears quickly when the infusion is discontinued. The blood pressure may fluctuate rapidly, so the rate of administration and blood pressure must be monitored constantly. The patient should be placed in reverse Trendelenburg's position with the head of the bed on blocks to allow gravity to increase venous pooling.

Side Effects
Side effects of autonomic blockade include dry mouth, blurred vision, constipation or paralytic ileus, impotence, and urinary retention. The drug is contraindicated in respiratory insufficiency and glaucoma.

Clonidine
Clonidine is a centrally acting drug of moderate potency available for oral administration. The drug appears to activate receptors in a cardiovascular control center in the medulla oblongata, resulting in a decrease in sympathetic neuronal stimulation of the heart, kidney, and peripheral vasculature. Renin release is decreased because of depressed adrenergic tone to the juxtaglomerular apparatus through the renal nerves.

Clonidine has an onset of action within 30 minutes after administration. It often is used with a diuretic agent to prevent fluid retention and loss of antihypertensive effectiveness. The action of clonidine is additive to that of a vasodilator and β-adrenergic blocking agent combination.

Dosage
Oral clonidine can be used for rapid reduction of blood pressure in a semi-emergency situation in which it is felt that blood pressure control can be achieved within a few hours rather than within minutes, as may be achieved with other agents [1]. Clonidine can be given with an initial oral dose of 0.1 to 0.2 mg, followed by 3 to 4 further doses if needed at 2-hour intervals. A number of patients may have an exaggerated hypotensive response that may require volume and/or pressors for blood pressure support.

After initial blood pressure control, long-term therapy can be undertaken, with clonidine being given primarily at bedtime (to minimize side effects); alternatively, transdermal clonidine can be used. The slow onset of action of the transdermal preparation makes it unsuitable for emergency situations.

Side Effects
Sedation and dry mouth are the major dose-related adverse effects of clonidine. Impotence and orthostatic hypotension occur with a frequency similar to that observed with methyldopa.

Patients should not abruptly discontinue clonidine therapy. Blood pressure may rise rapidly to pretreatment levels and possibly higher. A syndrome of adrenergic overactivity has been described after clonidine discontinuation. The syndrome can be treated by reinstitution of clonidine or by α-adrenergic blocking agents such as phentolamine. Clonidine is best avoided in unreliable patients. To prevent occurrence of this adrenergic overactivity in the perioperative period, clonidine should be withdrawn gradually prior to elective surgical procedures that will prohibit oral administration of clonidine. Alternatively, the postoperative patient can be managed with transdermal clonidine.

Prazocin
Prazocin is a quinazoline derivative that results in vasodilation through peripheral α-adrenergic blockade. Reflex tachycardia does not occur. Prazocin has been used in combination with a diuretic in mild-to-moderate hypertension. It has been used in association with a β-adrenergic blocking agent in more severe hypertension and has been shown to have an effectiveness similar to hydralazine in this role.

Dosage
To avoid a first-dose effect of syncope probably related to orthostatic hypotension, the drug should be initiated at a dose of 1 mg at a time when the patient can remain supine for at least 3 hours—e.g., bedtime. Dosage titration should be gradual to a maximum of 20 mg per day in 2 divided doses.

Side Effects
Postural hypotension with syncope, drowsiness, weakness, and anticholinergic effects may limit the use of prazocin.

α-Adrenergic Blocking Agents
Phentolamine is an α-adrenergic blocker that is used in the treatment of hypertensive crisis in the setting of pheochromocytoma. It may also be useful in therapy of hypertensive crisis associated with tyramine ingestion in patients taking MAO inhibitors and in the hypertension of clonidine withdrawal.

The drug is given intravenously in a dose of 2 to 5 mg every 5 minutes until the blood pressure is controlled. The head of the bed should be elevated. If tachycardia produces symptoms, β-adrenergic blockers can be used. However, β-adrenergic blockers should not be used alone because blood pressure may become further elevated due to unopposed α-adrenergic vasoconstriction.

Phenoxybenzamine can be given at a dose of 20 mg per day in 2 divided doses as an oral α-adrenergic blocker. Doses can be titrated upward slowly; the drug has a prolonged half-life and tends to accumulate. Phenoxybenzamine is used for the treatment of pheochromocytoma during stabilization for surgery or in patients with metastatic pheochomocytoma. It has limited usefulness in the treatment of patients with essential hypertension resistant to conventional therapy.

Minoxidil

Minoxidil is a potent oral vasodilator. It has a direct effect on smooth muscle of arterial resistance vessels. Cardiovascular reflexes are brought into play, and tachycardia and increased cardiac output occur.

Minoxidil is used in combination with propranolol for the treatment of severe hypertension refractory to conventional antihypertensive therapy. This combination will lead to vigorous sodium retention. Diuretics, generally furosemide, are required, sometimes in high doses. The potency of minoxidil exceeds that of hydralazine. In patients with renal disease and refractory hypertension, minoxidil may offer an alternative to bilateral nephrectomy.

In those instances in which it is acceptable to lower blood pressure within hours, therapy can be initiated with oral minoxidil, a β-blocker, and a diuretic. If a β-blocker is contraindicated, clonidine or α-methyldopa can be used to decrease the reflex tachycardia induced by the minoxidil-induced vasodilation.

Dosage

The antihypertensive effect of minoxidil begins in 30 to 60 minutes and reaches a maximum in 2 to 4 hours. In a semi-emergency situation, minoxidil can be initiated in an oral dose of 2.5 mg, followed by doubling of the dose every 6 hours up to a dose of 20 mg per dose until adequate blood pressure control is obtained.

In a nonemergent situation, minoxidil is initiated in doses of 2.5 mg twice daily, with increases of 5 mg per day every 2 to 3 days as needed to a maximum of 40 mg daily. Heart rate and weight must be monitored to allow for proper adjustment in dosages of the sympatholytic agent (usually a β-blocker) and the diuretic (usually a loop diuretic), respectively.

Side Effects

Hirsutism makes the drug almost unusable in the chronic situation in females unless the dose is kept very low. Male patients have few complaints about increased hair growth. Although edema may be a major problem, this is controllable in most instances with the proper amount of diuretic. In rare instances pericardial effusion has been seen with chronic minoxidil therapy. Reflex tachycardia with inadequate sympathetic blockade can lead to palpitations, angina, or an acute myocardial infarction in a susceptible patient.

Calcium-Channel Blockers

The antihypertensive action of calcium-channel blockers results from vasodilation. This effect occurs as a consequence of reduced movement of calcium into cells and the release of calcium from sarcoplasmic reticulum into the cell cytoplasm. Although calcium-channel blockers have some negative inotropic effects, this is more pronounced with verapamil and diltiazem than it is with nifedipine. The diminished afterload from vasodilation with nifedipine results in an increase in cardiac output and a variable tendency toward an increase in heart rate. Intravenous verapamil has been used to reduce blood pressure. However, its use is limited by its negative inotropic effect in patients with impaired cardiac function, and its prolongation of cardiac conduction that can result in varying degrees of heart block. It is used extensively in treating supraventricular arrhythmias but may lower blood pressure excessively in this setting.

Nifedipine is by far the most useful calcium-channel blocker in the treatment of hypertensive emergencies. In many centers, sublingual nifedipine is the treatment of choice for patients requiring prompt reduction of blood pressure. In a sublingual dose blood pressure will fall within 10 to 15 minutes, with a peak response in 15 to 30 minutes and duration of action of 3 to 5 hours. If the effect on blood pressure is inadequate the dose can be repeated in 30 to 60 minutes as needed. Hypotension or too-rapid lowering of blood pressure may occur, especially if the patient is hypovolemic [7].

Although excessive hypotension is unusual with nifedipine, the use of this agent sublingually in a patient with evolving cerebral or coronary ischemia has the disadvantage of not allowing minute-to-minute titration of blood pressure that is possible with drugs, such as nitroprusside, that are continuously infused. Calcium-channel blockers have broad application in the ongoing care of hypertensives. They are well tolerated and appear to be particularly effective in patients 50 years of age and older and in black patients.

Dosage

In an emergency situation, sublingual nifedipine in a dose of 10 to 20 mg may be effective within 10 to 15 minutes, with a peak response in 15 to 30 minutes and a duration of action of up to 6 hours. The dose can be repeated by mouth or sublingually in 30 to 60 minutes until the desired effect is seen. Orally the drug is effective in 1 hour and may be maintained in a dose of 10 to 30 mg every 6 hours.

Long-term therapy with oral verapamil in a dose of 80 to 120 mg every 8 hours or once or twice daily in the form of a sustained-release 240-mg tablet may be effective as monotherapy or with other agents such as diuretics or angiotensin-converting enzyme inhibitors.

Diltiazem is an excellent agent for long-term use but must generally be given in doses of 120 to 360 mg daily in divided doses.

Side Effects

Conduction disturbances, excessive bradycardia, and negative inotropic effect seen primarily with verapamil and diltiazem limit their use in certain patients. Patients with the above problems may do well on nifedipine. Constipation may be a troublesome side effect and is seen mostly with verapamil. Although salt restriction is not necessary for the hypotensive effect of calcium blockers, some patients may develop edema that requires salt restriction and/or diuretics. Palpitations, flushing, and postural hypotension are most common with nifedipine.

Angiotensin-Converting Enzyme Inhibitors

The renin-angiotensin-aldosterone system plays a key role in regional organ perfusion and blood pressure control. Angiotensin-converting enzyme (ACE) converts the inactive angiotensin I to the vasoconstricting and aldosterone-stimulating angiotensin II. Also, ACE also inactivates the vasodilator bradykinin. An ACE inhibitor causes peripheral vasodilation primarily by inhibiting formation of angiotensin II. In states of high plasma renin activity, such as is often seen in accelerated hypertension, an ACE inhibitor may have a particularly dramatic effect upon blood pressure.

Although ACE inhibitors are not regarded as a treatment of choice for hypertensive emergencies, the onset of action is relatively short, making them useful in certain patients when immediate lowering of blood pressure is not needed. Furthermore, for long-term maintenance of the cardiac patient these agents have been the most effective as unloading agents.

The ACE inhibitors must be used with caution in patients with impaired renal function. The intrarenal effects of ACE inhibitors include a loss of autoregulation of glomerular hemodynamics, in that the efferent arteriole is dilated. This leads to a fall in glomerular filtration if there is renal artery occlusive disease. Thus, the patient with intrinsic renal vascular disease may develop azotemia or acute renal failure when placed on an ACE inhibitor.

Maintenance therapy with ACE inhibitors is generally well tolerated and may be effective as monotherapy or may be combined with calcium-channel blockers, diuretics, or β-blockers to augment their effectiveness. They are not very effective when used alone in black patients and may be somewhat less effective in older patients than calcium-channel blockers as monotherapy.

By prevention of glomerular hypertension, ACE inhibitors offer some promise of being useful in prevention of progressive renal insufficiency in patients with glomerular hyperfiltration. This may include patients with diabetes mellitus and certain patients with chronic renal failure.

Dosage

Orally, ACE inhibitors are available as captopril, enalapril, and lisinopril. Captopril has the most rapid onset of action and the shortest half-life. The onset of action of captopril after oral ingestion is 15 minutes, with the dosing interval usually being 1 to 4 times daily. In an unstable cardiac patient, captopril is usually started in a dose of 6.25 to 12.5 mg with careful monitoring of blood pressure to look for excessive hypotension.

The longer-acting enalapril and lisinopril are usually given 1 to 2 times daily. Intravenous enalaprilat is available and is given in a dose of 1.25 to

5.0 mg each 6 hours. Blood pressure reduction in those patients respond-ing occurs with 30 to 60 minutes. Experience with this in hypertensive emergencies is limited.

The predominant renal excretion of ACE inhibitors requires a dose mod-ification in patients with impaired renal function.

Side Effects
By inhibiting aldosterone, ACE inhibitors may cause hyperkalemia, espe-cially in patients with impaired renal function. This may be counteracted by diet, diuretics, or in certain instances, by the use of the ion exchange resin kayexalate.

Chronic cough has been a troublesome side effect in a small group of patients and may require discontinuing the medication.

An unacceptable degree of rise in serum creatinine may require discontinuing the drug, particularly in patients with renal arterial occlu-sive disease. This is generally a reversible problem. Proteinuria with membranous nephropathy has been seen rarely with long-term high-dose captopril therapy.

Neutropenia, rash, fever, and ageusia (with captopril) are unusual side effects that may require discontinuing the drugs.

Labetalol
Labetalol is a unique agent in that it blocks both α- and β-adrenergic re-ceptors. Although it blocks both β_1- and β_2-receptors, there are also some β_2-agonist effects that contribute to peripheral vasodilation. It can be used for therapy of ambulatory patients with mild-to-severe hypertension, and because of rapid onset of action, it is useful as a parenteral agent in hyper-tensive emergencies [17]. It has been reported to be used successfully in patients with hypertension and acute myocardial infarction, dissecting aneurysms, hypertensive emergencies in pregnancy, and hypertensive en-cephalopathy. The ratio of β- to α-blocking potency is 7 : 1 for intravenous labetalol and 3 : 1 for oral labetalol. The primary blood pressure–lowering effect relates mostly to a decrease in systemic vascular resistance without much decrease in cardiac output. Venodilation from α-blockade may con-tribute to the postural hypotension observed with intravenous labetalol.

Dosage
For prompt lowering of blood pressure, intravenous bolus therapy is ini-tiated with 20 mg administered over 2 minutes. The major blood pressure reduction occurs 5 minutes after injection. Additional boluses can be ad-ministered in doses of 40 to 80 mg at 10-minute intervals until a satisfac-tory reduction of blood pressure has been achieved or until a maximal dose of 300 mg has been administered.

With intravenous bolus therapy, blood pressure can usually be satisfac-torily controlled within 30 minutes and will be maintained for 6 hours. When the blood pressure begins to rise, oral labetalol can be initiated in a dose of 200 mg twice daily with a maximal dose of 600 mg twice daily if needed.

An alternative to intravenous bolus therapy is continuous-infusion therapy at 2 mg per minute given until a maximum total dose of 300 mg is given. Then, oral therapy can be initiated as above following bolus therapy.

Side Effects
Intravenous labetalol can lead to hypotension, especially if excessive doses are administered. This may lead to cerebral or cardiac ischemia. Fluid administration will help to restore a more desired blood pressure in this situation. The nonselective β-blockade capacities make the drug contraindicated in bradycardic states, congestive heart failure, heart block, and asthma. Less-critical side effects with intravenous therapy include paresthesias, sweating, dizziness, headaches, flushing, and nausea.

Diuretics
Diuretics, a firmly established component of the management of most hypertensive disorders, are useful in the therapy of patients with mild-to-moderate hypertension and may suffice as single-agent therapy. Diuretics potentiate the effects of most antihypertensive medications. In addition, diuretics can control sodium retention that occurs when blood pressure is reduced with other agents. Sodium retention of this type often leads to recurrence of hypertension after a period of initial blood pressure control.

There is some evidence that thiazide diuretics produce a decrease in peripheral vascular resistance. Interestingly, it is thought that the sodium content of the arteriolar wall may be a factor in determining vascular resistance. It may be that some of the effect diuretics have on peripheral vascular resistance is mediated by a decrease in the sodium content of the vessel wall. The major mode of action of diuretics in hypertensive emergencies, however, stems from the ability of these agents to reduce plasma volume.

Diuretics have their effect by interfering with reabsorption of filtered sodium. Thiazide diuretics work at a site in the distal cortical diluting segment. Furosemide, ethacrynic acid, and butethamide are diuretics with action in the thick ascending limb of Henle's loop. They are of higher potency than thiazides and can be given intravenously. Aldosterone antagonists, triampterine, and amiloride act on the distal nephron to inhibit the reabsorption of sodium and secretion of potassium and hydrogen ions. Since other factors can produce sodium retention even in the absence of aldosterone, agents acting in this segment of the nephron may lack sufficient potency.

Appropriate use of diuretics is an important skill in the management of hypertension, especially of hypertensive emergencies. No predetermined dose of a diuretic may be invariably relied on. The dose of each diuretic must be adjusted on the basis of underlying cardiac and renal function, sodium intake, and clinical evidence of hypervolemia. Assessment of the effect of the diuretic dose must be made by serial evaluation of edema, diuresis, body weight, and orthostatic blood pressure change. Since significant plasma volume expansion may be present and may contribute to hypertension even in the absence of detectable edema, it may be necessary to augment diuretic dosage to achieve a negative sodium balance in a patient who appears refractory to antihypertensive therapy. Observations must then be made to see if blood pressure control improves without the development of diuretic complications. If plasma volume is reduced excessively with diuretics, patients may develop weakness, orthostatic dizziness, and unacceptable degrees of azotemia. In some patients, blood pressure may actually become more labile because of stimulation of the renin-angiotensin system and catecholamines in response to the stress of volume depletion.

The thiazide diuretics all have a similar site of action and at equivalent natiuretic doses have equal antihypertensive action. In mild hypertension a dose of hydrochlorothiazide of 12.5 to 25 mg daily may be satisfactory. At a daily dose of 100 mg of hydrochlorothiazide, the dose-response curve flattens and further dosage increase will add little to blood pressure control. Patients with diastolic blood pressures greater than 100 mm Hg will rarely be controlled with a thiazide diuretic alone.

Metolazone is a unique diuretic that retains its natiuretic potency even when renal function is significantly impaired.

The loop diuretics furosemide, ethacrynic acid, and butethamide have considerable potency as natiuretic agents. The dose of the drug can be titrated upward as needed to achieve the desired negative sodium balance even in patients who are refractory to thiazide diuretics or who have renal insufficiency. Because of the potency of these drugs, inappropriate plasma volume depletion and prerenal azotemia may occur with loop diuretics. Although thiazide diuretics are preferred for routine use in uncomplicated essential hypertension, furosemide in doses of 20 to 200 mg may frequently be useful in the management of hypertensive emergencies. When needed there is a synergistic effect between the thiazide diuretics or metolazone and the loop diuretics.

Ototoxicity can occur with loop diuretics. High doses and rapid intravenous administration may predispose to hearing loss in some patients. The toxicity may be temporary, although with ethacrynic acid, permanent hearing loss has been reported. Allergic reactions of a hypersensitivity nature occur occasionally and may require change to an agent that does not have cross-reactivity.

A variety of metabolic problems may develop with diuretic therapy. Hypokalemia occurs frequently. Symptomatic gout or asymptomatic hyperuricemia may occur during diuretic therapy. The thiazide diuretics may induce hyperglycemia and hyperlipidemia. Another problem that has been seen with the various diuretic agents is hyponatremia related to a water excretion defect, with inability to dilute the urine appropriately.

Spironolactone may be successful in entirely correcting hypertension in primary hyperaldosteronism and in some metabolic disorders associated with mineralocorticoid excess. Its main use in the treatment of hypertensive states, however, is to control potassium wasting that can occur in association with the use of other diuretics. Spironolactone in doses up to 100 mg per day can be given for this purpose. It has a steroid nucleus, and estrogenic side effects such as gynecomastia can occur with prolonged use. Triamterene is a nonsteroidal drug that blocks sodium reabsorption in the distal nephron independently of aldosterone. It can be used in a similar fashion in doses of 100 to 300 mg per day to control potassium loss caused by other diuretic agents. Fatal hyperkalemia can occur with either spironolactone or triamterene if given to patients with high potassium intake or with underlying renal failure.

The most potent distal blocking agent is amiloride. This can be administered in doses of 5 to 20 mg daily. As with the other distal-acting agents, the major risk of this agent is serious hyperkalemia.

REFERENCES

1. Anderson, R. J., Hart, G. R., Crumpler, C. P., et al. Oral clonidine loading in hypertensive urgencies. *J.A.M.A* 246:848, 1981.
2. Blackwell, B., Marley E, Price, E. J., et al. Hypertensive interactions between monoamine oxidase inhibitors and food stuffs. *Br. J. Psychiatry* 113: 349, 1967.
3. Chiarieelo, M., Gold, H. K., Leinbach, R. C., et al. Comparison between the effects of nitroprusside and nitroglycerin on ischemic injury during acute myocardial infarction. *Circulation* 53:766, 1976.
4. Cressman, M. D., and Gifford, R. W., Jr. Hypertension and stroke. *J. Am. Coll. Cardiol.* 1:521, 1983.
5. Dequattro, V. Treating hypertensive crises: Which drug for which patient? *J. Crit. Illness* 2(7):24, 1987.
6. Esler, M. Mild high-renin essential hypertension. *N. Engl. J. Med.* 296: 405, 1977.
7. Frishman, W. H., Weinberg, P., Pedod, H. B., et al. Calcium entry blockers for the treatment of severe hypertension and hypertensive crises. *Am. J. Med.* 77(2B):35, 1984.
8. Haddy, F. J. Ionic control of vascular smooth muscle cells. *Kidney Int.* 34 (Suppl. 25):S2, 1988.
9. Laragh, J. H. Vasoconstrictor-volume analysis for understanding and treating hypertension: The use of renin and aldosterone profiles. *Am. J. Med.* 55: 261, 1973.
10. Laragh, J. H., and Atlas, S. A. Atrial natriuretic hormone: A regulator of blood pressure and volume homeostasis. *Kidney Int.* 34 (Suppl. 25):S64, 1988.
11. Lindheimer, M. D., and Katz, A. I. Hypertension in pregnancy. *N. Engl. J. Med.* 313:675, 1985.
12. Nolan, C. R., and Linas, S. L. Accelerated and Malignant Hypertension. In R. W. Schier and L. W. Gottochalk (eds.), *Diseases of the Kidney* (4th ed.). Boston and Toronto: Little, Brown, 1988. Chapter 59.
13. Strangaard, S., et al. Autoregulation of brain circulation in severe arterial hypertension. *Br. Med. J.* 1:507, 1973.
14. Tarazi, R. C. Clinical import of systolic hypertension. *Ann. Intern. Med.* 88:426, 1978.
15. Weiss, N. S. Relation of high blood pressure to headache, epistaxis, and selected other symptoms. *N. Engl. J. Med.* 287:631, 1972.
16. Wheat, M. W., Jr. Acute dissecting aneurysms of the aorta: Diagnosis and treatment. *Am. Heart J.* 99:373, 1980.
17. Wilson, D. J., Wallen, J. D., Vlachakis, N. D., et al. Intravenous labetalol in the treatment of severe hypertension and hypertensive emergencies. *Am. J. Med.* 75 (Suppl.):95, 1983.
18. Woods, J. W., et al. Renin profiling in hypertension and its use in treatment with propranolol and chlorthalidone. *N. Engl. J. Med.* 294:1137, 1976.

Management of Acute Coronary Occlusion

Warren Sherman
Richard Gorlin

PATHOPHYSIOLOGY

This discussion will be divided between the consideration of the vascular lesion leading to myocardial ischemia and necrosis and the myocardial lesion itself (Fig. 17-1). In virtually all instances, acute myocardial infarction results from occlusion of a coronary artery by sudden progression of an atherosclerotic plaque [5]. Aside from major coronary embolic diseases involving the coronary ostia and rare arteritis, the overwhelming majority of patients who have a myocardial infarction will have coronary atherosclerosis. It is the atherosclerotic lesion complicated by fissuring of the plaque that leads to occlusion [4]. If the break in the endothelium and intima is minimal, then this lesion may heal by reendothelialization and platelet aggregation with minimal change in the lumen. On the other hand, this fissuring, by exposing deep layers of the artery, leads to the attraction of platelets to the exposed collagen and lipid moieties. This is followed by fibrin infiltration and, finally, by accumulation of red and white blood cells. This results in an adherent thrombus that has a variable degree of attachment to the site of injury. The thrombus may propagate downstream, embolize to distal arteries, dissolve, or obstruct or occlude the lumen. It is this recognition of the complicated acute lesion resulting from rupture of an atheromatous plaque and the succeeding thrombosis that drives modern therapy. The arterial lesion may be complicated further in that changes in the intima may lead to reduction in endothelial relaxing factor and prostacyclin and to augmentation of the action of such vasoconstrictor hormones as platelet-derived thromboxane A_2 and serotonin. The result is that very often when an artery occludes, there is localized vasoconstriction, and even spasm, potentiated by the chemical events surrounding the abnormal segment of the artery. This complex lesion of the coronary artery causes occlusion that may last from as little as 15 minutes to as long as 10 or more days. In most instances, however, spontaneous recanalization occurs or the thrombus breaks off and embolizes downstream. The process of recanalization is so active that between 40 and 80 percent of all vessels occluded

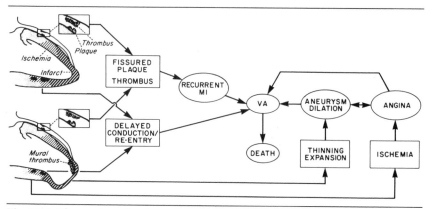

Fig. 17-1. The acute and subacute pathophysiologic changes that occur following plaque rupture and coronary artery occlusion. Each has its own effect on the cardiac-related consequences in the postinfarction period. Recurrent MI = recurrent myocardial infarction, VA = ventricular arrhythmias.

at the time of infarct are found to be patent some 2 weeks later. It is presumed that the extent of myocardial necrosis is dependent on the completeness and duration of the occlusion. This is modified, of course, if there have been preexisting collaterals to this segment. Collaterals would seem to modulate, but rarely eliminate, myocardial infarction. Furthermore, the very atherosclerotic plaque most likely to rupture or develop a fissure usually offers only mild intrusion into the lumen—i.e., it is not necessarily flow-limiting. As a consequence, in a large majority of patients there is no extensive collateral circulation present prior to the arterial occlusion. Collaterals result when there is a flow-limiting stenosis which leads to a pressure difference between the poststenotic segment and other tributaries. The effect is that preexisting collaterals are not adequate to prevent a major myocardial infarction when a mild lesion ruptures and thrombus or spasm, or both, develop. It is not known how significant downstream emboli are in the course of acute myocardial infarction (their role has been documented in patients with unstable angina). Furthermore, Kloner et al. [15] and Armiger et al. [2] have shown that the coronary capillaries are sensitive to ischemic insult, and within 1 hour (perhaps less) the endothelium of the capillaries swells and there is attachment of leukocytes to the capillary wall. This leads to further occlusion and probably underlies the "no reflow" phenomenon observed following elimination of the occlusion. With time, there is swelling and edema of the myocardium, as well as a rise in intramyocardial pressure. These forces tend to close the intramyocardial capillaries and complete the vascular lesion.

In response to this cessation of flow, the myocardium undergoes almost immediate changes. There is a reduction in high-energy phosphate that affects cyclic AMP levels and therefore cell function. Intracellular acidosis develops, with calcium and potassium accumulating in the perimyocyte space. The result is that hydrogen substitutes for calcium, bringing about a cessation of actin-myosin contractile effort, and that calcium accumulates in inappropriate areas such as the mitochondria and sacroplasmic reticulum. The ischemia also leads to the release of stored norepinephrine from cardiac nerve terminals, and there is also an increase of β-adrenergic receptors on the ischemic cell surface. The patient sustaining a myocardial infarction often has increased circulating norepinephrine and epinephrine levels from pain, anxiety, and altered perfusion dynamics. All these forces conspire to overdrive the myocardium and rapidly deplete the high-energy phosphate resources. The rapidity and uniformity with which changes take place relate to the suddenness and completeness of occlusion and the availability of collateral blood flow.

The subendocardial zone is least well supplied by preformed collaterals and usually suffers the earliest and most predictable necrosis; changes move in a wavefront fashion toward the more "protected" epicardial regions. Other changes depend on the availability of granulocytes and monocytes within the necrotic zone. These cells release leukotrienes and certain prostaglandins that enhance the inflammatory cell response of the myocardium to the ischemic insult. With passage of 6 to 12 hours, coagulation necrosis can be identified and loss of collagenous perimyocyte skeleton takes place.

While these complex biochemical changes are occurring, the affected zone of myocardium undergoes electrical or mechanical dysfunction. These occur within the Purkinje network of the two ventricles, and due to the irregular perfusion of different zones, one develops patterns of reentry as well as sites for increased automaticity. Similarly, edema and necrosis can lead to pacemaker dysfunction. All these factors account for the well known alterations in rate and rhythm that are part of the course of an acute myocardial infarction.

A change in myocardial contraction occurs within seconds following cessation of blood supply, often accompanied if not preceded by an alteration in diastolic function. Increased passive stiffness is ultimately superseded by *decreased* segmental stiffness and relaxation. Concomitantly, there occurs a decrease in contractile effort, leading to a zone of akinesis or dyskinesis. As time passes, this zone will show expansion or extension, or both, during the healing phase—a process that can be modified to some extent both through control of loading following the infarction and through limitation of the extent of the infarction. As a consequence of these mechanical changes, most patients with a large myocardial infarction will develop hemodynamic alterations characterized by an elevation in left ventricular filling pressure and a reduction in effective cardiac output. Similar pathophysiology applies to the right side of the heart when the right ventricle is extensively involved in inferior wall infarction. It should be recognized that the extent of the hemodynamic abnormality relates not only to the size of the infarction, but also to its location. For example, if an infarct involves the base of a papillary muscle leading to major dysfunction or rupture, then mitral regurgitation will be an important consequence. Similarly, if the septum is perforated during septal infarction, this will lead to major left-to-right shunting. For the most part, however, the serious consequences of an acute myocardial infarction result when the infarction is large, usually anterior and septal in location, such that there is major compromise of the contractile pattern. Cardiogenic shock most often occurs when at least one-third of the left ventricular mass has been either infarcted or involved in severe myocardial ischemia. When the right ventricle is involved, dramatic cardiac failure may occur, with elevated venous pressure and systemic hypotension. Yet the administration of volume can often reestablish the circulation and, quite surprisingly, lead to virtually complete recovery of right ventricular function.

These complex processes imply that the speed of application of therapy at the inception of infarction will govern the success or failure of a given acute intervention. How interventions are applied during the different stages of infarct will be discussed in subsequent sections.

DIAGNOSIS OF ACUTE CORONARY OCCLUSION

The hallmarks of acute coronary occlusion are the presence of myocardial ischemic chest pain for greater than 20 minutes and electrocardiographic changes of greater than 1-mm (0.1-mV) S–T segment elevation in any combination of regional (I, aVL or II, III, aVF or V_4–V_6) leads, or greater than 2 mm (0.2 mV) in leads V_1–V_3, the latter taking into account the high J-point normally present in these leads. The combination of these clinical findings yields a diagnostic specificity of greater than 90 percent for total obstruction of the coronary artery. With lesser criteria, such as shorter duration of pain, less S–T segment elevation, any amount of pure S–T segment depression, or pure T-wave inversion, the specificity declines rapidly. The sometimes rapid evolution of the electrocardiographic changes of acute coronary occlusion may also lead to its misinterpretation as a chronic abnormality. Q-waves can appear early (within hours) in acute coronary occlusion. However, they are nearly always associated with persistent S–T segment elevations when the occlusion is persistent. Other symptoms often associated with acute coronary occlusion, such as vomiting or diaphoresis, are unreliable signs.

Since knowing whether the coronary artery is patent is important, at least theoretically, in the choice of therapeutic modalities, much effort has been applied to understanding the clinical markers of "spontaneous reperfusion." A full 25 percent of patients with acute myocardial infarction undergoing early angiography (within hours of presentation to the emergency room) will have a patent infarct-related coronary artery. In such patients, one might choose a more conservative approach in terms of thrombolytic agents and, possibly, a more aggressive, interventional approach. Unfortunately, the ability to determine the patency status of a coronary artery noninvasively is limited [3]. The resolution of chest pain in combination with the return of the S–T segments to an isoelectric position is very specific (>90%) for infarct-related artery patency but is seen in relatively few patients.

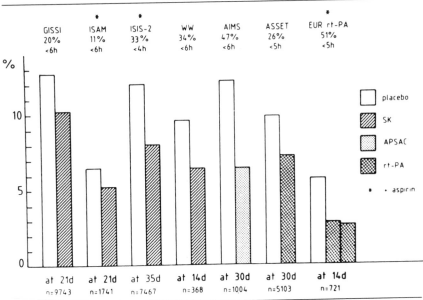

Fig. 17-2. The early mortality rates in the larger controlled trials with intravenous thrombolytic therapy. The top three lines depict the particular trial, the observed reduction in mortality, and the time window for treatment. The two lines beneath the graph indicate the time of end point measurement and total number of patients enrolled in each trial. GISSI = GISSI trial [6], ISAM = ISAM trial [10], ISIS-2 = ISIS-2 trial [12], WW = Western Washington trial [14], AIMS = AIMS trial [1], ASSET = ASSET trial [25], EUR rt-PA = European Cooperative trials [24, 22]. ([24] Reprinted with permission from the American College of Cardiology [*Journal of the American College of Cardiology* 12:14A, 1988].)

MANAGEMENT OF ACUTE CORONARY OCCLUSION

Since the clinical course of patients with acute coronary occlusion is time-dependent, so must be its management (Fig. 17-2). We have therefore chosen to divide our recommendations regarding management according to a chronologic scale following the presumed occlusive event: stage 1, 0 to 3 hours; stage 2, 3 to 6 hours; stage 3, 6 to 24 hours; stage 4, 1–3 days; and stage 5, 3 to 10 days (or average time of discharge). Of note, since the onset of coronary occlusion does not always result in chest pain, we use here the term *presumed occlusion*. Chest pain is, however, the only available clinical marker for the onset of occlusion.

At each stage we will address 3 areas of management: (1) reduction of myocardial oxygen demand, (2) increase in myocardial oxygen supply, and (3) prevention of subsequent events. Recently, the importance of the reduction of myocar ial oxygen demand has been lessened by vast research efforts into me hods of increasing myocardial oxygen supply and into the medical approaches of reducing cellular lysis, independent of changing myocardial oxygen supply. Nonetheless, the reduction of myocardial oxygen demand holds a primary role in the early management of acute coronary artery occlusion. Likewise, although less so, medical approaches aimed at preventing subsequent events have been somewhat ignored in the rush to tackle the myocardial oxygen supply problem. Fortunately, much has been learned from early, large trials of secondary prevention and can be easily summarized at each stage of the chronologic scale.

The methods for assessing the various treatments to be described in this chapter include measuring infarct size, left ventricular function, and patient survival. The most significant data from randomized drug trials are for in-hospital mortality: It is a finite and unambiguous end point, even though the causes may be manifold. Due to our inability to measure small differences in infarction size and left ventricular ejection fraction, larger randomized trials have avoided these parameters as end points.

Other management issues regarding myocardial infarction—i.e., acute and chronic arrhythmias, and congestive heart failure—are addressed in other chapters of this text and will only be highlighted here.

Stage 1: 0 to 3 hours

The greatest opportunities for salvaging myocardium occur when patients present to a medical facility during this stage. Unfortunately, the average time to presentation to an emergency room following the onset of an acute coronary occlusion is between 2 to 4 hours, and the average time to the initiation of therapy is 3 to 6 hours. Nonetheless, despite the time of presentation, certain medical approaches to the management of acute coronary occlusion described here are time-independent and will clearly apply to other stages.

Myocardial oxygen demand is at its highest during stage 1. Its primary determinants—heart rate, systolic blood pressure, and contractility—are variably affected by factors individual to each patient. A history of hypertension, medical treatment with antihypertensive or antianginal agents, and the adrenergic or vagal response of each patient to chest pain and to the overall medical situation all influence myocardial oxygen consumption. In this respect, the heart of the patient sustaining a myocardial infarction is overstimulated and possibly sensitized to elevated local and systemic catecholamine levels. Each patient responds differently to the complex set of conditions initiated by acute coronary occlusion. Cardiac output should be maintained at a level consistent with adequate tissue perfusion (urine volume, cerebration, etc.). Cardiac output is only a minimal indirect determinant of myocardial oxygen consumption. Emphasis needs to be placed on *net* myocardial perfusion pressure (diastolic blood pressure minus left ventricular filling pressure). Thus, it may be reasonable to lower blood pressure to reduce afterload and contractile tension and myocardial oxygen consumption, provided filling pressure is reduced pari passu. The balance between perfusion volume and pressure and filling pressure is complex and must be watched carefully and managed individually. Parallel treatment is very important at every stage.

In most cases, the assessment of cardiac output and loading conditions can be made quickly at the bedside by a combination of physical examination, chest radiography, and echocardiography. In patients in whom there is hemodynamic derangement, early and rapid reversal is required. The therapeutic options range from volume expansion (for the replacement of undetected losses or to raise ventricular filling pressures above normal to augment stroke work) to the medical and mechanical measures described in Chapter 15) for the treatment of acute heart failure. Volume expansion has a role in two types of patient. Many patients arrive at the hospital relatively volume-depleted, due to diaphoresis and vomiting. Additionally, volume expansion is particularly important in patients with right ventricular infarction, in which tissue perfusion can be severely impaired by underfilling of the left ventricle secondary to a sudden reduction in right ventricular stroke volume. One of the most important effects to be reversed is that of the sympathetic nervous system on myocardial dynamics. In particular, increases in adrenergic tone (such as is induced by anxiety) raise heart rate, myocardial contractility, myocardial irritability (possibly), and peripheral vascular resistance. The effects of such levels of adrenergic tone on coronary vascular resistance are unknown. However, in light of these effects, it is of critical importance to diminish chest pain and anxiety with an analgesic (morphine sulfate) and graduated doses of a sedative. It is here, also, that the role of β-blocking agents is most clear. In patients who are acutely hypertensive, tachycardic, and with no more than moderate left ventricular dysfunction, this class of drugs is of extreme value. If cardiac output is deemed adequate, anxiety is well controlled, and the patient remains hypertensive, peripheral vasodilators or α-adrenergic blockers must be used.

In patients who are stable and without hemodynamic derangement, the value of reducing adrenergic tone is less clear. Intravenous β-blockers clearly have a role when given early (within 4 hours) and when no contraindications are present. β-blockers examined for this purpose include metoprolol (15 mg IV in three equal doses at 2-minute intervals within 4 hours of pain) [8], atenolol (10 mg IV within 11 hours of pain onset) [11], timolol (2 mg IV in two doses over 10 minutes, followed by a 0.6 mg/hr infusion for 24 hours, within 5 hours of pain onset), and propranolol (0.1 mg/kg IV over 10 minutes). Any of these (especially metoprolol) may be used in combination with thrombolysis. Before using these agents, it is important to understand left ventricular systolic function, heart rate, atrioventricular conduction, and other contraindications to β-blockers (i.e., asthma).

The next class of drugs to be considered in the stage 1 patient is the nitrates, which, in addition to their effects on preload and afterload, may also improve coronary collateral flow. Equally important, due to the coronary vasospasm or, at least, enhanced coronary vasotonia in many patients with acute coronary occlusion [7], sublingual nitroglycerin may resolve this entirely and should be given to all patients in stage 1. One must be prepared to treat the hypotension that may infrequently result from giving such a drug by the administration of a small fluid load. The benefits outweigh the risks, and an occasional patient treated early in this manner may recanalize the coronary artery and lose all electrocardiographic measures of acute myocardial injury. Beyond sublingual nitroglycerin, intravenous nitroglycerin has been advocated for its reduction of infarct size, as measured indirectly by electrocardiographic, enzymatic, and radionuclide techniques. When given continuously to reduce the systolic blood pressure by 10 percent (and not less than 95 mm Hg systolic) for the 48 hours following the onset of chest pain, infarct size appears to be lessened, and the incidence of infarct expansion is reduced [13]. However, the effect of this drug on survival after an infarct is unknown, and its use with other drugs—i.e., thrombolytics—has been only partially examined [19].

Other treatment modalities of stage 1 patients might include intra-aortic balloon counterpulsation [16], calcium-channel blockers [18], and the combination of glucose, insulin, and potassium [20]. Based on available data, one cannot recommend the routine use of any of these therapies.

Once a feeling for the hemodynamic state of the patient is gained, a decision regarding the need to recanalize the occluded coronary artery must be made. In this stage, the persistence of chest pain and electrocardiographic changes (as described above), almost invariably means the persistence of coronary occlusion. Since virtually all patients presenting within 1 hour of coronary occlusion have an element of reversibility to their myocellular damage, medical approaches to recanalization should be begun immediately. The medical agents that are useful (and easily available) for this purpose are listed in Table 17-1. The issues relevant to the choice(s) of such agents include (1) the effectiveness (recanalization rate), (2) the time to recanalization from the beginning of treatment, (3) the ease with which the agent may be given, and (4) the frequency of side effects.

The highest recanalization rates during this or any other stage of coronary occlusion are achieved with the intracoronary administration of any of the thrombolytic agents listed in Table 17-1. The earlier the presentation of the patient, the higher the recanalization rate. When the duration of pain is less than 1 hour, the recanalization rate is in excess of 85 percent with intracoronary thrombolysis—unlike that for patients who present with between 3 and 6 hours of pain, in whom a recanalization rate of 75 percent is expected. One must keep in mind, however, that these rates are based on calculations in patients who recanalize arteries that initially are totally occluded; patients who present with infarct-related arteries that are subtotally occluded are excluded from such calculations. Therefore, the overall patency rate (not recanalization rate) with intracoronary streptokinase is in excess of 85 percent during stage 1. There is a cost to using intracoronary infusion of thrombolytic agents during this or any other stage. In having to perform a cardiac catheterization with this approach, the time to recanalization is prolonged, the ease of drug administration is complicated, and the frequency of severe side effects (catheter-induced cardiac and peripheral vascular complications) is increased. Additionally, the actual cost in dollars is obviously in excess of the intravenous approach. For these reasons, the currently popular and more practical route of administration of thrombolytic agents is by way of intravenous infusion.

Table 17-1. Thrombolytic agents

	Dose	Recanalization rate	Approved for use in U.S.
Streptokinase			
Intracoronary	240,000 units over 2 hr	75%	Yes
Intravenous	1.5 million units over 1 hr	40–60%	Yes
Urokinase			
Intracoronary	500,000 units over 2 hr	75%	Yes
Intravenous	3 million units over 90 min	40–60%	No
Tissue plasminogen activator	100 mg (or 1.25 mg/kg) over 3 hr	60–70%	Yes
Anisoylated plasminogen streptokinase complex	30 mg over 15 min	65%	Yes

Recanalization rates during intravenous administration of the various thrombolytic agents now (or soon to be) available are listed in Table 17-1. These data have been summarized from studies in which coronary angiography was performed prior to the intravenous infusion of the given agent and therefore conform to the above definition of recanalization rate. The agents listed, streptokinase (SK), urokinase (UK), anisoylated streptokinase plasminogen activator (APSAC), and tissue plasminogen activator (tPA), have been chosen because of the abundance of scientific data available and because of their roles as prototypes of subsequent generations of thrombolytic agents. SK, tPA, and APSAC have been approved for use in myocardial infarction in the United States.

The recanalization rates for SK and tPA when used in stage 1 appear to be similar. As with intracoronary SK use, the recanalization rate for intravenous SK is higher the earlier it is given. We currently recommend that patients presenting during stage 1 be given 1.5 million units of intravenous SK.

The benefit of thrombolytic therapy on in-hospital mortality is the clearest for stage 1 patients (Fig. 17-2). Two major intravenous SK trials [6, 12], one tPA trial [25], and one APSAC trial [1] describe up to 50 percent reductions in mortality. For a number of reasons, including differences in patient populations both before (i.e., age) and after (i.e., medical treatment in addition to thrombolytics) entry, the mortality data between trials are not comparable. In this regard, aspirin, which has value both alone and as an adjunct to thrombolytic therapy [6], was used variably in the large intravenous trials. Heparin may also offer similar benefits. These two drugs may account for a significant beneficial effect on postinfarction survival in control groups alone (Fig. 17-3). Unfortunately, mortality data directly comparing SK and tPA are lacking. Two major trials currently underway will address this issue: one comparing SK and tPA, and the other comparing SK, tPA, and APSAC.

In terms of salvaging myocardium and preserving left ventricular function, the available data are not compelling, even in the stage-1 patient. Despite this, when one looks at the overall results of thrombolytic therapy during stage 1, the resultant increase in survival is highly significant and stands ahead of that achievable by any other therapy.

Although the mortality data for thrombolytic therapy during stage 1 are convincing, several caveats apply to such therapy at any stage. First, a certain morbidity is introduced with thrombolytic therapy, even by intravenous infusion. The incidence of intracranial bleeding, even though rarely life-threatening, is measurable (<1.0% with tPA) and diminishes the benefits of thrombolytic therapy. Second, the mechanism(s) by which thrombolytic therapy enhances survival is (are) not clear. Even though their primary action is thrombolysis, other actions, such as blood pressure reduction and an improvement in the rheologic properties of the blood (as seen with SK), may account for some of the beneficial effects on survival. Diminished propensity to arrhythmias, reduction in late potentials, and lessened likelihood of infarct expansion irrespective of size may all play a role. Third, in the setting of an acute myocardial infarction, a patent cor-

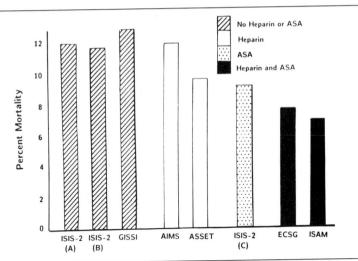

Fig. 17-3. Control group mortality in relation to concomitant heparin and/or ASA therapy.

onary artery is an unstable one. It is likely to reocclude (in 25% of patients), leading to any one or more of the sudden clinical events known to befall post-MI patients. Among these are unstable angina, reinfarction, further myocardial dysfunction, and, although never proven, ventricular arrhythmias and infarct expansion. One must therefore be prepared to manage the consequences of reperfusion if one is contemplating reperfusion therapy.

The other methods of acutely increasing myocardial oxygen supply are emergency coronary angioplasty, either with or without concomitant thrombolysis; surgical revascularization; and coronary sinus retroperfusion of oxygenated blood. Despite its attractiveness in resolving the underlying coronary lesion, angioplasty alone has limited value in acute coronary occlusion, in that the reocclusion rate appears to be higher than that for thrombolysis alone. When the two are combined, as was done in the Thrombolysis in Myocardial Infarction Trial (TIMI) [23], there was no statistically significant difference in survival when compared with thrombolysis (with tPA) alone. Similarly, surgical revascularization has seen limited use, none of which has come in a randomized trial. The patients who appear to benefit from this approach are those in whom severe three-vessel or left main coronary artery disease has been uncovered, especially in the setting of severe left ventricular failure or cardiogenic shock. And lastly, coronary retroperfusion is thus far in a very early experimental stage clinically. It clearly will require an additional intervention (i.e., thrombolysis, coronary angioplasty, or surgical revascularization) to be of any value and in fact may only be supportive of these other interventions.

The reduction of cellular lysis and fibrosis by medical means has received little positive clinical attention for patients of any stage but offers some provocative therapeutic approaches. The methods thus far tested include limitation of the inflammatory response with steroidal or nonsteroidal anti-inflammatory agents, reduction in the laying down of fibrotic tissue (hyaluronidase), and reduction of free-radical–induced cell lysis by use of free-radical scavengers (supraoxide dismutase, etc.). To date, none of these therapies has found a solid position at the bedside.

The prevention of subsequent events is necessarily related to all of the above treatment strategies. As previously stated, some of these strategies (i.e., thrombolysis) may in fact increase the incidence of certain (especially coronary-related) postinfarction events. They also decrease the incidence of other, noncardiac events, especially when combined with aspirin [25]. Equally important is the administration of heparin, with or without thrombolysis, for prevention of peripheral venous thromboembolism and mural thrombus formation in patients with large (anterior wall) infarctions.

The prevention of arrhythmias (ventricular tachycardia and fibrillation) by the routine use of antiarrhythmic agents (lidocaine) has been studied [17,26]. Patients who are not susceptible to the toxic effects of such agents (i.e., patients less than 70 years of age and without chronic liver disease) benefit from the prophylactic use of lidocaine, especially if, when monitored, a timely response to sudden ventricular arrhythmias is not optimal. In this case, an adequate loading and infusion (3 mg/min) dose is important. A recent meta analysis suggests that although frequency of ventricular fibrillation is decreased, survival may actually be adversely affected [17]. The routine injection of lidocaine by paramedical personnel in the preadmission (ambulance) phase has not been conclusively shown to be of value. It should be mentioned that β-blockers may play a comparable, if not more useful, role in the prevention of arrhythmias in acute myocardial infarction [21].

The prevention of bradyarrhythmias in high-risk patients has also been well studied [9]. For all patients with symptomatic bradycardia unresponsive to medical (atropine) management, temporary pacemaking is warranted. For patients with inferior wall myocardial infarctions, only those with high-degree atrioventricular (AV) block and an infranodal escape rhythm should receive a temporary pacemaker. In patients with fascicular block (usually in anterior wall infarctions) who fall into a high-risk category (prolonged P–R interval or bifascicular or bilateral bundle branch block, any of which are new) the incidence of progression to complete AV block is substantial (approximately 20%) and temporary pacemaking is advised. With the advent of transcutaneous pacemaking, the management of all patients with or at risk for severe bradyarrhythmias has been made easier, although the reliability of these devices varies from patient to patient.

Stage 2: 3 to 6 hours

The management of stage-2 patients resembles that of stage-1 patients (Table 17-2) in nearly all respects. This is still a very acute stage in the pathophysiology of the infarction. Therefore, the derangements and imbalances in cardiovascular function and loading conditions affecting a patient are

Table 17-2. Treatment recommendations

Stage	Time	Optimization of hemodynamics	Thrombolysis	Routine revascularization	β-blockers	Intravenous nitroglycerin	Calcium-channel blockers
1	0–3 hr	Y	Y	N	Y	Y	?
2	3–6 hr	Y	Y	N	Y	Y	?
3	6–24 hr	Y	?	N	?	?	?
4	1–3 days	Y	N	N	?	?	?
5	3–10 days	Y	N	N	Y	?	?

Y = yes, N = no, ? = unknown.

equally relevant and demand stabilization, as described in the previous section. In this regard, the use of intravenous β-blockers is still advised for the patient whose left ventricular systolic performance is not severely impaired and whose atrioventricular conduction is electrocardiographically normal. Nearly all intravenous β-blocker trials have included patients in stage 2.

The major differences in treatment between stages 1 and 2 relate to the efficacy of thrombolytic therapy. First, recanalization rates appear to be higher for tPA than the nonspecific agents such as streptokinase. Second, the magnitude of reduction in mortality for thrombolytic therapy is less for stage-2 than for stage-1 patients. This appears to be independent of the agent used; that is, all thrombolytic agents that have been shown to reduce mortality do so less effectively the later they are given. Thus, streptokinase, tPA, and APSAC have all been demonstrated to decrease mortality in stage-2 patients.

As with stage 1 treatment, aspirin and heparin are of considerable value, especially in patients given thrombolytic therapy. These medicines must be continued to preserve the patency (presumably) and clinical benefit afforded by the thrombolytic agent. The only reasons to terminate them are bleeding or other adverse effects directly attributable to the drugs.

Stage 3: 6 to 24 hours

For the reasons cited in the above discussion on pathophysiology, and for reasons partially borne out in clinical trials, a major breakpoint in the efficacy of treatment of acute coronary occlusion occurs during this stage. The reversibility of myocardial cellular damage and of overall myocardial performance reaches a rather sudden halt after 6 hours of coronary occlusion. These facts have major implications for the aggressive treatment of acute coronary occlusion.

Most patients who tolerate the initial hemodynamic alterations imposed by the myocardial infarction remain stable throughout this stage. Therefore, in terms of medical treatment, for patients presenting during an earlier stage, maintenance of the status quo with β-blockers, nitrates, and other therapies is generally advised. However, for patients presenting to the hospital during this stage, the treatment is often considerably different.

First, patients with severe compromise in hemodynamic status generally present during earlier stages. Such patients do not survive a prolonged (>6 hours) prehospital phase. It is unusual, therefore, for a patient presenting in stage 3 to require aggressive hemodynamic support for cardiogenic shock. Second, the efficacy of starting β-blockers or intravenous nitrates during this stage is much less clear than for earlier stages, as was alluded to above. And third, only one randomized trial of thrombolytic therapy [25] has shown benefit to patients presenting beyond 6 hours. The difference in cardiovascular morbidity and mortality was small in these patients given SK and/or aspirin, but due to the massive numbers of patients enrolled in this study, the 2 percent difference in mortality achieved statistical significance. Therefore, thrombolytic therapy is of questionable value in patients presenting during stage 3. Unfortunately, intravenous thrombolytic trials now underway are designed to measure clinical differences between two or more thrombolytic agents: control groups are not included.

As with patients at any stage, but particularly stages 3 and 4, when chest pain recurs and is accompanied by new deviations (especially elevations) in S–T segments (generally in the infarct region), strong evidence for reocclusion is present. If these clinical findings are transient and associated with either no change or only a small increase in serum creatine kinase, then urgent coronary arteriography and revascularization are warranted. This approach is advocated regardless of the type or intensity of medical therapy (i.e., heparin and/or aspirin) in place prior to the recurrent ischemia.

If the recurrent chest pain and electrocardiographic changes persist for greater than 30 minutes, a more lasting reocclusion and, therefore, reinfarction is in progress. In certain respects, reinfarction is a surprisingly different clinical event when compared to the initial infarction. Even though the cause(s) (primary rethrombosis, or vasospasm plus thrombosis) are probably identical, some patients tolerate the second event much more poorly than the first. Greater hemodynamic embarrassment is not uncommon in such patients. The reasons for this are unclear but may include infarct expansion. The treatment also may be different. First, as with the first coronary occlusion, thrombolytic therapy may be helpful in reestablishing coronary flow. The choices of agents, however, are more restricted. Neither streptokinase nor APSAC can be given to the same patient twice over such a short period of time, due to their antigenicity. On the other hand, tPA can be and has been given twice in this setting, the recanalization rate reportedly being similar for both first and second usages. And second, the role of urgent coronary revascularization during a hemodynamically stable reinfarction is not clear, although such a strategy has been advocated. Patients who are hemodynamically unstable or who have evidence for recanalization probably benefit from urgent revascularization.

Aspirin is also useful [25] for most stage-3 patients, as is heparin, in reducing cardiovascular morbidity and mortality, regardless of whether thrombolytic therapy was applied. As with stage-1 and -2 patients, the value of revascularization in patients without recurrent ischemia is unproven.

In general, then, patients presenting to the hospital during stage 3 warrant the same medical treatment as those presenting during stages 1 and 2, with the exception, perhaps, of those presenting within 6 to 12 hours after onset of pain, in whom thrombolytic therapy is only conditionally (persistence of chest pain) advised. Patients who presented to the hospital during stages 1 or 2 and have now advanced to stage 3 deserve to be maintained on the medical regimen initiated in the earlier stage, provided that their clinical course has been a stable one. Urgent, often invasive measures are frequently required for unstable stage-3 patients.

Stage 4: 1 to 3 days

It is unusual for a patient with an acute coronary occlusion to first present for medical care during stage 4. Such patients represent a select group who, depending on the presence of other medical diseases, have a generally good prognosis. We will therefore restrict our discussion to stage-4 patients who have endured one or more of the first three stages.

As with stages 2 and 3, medical regimens in stable patients should not be altered. The logic for extending this advice hinges primarily on the still significant reocclusion rates observed during stage 4. Therefore, antithrombotic treatment, including aspirin and heparin, should be continued, and vigilance for recurrent chest pain must be maintained. Very stable patients on arrhythmia prophylaxis and intravenous nitroglycerin can be withdrawn from these drugs. β-blockers, depending on one's approach to chronic therapy, should also be continued. Where stage-4 patients begin to deviate from those of previous stages is in the development of the mechanical complications of myocardial infarction.

Although the most common mechanical impairment brought on by an acute myocardial infarction occurs during stages 1 or 2 and relates to the extent of myocardial damage, other processes, often occurring suddenly, develop primarily in stage 4. Rupture of the left ventricular free wall, interventricular septum, papillary muscle, or a combination of these leads most often to immediate or steadily progressive failure of cardiac performance and death. The variables that relate to such events are hypertension, female sex, and the absence of coronary collateral flow to the infarcted region. The only premonitory symptom may be a recurrence of chest pain, especially in the case of free-wall rupture.

The diagnosis of these entities is all too often delayed and difficult. The physical examination is helpful only in interventricular septal or papillary rupture, in which the occurrence of a new systolic murmur signals the onset of such a process. The most rapid and useful tool in diagnosing these entities is Doppler echocardiography, which should be used at the earliest suspicion of a rupture. If this tool is unavailable and/or if the diagnosis of interventricular septal versus papillary muscle rupture is the issue, then a right heart catheterization with oximetry must be performed.

The treatment for all but the smallest, hemodynamically tolerated ventricular septal defect (and there is some disagreement even on this point) is urgent surgical repair. The urgency is highlighted by the recommendation to ignore the status of the coronary arteries (i.e., not to perform coronary angiography or, therefore, revascularization) during the repair. Of course, temporizing measures, including intra-aortic balloon counterpulsation, are advocated prior to surgery. The aggressive use of surgical repair seems to offer the only hope for survival.

Aside from these mechanical events, the other serious problems which may arise during stage 4 are (1) recurrent ischemia (as described above), and (2) new ventricular arrhythmias. Both of these entities are prognostic signs of a poor outcome and should be treated aggressively. Treatment should include medical and surgical approaches.

Stage 4, then, represents a transition period from the early treatment efforts to maintain coronary artery patency and prevent early complications (stages 1–3) to the later phase of preparing for chronic medical management (stage 5). Unfortunately, possible complications of the infarction, infrequent but potentially devastating in outcome, warrant the continuation of careful observation.

Stage 5: 3 to 10 days

The major risks after leaving the coronary care unit (and step-down unit) are (1) recurrent myocardial infarction, (2) recurrent ischemia, (3) life-threatening arrhythmia, and (4) heart failure. Thromboembolic events, either pulmonary or systemic, occur, but at reduced frequency.

The use of thrombolytic and antithrombotic agents seems to reduce arrhythmias, thromboembolic events, and, in combination perhaps, recurrent myocardial infarction. There may also be a reduction in heart failure due to less loss of myocardium. Aspirin will become a chronic therapy from day 1 on. Chronic anticoagulation with coumarin derivatives may be indicated in some patients even as heparin is stopped. Such therapy would be appropriate when a large mural thrombus has been identified, when severe cardiomegaly is present, when there have been multiple prior myocardial infarctions, and when thromboembolism or persistent atrial fibrillation have manifested themselves.

β-blockers should be continued unless contraindicated, for their putative antiarrhythmic or ischemic action, or both, and for their proven ability to reduce recurrent myocardial infarction and death. In titrating the dose, all trials to date indicate that the lower the achieved heart rate on blockade, the greater the cardioprotective effect.

Nitrates also should be continued. These agents have favorably affected infarct size and left ventricular volume, and there are two reports suggesting a favorable effect on post-MI mortality.

Finally, angiotensin-converting enzyme inhibitors given post-MI beginning during the early- to mid-hospital phase attenuate the progressive increase in left ventricular size and filling pressure seen in the majority of patients. This effort begins during the acute phase (3–5 days), when about one-third of all MIs will exhibit frank expansion and thinning, which is usually progressive. Whether this intervention will further improve survival is unknown at present.

SUMMARY

Care for patients with acute coronary occlusion must be based on a full understanding of the pathophysiology of the atherosclerotic plaque, as well as the myocardial and systemic effects that result therein. A time-related therapeutic regimen is recommended (Table 17-2, Fig. 17-4) due to the dynamic nature of the pathophysiologic processes involved. What is done in the first 4 to 48 hours influences the long-term result. Furthermore, several pharmacotherapies used acutely find application in the chronic phase, all aimed at minimizing the electrical and mechanical consequences of myocardial infarction. With the guidelines described in Table 17-2, the number of lives saved—and quite possibly, myocardium salvaged—will be maximized.

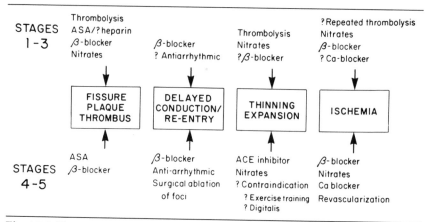

Fig. 17-4. Time-, stage-, and lesion-related treatment options of the consequences of acute coronary occlusion. ASA = aspirin, Ca blocker = calcium-channel blocker, ACE inhibitor = angiotensin-converting enzyme inhibitor, ? = unknown.

REFERENCES

1. AIMS Trial Study Group. Effect of intravenous APSAC on mortality after acute myocardial infarction: Preliminary report of a placebo-controlled clinical trial. *Lancet* 1:545, 1988.
2. Armiger, L. C., and Gavin, J. B. Changes in the microvasculature of ischemic and infarcted myocardium. *Lab. Invest.* 33:51, 1975.
3. Califf, R. M., O'Neil, W., Stack, R. S., et al. Failure of simple measurements to predict perfusion status after intravenous thrombolysis. *Ann. Intern. Med.* 108:658, 1988.
4. Davies, M. J., and Thomas, A. C. Plaque fissuring—The cause of acute myocardial infarction, sudden ischaemic death, and crescendo angina. *Br. Heart J.* 53:363, 1985.
5. Factor, S., and Kirk, E. S. Pathophysiology of myocardial infarction. In J. W. Hurst (ed.), *The Heart.* New York: McGraw-Hill, 1982.
6. Gruppo Italiana per Lo Studio della Streptochinasi nell'Infarcto Myocardico (GISSI). Effectiveness of intravenous thrombolytic treatment in acute myocardial infarction. *N. Engl. J. Med.* 308:1305, 1983.
7. Hackett, D., Davies, G., Chierchia, S., Maseri, A. Intermittent coronary occlusion in acute myocardial infarction. *N. Engl. J. Med.* 317:1055, 1987.
8. Hjalmarson, A., Herlitz, J., Malek, I., et al. Effect on mortality of metoprolol in acute myocardial infarction. *Lancet* 1:823, 1981.
9. Hindman, M. C., Wagner, G. S., Jaro, M., et al. The clinical significance of bundle branch block complicating acute myocardial infarction. *Circulation* 58:679, 1978.
10. ISAM Study Group. A prospective trial of intravenous streptokinase in acute myocardial infarction (ISAM). Mortality, morbidity and infarct size at 21 days. *N. Engl. J. Med.* 314:1456, 1986.
11. ISIS-1 (First International Study of Infarct Survival) Collaborative Group. Randomised trial of intravenous atenolol among 16,027 cases of suspected acute myocardial infarction: ISIS-1. *Lancet* 2:57, 1986.

12. ISIS-2 (Second International Study of Infarct Survival) Collaborative Group. Randomised trial of intravenous streptokinase, oral aspirin, both, or neither among 17,187 cases of suspected acute myocardial infarction: ISIS-2. *Lancet* 2:349, 1988.
13. Jugdutt, B. I., and Warnica, J. W. Intravenous nitroglycerin therapy to limit myocardial infarct size, expansion, and complications. *Circulation* 78:906, 1988.
14. Kennedy, J. W., Martin, G. V., Davis, K. B., et al. The Western Washington intravenous streptokinase in acute myocardial infarction randomized trial. *Circulation* 77:345, 1988.
15. Kloner, R. A., Rude, R. E., Carlson, N., et al. Ultrastructural evidence of microvascular damage and myocardial cell injury after coronary artery occlusion: Which comes first? *Circulation* 62:945, 1980.
16. Leinbach, R. C., Gold, H. K., Harper, R. W., et al. Early intraaortic balloon pumping for anterior myocardial infarction without shock. *Circulation* 58:204, 1978.
17. McMahon, S., Collins, R., Peto, R., Koster, R. W., Yusuf, S. Effects of prophylactic lidocaine in suspected acute myocardial infarction. An overview of results from the randomized controlled trials. *J.A.M.A.* 260:1910, 1988.
18. The Multicenter Diltiazem Postinfarction Trial Research Group. The effect of diltiazem on mortality and reinfarction after myocardial infarction. *N. Engl. J. Med.* 319:385, 1988.
19. Rentrop, P., and Feit, F. Reperfusion Study Group. The Second Mount Sinai-NYU Reperfusion Trial: Main endpoints. *J. Am. Coll. Cardiol.* 9:239A, 1987.
20. Rogers, W. J., McDaniel, H. G., and Mantle, J. A., et al. Prospective randomized trial of glucose-insulin-potassium in acute myocardial infarction: Effects on hemodynamics, short- and long-term survival [abstract]. *J. Am. Coll. Cardiol.* 1:628, 1983.
21. Ryden, L., Ariniego, R., Arnman, K., et al. A double-blind trial of metoprolol in acute myocardial infarction: Effects on ventricular tachyarrhythmias. *N. Engl. J. Med.* 308:614, 1983.
22. Simoons, M. L., Arnold, A. E. R., Betriu, A., et al. Thrombolysis with rt-PA in acute myocardial infarction: No additional benefit of immediate PTCA. *Lancet* 1:197, 1988.
23. The TIMI Study Group. Preliminary results of TIMI 2A. Presented at the Scientific Sessions, American Heart Association, Washington, D.C., November 1988.
24. Van de Werf, F. Lessons from the European cooperative recombinant tissue-type plasminogen activator (rt-PA) versus placebo trial. *J. Am. Coll. Cardiol.* 12:14A, 1988.
25. Wilcox, R. G., von der Lippe, G., Olson, C. G., et al. Trial of tissue plasminogen activator for mortality reduction in acute myocardial infarction: The Anglo-Scandinavian Study of Early Thrombolysis (ASSET). *Lancet* 2:525, 1988.
26. Yusuf, S., Sleight, P., Rossi, P., et al. Reduction in infarct size, arrhythmias and chest pain by early intravenous beta blockade in suspected acute myocardial infarction. *Circulation* 67(Suppl I):I-32, 1983.

Surgical Management of Acute Heart Failure

Pamela S. Peigh
Lawrence H. Cohn

DEFINITION

Acute congestive heart failure can be broadly defined as an abnormality of cardiac function that is responsible for failure of the heart to pump blood at a rate equal to the requirements of the metabolizing tissues. The pathophysiology of congestive heart failure involves a failure of the body's three important compensatory mechanisms: (1) the Frank-Starling mechanism (increased preload maintains cardiac output); (2) heightened release of catecholamines, which in turn increases myocardial contractility and heart rate; (3) myocardial hypertrophy. Clinically, we can manipulate the first two of these mechanisms.

ETIOLOGY

The surgically-treatable etiologies of acute congestive heart failure include

1. Cardiac tamponade.
2. Acute myocardial infarction with ventricular dysfunction.
3. Mechanical complications of myocardial infarction—acute mitral regurgitation and ventricular septal defect.
4. Acute aortic insufficiency—infective endocarditis and aortic dissection.
5. Pulmonary embolus.
6. Postcardiotomy cardiogenic shock in patients who have recoverable ventricular function.

The surgically-treatable etiologies of subacute congestive heart failure include

1. Cardiomyopathies.
2. Cardiomyopathies listed for transplantation with deterioration in heart failure.

INITIAL EVALUATION

The initial evaluation of a patient in acute congestive heart failure with a potential surgical etiology should begin with a directed history and physical examination. Chest x-ray, electrocardiogram (ECG), and echocardiogram should be obtained shortly thereafter. Based on this initial evaluation, the decision to proceed to cardiac catheterization will likely be made.

INITIAL MANAGEMENT

The initial management of the several subgroups of patients is similar in many regards. All require placement of an intra-arterial catheter for monitoring blood pressure and following systemic blood gases. As soon as this is placed, correction of contributing factors such as acidosis, hypoxemia, anemia, and hypokalemia can be started as necessary.

Placement of a pulmonary artery catheter early in the patient's course provides important management data. The current triple-lumen catheters (Fig. 18-1) can provide the following information: right atrial pressure, pulmonary artery pressure and blood for pulmonary artery oxygen saturation determination, pulmonary capillary wedge pressure, cardiac output (and consequently, by calculation, cardiac index and systemic vascular resistance). Thus, intelligent manipulation of preload and afterload is made possible. Also available are pulmonary artery catheters that, operating via reflectance spectrometry, can give continuous readout of pulmonary artery oxygen saturation and are quite useful for the management of the several factors contributing to pulmonary artery oxygen saturation (hematocrit, systemic oxygen saturation, and cardiac output). Further, there are modified pulmonary artery catheters in which right atrial and right ventricular pacing electrodes have been placed, both for pacing and for recording electrograms to diagnose arrhythmias. Pulmonary artery catheters can be safely inserted at the bedside, using pressure waveforms to guide placement (Fig. 18-2). Once the initial measurements have been made, the four important hemodynamic determinants of cardiac output can be maximized: heart rate, preload, afterload, and, finally, contractility. Despite pacing, volume therapy, and vasodilator and inotropic therapy, these patients may still remain in a low cardiac output state secondary to ischemia or elevated afterload (relative to intrinsic contractility).

At this point the use of an intra-aortic balloon should be considered if the heart failure is due to severe left ventricular failure. The mechanism of action of the intra-aortic balloon is that of inflation during diastole and deflation during systole (Fig. 18-3). This improves hemodynamics in two ways: by diastolic pressure augmentation, thus improving coronary artery blood flow; and by systolic unloading, thus decreasing myocardial work and oxygen demand (Fig. 18-4).

Contraindications to the use of the intra-aortic balloon are few. They include irreversible brain damage, end-stage congestive heart failure (not a transplant candidate), and incompetent aortic valve (the intra-aortic balloon cannot augment flow retrograde with the aortic valve open in diastole).

CARDIAC TAMPONADE

When cardiac tamponade is the etiology for congestive heart failure, it is important to ask if there is a history of trauma, previous heart surgery with

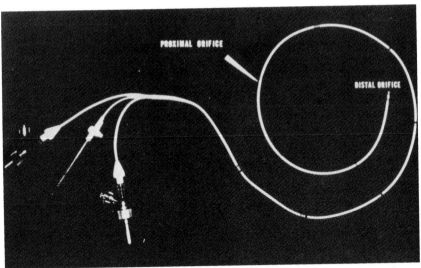

Fig. 18-1. Flow-directed triple-lumen balloon catheter for measurement of cardiac output by thermodilution. Distance from tip is marked in 10-cm intervals. Position of thermistor proximal to inflated balloon is indicated by arrow. Proximal end of catheter contains two thermistor leads, lumen for inflation of balloon (small syringe), lumen for injection of the cold liquid (large syringe), and distal lumen, connected to a pressure transducer. (From J. S. Forrester et al., Thermodilution cardiac output determination with a single flow-directed catheter. *Am. Heart J.* 83:306, 1972. Reproduced by permission.)

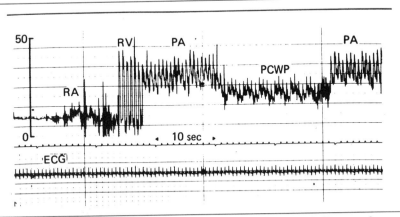

Fig. 18-2. Pressure recorded during insertion of flow-directed balloon catheter. RA = right atrial pressure; RV = right ventricular pressure; PA = pulmonary artery pressure; PCWP = pulmonary capillary wedge pressure. Pressure scale: 50 mm Hg. (From K. Chatterjee, Acute Heart Failure. In J. L. Berk and J. E. Sampliner (eds.), *Handbook of Critical Care* (2nd ed.). Boston: Little, Brown, 1982. P. 206.)

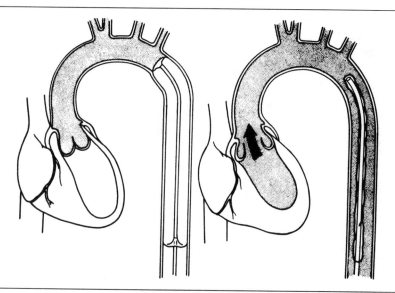

Fig. 18-3. Intra-aortic balloon performance is sequenced so that balloon suddenly deflates immediately before the onset of mechanical ventricular systole (right) and inflates at the onset of diastole (left). (From R. S. Litwak, Analysis, Maintenance, and Support of Cardiac Function After Cardiac Surgery. In R. S. Litwak and R. A. Jurado (eds.), *Care of the Cardiac Surgical Patient,* Norwalk, CT: Appleton-Century-Crofts, 1982. P. 224. Reproduced by permission.)

postoperative anticoagulation, chronic renal failure, cancer, or tuberculosis. Physical examination should be directed to looking for a small heart with diminished heart sounds, increased jugular venous pressure, decreased systemic arterial blood pressure, and a pulsus paradoxus (an inspiratory decrease in arterial systolic blood pressure greater than 10 mm Hg during quiet respiration). Chest x-ray generally will demonstrate an enlarged cardiac silhouette. Echocardiogram will show pericardial fluid and collapse of the right ventricular free wall in diastole (Fig. 18-5).

If tuberculosis is the etiology, surgery is better delayed for 6 to 12 weeks, until antituberculous therapy is given—assuming the patient's hemodynamics will allow this. Unless trauma is the etiology, the first therapeutic maneuver in the remainder of cases can be ultrasound-guided aspiration with the potential for placement of a catheter in the pericardial space. If trauma is the etiology, all wounds need to be explored in the operating room immediately.

With regard to preoperative preparation, the best plan is to make sure the patient is not volume-depleted. Then, if the patient begins to deteriorate prior to initiation of one of the above procedures, pericardiocentesis should be done at the bedside. This can be easily accomplished using a 19-gauge spinal needle, a stopcock, and a 60-cc syringe. If available, an alligator clamp attached to an ECG electrode can be used to determine

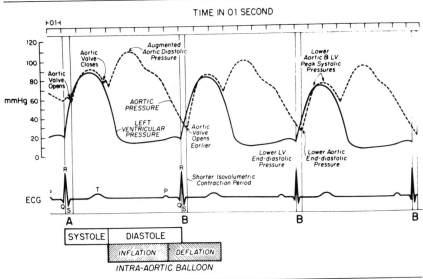

Fig. 18-4. Schematic representation of the relationships of the electrical and mechanical events of the cardiac cycle during intra-aortic balloon (IAB) counterpulsation. IAB inflation early in diastole augments aortic diastolic and coronary perfusion pressure, whereas IAB deflation in late diastole lowers aortic diastolic pressure and shortens the duration of isovolumetric contraction by allowing the aortic valve to open earlier (B versus A) and at a lower level of developed left ventricular pressure. Properly synchronized IAB counterpulsation eventually results in lower left ventricular and aortic peak systolic and end-diastolic pressures (IAB inflation and deflation indicators shown in only one cardiac cycle.) (From R. S. Litwak, Analysis, Maintenance, and Support of Cardiac Function After Cardiac Surgery. In R. S. Litwak and R. A. Jurado (eds.), *Care of the Cardiac Surgical Patient.* Norwalk, CT: Appleton-Century-Crofts, 1982. P. 224. Reproduced by permission.)

when the needle has touched the ventricle. A premature ventricular contraction will be seen on the tracing. The needle should be inserted just left of the xiphoid process at approximately a 45-degree angle to the skin and angled toward the patient's left shoulder (Fig. 18-6).

If the effusion reoccurs, after a trial of catheter placement, operative intervention is indicated. In a patient with a limited life expectancy, such as a cancer patient, a partial pericardiectomy through a left thoracotomy is appropriate. This procedure involves removal of all of the pericardium within the operative field from phrenic nerve to the anterior pericardium. In patients with a normal life expectancy, the more definitive anterior pericardiectomy through a median sternotomy is indicated. This procedure involves removal of the pericardium from the great vessels to the diaphragm and phrenic nerve to phrenic nerve (Fig. 18-7). Rarely, cardiopulmonary bypass is necessary.

The most important prognostic indicator seems to be preoperative func-

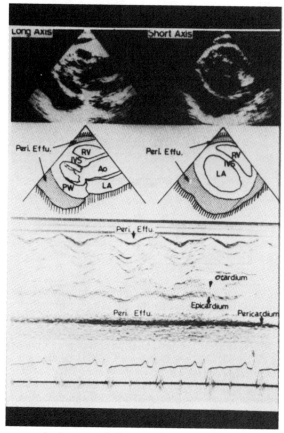

Fig. 18-5. Upper panels: long- and short-axis views of a large pericardial effusion on a two-dimensional echocardiogram. Lower panel: M-mode echocardiogram at the midventricular level, showing echo-free spaces that denote anterior and posterior pericardial effusions. Peri. Effu. = pericardial effusion; RV = right ventricle; IVS = interventricular septum; Ao = aorta; PW = left ventricular posterior wall; LA = left atrium. (From P. M. Shah, Echocardiography in Pericardial Diseases. In P. S. Reddy et al. (eds.), *Pericardial Disease,* New York: Raven Press, 1982. P. 133. Reproduced by permission.)

tional class. Operative mortality is essentially 0 percent for patients in New York Heart Association classes I or II, 10 percent for those in New York Heart Association class III, and 46 percent for those in New York Heart Association class IV.

ACUTE MYOCARDIAL INFARCTION WITH VENTRICULAR DYSFUNCTION

If one suspects acute myocardial infarction as the etiology for congestive heart failure, a history of previous myocardial infarction or angina may be elicited. Physical examination will support the diagnosis of cardiogenic

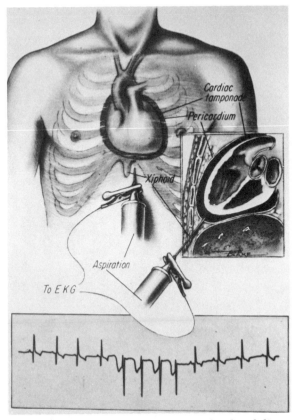

Fig. 18-6. The needle is inserted to the left of the xiphoid and directed toward the midscapular area. The electrocardiogram is attached to the needle, and the negative deflection of the QRS complex represents contact with the heart surface. The needle is slowly withdrawn, and the electrocardiogram reverts to normal when the needle loses contact with the myocardium. (From P. A. Ebert, The Percardium. In D. C. Sabiston and F. C. Spencer, *Gibbon's Surgery of the Chest.* Philadelphia: Saunders, 1983. P. 996. Reproduced by permission.)

shock, which is defined as a systemic arterial blood pressure of less than 80 mm Hg or of 30 mm Hg less than basal level and a cardiac index (CI) less than 2 liters/min/m^2 in the presence of adequate filling pressures. Furthermore, there is evidence of decreased blood flow, as indicated by low urine output (less than 20 ml/hour), impaired mentation, and signs of decreased peripheral perfusion—i.e., peripherally cool and diaphoretic. The patient may have an S3 gallop on cardiac examination, with bibasilar rales on pulmonary examination. Chest x-ray will show a normal-sized heart with pulmonary vascular redistribution. ECG will show the classic S–T segment depressions with Q waves depending on the time course of the event. Echocardiogram will likely demonstrate wall motion abnormalities. Immediate cardiac catheterization should be performed if the patient pre-

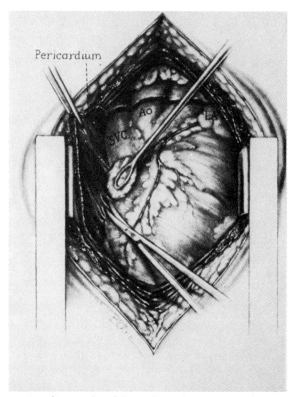

Fig. 18-7. The pericardium is freed from the right atrium and venae cavae.
These very thin-walled structures are easily torn, and adequate exposure is
mandatory for this part of the dissection. (From P. A. Ebert, The Pericardiums.
In D. C. Sabiston and F. C. Spencer, *Gibbon's Surgery of the Chest.*
Philadelphia: Saunders, 1983. P. 1007. Reproduced by permission.)

sents within the first 6 hours of the onset of symptoms, to delineate coronary anatomy. Revascularization currently can be attempted by percutaneous transluminal coronary angioplasty (PTCA) or surgery. We will
assume, for the purposes of this chapter, that the patient's anatomy dis-
qualifies him/her for PTCA. The indication to proceed to surgery in the
face of an acute evolving myocardial infarction is duration of symptoms of
less than 6 hours with (1) unstable hemodynamics or (2) postinfarction
angina and double- or triple-vessel coronary artery disease.

The rationale for proceeding to revascularization in this setting is twofold. First, a new occlusion may interrupt collaterals to other compromised
vessels, yielding "ischemia at a distance." Second, left ventricular subendocardial ischemia can occur in cardiogenic shock secondary to increased
left ventricular cavity pressure and decreased coronary perfusion pressure.

Time is obviously of the essence, but while the patient is still in the catheterization laboratory and the operating room is being readied, guided
placement of an intra-aortic balloon is indicated, to improve coronary artery perfusion pressure as well as to unload the heart.

Coronary artery bypass grafting is the operation performed. Most would agree that the use of the internal mammary artery under these circumstances is not advisable, because of the slight increase in the amount of time required to provide revascularization and, more importantly, because it is a lower flow conduit than is the saphenous vein graft.

Results with this approach have been gratifying. DeWood and associates studied two groups of patients with acute anterior transmural myocardial infarction. In the group undergoing reperfusion within 6 hours of symptoms' onset, there was a significant improvement in global and regional ventricular function. Berg and associates reported their results in 227 patients with acute evolving myocardial infarction who had coronary artery bypass grafting performed in less than 6 hours after the onset of symptoms. Their in-hospital mortality was 1.7 percent and first-year mortality was 1.4 percent. In comparison, there was a hospital mortality of 11.5 percent in 200 patients treated conventionally in their hospital for acute evolving myocardial infarction.

MECHANICAL COMPLICATIONS OF ACUTE MYOCARDIAL INFARCTION: VENTRICULAR SEPTAL DEFECT AND MITRAL REGURGITATION

The classic history for development of one of the mechanical complications of acute myocardial infarction is sudden hemodynamic deterioration, frequently leading to cardiogenic shock in days to 2 weeks after the diagnosis of myocardial infarction. This is accompanied by a physical examination that reveals a new systolic murmur. Frequently, the heart failure is more right-sided for ventricular septal defect (VSD), versus mostly left-sided failure for acute mitral regurgitation (MR). Chest x-ray will likely show pulmonary vascular redistribution. ECG will show recent myocardial infarction. In this setting the immediate next step in the workup should be placement of a pulmonary artery catheter. This will make the diagnosis of postinfarction VSD (oxygen saturation step-up in the right atrium compared with the pulmonary artery greater than or equal to 5 volumes percent) versus postinfarction MR (V waves on pulmonary capillary wedge tracing greater than 10 mm Hg above the mean). While the catheterization laboratory is being readied, urgent echocardiogram will help substantiate and typify the diagnosis—specifically, the location of the VSD can be ascertained and the anatomy of the MR visualized (chordal rupture versus papillary muscle dysfunction).

The very next step should be placement of the intra-aortic balloon in the catheterization laboratory prior to cardiac catheterization with left ventriculography. The intra-aortic balloon helps to reduce the left-to-right shunt of the VSD by its unloading of the left ventricle. With postinfarction MR the intra-aortic balloon helps to unload the acutely volume-overloaded left ventricle. These hemodynamic benefits frequently are enough to allow stabilization of the patient long enough for cardiac catheterization.

Postinfarction Ventricular Septal Defect

When the diagnosis of postinfarction VSD is confirmed, the patient should be taken to surgery as soon as an operating room can be made available.

On rare occasions (less than 5 percent of the time) the patient is hemodynamically stable without any signs of end-organ dysfunction and will benefit from maturation and fibrosis of the area of injury prior to repair. These few patients need to be monitored very closely in the hospital, however, for any change in status. Contraindications to proceeding immediately to surgery in the vast majority of patients would be a history of prolonged shock with end-organ dysfunction, such as acute renal failure, a history of metastatic carcinoma, or irreversible brain damage.

The operation performed, in general, requires infarctectomy through a left ventriculotomy and septal patching. If the defect is in the posterior septum, prosthetic replacement of the posterior left ventricular (LV) free wall is indicated. Major coronary artery obstructions are bypassed (Fig. 18-8).

Hospital mortality is influenced by several factors. If right ventricular (RV) contractility is good, 80 percent operative survival can be expected, but if RV contractility is poor, there is only 24 percent operative survival. In patients with anterior defects, there is an 85 percent hospital survival rate, but in patients with posterior defects there is only a 67 percent hospital survival rate. Of hospital survivors, approximately 75 percent are alive 5 years later.

Postinfarction Mitral Regurgitation

The indications for proceeding to urgent surgery are quite similar to those for VSD. This population of patients is clearly among the sickest of the patients discussed in this chapter, as their presentation is that of florid pulmonary edema. Clearly, surgery needs to be done prior to any signs of LV decompensation, but this is rarely possible unless the patient is in the hospital when he/she infarcts. Clearly, if the diagnosis of papillary muscle rupture can be made on echocardiogram, there is no virtue to temporizing.

The operation performed depends on the lesion of the mitral valve. Papillary muscle rupture requires mitral valve replacement. Chordal rupture, in selected circumstances (involving less than or equal to half of the circumference of the posterior leaflet) may be best treated by mitral valvuloplasty, which has the added benefit of better preservation of LV function (Fig. 18-9). Barratt-Boyes reported a 17 percent hospital mortality rate for mitral valve replacement performed less than 6 weeks after myocardial infarction and a 6 percent hospital mortality for that performed more than 6 weeks after myocardial infarction. In his acute series (less than 6 weeks), there was 100 percent survival at 4 years.

ACUTE AORTIC INSUFFICIENCY

Aortic Infective Endocarditis

The most common cause of acute aortic insufficiency requiring surgical attention is infective endocarditis. In Barratt-Boyes' series, 29 percent of the patients had aortic insufficiency requiring surgery on this basis. The pathophysiology of aortic insufficiency secondary to infective endocarditis is that of destruction of the aortic valve leaflets and, frequently, the occurrence of vegetations, both of which often do not allow apposition of the aortic valve leaflets. Further destruction can result in the formation of an

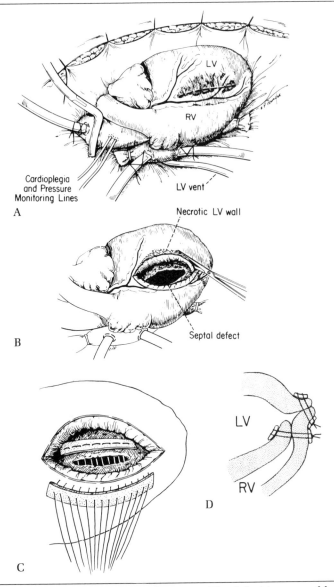

Fig. 18-8. A. Approach to anterior septal rupture. The defect is exposed by an incision (dashed line) through the center of the infarcted area of the left ventricle (LV). B. Necrotic left ventricular wall is debrided, improving exposure of the septal defect and avoiding later difficulty with sutures pulling out through this friable tissue. RV = right ventricle. C. Closure of a small anterior septal defect by approximation of the septum to the right ventricular free wall. Strips of Teflon felt are used to buttress interrupted mattress sutures of 0-Tevdek. D. All sutures are placed before any are tied. The ventriculotomy is closed in a similar manner. A cross-section of the completed repair is shown. LV = left ventricle; RV = right ventricle. (From S. W. Guyton and W. M. Daggett, Surgical repair of postinfarction ventricular septal rupture. In L. H. Cohn (ed.), *Modern Technics in Surgery/Cardiac Thoracic Surgery*. Mt. Kisco, NY: Futura, 1983. Pp. 61–64. Reproduced by permission.)

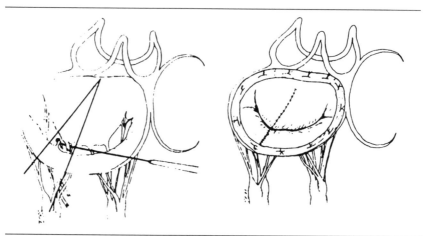

Fig. 18-9. Chordal ruptures. Segmental resection of the anterior leaflet is
triangular in shape, with the apex pointing toward the aortic valve. Posterior
leaflet resections are trapezoidal. All segmental resections must be followed by
ring annuloplasty. (From G. C. Duran, Reconstructive Procedures of the Mitral
Valve Including Ring Annuloplasty. In L. H. Cohn (ed.), *Modern Technics in
Surgery/Cardiac Thoracic Surgery*. Mt. Kisco, NY: Futura, 1979. Pp. 20–25.
Reproduced by permission.)

aneurysm of the sinus of Valsalva, fistulae between the aorta and atria or
ventricles, and myocardial abscess that can result in heart block. When one
suspects this diagnosis, it is important to ask if there is a history of a known
heart murmur, intravenous drug abuse, or any recent invasive procedures,
such as dental work or cystoscopy. Physical examination may reveal water
hammer pulses and a holodiastolic murmur with radiation to the apex.
Chest x-ray may show increased pulmonary vascular markings and LV
prominence. ECG demonstrates LV strain. Echocardiogram visualizes the
insufficient valve, as well as giving a picture of LV function; it may also
show vegetations on the valve. If one is planning surgery in the under-40
age group, cardiac catheterization is not necessary as long as there is no
history of coronary artery disease; however, cardiac catheterization is important in those over 40 years of age, due to the increasing incidence of
coronary artery disease with age.

   Of course, the primary treatment for infective endocarditis is antibiotics.
However, surgery is indicated in several specific instances. Failure of medical therapy resulting in congestive heart failure, signs of persistent sepsis
after 1 week of antibiotics, or recurrent episodes of thromboembolism are
regarded as clear indications for surgical therapy. Further, staphylococcal
endocarditis not responding early on to antibiotics is an indication for earlier surgery. Finally, fungal endocarditis is an indication for urgent surgery,
due to nearly uniformly-fatal results with medical therapy.

   It may be that unloading agents and digitalis are needed to stabilize the
patient long enough to obtain several days of sustained adequate antibiotic

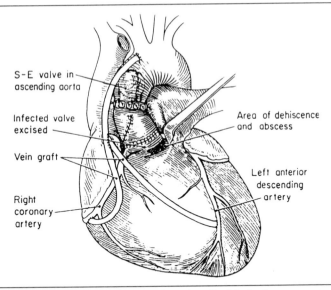

S-E valve in ascending aorta

Infected valve excised

Vein graft

Right coronary artery

Area of dehiscence and abscess

Left anterior descending artery

Fig. 18-10. Diagram of aortic valve translocation. In this instance, coronary artery bypass originated as a Y-graft from the ascending aorta. S-E = Starr-Edwards valve. (From G. K. Danielson et al. Successful treatment of aortic valve endocarditis and aortic root abscesses by insertion of prosthetic valve in ascending aorta and placement of bypass grafts to coronary arteries. *J. Thorac. Cardiovasc. Surg.* 67:443, 1974. Reproduced by permission.)

levels. The most important concern with regard to preoperative timing is that the patient be operated upon prior to LV decompensation.

An important principle in this type of surgery is that of meticulous debridement. If infection is confined to the leaflets, the surgical procedure is aortic valve replacement. There is some controversy regarding which valve has the least chance of becoming reinfected. However, if homograft placement is possible, this approach probably has the lowest rate of prosthetic valve endocarditis. If there is extensive annular destruction, the procedure required may be placement of the valve in the supra-annular position with coronary artery bypass of the excluded coronary ostia (Fig. 18-10). For a sinus of Valsalva aneurysm with perforation, a pledgetted closure or patch closure of the perforation may be required. If the process has advanced to the point of aorto-LV discontinuity, a patch repair is required.

In general, operative mortality is 2 percent, with a 5-year survival of 85 percent. Reinfection rate is 10 percent.

Acute Ascending Aortic Dissection

Aortic insufficiency secondary to acute dissection is another cause of acute congestive heart failure requiring immediate surgical attention. The pathophysiology of this process involves blood suddenly leaving the normal aortic channel through an intimal tear and dissecting the inner from the outer layer of the media. This process then causes a disruption of the support structures of the aortic valve, leading to acute incompetence. This can be seen with types I or II dissection (also known as type A). Predisposing factors include cystic medial necrosis, Marfan's syndrome, bicuspid aortic valve, and a history of hypertension. Presentation is usually dramatic: sudden death, hypovolemic shock, acute aortic insufficiency, or cardiac tamponade. Further, the patient may complain of severe intrascapular pain with a feeling of impending death. Major vessel occlusion may be the mode of presentation manifesting as stroke, a numb pulseless extremity, paraparesis/paraplegia, or oliguria/anuria. If pain is the only symptom, an important differential diagnosis is myocardial infarction.

Chest x-ray will demonstrate an enlarged mediastinal silhouette, possibly with cardiomegaly or pleural effusion (left more frequently than right). Echocardiogram is accurate in demonstrating a false lumen, although in the setting of an acutely ill patient as described above, the time is better spent in obtaining aortography (Fig. 18-11).

During the evaluation phase of the patient's course, intravenous vasodilator therapy along with β-blockade (to diminish dp/dt) is important to help arrest progression of the dissection.

The purpose of surgery for this problem is twofold: first, to prevent death from exsanguination; and second, to reestablish flow. In view of this, once the patient has undergone aortography, emergency surgery is indicated. The only real contraindications would be metastatic carcinoma and brain death. Paraplegia cannot be expected to be reversed, but death from exsanguination can still be prevented. Paraparesis, on the other hand, may recede.

The surgical procedures available include interposition graft replacement of the ascending aorta with resuspension of the aortic valve leaflets at the commissures (Fig. 18-12), valved conduit replacement of the aortic root, and aortic valve replacement with interposition graft replacement of the ascending aorta.

Miller's series showed that a minority (11 percent) of patients required aortic valve replacement.

Results from surgical treatment of this problem in Miller's series and in those of others revealed a 35 percent operative mortality (unaffected by the need for aortic valve replacement) and an actuarial survival of 66 percent at 5 years and of 37 percent at 10 years.

PULMONARY EMBOLISM

When one is considering the diagnosis of pulmonary embolus, the basic historical questions include a history of immobilization or cancer. On physical examination, the finding for massive pulmonary embolus may be that of cardiogenic shock with acute right heart failure and tachypnea. Hypoxemia is a helpful and sensitive sign. Chest x-ray may show signs of pulmonary infarct, but this is present in a minority of cases. ECG is important to exclude myocardial infarction. Echocardiogram is not helpful in the evaluation of this problem. Of the salvageable subset, approximately 50 percent die within 2 hours of the acute episode. Consequently, it is im-

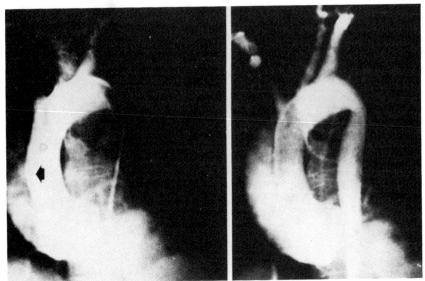

Fig. 18-11. Retrograde aortic root injection of contrast medium demonstrates aortic regurgitation secondary to dissection originating in the proximal ascending aorta. The arrow points to the partition between the true lumen (medial) and false channel (lateral). The picture on the right shows the characteristically narrow true lumen in the descending arota. The distal false channel has not as yet opacified. (From CCCETS, *SESATS Syllabus.* Copyright © 1980 by Kendall/Hunt Publishing Company. Reprinted with permission.)

portant to move the patient quickly to the angiography suite for pulmonary arteriography. Berger and associates have recommended giving 10,000 to 15,000 units of heparin to the patient as one is making arrangements to study the patient angiographically. Inotropes to maintain blood pressure are used as needed to support the patient during pulmonary arteriography.

Intervention without a pulmonary angiogram is deemed imprudent in the overwhelming majority of cases, as this is a difficult clinical diagnosis to make and is missed easily 50 percent of the time.

Indications for intervention (be it lytic therapy or pulmonary embolectomy) are generally felt to be (1) occlusion of the major trunks that involve greater than 50 percent of the pulmonary vasculature, as documented by angiography; (2) shock; (3) failure to reverse shock with moderate doses of inotropic support promptly after the onset of the event. Patients with contraindications for lytic therapy would include those with active bleeding, central nervous system damage within the last 2 months, a history of surgery within the last 10 days, inflammatory bowel disease, diverticular disease, a history of a recent intra-arterial procedure, malignant hypertension, and renal or hepatic insufficiency, as well as those who are pregnant or who are less than 10 days postpartum. This list of patients would clearly be better managed by operative pulmonary embolectomy. To this list

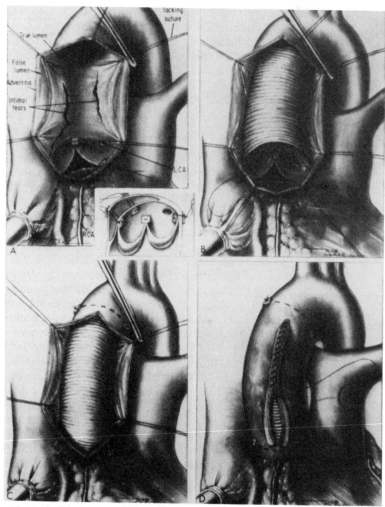

Fig. 18-12. A. Diagram of the open ascending aorta demonstrating initial tear and dissection, as well as techniques of resuspension of the aortic valve. B. Suturing of the woven Dacron graft inside the aorta. C. The graft sutured within the ascending aorta. D. Closure of the adventitia over the Dacron graft. (From W. G. Wolfe, Acute ascending aortic dissection. *Ann. Surg.* 192:658, 1980. Reproduced by permission.)

should be added patients who suffer a cardiac arrest in the initial phases of lytic therapy or at the time of pulmonary arteriography. Operative intervention in this last population not only deals with the pulmonary embolus, but also allows for resuscitation with the institution of cardiopulmonary bypass by the femoral artery/femoral vein route.

The operative procedure involves the utilization of cardiopulmonary bypass and then opening the main pulmonary artery and manually extracting

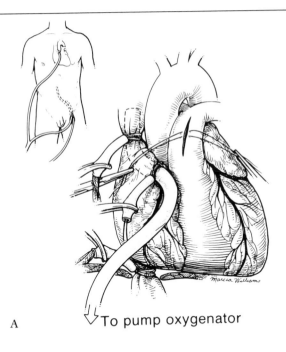

A   ⤵ To pump oxygenator

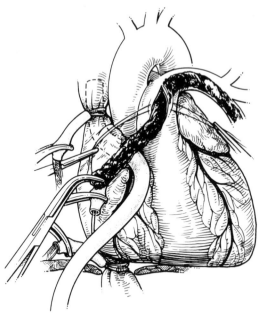

B

Fig. 18-13. A. The superior vena cava is cannulated through the right atrial appendage and total cardiopulmonary bypass is established. A longitudinal pulmonary arteriotomy is made between two stay sutures. B. The clot is engaged, the instrument is slowly withdrawn, and with it the clot is extracted. (From R. Berger and Z. Davis, Pulmonary Embolectomy. In L. H. Cohn (ed.), *Modern Technics in Surgery/Cardiac Thoracic Surgery.* Mt. Kisco, NY: Futura, 1980. Pp. 32–37 and 32–39. Reproduced by permission.)

thrombus from the affected side, as well as "milking" peripheral thrombi out through the main pulmonary artery (Fig. 18-13).

With the current state of the art, operative mortality is 25 to 30 percent.

POSTCARDIOTOMY CARDIOGENIC SHOCK

The usual scenario involved in this case is that of a technically perfect open heart operation in a patient who then cannot be weaned from bypass despite inotropes, vasodilators, or the intra-aortic balloon. The incidence of this occurrence is approximately 1 percent of open heart procedures performed with hyperkalemic cardioplegia. The usual criteria for patient selection are age less than 70 years, CI less than 1.8 liters/min/m^2, systemic blood pressure less than 90 mm Hg, and left atrial pressure greater than 25 mm Hg. (If RV failure is involved, the left atrial pressure will remain less than 15 mm Hg despite volume-loading the right side to 25 mm Hg.)

Several assist devices are available for support of the heart under these circumstances. The theory behind their use is that they will allow for diminished myocardial oxygen consumption and work, thereby allowing time for recovery of the "stunned" myocardium. Three different pump types are currently available—roller, centrifugal, and pneumatic. For LV assist, they are attached to the left atrium and aorta; for RV assist, they are attached to the right atrium and pulmonary artery. Patients needing biventricular support can have either implantation of two separate ventricular assist devices (VAD) or implantation of the total artificial heart (TAH). This is an area of debate, in theory; and in practical terms, sometimes RV failure is not apparent until the LV has been unloaded by an assist device. Also, total artificial heart commits the patient to either a lifetime with a TAH or a transplantation.

Survival ranges from 25 to 45 percent in most series, with greater than 90 percent of patients in NYHA I and II.

CARDIOMYOPATHIES

In patients who present in profound congestive heart failure *de novo*, a history of a viral syndrome, alcohol abuse, pregnancy, hypertension, or amyloidosis should be sought. Physical examination may reveal signs of univentricular or biventricular heart failure. Chest x-ray will show an enlarged cardiac silhouette. Cardiac catheterization will reveal a markedly diminished ejection fraction (usually less than 15 percent). Endomyocardial biopsy is infrequently helpful as to the etiology of the cardiomyopathy.

Candidates for transplantation are those patients with cardiomyopathy for whom there is no other treatment and whose prognosis is presumed at approximately 6 months.

Preoperative preparation includes recipient screening. This means that patients should be no older than 60 years (as a rule); be psychologically stable; have no infection, insulin-dependent diabetes mellitus, peptic ulcer disease, or recent history of pulmonary embolus; and have a pulmonary vascular resistance less than 7 wood units/m^2. When a donor heart becomes available, the recipient and donor must be ABO compatible, and their sizes should be comparable (within 10 to 15 kg of each other). A lymphocyte cross-match is performed between donor and recipient only if a preexisting recipient antibody screen is highly positive.

Distant procurement is the rule these days. Most authorities feel that there are 4 hours available from time of harvest to implant in order to expect a well-functioning heart.

Prognosis continues to improve. Currently, there is an 80 percent 1-year survival and a 50 to 60 percent 5-year survival. Most all of these patients function in NYHA class I.

Cardiomyopathies Listed for Transplantation with a Deterioration in Their Heart Failure

In this set of circumstances the patient has failed outpatient and inpatient medical management, as well as intra-aortic balloon support. This is the setting for VAD as a "bridge to transplant." A left or right VAD or both can be implanted until a heart becomes available, at which time transplantation would be performed as long as an absolute contraindication to transplantation did not develop in the interim.

Overall survival with this approach has been 48 percent, although the numbers are small.

SELECTED READINGS

Berg, R., Selinger, S. L., Leonard, J. J., et al. Immediate coronary artery bypass for acute evolving myocardial infarction. *J. Thorac. Cardiovasc. Surg.* 81:493, 1981.

Berger, R. L., and Davis, Z. Pulmonary Embolectomy. In L. H. Cohn (ed.), *Modern Technics in Surgery/Cardiac Thoracic Surgery,* Mt. Kisco, NY: Futura, 1980. Pp. 32–31.

Berger, R. L., Gibson, H., and Faris, E. J. Reappraisal of the indications of pulmonary embolectomy. *Am. J. Surg.* 116:403, 1968.

Braunwald, E. *Heart Disease: A Textbook of Cardiovascular Medicine* (2nd ed.). Philadelphia: Saunders, 1984.

Cohn, L. H., and DiSesa, V. J. *Aortic Regurgitation: Medical/Surgical Management.* New York: Marcel Dekker, 1986.

Daggett, W. M., et al. Improved results of surgical management of postinfarction ventricular septal rupture. *Ann. Surg.* 196:269, 1982.

DeWood, M. A., Heit, J., Spores, J., et al. Anterior transmural myocardial infarction: Effect of surgical coronary reperfusion on global and regional left ventricular function. *J. Am. Coll. Cardiol.* 1:1223, 1983.

Fananapazir, L., et al. Right ventricular dysfunction and surgical outcome in postinfarction ventricular septal defect. *Eur. Heart J.* 4:155, 1983.

Fragomeni, L. S., and Kaye, M. P. The Registry of the International Society for Heart Transplantation: Fifth Official Report—1988. *J. Heart Transplant.* 7:249, 1988.

Holmes, J., Kubo, S. H., Cody, R. J., et al. Arrhythmias in ischemic and non-ischemic dilated cardiomyopathy: Prediction of mortality by ambulatory electrocardiography. *Am. J. Cardiol.* 55:146, 1985.

Kay, P. H., Oldershaw, P. J., Dawkins, K., et al. The results of surgery for active endocarditis of the n tive aortic valve. *J. Cardiovasc. Surg.* 23:321, 1984.

Kirklin, J. W., and Barr tt-Boyes, B. G. *Cardiac Surgery.* New York: Churchill Livingston, 1986.

Miller, D. C., Stinson, E. B., Oyer, P. E., et al. Operative treatment of aortic dissection: Experience with 125 patients over a 16-year period. *J. Thorac. Cardiovasc. Surg.* 78:365, 1979.

Pae, W. E. Temporary ventricular support—Current indications and results. *Trans. Am. Soc. Artif. Intern. Organs* 33:4, 1987.

Pae, W. E., Pierce, W. S., Pennock, J. L., et al. Long-term results of ventricular assist pumping in postcardiotomy cardiogenic shock. *J. Thorac. Cardiovasc. Surg.* 93:434, 1987.

Pae, W. E., and Pierce, W. S. Combined Registry for the Clinical Use of Mechanical Ventricular Assist Pumps and the Total Artificial Heart. First Official Report—1986. *J. Heart Transplant.* 6:68, 1987.

Pennock, J. L., Pierce, W. S., Campbell, D. B., et al. Mechanical support of the circulation followed by cardiac transplantation. *J. Thorac. Cardiovasc. Surg.* 92:994, 1986.

Roberts, A. J. *Difficult Problems in Adult Cardiac Surgery.* Chicago: Year Book, 1985.

Robinson, R. J., Fehrenbacher, J., Brown, J. W., et al. Emergent pulmonary embolectomy: The treatment for massive pulmonary embolism. *Ann. Thorac. Surg.* 42:54, 1986.

Sabiston, D. C., and Spencer, F. C. *Gibbon's Surgery of the Chest* (4th ed.). Philadelphia: Saunders, 1983.

Unverferth, D. V., Magorien, R. D., Moeschberger, M. L., et al. Factors influencing the one-year mortality of dilated cardiomyopathy. *Am. J. Cardiol.* 54:147, 1984.

Volgesang, G. B., and Bell, W. R. Treatment of pulmonary embolism and deep vein thrombosis with thrombolytic therapy. *Clin. Chest Med.* 5:489, 1984.

19

Pathophysiology, Monitoring, Outcome Prediction, and Therapy of Shock and Trauma States

William C. Shoemaker
Harry B. Kram

In shock states, treatment should be given promptly and in the early stages, when it is most effective; it should be given aggressively and adequately to correct the primary underlying circulatory problem; and it should be titrated to achieve optimal physiologic goals. The clinical problem is that shock is a syndrome—a symptom complex. Therefore, it is recognized clinically by symptoms and signs that are subjective and imprecise. Moreover, the traditional approach is based on these subjective signs and symptoms as therapeutic criteria. Although most patients eventually get all the therapy they need by this approach, it is not necessarily at the right time, in the right amount, or in the right order. The result is often less than optimal.

This chapter describes the physiologic natural history of various shock syndromes in terms of their circulatory physiology, contrasts the hemodynamic and oxygen transport patterns of survivors and nonsurvivors, describes outcome predictors, defines objective physiologic criteria for therapeutic goals based on survival patterns, and proposes therapeutic regimens that improve survival rates and minimize complications.

Misconceptions that have obscured our understanding of the essential nature of acute circulatory failure are as follows. First, there is the misconception that the shock state is primarily hypotension, low flow, and high resistance. This concept arose from experimental studies on hemorrhagic and early clinical studies of cardiogenic, accidental traumatic, and postoperative shock [2–4, 6–8, 11, 13–21, 28–30]. However, the anesthetized, exsanguinated dog and the patient with hypovolemia or myocardial infarction are not representative of most clinical shock syndromes, particularly postoperative conditions [2, 3, 7, 8, 11, 13–15, 28, 30]. Second, shock was often regarded as a single physiologic entity rather than a widely diverse group of life-threatening circulatory conditions whose multifactorial physiologic patterns ·volve in time [3, 14, 16]. A third misconception is that therapeutic goal· are to restore blood pressure (BP), heart rate (HR), and cardiac output values to their normal range. The dangerous assumption of this approach is that normal or high cardiac values indicate no further volume therapy is needed and that vasopressors are appropriate to maintain pressure. Therapy based on these and other simplistic notions is likely to be suboptimally effective [16].

THE CONVENTIONAL APPROACH BY ETIOLOGIES
Traditionally, shock is analyzed and classified by etiology: i.e., hemorrhagic, cardiogenic, traumatic, and septic shock syndromes. Each of these etiologic categories of shock are then described by their clinical signs and symptoms, laboratory findings, and primary pathophysiologic derangements. Therapeutic principles based on this approach were developed for each etiologic type of shock (Table 19-1).

This approach is simple, easily understood, and generally accepted—but wrong. The real problem is that this approach is a simplistic answer to a complex problem; in real life, each primary etiologic event does not begin and end with a single pathophysiologic alteration that when therapeutically corrected, necessarily reverses the primary cause. This is because the primary alteration of each etiologic type of shock produces complex sets of neural and hormonal compensatory reactions that on decompensation, lead to circulatory failure and complications. Some of these physiologic interactions are obvious: in hemorrhage, reduced blood volume decreases flow and oxygen transport; in cardiogenic shock, the reduced flow decreases BP and oxygen transport; in traumatic and septic shock, flow increases, but these increases may not be sufficient for the concomitantly increased metabolic requirements. Thus, interacting changes in volume, flow, and oxygen transport irrespective of the initiating event lead to the characteristic patterns of survival or circulatory failure and death [15].

DIMENSIONS OF CIRCULATORY FUNCTION
Circulatory function may be expressed in terms of cardiac hemodynamics, but these cardiac functions reflect only one aspect of circulatory function. Overall evaluation of circulatory function includes the fundamental dimensions that physically characterize fluid systems: pressure, volume, flow, and function. The function of the circulation may be described by oxygen transport and consumption ($\dot{V}O_2$) [22].

Figure 19-1 schematically represents the four dimensions of the normal circulation, with 100 percent as the normal value of each dimension. This representation can illustrate changes in these principal dimensions and their interactions. For example, Figure 19-2 illustrates average changes observed in a large series of patients with compensated septic shock. The normal values (shown by the fine lines of the square) may be compared to the thick lines representing decreased arterial pressure and blood volume from dehydration and fever, as well as increased flow and $\dot{V}O_2$. The lower horizontal dimension, representing $\dot{V}O_2$, shows the normal value, the actual observed mean value, and the needed $\dot{V}O_2$ values that are found in compensated septic patients [15].

Figure 19-3 illustrates the evolving pattern of circulatory dimensions in hemorrhagic (upper tier), cardiogenic (second tier), traumatic (third tier),

Table 19-1. Approach to various etiologic types of shock

	Hemorrhagic	Cardiogenic	Traumatic	Septic
Signs and symptoms	Pallor, fainting	Pallor, fainting	History of injury	Fever, chills
	Skin clammy, cold	Skin clammy, cold	Physical evidence of injury, fractures	Skin warm
	Tachycardia	Arrhythmias	Oliguria	Tachycardia
	Oliguria	Oliguria	Tachycardia	Oliguria
	Collapse	Collapse	Collapse	Altered mental status
				Collapse
Laboratory	↓ Hct, Hgb	↑ Cardiac enzymes	X-rays, CT scan, angiograms for organ and vascular injury	Positive smears and cultures
		ECG		
Pathophysiology	↓ Blood volume	↓ Cardiac output	Direct injury to organs and tissue	Peripheral resistance
Therapy	1. Fluids	1. Antiarrhythmics	1. Repair injuries	1. Antibiotics
	2. Blood	2. Vasopressors	2. Fluids	2. Fluids
	3. Control bleeding	3. Vasodilators	3. Blood	3. Drain abscesses

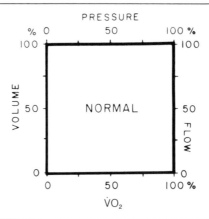

Fig. 19-1. Normal circulatory dimensions representing pressure, volume, flow, and function ($\dot{V}O_2$). The dimensions are drawn to a scale in which the normal values are shown as 100 percent and changes of each dimension above or below the normal expressed as percentage changes of that scale.

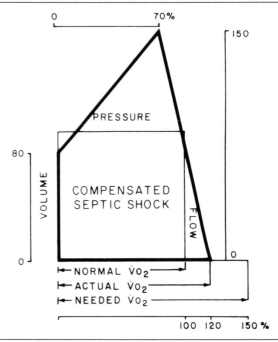

Fig. 19-2. Average values of patients with compensated septic shock showing 20 percent reduction in volume and 30 percent drop in pressure, but 75 percent increase in flow and 20 percent increase in $\dot{V}O_2$. Although the observed $\dot{V}O_2$ values are greater than normal, they are considerably less than needed.

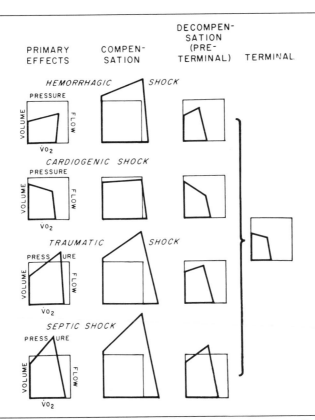

Fig. 19-3. Circulatory dimensions of patients with hemorrhagic, cardiogenic, traumatic, and septic shock. The primary effects of each etiologic type, their compensatory responses, their decompensations, and their terminal state are shown.

and septic shock (lowest tier) syndromes. The initial primary changes of each etiologic type of shock at the time of the initial hypotensive crises are shown in the left column; the mean values of compensated shock are shown in the second column; the decompensated state in the third column; and the terminal state, which is often very similar in each etiologic type of shock, is shown on the extreme right. The figure shows interactions of circulatory dimensions: (a) produced by the primary etiologic event, (b) the body's compensatory responses usually represented by increased flow, (c) decompensation, and (d) terminal state result from inadequate flow, $\dot{D}O_2$, and $\dot{V}O_2$ [2–4, 15–22].

THE CLINICAL PROBLEM
In critical illness, circulatory status largely depends on the nature and severity of the primary event, the severity of hypotension, the duration of the

shock state, the presence of associated medical illnesses, the patient's physiologic reserve capacities, and the influence of therapy, as well as many
other associated clinical factors. Uncontrolled anecdotal observations of
patients with widely differing etiologies, degrees of shock, durations of
shock, and associated conditions have led to confused therapeutic priorities. Nevertheless, the most important factor is time; rapid, expeditious
therapy in the early stages may lead to good results, but adequate therapy
that is delayed may be ineffective.

Shock usually is first recognized clinically by hypotension, tachycardia,
and oliguria, after which vigorous therapy is begun. When hypotension is
prevented or treated by vasopressors, the underlying physiologic problem
does not go away, it is just not apparent until lethal complications such as
shock lung, renal failure, overwhelming sepsis, and multiple organ failure
subsequently occur. Therapy must then be redirected toward myriad terminal mechanisms.

The conventional approach to shock therapy consists of a search for specific defects, their documentation, and their correction. This one-at-a-time
search for defects followed by their normalization unfortunately leads to
fragmented, episodic patient care [15]. The most serious flaw in this simplistic unidimensional approach is that it leads to simplistic unidimensional therapy. The primary event, its compensatory reactions, and its decompensations should be considered in the development of therapeutic
plans. Therapy of shock should address the major components of the disturbed circulation, not just the primary initiating event. An automobile
wreck produced by a tire blowout is not correctable by the tire's replacement.

PHYSIOLOGIC MONITORING
The Traditional Approach
The monitoring of patients in shock has conventionally been focused on
the superficial manifestations of shock that are conveniently available,
such as the vital signs, hematocrit (Hct), and urine output. Moreover, even
when invasive physiologic measurements are made, the conventional approach is to correct monitored deficiencies soon after they are discovered.
Commonly monitored variables were evaluated in a series of critically ill
postoperative survivors and nonsurvivors (Table 19-2) [30]. With therapy,
mean arterial pressure (MAP), heart rate (HR), central venous pressure
(CVP), pulmonary artery wedge pressures (WP), and cardiac output were
returned to the normal range in 76 percent of nonsurvivors, who nevethe-
less still went on to die despite return to normal values. By comparison,
75 percent of the survivors also had two or more values in the normal
range, indicating no essential differences between survivors and nonsurvivors. The commonly monitored variables are useful descriptors of the
end stage of circulatory failure, but they are not sensitive or accurate for
early warning of death in acutely ill surgical patients. Clearly, it is inappropriate to select variables because they are convenient to measure and
to select normal ranges as therapeutic goals. Objective criteria relevant to

Table 19-2. Number and percent of patients with
two or more values in the normal range

	Nonsurvivors		Survivors	
	Number	%	Number	%
Mean arterial pressure	29	78	68	89
Heart rate	30	81	66	87
Central venous pressure	35	95	72	95
Pulmonary wedge pressure	11	30	21	28
Cardiac index	35	95	64	84
Mean of all variables		76		75

outcome, not traditional ideas, are needed to select the appropriate physiologic variables to monitor, as well as the appropriate goals of therapy [15].

Invasive Monitoring of Hemodynamic and Oxygen Transport Variables

Repeated monitoring with systemic arterial and pulmonary arterial catheters (Table 19-3) provides frequent measurements of arterial and venous pressures in the systemic and pulmonary circulations, cardiac output, arterial and mixed venous gases and saturations, core temperature, hemoglobin (Hgb), and Hct [2, 3, 14–16]. A variety of hemodynamic values may be derived from these, including cardiac index (CI), systemic (SVRI) and pulmonary (PVRI) vascular resistance indexes, left (LVSWI) and right (RVSWI) ventricular stroke work indexes, and left (LCWI) and right (RCWI) cardiac work indexes. When arterial and mixed venous gases, saturation, and Hgb are measured simultaneously with cardiac output, oxygen delivery ($\dot{D}O_2$), oxygen consumption ($\dot{V}O_2$), oxygen extraction, pulmonary venous admixture or shunting ($\dot{Q}sp/\dot{Q}T$), and the alveolar-arterial oxygen gradient [P(A-a)O_2] can be calculated. Flow- and volume-related variables are indexed according to body surface area. The variables, abbreviations, units, formulas, normal values, and optimal values are shown in Table 19-3. These variables can be readily calculated on a computer or a hand-held programmable calculator [13, 15, 16, 21, 22].

PATHOPHYSIOLOGY: THE PHYSIOLOGIC NATURAL HISTORY OF SHOCK

The physiologic natural history of clinical shock produced by hemorrhage, accidental or surgical trauma, sepsis, cardiac problems, and various combinations of these etiologies was described by sequential changes obtained during periods remote from therapy: i.e., before therapy was begun or after the immediate direct effects of therapy were over. Distinctive patterns characterize the physiologic natural histories of the shock syndromes of various clinical etiologies [2, 3, 14–16].

Table 19-3. Cardiorespiratory variables: abbreviations, units, calculations, normal values, preferred values, and predictive capacity

Variables	Abbre-viations	Units	Measurements or calculations	Normal values	Preferred values	Percent correct
Volume-related						
Mean arterial pressure	MAP	mm Hg	Direct measurement	82–102	>84	76
Central vent pressure	CVP	cm H$_2$O	Direct measurement	1–9	<5	62
Central blood volume	CBV	ml/M^2	CBV = MTT × CI × 16.7	660–1,000	>925	61
Stroke index	SI	ml/M^2	SI = CI/HR	30–50	>48	67
Hemoglobin	Hgb	gm/dl	Direct measurement	12–16	>12	66
Mean pulmonary artery pressure	MPAP	mm Hg	Direct measurement	11–15	<19	68
Wedge pressure	WP	mm Hg	Direct measurement	0–12	>9.5	70
Blood volume	BV	ml/M^2	BV = PV/(1 − Hct)* × surface area	Men 2.74 Women 2.37	>3.0 2.7	76
Red cell mass	RCM	ml/M^2	RCM = BV − PV	Men 1.1 Women 0.95	>1.1 >0.95	85
Flow-related						
Cardiac index	CI	liter/min/M^2	Direct measurement	2.8–3.6	>4.5	70
Left vent stroke work	LVSW	gm·M/M^2	LVSW = SI × MAP × 0.0144	44–68	>55	74
Left cardiac work	LCW	kg·M/M^2	LCW = CI × MAP × 0.0144	3–4.6	>5	76
Right vent stroke work	RVSW	g·M/M^2	RVSW = SI × MPAP × 0.0144	4–8	>13	70
Right cardiac work	RCW	kg·M/M^2	RCW = CI × MPAP × 0.0144	0.4–0.6	>1.1	69

Stress-related						
Systemic vasc resist	SVR	dyne·sec/cm⁵·M²	$SVR = 79.92 \ (MAP\text{-}CVP)$†$/CI$	1,760–2,600	>1450	62
Pulmonary vasc resist	PVR	dyne·sec/cm⁵·M²	$PVR = 79.92 \ (MPAP\text{-}WP)$†$/CI$	45–225	<226	77
Heart rate	HR	beat/min	Direct measurement	72–88	<100	60
Rectal temperature	temp	°F	Direct measurement	97.8–98.6	>100.4	64
Oxygen-related						
Hemoglobin saturation	SaO_2	%	Direct measurement	95–99	>95	67
Arterial CO_2 tension	$PaCO_2$	torr	Direct measurement	36–44	>30	69
Arterial pH	pH	...	Direct measurement	7.36–7.44	>7.47	74
Mixed venous O_2 tension	$P\bar{v}O_2$	torr	Direct measurement	33–53	>36	68
Arterial-mixed venous O_2 content difference	$C(a - \bar{v})O_2$	ml/dl	$C(a - \bar{v})O_2 = CaO_2 - C\bar{v}O_2$	4–5.5	<3.5	68
O_2 delivery	$\dot{D}O_2$	ml/min/M²	$\dot{D}O_2 = CaO_2 \times CI \times 10$	450–600	>600	76
O_2 consumption	$\dot{V}O_2$	ml/min/M²	$\dot{V}O_2 = C(a - \bar{v})O_2 \times CI \times 10$	100–150	>167	69
O_2 extraction rate	O_2 ext	%	$O_2 \ ext = (CaO_2 - C\bar{v}O_2)/CaO_2$	22–30	<31	69

*Hematocrit (Hct) value corrected for packing fraction and large vessel hematocrit to total body hematocrit ratio.
†Venous pressures expressed in mm Hg.
Vasc resist = vascular resistance.
(From Shoemaker, W. C., Czer, L., Chang, P., et al. Cardiorespiratory monitoring in postoperative patients. I. Prediction of outcome and severity of illness. *Crit. Care Med.* 7:237, 1979. With permission.)

Hemodynamic and Oxygen Transport Patterns of Survivors and Nonsurvivors

Surgical trauma provides a unique opportunity to analyze shock, because physiologic measurements may be obtained in a preillness control period, during the hemodynamic crisis, and throughout the subsequent periods leading to recovery or death. Postoperative shock, therefore, serves as a model for other etiologic types of shock syndromes.

Circulatory patterns of a large series of critically ill surgical patients were observed over their temporal course preoperatively, intraoperatively, and postoperatively to characterize the effects of surgical trauma in actual time elapsed [2, 3, 14–16]. Despite the wide variety of surgical diseases and surgical operations, there were rather consistent physiologic patterns in postoperative survivors that were different from the patterns of nonsurvivors. Nevertheless, many preoperative conditions, including age, sepsis, accidental trauma, stress, hypovolemia, cirrhosis, and cardiac failure, affect these patterns [3]. There are a limited number of physiologic compensatory responses; physiologic patterns of the survivors compared with the patterns of those who died provide the basis for analyzing the nature and biologic importance of circulatory compensations.

Departures from the normal range may indicate compensatory responses, unrecognized complications, new physiologic processes, or cardiorespiratory deterioration of the patient; the basis for these alterations is not always apparent. Therefore, it is important to examine the pattern of responses in patients with relatively normal preoperative states, to identify the basic physiologic response to surgical trauma with and without the confounding influences of associated medical problems. Data from patients with specific diseases and complications also reveal important information about pathophysiology.

Although it may be impossible to survive carcinomatosis or random catastrophic events such as major transfusion reactions or pulmonary emboli, the great majority of nonsurvivors die of complications that may be directly or indirectly attributed to inadequate circulatory compensations or overwhelming surgical trauma [22].

Critically Ill Patients with Normal Preoperative Cardiac Output

To characterize the circulatory effects of operative trauma per se, circulatory patterns were observed in critically ill patients who preoperatively had normal cardiac output and no evidence of associated conditions that would affect baseline hemodynamic values (Figs. 19-4 through 19-7). Intraoperatively, CI, $\dot{D}O_2$, and $\dot{V}O_2$ fell from normal preoperative values in both survivors and nonsurvivors, but this fall was greater in the nonsurvivors. Postoperatively, there were minimal variations in the routine vital signs of both groups, but in survivors the $\dot{D}O_2$, $\dot{V}O_2$, and oxygen extraction steadily increased during the first 12 postoperative hours. There was an early partial recovery of these variables toward preoperative control values in those who died. The cardiorespiratory responses of nonsurvivors were similar but less pronounced than those of the survivors; the nonsurvivor pattern was characterized by early compensatory stress responses that

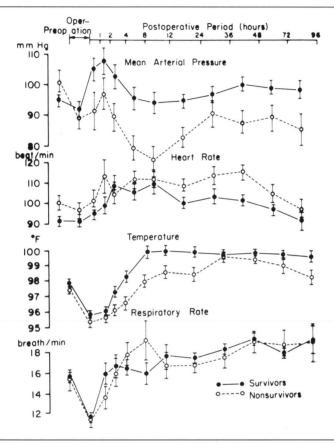

Fig. 19-4. Temporal patterns of the vital signs, mean arterial pressures, heart rates, temperatures, and respiratory rates of survivors (solid line) and nonsurvivors of life-threatening surgical illnesses. Dots represent mean values; vertical bars represent SEM in the preoperative control period, intraoperative period, and at various time intervals in the postoperative period. From Bland, Shoemaker, Abraham, et al. [2].

failed to achieve the magnitude of the survivors' responses. The nonsurvivors were often unable to maintain normal, much less elevated, cardiac function despite elevated venous filling pressures; their $\dot{D}O_2$ and $\dot{V}O_2$ values fell below those of survivors, while oxygen extraction rose in partial compensation. Despite normal blood gases, nonsurvivors' $\dot{Q}SP/\dot{Q}T$ and $P(A-a)O_2$ increased intraoperatively and remained elevated postoperatively [2].

Patients with Low and High Preoperative Cardiac Output
Patients who were elderly, were in cardiac failure, or were in hemorrhagic shock with low preoperative cardiac output developed postoperative stress responses that were similar but less intense than those developed by pa-

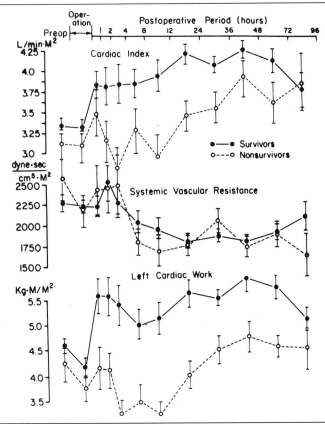

Fig. 19-5. Temporal patterns of systemic hemodynamic variables, cardiac index, systemic vascular resistance index, and left cardiac work index. See Figure 19-4 for explanation. From Bland, Shoemaker, Abraham, et al. [2].

tients with normal preoperative CI values. Survivors' CI, $\dot{D}O_2$, and $\dot{V}O_2$ values increased in the postoperative period from their low preoperative baseline values. The nonsurvivors had lower postoperative CI, $\dot{D}O_2$, and $\dot{V}O_2$ values despite high WP: i.e., less postoperative responses compared with the survivors. The nonsurvivors also had significantly greater increases in PVRI and $\dot{Q}SP/\dot{Q}T$ [2].

Septic patients, patients severely stressed by major preoperative trauma, and patients with advanced cirrhosis usually have high CI values, indicative of a preoperative compensatory circulatory stress response. The mean CI, $\dot{D}O_2$, and $\dot{V}O_2$ values increased postoperatively above their preoperative baseline; this increase was greater in the survivors than in the nonsurvivors, whereas the WP, PVRI, and $\dot{Q}SP/\dot{Q}T$ were higher in the nonsurvivors. Both groups maintained intravascular pressures and other nonflow-related variables in relatively normal ranges [2].

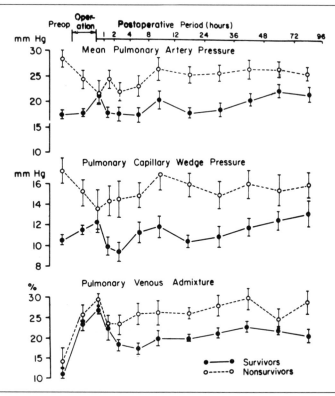

Fig. 19-6. Temporal patterns of pulmonary hemodynamics in survivors and nonsurvivors. See Figure 19-4 for explanation. From Bland, Shoemaker, Abraham, et al. [2].

Physiologic Differences Between Survivor and Nonsurvivor Patterns

Inadequate $\dot{D}O_2$ and $\dot{V}O_2$ leading to tissue hypoxia and oxygen debt is the basic physiologic problem of accidental or surgical shock and trauma. The type of surgical illness or operation is not important to the survivor-nonsurvivor patterns, but the degree of tissue hypoxia due to the patients' inability to compensate with increased CI, $\dot{D}O_2$, and $\dot{V}O_2$ is a major determinant of outcome.

Unevenly maintained local vascular tone leads to uneven distribution of flow that compromises local tissue perfusion and metabolism. Hypovolemia produced by hemorrhage, as well as by leakage of plasma volume from the intravascular to the interstitial compartment, reduces the capacity of the heart to compensate with increased CI and $\dot{D}O_2$. Anesthesia is also a stress on the cardiovascular system; inhalation anesthetics depress myocardial function and reduce neural control of peripheral vascular tone. In addition, anesthesia inhibits cellular function and further reduces $\dot{V}O_2$. Many surgical patients with preoperative complications, associated severe

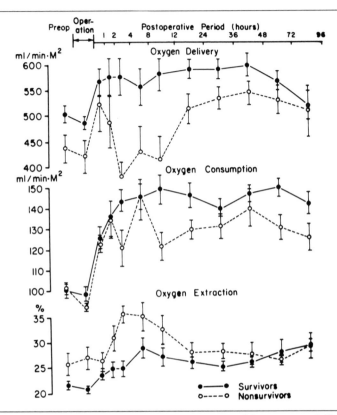

Fig. 19-7. Temporal patterns of oxygen transport variables, oxygen delivery index, oxygen consumption index, and oxygen extraction for survivors and nonsurvivors. See Figure 19-4 for explanation. From Bland, Shoemaker, Abraham, et al. [2].

medical illnesses, or cardiorespiratory problems have altered preoperative values, but their postoperative biphasic cardiorespiratory patterns are similar, except they begin from different baselines. Furthermore, both survivors and nonsurvivors may have compensatory responses, but survivors have smaller intraoperative $\dot{V}O_2$ decreases and greater postoperative $\dot{V}O_2$ increases, whereas nonsurvivors have greater intraoperative $\dot{V}O_2$ reductions and smaller postoperative compensatory increases. Diminished $\dot{V}O_2$ produces a cumulative tissue oxygen debt that must be paid by compensatory increases during the immediate postoperative period for survival to occur. The greater the reduction in $\dot{V}O_2$ and the longer the operation, the greater must be the postoperative compensatory increase of $\dot{V}O_2$.

Significance of Hemodynamic and Oxygen Transport Patterns
The compensatory responses to tissue hypoxia from low $\dot{V}O_2$ include increased HR, increased myocardial contractility, increased cardiac output,

increased oxygen extraction rate, hyperpnea, tachypnea, and altered vascular tone. These compensatory reactions to inadequate $\dot{V}O_2$ are the most apparent early manifestations of shock; they are often the first recognized clinical features that suggest something is wrong. Unfortunately, only the most superficial manifestations of shock usually are routinely monitored. Even more disastrously, when these superficial vital signs are misconstrued as the major problem of shock, therapy is inappropriately directed against them rather than against the primary physiologic problem.

The pathophysiology may be summarized as follows. (a) The transport of blood constituents, particularly oxygen, is the major function of the circulation. (b) Oxygen has the highest extraction ratio and is the most flow-dependent blood constituent. (c) Since oxygen cannot be stored, the rate at which oxygen is transported across the alveolar-capillary membrane in steady-state conditions is equivalent to the rate at which oxygen is consumed by the tissues. (d) The overall circulatory function is best evaluated in terms of the $\dot{D}O_2$. (e) The rate of oxygen utilization ($\dot{V}O_2$) reflects the sum of all oxidative metabolic reactions and measures the body's overall metabolic state. (f) $\dot{V}O_2$ may be rate-limited by hypovolemia, reduced supply ($\dot{D}O_2$), or flow maldistributions produced by accidental trauma, surgical operations, anesthetic agents, sepsis, postoperative states, endocrine and metabolic disorders, capillary leak, and other forms of acute illness. (g) The pattern of changes in the values of these variables and their responses to various therapeutic interventions provide the most sensitive and specific criteria of overall circulatory status and its compensatory capacities. (h) Direct microscopic observations have shown wide variations in microcirculatory flow, with dilated metarteriolar capillary networks next to vasoconstricted networks; the tissue supplied by free-flowing microcirculation may be adequately nourished, whereas cells surrounding vasoconstricted networks will be hypoxic. (i) The patterns of $\dot{D}O_2$ and $\dot{V}O_2$ are strongly related to survival or death.

$\dot{D}O_2$ and $\dot{V}O_2$ provide the best available measure of the functional adequacy of both circulation and metabolism. As such, these two oxygen transport variables represent an important method for evaluating both circulatory and metabolic functions. $\dot{V}O_2$ may be reduced by rate-limited $\dot{D}O_2$ (the supply side). The inadequate $\dot{V}O_2$ is greater and more prolonged in patients who die than in those who survive. Inadequate $\dot{V}O_2$ is not just associated with shock—it is the major pathogenic mechanism of shock syndromes and a major determinant of outcome [2–5, 14–23].

From serial measurements, basic patterns have emerged. The common physiologic alteration is reduced or inadequate $\dot{V}O_2$, which occurs at or before the initial hypotensive crisis, produces tissue hypoxia, limits body metabolism, and therefore compromises survival. It may be produced by (a) low cardiac output from hemorrhage or other causes of hypovolemia; (b) maldistribution of flow, particularly at the microcirculatory level, from uneven vasoconstriction, neurohormonal mechanisms, and various mediator-induced responses; and (c) increased metabolic demand that exceeds the supply. The basic problem is an inadequate transport function of the circulation for oxygen and other nutrients transported by the circulation.

Blood Volume and Fluid Status

The most important goal in the treatment of hemorrhagic, traumatic, and septic shock is to restore blood volume. However, the criteria for achieving this goal are ill-defined. Tachycardia and reduced MAP, CVP, WP, and Hct values are often used based on experimental and clinical studies immediately after sudden acute hemorrhage. Unfortunately, these values, including WP, do not reflect the blood volume status throughout the subsequent course of these patients in the ICU. Moreover, in critically ill postoperative patients, these commonly used clinical criteria were found to be unreliable when compared with careful measurements of blood volume [12].

Surgeons are often accused of protagonizing overly aggressive fluid administration on minimal clinical indications—especially in patients with surgical or accidental trauma—contrary to the approach of many internists. Medical patients, especially those with chronic cardiac, renal, pulmonary, and hepatic disorders, often have too much salt and water; they may require diuretics and fluid restriction. In shock, however, fluid therapy should be based on objective physiologic criteria that can be reliably used for therapeutic goals.

This fluid controversy arises from a common misconception: the failure clinically to differentiate among total body water, extracellular water, and plasma volume. For example, the patient with peripheral edema obviously has too much total body water but also may be hypovolemic. Frequently, patients have maldistributed extracellular water with contracted plasma volume but expanded interstitial water. This is the most common situation in the partially resuscitated surgical or trauma patient [25]. Therapy should improve circulatory function by restoring plasma volume, not overload an already expanded interstitium.

Since the most important correctable clinical problem in acute circulatory shock is replacement of blood volume losses, it is essential to have a reliable assessment of volume. Measurement of plasma volume by ^{125}I-labeled albumin or red cell mass by [55]Cr-labeled red cells is time-consuming, expensive, and usually only performed in research centers. The CVP and WP, which can be repeated at frequent intervals or monitored continuously, have been thought to have the needed accuracy and have largely replaced blood volume measurements in most clinical centers. CVP and WP rapidly decrease with acute hemorrhage and increase with fluid therapy in the immediate posttransfusion–and–fluid-restoration period. High venous pressures are associated with both acute blood volume overload in the initial resuscitation or in the immediate postoperative period and cardiac failure at any time. However, venous pressures are notably unreliable indicators of blood volume status in ICU patients [12]. This is because of compliance changes in venous wall tensions that occur over time after stress-induced neurohormonal responses. In the postresuscitation, postoperative ICU period, venous pressures accommodate to either high or low blood volumes with values that usually remain in the range of about 10 to 15 mm Hg. Figure 19-8 illustrates the values of over 1700 precisely measured blood volumes relative to the commonly monitored variables [12]. The latter fail to reflect blood volume changes over a wide range of values.

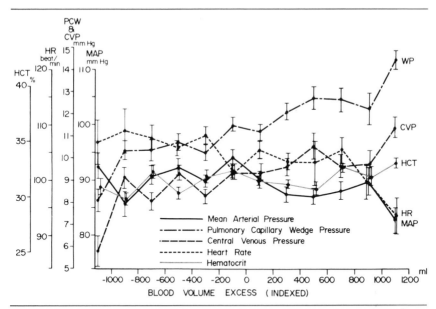

Fig. 19-8. Blood volume index values plotted against Hct, HR, CVP, WP, and MAP on the *Y* axis. Blood volume values are expressed as ml excess (+) or deficit (−) from the patient's predicted norm indexed to BSA. Note the very poor correlation of the commonly monitored variables. From Shippy, Appel, and Shoemaker [12], with permission.

Figure 19-9 illustrates the scatter of blood volume values relative to their corresponding CVP values.

Although CVP and WP measure venous pressures but do not accurately reflect blood volume in most ICU patients, they are useful to prevent acute volume overload during rapid fluid restoration and subsequent fluid challenges; that is, with rapid volume loading, the CVP and WP reflect the capacity of the vascular system to accept more volume without producing pulmonary edema. It must also be clearly stated that peripheral as well as pulmonary edema may result from massive crystalloid infusions that expand the interstitial space without fully restoring plasma volume or exceeding "safe" venous pressures.

Daily weight and fluid balance measurement are used to monitor fluid management, but both of these measure body water or changes in body water, not blood volume. The distribution of body water among the plasma, interstitium, and intracellular compartments can be measured definitively only by isotopic body composition studies.

Therapeutic Goals

Therapeutic goals for high-risk postoperative patients are best defined by the values of survivors of life-threatening critical illnesses. Criteria established by two large retrospective series [15, 18, 23] and several prospective

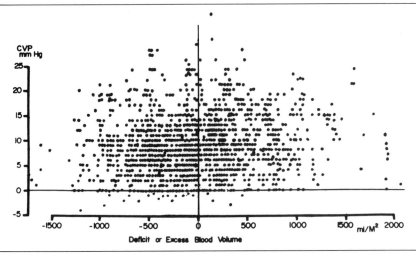

Fig. 19-9. Blood volume index values plotted against their simultaneously measured CVP values. From Shippy, Appel, and Shoemaker [12], with permission.

series [2, 3, 21, 22] include (a) CI 50 percent greater than normal (4.5 liters/min/M²); (b) $\dot{D}O_2$ slightly greater than normal (>600 ml/min/M²); (c) $\dot{V}O_2$ about 30 percent greater than normal (>170 ml/min/M²); and (d) blood volume 500 ml in excess of the norm—i.e., 3.2 liters/M² for males, 2.8 liters/M² for females [2, 3, 14, 21]. These increments are needed to overcome poorly distributed blood volume and blood flow, as well as to supply the increased metabolism associated with wound healing, fever, and the accumulated oxygen debt. Severely traumatized, septic, and burn patients may require even higher values [2, 3, 16].

PREDICTION OF OUTCOME

Relative Importance of Hemodynamic and Oxygen Transport Variables

Frequently, hemodynamic and oxygen transport measurements provide crucial information on underlying physiologic mechanisms relevant to survival and death. The biologic importance of each cardiorespiratory variable may be based on its ability to predict outcome. The relationship of a given variable to survival or death is also the best criterion of its usefulness in making clinical decisions. If a variable does not reflect outcome, it may not be relevant. However, if it does predict outcome, it may reflect important pathophysiology and, therefore, provide a useful criterion for therapeutic decisions.

The percentages of correctly predicted outcomes for each monitored variable were calculated at each stage and for all stages in a series of postoperative patients (Table 19-3) [19]. The commonly measured variables, which were the poorest predictors, track where the patient has been, not where the patient is headed. In contrast, oxygen transport-related variables were good outcome predictors and, therefore, are clinically important. Recently, this concept has been corroborated in surgical and medical patients [9].

Outcome Prediction from Survivors and Nonsurvivors' Patterns

Multivariate nonparametric statistical analyses have been used to predict outcome early in the postoperative period [4, 16, 18]. These analyses also provide an objective, physiologic, and heuristic basis for therapeutic decisions. The sole criterion of this type of empiric physiologic analysis is survival. More important, predictors objectively measure severity of illness and express this in quantitative terms.

Outcome prediction for each hemodynamic and oxygen transport variable varies from stage to stage as the patient's shock syndromes evolve: i.e., predictors are stage-specific. For example, $\dot{D}O_2$ and PVRI are good early predictors but not late predictors, and MAP is a poor early predictor but a good late predictor. Most variables predict outcome well in the late stage, but clinical judgment at this time is also excellent while the predictor usefulness is minimal [5].

Recently, a greatly simplified predictor was developed based on the survival rate calculated for values in each of 10 equally spaced divisions of the total range of values for each cardiorespiratory variable. The average score of each variable's prediction was computed to give an overall predictive index for the patient during each postoperative period [4, 16]. For example, Figure 19-10 illustrates the survival rates of patients whose left ventricular stroke work index values ranged from 15 to 90 gm·M/M² in the first 8 hours postoperatively in our initial retrospective series of critically ill postoperative patients. Survival rates progressively increase from the low values until a plateau is reached; the height of the plateau measures how well the variable predicts outcome and the width of the plateau defines the optimal values based on survival for this variable. Figure 19-11 illustrates $\dot{D}O_2$ and $\dot{V}O_2$ values in the same series and demonstrates a wide, high plateau for $\dot{D}O_2$, indicating that this variable is one of the best variable predictors and that optimal values for survival were over 600 ml/min/M²; the $\dot{V}O_2$ pattern shows that survival increases with increasing values of $\dot{V}O_2$. Figure 19-12 illustrates the survival rates of patients for HR and PVRI values. Survival rates were approximately 50 percent for HR values throughout the observed spectrum, indicating poor prognostic capability for this variable. The low PVRI plateau indicated poor prediction of survival, but the decrease to 0 percent survival above values of 500 dyne·cm/sec⁵·M² indicated that this variable was a good predictor of death in the early postoperative period. This recently developed predictor was also prospectively tested in a fresh series of patients and found to be 94 percent correct. Figure 19-13 shows significant separation between survivors and nonsurvivors in the prospective series beginning 2 to 4 hours postoperatively [4].

These predictors objectively analyze the complex physiologic problems with no preconceptions and a minimum number of assumptions. The criteria are determined solely by the observed values of critically ill surgical

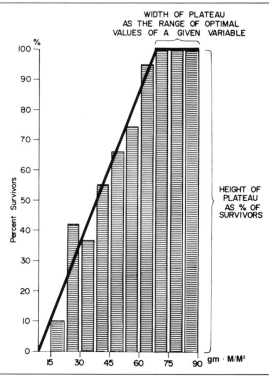

Fig. 19-10. Distribution of observed values for left ventricular stroke work in the first 8 hours postoperatively in our first series [14]. The survival rates were calculated for the patients whose values fell into each of the 10 divisions, from the lowest to the highest value. Note the plateau at the top; the height of this plateau reflects how good the variable is as a predictor. The width reflects the values that are associated with good outcome. From Shoemaker, Bland, and Appel [16].

patients who survived as compared with the values of those who subsequently died. Therapeutic goals were defined empirically from the median values for each cardiorespiratory variable of the survivors and were confirmed by the predictors [2, 9, 16, 19].

Predictive Index as a Measure of the Severity of Illness

Critically ill postoperative patients have a substantial incidence of postoperative shock and its sequelae. An accurate, reproducible predictive index based on survival statistics also may be used to evaluate the severity of illness. Such a predictive or severity index may be also used as a "proxy outcome," to evaluate the patient's progress from hour to hour, as well as before and after specific therapies, to assess therapeutic effectiveness. Changes in the predictive index provide an objective physiologic criterion for evaluating the relative efficacy of alternative therapies.

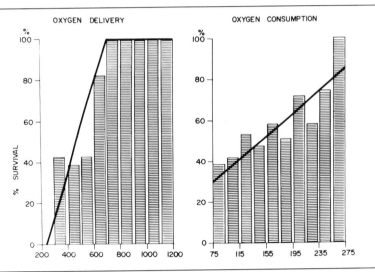

Fig. 19-11. Distribution of values for oxygen delivery (left) and oxygen consumption (right). (Format as in Figure 19-10.) From Shoemaker, Bland, and Appel [16].

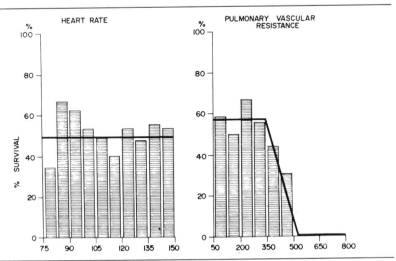

Fig. 19-12. Distribution of values for heart rate (left) and pulmonary vascular resistance index (right). (Format as in Figure 19-10.) From Shoemaker, Bland, and Appel [16].

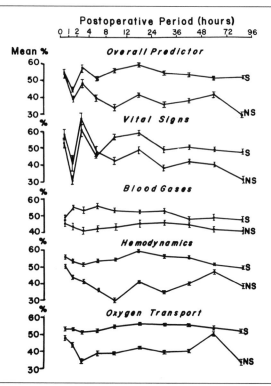

Fig. 19-13. Top section: overall predictor for survivors (S) and nonsurvivors (NS) at each time interval postoperatively. Second section: predictions calculated from the vital-signs variables for S and NS. Third section: predictions calculated from the blood gas variables for S and NS. Fourth section: predictions calculated from the hemodynamic variables for S and NS. Bottom section: predictions calculated from the oxygen transport variables for S and NS. Dots represent mean values, vertical bars SEM. From Bland and Shoemaker [4].

Therapeutic Implications of Physiologic Compensations

Physiologic compensatory responses maintain overall circulatory function and integrity after trauma, hemorrhage, sepsis, and other types of shock. Complications occur when these responses fail to compensate adequately; for example, increased cardiac output may compensate for reduced hematocrit, low PaO_2, or inadequate tissue oxygenation. Since this compensatory flow increase has survival value, therapy should augment cardiac output; the use of β-blockers to reduce HR or to lower high cardiac output values to the normal range in patients with traumatic or septic shock may result in precipitous circulatory and metabolic deterioration. The understanding of cardiorespiratory responses to stress in mechanistic terms is essential, since augmentation of compensatory responses may be needed for survival. If the physiology is not understood and monitoring is not appropriate, death will be attributed to the patient's disease rather than to inappropriate therapy.

THERAPY
The standard conventional approach to therapy is to search for specific defects, document their presence, and then correct them. Essentially this means a one-at-a-time search for an abnormality, bringing the values into the normal range, and then going on to search for another defect. This approach results in a fragmented, episodic plan. The alternative is to base early therapy on survivors' patterns and underlying circulatory mechanisms that determine survival.

A Therapeutic Plan Using a Branched-Chain Decision Tree
Strategies for achieving therapeutic goals were determined empirically by evaluating the relative effectiveness of each therapy to produce the desired goals. Decision rules were generated from survivor or nonsurvivor patterns and from these patients' responses to specific therapeutic interventions. A branched-chain decision tree was developed based on these criteria and priorities (Fig. 19-14).

Vigorous and rapid volume loading without exceeding WP values greater than 18 mm Hg is the first therapy. It is easier to achieve the therapeutic goals with colloids that expand the plasma volume without overexpansion of the interstitial water [12, 25]. Plasma volume restoration cannot be assumed in patients with pitting edema who have received large volumes of crystalloids, because hypovolemia frequently occurs in the presence of expanded interstitial water. In these conditions, we prefer to give concentrated (25%) albumin, which expands plasma volume by shifting interstitial water back into the plasma volume [1, 10, 26, 27].

After the maximum effect of fluids has been obtained, an inotropic agent such as dobutamine may be started at about 2 μg/kg/min; the appropriate dose is obtained by titration to achieve the optimal goals in terms of CI, $\dot{D}O_2$, and $\dot{V}O_2$. If the patient has normal or high MAP with high systemic vascular resistance index (SVRI), vasodilation with nitroglycerin, nitroprusside, or labetalol is considered; the optimal dose is obtained by titration to achieve improved cardiac index without producing hypotension (i.e., MAP > 80, systolic arterial pressure (SAP) > 100 mm Hg). If fluids, inotropic agents, and vasodilators fail to achieve optimal goals, vasopressors such as dopamine may be given at the lowest dose needed to maintain MAP. Vasopressors are given as a last resort, because they increase venous pressures, pulmonary venous shunt, and lactic acidemia. Moreover, the increased venous pressure produced by vasopressors may limit optimal fluid administration.

Treatment of Postoperative Shock and Other Etiologic Types of Shock
The advantage of studying surgical traumatic shock is that one can obtain preillness control measurements as well as serial measurements during the

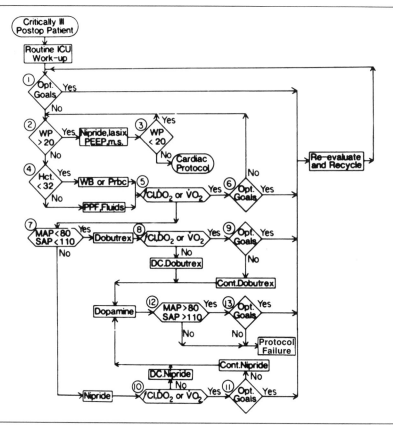

Fig. 19-14. Branched-chain decision tree for postoperative ICU patients.
Preliminary evaluation of high-risk critically ill patients by routine ICU workup that includes arterial blood gases, chest x-ray, routine blood chemistries,
ECG, and coagulation studies. These tests should either have been performed
or be in process, and the observed defects corrected. *Step 1.* Measure CI, $\dot{D}O_2$,
$\dot{V}O_2$, and blood volume (BV) to determine if the patient has reached the optimal
goals. If CI < 4.5 liters/min/M^2, $\dot{D}O_2$ < 600 ml/min/M^2, $\dot{V}O_2$ < 160 ml/min/M^2,
or BV < 3 liters/M^2 for men or 2.7 liters/M^2 for women, proceed to step 2; but if
the goals are reached, the objective of the algorithm has been achieved.
Reevaluate and recycle at intervals to maintain these goals. *Step 2.* Take
pulmonary artery wedge pressure (WP). If > 20 mm Hg, proceed to step 3; if <
20, proceed to step 4. *Step 3.* If WP > 20, give furosemide intravenously at
increasing dose levels (20, 40, 80, 160 mg) if there is clinical or x-ray evidence
of salt and water overload or clinical findings of pulmonary congestion. If not,
consider vasodilators, nitroprusside, or nitroglycerin if MAP > 80 and systolic
pressure > 100 mm Hg. Recycle to titrate the dose as needed to reduce WP <
15 mm Hg but maintain MAP > 80 mm Hg. If unsuccessful, place on cardiac
protocol. *Step 4.* If Hct < 32 percent, give 1 unit of whole blood (WB) or 2 units
of packed red blood cells (Prbc). If Hct > 32 percent, give a fluid load (volume
challenge) consisting of one of the following (depending on clinical indications
of plasma volume deficit or hydration): 500 ml of 5% PPF, 500 ml of 5%

hemodynamic crisis and throughout the postoperative period leading to recovery or death. This permits objective definition of physiologic criteria for therapy. Similar underlying physiologic alterations occur in accidental trauma and sepsis, but the optimal goals are not necessarily the same: That is, the defects may be qualitatively similar and the metabolic requirements greater, but therapy may differ quantitatively. The strategy in each case is to open up unevenly vasoconstricted metarteriolar-capillary networks. This may be done by volume loading and by increasing flow with inotropic agents and vasodilators to force open the constricted circuits. Volume is given until optimal goals are achieved or WP reaches 18 mm Hg. In this approach, WP is not used as a measure of blood volume, because it clearly does not reflect blood volume [12]. Rather, WP is used as an upper limit for volume therapy in order to avoid pulmonary edema. The optimal values after trauma and sepsis cannot be evaluated directly, because widely varying increases in metabolism require a wide range of circulatory function to supply these increased needs. The answer to this dilemma is an operational definition of goals: Continue to give each therapy as long as it improves CI, $\dot{D}O_2$, and $\dot{V}O_2$, unless limited by WP in fluid therapy, tachycardia greater than 130 with inotropic agents, and hypotension less than 80 MAP or 110 SAP with vasodilators. Vasopressors are used as a last resort to maintain sufficient MAP to provide for coronary and cerebral perfusion.

---

albumin, 100 ml of 25% albumin (25 g), 500 ml of 6% hydroxyethyl starch, 500 ml of 6% dextran-60, or 1000 ml of D5RL. *Step 5.* If the blood or fluid load improved any of the optimal therapeutic goals defined in step 1, proceed to step 6; if none is improved, proceed to step 7. *Step 6.* If goals are not reached, recycle steps 2 through 6 until these goals are met or WP > 20 mm Hg. *Step 7.* If MAP > 70 or systolic arterial pressure (SAP) < 100 mm Hg, give dobutamine by constant intravenous infusion in increasing doses to increase CI, $\dot{D}O_2$, and $\dot{V}O_2$. *Step 8.* Titrate dobutamine beginning with 2 μg/min/kg and gradually increasing doses up to 10 μg/min/kg, provided there is improvement in CI, $\dot{D}O_2$, or $\dot{V}O_2$ without further lowering of arterial pressure until goals are met. *Step 9.* If goals are reached, reevaluate and recycle. If goals are not reached or it becomes evident that higher doses of the drug are not more effective or that they produce hypotension and tachycardia, continue dobutamine at its most effective dose range. *Step 10.* If MAP > 80 mm Hg and SAP > 110 mg Hg, give sodium nitroprusside or nitroglycerin in gradually increasing doses, provided there is improvement in CI, $\dot{D}O_2$, or $\dot{V}O_2$. *Step 11.* If there is no improvement in CI, $\dot{D}O_2$, or $\dot{V}O_2$ with the vasodilator, or if hypotension (MAP < 80 mm Hg, SAP < 110 mm Hg) ensues, discontinue the vasodilator. If there is improvement in CI, $\dot{D}O_2$, or $\dot{V}O_2$, titrate the vasodilator to its maximum effect consistent with satisfactory arterial pressures. *Step 12.* If optimal goals are reached, reevaluate and recycle at intervals. If these goals are not reached and MAP < 80 mm Hg, and SAP < 110, give vasopressor, dopamine, or if ineffective, norepinephrine. *Step 13.* Titrate doses of vasopressor in the lowest doses possible to maintain arterial pressures, MAP > 80, SAP > 110. If the goals and pressures cannot be maintained, the patient is considered to be a protocol failure. From Shoemaker, Appel, and Bland [21].

Therapeutic Goals and Strategies in Elderly and Cardiac Patients
Patients with primary cardiac disease have considerably different physiologic problems and different potential mechanisms for death than do patients with normal hearts but multiple vital organ failures. The heart may be the weak link in the former, but circulatory transport functions are likely to limit survival in the latter. An appropriate strategy in cardiac patients may be to reduce cardiac work by afterload reduction with vasodilators. Hemodynamic aspects of cardiac patients have been well studied and therapies extensively evaluated.

Unfortunately, critically ill patients do not always fall neatly into cardiac and noncardiac categories. More often, the elderly patient and the patient with preexisting cardiac problems also have life-threatening multiple organ failures. Under these conditions, rigid interpretation with the decision tree is not really appropriate. Volume therapy with concentrated (salt-poor) albumin may be given, but salt should be avoided. Inotropic agents such as dobutamine may be tried in the lowest effective dose, whereas isoproterenol and vasopressors that increase cardiac work should be avoided. Vasodilators may be effective after plasma volume is adequately restored by volume therapy. The hemodynamic effectiveness of each agent given separately should be established before combining agents. The most important principles in these complex clinical conditions are to (a) document baseline hemodynamic and oxygen transport variables, (b) measure changes with each appropriate agent, and (c) titrate the dose to achieve optimal or near optimal values.

Therapy of Surgical Patients with High Cardiac Output Preoperatively
Increased $\dot{V}O_2$ in preoperative and postoperative patients with severe trauma, stress, sepsis, and hypercatabolic states indicates increased metabolic requirements. However, the increased metabolism should not be interpreted to mean that all metabolic needs have been met. With increased metabolism, therapeutic goals cannot be defined precisely, and therapeutic adequacy cannot be determined directly. However, tissue oxygen demand may be inferred indirectly by an empirical trial of therapy. If therapy increases cardiac output and $\dot{V}O_2$, it may be assumed that it opened up additional microcirculatory channels that perfused relatively hypoxic tissues, which then extracted more oxygen. Since tissues cannot take up more oxygen than they use, the increased $\dot{V}O_2$ after fluid challenge indicates an oxygen debt that was at least partially satisfied.

Prospective Clinical Trials
A therapeutic plan that used the empirically defined median values of survivors as therapeutic goals was prospectively tested in clinical trials against a control group that used normal values as the therapeutic goals [16, 20, 21]. Both protocol and control groups had the same availability of x-rays and lab tests, monitoring, nursing care, ancillary facilities, and therapy; both groups were prospectively allocated from patients whose critical illnesses were specified by prearranged criteria; and both were managed

by the same pool of attending staff and residents. Comparison of the clinical data, clinical diagnosis, operations, and associated medical conditions demonstrated that the patients in the protocol group were at least as ill as, and probably more ill than, the control group. The only real difference was that the control patients had normal hemodynamic and oxygen transport values as their therapeutic goals, whereas the protocol group had the median values of the survivors as their therapeutic goals. The results of this study demonstrated marked reduction in morbidity and mortality in the protocol patients [20, 21].

Recently, we have tested the hypothesis that survivors' values are optimal goals in an additional three-leg trial of (a) CVP catheter, (b) pulmonary artery catheter with normal values as goals, and (c) pulmonary artery catheter with optimal values as goals of therapy [22]. This trial was begun preoperatively and was strictly randomized using sealed envelopes containing cards identifying one of the three monitoring/therapeutic approaches. The results showed no statistically significant difference between the mortality of patients managed with a CVP catheter (23%) and those of the pulmonary artery catheter with normal values as therapeutic goals (33%). However, use of optimal goals with the pulmonary artery catheter led to significantly reduced (4%) mortality. Moreover, the number of complications, hospital days, ICU days, ventilator days, and hospital costs were reduced [22]. Thus, when the survivors' oxygen transport values were achieved with rapid vigorous therapy, mortality, morbidity, and hospital costs significantly decreased.

These prospective clinical trials suggest that at least half of all postoperative deaths are due to physiologic problems that can be identified, described, predicted, and prevented. Therefore, therapy for the critically ill postoperative patient should be defined by physiologic criteria. Therapy should be monitored prophylactically to obtain promptly and aggressively optimal physiologic goals rather than merely to attain normal values after the predictable deficit has occurred [22].

A branched-chain decision tree helps to achieve these therapeutic goals expeditiously by providing a coherent organized patient management plan. The plan aims to prophylactically maintain the patient in the optimal hemodynamic state and does not allow the development of tissue hypoxia from blood volume, hemodynamic, and oxygen transport deficits. One should not wait for patients to develop cardiorespiratory deficits before initiating therapy. Therapy should be started promptly, to optimize the important variables as soon as possible after the onset of accidental trauma as well as before, during, and immediately after surgery in the high-risk patient [16].

This approach to fluid and pharmacologic management of shock obviously will not correct diagnostic errors, anatomic problems, surgical misadventures, transfusion reactions, idiosyncratic drug reactions, iatrogenic ineptitudes, or the lack of the patient's motivation to live. Moreover, even if physiologic variables are optimized, success is not guaranteed when the patient's cardiac and pulmonary reserve capacities are not adequate or the stress is overwhelming [15, 16, 20, 22].

SUMMARY

The conventional approach to monitoring of readily available variables has severe limitations because of subjective criteria that lead to suboptimal therapy. An alternative approach is provided by descriptions of the hemodynamic and oxygen transport patterns of the survivors and nonsurvivors of life-threatening illness. The differences between survivor and nonsurvivor patterns provide (a) data for early prediction of outcome, (b) the basis for analysis of pathophysiologic mechanisms seen from the nonsurvivors' pattern, (c) elucidation of compensatory responses with survival value from the survivors' patterns, and (d) definition of therapeutic goals empirically determined from the predictions and the physiologic patterns of survivors. When these goals were prophylactically achieved and maintained, there was marked reduction in mortality, morbidity, hospital days, ICU days, ventilator days, and hospital costs.

REFERENCES

1. Appel, P. L., and Shoemaker, W. C. Fluid therapy in adult respiratory failure. *Crit. Care Med.* 9:862, 1981.
2. Bland, R. D., Shoemaker, W. C., Abraham, E., et al. Hemodynamic and oxygen transport patterns in surviving and nonsurviving postoperative patients. *Crit. Care. Med.* 13:85, 1985.
3. Bland, R. D., and Shoemaker, W. C. Common physiologic patterns in general surgical patients. Hemodynamic and oxygen transport changes during and after operation in patients with and without associated medical problems. *Surg. Clin. North Am.* 65:793, 1985.
4. Bland, R. D., and Shoemaker, W. C. Probability of survival as a prognostic and severity of illness score in critically ill surgical patients. *Crit. Care Med.* 13:91, 1985.
5. Bland, R., Shoemaker, W. C., and Shabot, M. M. Physiologic monitoring goals for the critically ill patient. *Surg. Gynecol. Obstet.* 147:833, 1978.
6. Cournand, A., Riley, R. L., Bradley, S. E., et al. Studies of the circulation in clinical shock. *Surgery* 13:964, 1943.
7. Clowes, G. H. A., Jr., and Del Guercio, L. R. M. Circulatory response to trauma of surgical operations. *Metabolism* 9:67, 1960.
8. Del Guercio, L. R. M., Commarswamy, R. F., Feins, N. R., et al. Pulmonary arteriovenous admixture and the hyperdynamic state in surgery for portal hypertension. *Surgery* 56:57, 1964.
9. Hankeln, K., Senker, R., Schwarten, J. M., et al. Evaluation of prognostic indices based on hemodynamic and oxygen transport variables in shock patients with adult respiratory distress syndrome. *Crit. Care Med.* 15:1, 1987.
10. Hauser, C. J., Shoemaker, W. C., Turpin I., et al. Hemodynamic and oxygen transport responses to body water shifts produced by colloids and crystalloids in critically ill patients. *Surg. Gynecol. Obstet.* 150:811, 1980.
11. Heilbrunn, A., and Allbritten, F. F. Cardiac output during and following surgical operation. *Ann. Surg.* 152:197, 1960.
12. Shippy, C. R., Appel, P. L., and Shoemaker, W. C. Reliability of clinical monitoring to assess blood volume in critically ill patients. *Crit. Care Med.* 12:107, 1984.
13. Shoemaker, W. C., Printen, K. J., Amato, J. J., et al. Hemodynamic patterns after acute anesthetized and unanesthetized trauma. *Arch. Surg.* 95:492, 1967.

14. Shoemaker, W. C., Montgomery, E. S., Kaplan E., et al. Physiologic patterns in surviving and nonsurviving shock patients. *Arch. Surg.* 106:630, 1973.
15. Shoemaker W. C. Shock States: Pathophysiology, Monitoring, Outcome Prediction, and Therapy. In W. C. Shoemaker, S. M. Ayres, A. Grenvik, P. R. Holbrook, and W. L. Thompson (eds.), *Textbook of Critical Care* (2nd ed.). Philadelphia: Saunders, 1989.
16. Shoemaker, W. C., Bland, R. D., and Appel, P. L. Therapy of critically ill postoperative patients based on outcome prediction and prospective clinical trials. *Surg. Clin. North Am.* 65:811, 1985.
17. Shoemaker, W. C. Circulatory mechanisms of shock and their mediators. *Crit. Care Med.* 15:787, 1987.
18. Shoemaker W. C., Czer, L., Chang, P., et al. Cardiorespiratory monitoring in postoperative patients. I. Prediction of outcome and severity of illness. *Crit. Care Med.* 7:237, 1979.
19. Shoemaker W. C., Appel, P. L., Bland, R., et al. Clinical trial of an algorithm for outcome prediction in acute circulatory failure. *Crit. Care Med.* 10:390, 1982.
20. Shoemaker, W. C., Appel, P. L., Waxman, K., et al. Clinical trial of survivors' cardiorespiratory patterns as therapeutic goals in critically ill postoperative patients. *Crit. Care Med.* 10:398, 1982.
21. Shoemaker, W. C., Appel, P., and Bland, R. Use of physiologic monitoring to predict outcome and to assist in clinical decision in critically ill postoperative patients. *Am. J. Surg.* 146:43, 1983.
22. Shoemaker, W. C., Appel, P. L., Kram, H. B., et al. Prospective trial of supranormal values of survivors as therapeutic goals in high risk surgical patients. *Chest* 94:1176, 1988.
23. Shoemaker, W. C., and Czer, L. S. C. Evaluation of the biologic importance of various hemodynamic and oxygen transport variables. *Crit. Care Med.* 7:424, 1979.
24. Shoemaker, W. C., Appel, P. L., Kram, H. B., et al. Multicomponent noninvasive physiologic monitoring of circulatory function. *Crit. Care Med.* 16:482, 1988.
25. Shoemaker, W. C., Bryan-Brown, C. W., Quigley, L., et al. Body fluid shifts in depletion and post stress states and their correlation with adequate nutrition. *Surg. Gynecol. Obstet.* 136:371, 1973.
26. Shoemaker, W. C., and Monson, D. O. Effect of whole blood and plasma expanders on volume-flow relationships in critically ill patients. *Surg. Gynecol. Obstet.* 137:453, 1973.
27. Shoemaker, W. C., Matsuda, T., and State, D. Relative hemodynamic effectiveness of whole blood and plasma expanders in burn patients. *Surg. Gynecol. Obstet.* 144:909, 1977.
28. Siegel, J., Goldwyn, P. M., and Friedman, H. P. Pattern in process in the evolution of human septic shock. *Surgery* 70:232, 1971.
29. Wiggers, C. J. *Physiology of Shock.* New York: Commonwealth Fund, 1940.
30. Wilson, R. F., Thal, A. P., Kinding, P. H., et al. Hemodynamic measurements in shock. *Arch. Surg.* 91:124, 1965.

Critical Care of the Neurosurgical Patient

William T. Couldwell
Martin H. Weiss

Once cardiopulmonary parameters have been stabilized in the critically ill patient, attention must be logically directed to assessment of the central nervous system (CNS), both brain and spinal cord, since its stability is essential in assuring true recovery. During normal conditions, the brain and spinal cord enjoy a biochemically and immunologically privileged status in being isolated from ordinary and even extraordinary variations in metabolic and toxic parameters by the blood-brain and blood–cerebrospinal fluid (CSF) barriers. This privileged status is required for maintenance of the excitable membrane potential, which must be carefully regulated if neural function is to be preserved. However, the barriers may be disrupted by external influences impacting directly upon the central nervous system or by systemic influences deviating widely from the norm, thus altering the barriers.

CLINICAL EVALUATION

The clinical evaluation of the patient with central nervous system disorder remains the single most important assessment that can be made to determine the extent of dysfunction and to provide a background upon which an evaluation of therapy may be established. In assessing intracranial function, the following parameters must be considered: level of consciousness, orientation, brain stem/cranial nerve function, motor coordination, motor evaluation of the four extremities, multimodal sensory examination, and assessment of normal as well as potential pathologic reflexes.

Far and away the most important clinical parameter in assessing any urgent intracranial process in the critically ill patient is evaluation of the level of consciousness. In performing such an evaluation, the examiner should avoid the use of such vague terms as *semicomatose, stuporous, comatose,* or *obtunded.* Although meaningful to the examiner at that particular time, such terms 'o not describe the patient precisely enough to allow for accurate follow-up ind assessment of therapy. Upon initial evaluation, one should accurately describe the patient's reactions with respect to ver-

balization, eye opening, orientation, and cranial nerve function, as well
as the extent of stimulation required to elicit a response. Jennett and
Teasedale's *Glasgow Coma Score* [16], a standardized coma grading system, is one with which all physicians concerned with the care of patients
with marked depression of consciousness should become familiar (Fig. 20-
1).

In the awake patient, a degree of confusion as indicated by the orientation evaluation may be the only clue to a disordered metabolic or hypoxic
state, if this dementia represents a recent change in behavior. It is, important, of course, to have a historical perspective on the patient's level of
mentation before a given ictus, since the dementia may have been long-
standing. Brain stem function can frequently be assessed through evaluation of cranial nerves relating to its given levels. The midbrain lends itself
best to evaluation by assessment of pupillary status and the conjugate relationship between globes. One may then evaluate projections from the
level of the vestibular nucleus all the way to the third nerve nucleus by
performance of ice water calorics. To perform this appropriately, one must
first evaluate the patency of the external canal and the integrity of the tympanic membrane. Once any impacted cerumen is removed, the head
should be elevated 30 degrees above the horizontal; the lateral semicircular
canal is then in a vertical position, so as to evoke a maximal response upon
stimulation. A small, red rubber catheter may be placed in the external
canal near the tympanic membrane and filled with cool water (30°C) or
small amounts of ice water, so as to bathe the tympanic membrane. In the
markedly obtunded patient, the conjugate deviation of both eyes toward
the side of the cold water stimulation provides evidence of anatomic integrity of the brain stem from the level of the midpons to the third nerve
nucleus in the midbrain. The lower brain stem may be assessed by evaluating the integrity of the gag reflex and evidence of swallowing. Medullary
compression may also be detected by assessment of vital signs. Slow, shallow respiration, bradycardia, and possible systolic hypertension are classic indexes of medullary dysfunction.

Motor examination provides a reasonable index of localization at all levels of cerebral function. This evaluation should include not only the assessment of power and strength, but also a careful consideration of tone.
Hyper- or hypotonicity may clearly point to a frontal or cerebellar lesion,
respectively, particularly in the patient lacking cooperation. The sensory
examination, on the other hand, generally provides an evaluation of the
sophisticated integration of the cerebrum and requires an extremely cooperative patient. It is, therefore, of little value in patients who have sustained significant depression of consciousness, except, of course, in the
evaluation of the response to deep pain (vis-à-vis above). In the patient
with a depressed level of consciousness, however, all four extremities
should be stimulated with sufficient intensity to evoke a motor response;
a coincident spinal cord injury may be clinically evident only by the finding of a flaccid paresis in one or more of the extremities.

Assessment of spinal cord injury takes on additional clinical dimensions. It would be a rare awake patient who failed to complain of signifi-

EYE OPENING	
Spontaneously	4
To verbal stimuli	3
To pain	2
Never	1
BEST VERBAL RESPONSE	
Oriented and converses	5
Disoriented and converses	4
Inappropriate words	3
Incomprehensible sounds	2
No response	1
BEST MOTOR RESPONSE	
Obeys commands	6
Localizes to pain	5
Flexion withdrawal	4
Flexor posture (decorticate)	3
Extensor posture (decerebrate)	2
No response	1
Total	3–15

Fig. 20-1. The Glasgow Coma Scale. (Adapted from Teasedale and Jennett [16].)

cant pain in the vertebral area involved by injury. Pain may also be elicited by careful palpation of the spinal axis. The clinical assessment of the patient's motor, sensory, and reflex responses remains the best index of the extent of spinal cord damage. In the awake patient, sensory modalities—including posterior column functions, as evidenced by vibration and position sense, and anterolateral quadrant function, as evidenced by pain and temperature sensation—should be meticulously evaluated. Voluntary motion at all joints in a given extremity must also be carefully assessed, as well as all reflexes in each extremity. Perianal sensation and the integrity of both the anal reflex and voluntary contraction of the anal sphincter should be assessed. Total absence of all of the above-mentioned parameters (complete sensorimotor areflexic paraplegia) establishes the state of spinal shock, with an extremely poor potential for functional recovery. Careful recording of any intact neurologic function provides a basis for optimism about potential recovery, as well as a baseline for assessment during ensuing management.

Monitoring

Monitoring of intracranial parameters provides the status of intracranial physical dynamics, as well as alterations in such parameters as affected by therapy. These factors call for continuous on-line monitoring of both intra-cranial and systemic arterial pressures. The continuous recording of sys-temic arterial pressure is well understood, but the simultaneous monitor-ing of intracranial pressure deserves additional comment.

Intracranial pressure monitoring is now an accepted part of interven-tional therapy in the management of patients with severe cranial disorders. The indications for monitoring intracranial pressure certainly are not ab-solute. In the acute head-injured patient, a significantly depressed level of consciousness (usually a Glasgow Coma score of 8 or less) is an indication for intracranial pressure monitoring for a period of at least 24 hours. This should help ascertain the role of intracranial hypertension in the cerebral dysfunction. In cases of CSF obstruction, placement of an intraventricular catheter enables the diversion of spinal fluid to lower intracranial pressure. In certain encephalopathic processes, such as Reye's syndrome, intracra-nial pressure may be a significant determinant of the neurologic outcome; accordingly, these disorders justify the insertion of an intracranial pressure monitoring device to offer early and aggressive treatment of intracranial hypertension.

Different Methods of Monitoring Intracranial Pressure

Techniques of monitoring intracranial pressure vary from direct cannula-tion of the lateral ventricles to recording of pressures measured through the extradural space. Each of these techniques represents an invasion of the cranial vault, although the preservation of the integrity of the dura ma-ter by using the extradural space may significantly reduce the potential risk for infection when such monitoring techniques are employed over a prolonged period of time. The measurement of intracranial pressure may be achieved from several different anatomic locations.

1. Epidural space
2. Subdural/subarachnoid space
3. Intraparenchymal
4. Intraventricular
5. Lumbar theca

Each of these sites offers attendant advantages and disadvantages. The epidural space was originally thought to offer recording accuracy with re-duced risk of significant intracranial infection. This is undoubtedly the largest advantage to its usage; the major disadvantage lies in the necessity of insertion and removal under direct vision in the operating room envi-ronment. There is also some evidence that true correlation with intradural pressures may falter at higher levels of intracranial pressure; this may be of critical importance in managing the patient with significant elevations in intracranial pressure.

The subdural or subarachnoid devices offer unquestionably greater ac-curacy than do the epidural systems. The price paid for this added accu-racy, however, is an increase in the infection rate in these systems inherent to the violation of the dura. In addition, the complexity of the monitoring system itself is greater, posing a greater chance of technical malfunction. The systems rely on a fluid "coupling" to allow accurate pressure recording. With the subarachnoid systems, in cases of markedly increased intracranial pressure from general cerebral swelling, the subarachnoid space may be obliterated, thus obviating the fluid interface necessary for proper transducer function and producing inaccurate readings at such time when ICP recording is critical. In general, we reserve the use of subarachnoid or subdural systems for those instances in which the ventricular anatomy is such that it precludes accurate placement of a ventricular catheter.

Recent technological advances have enabled the use of fiber-optic devices for pressure transduction, thus permitting the use of the parenchyma itself for pressure recording with no requisite for fluid coupling. The advantage of this system lies in those cases in which severe ventricular distortion or collapse would preclude proper ventricular catheter placement. Though currently not in widespread use, the placement of such devices offers the advantage of being technically simple; major disadvantages include expensive disposable parenchymal transducers, the necessity for initial accurate monitor calibration by a trained nursing staff, and the potential for serious intracranial infection or hemorrhage from the implanted device.

The indwelling ventricular catheter remains the gold standard for intracranial pressure monitoring. Bedside insertion is feasible in the intensive care unit setting. Ventricular catheters are most frequently placed via the frontal, coronal, or occipital routes, with ideal placement allowing monitoring with the catheter tip placed at the foramen of Monroe. The major advantage is the simultaneous access to ventricular fluid, thus enabling drainage of fluid for diagnostic purposes or reduction in intracranial pressure. Disadvantages include the potential for fouling of the catheter tip with the choroid plexus and the small (usually less than 2%) but potentially serious risk of ventricular or parenchymal infection. The risk of infection may be reduced by adherence to meticulous aseptic technique during insertion and maintenance of the catheter by medical staff, as well as by frequent changing of insertion site and catheter (usually, at least every 5 days). Repeated drainage of ventricular fluid may result in obliterated ventricular spaces and loss of fluid coupling necessary for accurate transduction. Similarly, inadequate placement in the parenchyma may offer false recordings; injection of small amounts of fluid to surround the catheter tip in this circumstance may actually result in transient falsely-high pressure readings. In experienced hands, placement of the catheter is usually possible in those instances in which ventricles are visible on computed tomography (CT) or magnetic resonance imaging (MRI); for this reason, we advocate ventricular catheter placement as the initial modality of choice for intracranial pressure monitoring in the majority of these cases.

If there is free communication between the intracranial cavity and the intraspinal space, the lumbar theca is a potential site for accurate intracranial pressure monitoring if the patient remains in the recumbent position. The presence of an intracranial mass, however, is a contraindication to lumbar puncture, for the induction of a pressure gradient between the intracranial and intraspinal space potentially can worsen the neurologic condition. Accordingly, lumbar monitoring is probably of no clinical use in the setting of head injury with suspected increased intracranial pressure. In addition, the recording of low lumbar thecal pressures does not preclude the possibility of tonsillar herniation, and the diagnosis of traumatic subarachnoid hemorrhage by lumbar cannulation is of no therapeutic assistance. Thorough imaging (CT or MRI) is of paramount importance to rule out any intracranial mass lesions prior to implementation of this technique.

A standardized reference to intracranial pressure in terms of millimeters of mercury has been adopted in order to make adequate comparisons of factors considered critical in intracranial dynamics. The generally accepted upper limit of normal for intracranial pressure is 15 mm Hg (approximately 225 mm H_2O), which requires comparison with systemic arterial pressures to determine the adequacy of cerebral perfusion. Because of this relationship, the concept of cerebral perfusion pressure (CPP) has been derived. The cerebral perfusion pressure expresses the differential between mean systemic arterial pressure and the mean intracranial pressure (SAP–ICP). A fall in CPP below 55 mm Hg is associated with significant cerebral ischemia. The objective of monitoring techniques is to assure maintenance of CPP to provide adequate cerebral circulation.

Spinal cord monitoring has generally revolved around the utilization of somatosensory-evoked responses in an effort to ascertain the physiologic integrity of the cord. Experience to date has shown that the utilization of such systems yields no more information than does clinical examination in the awake patient. A careful and detailed sensory and motor examination in an awake patient appears to document the anatomic and physiologic integrity of the cord, as well as somatosensory-evoked responses. However, this system, in addition to the newly developed motor-evoked–responses technique, has value in the operating room when the patient is asleep and spinal cord manipulation is being undertaken, particularly in the correction of scoliosis.

Diagnostic Tools

The development of CT and, more recently, MRI has virtually revolutionized diagnostic capacities for evaluation of intracranial mass lesions. In addition to mass effects, one may also detect acute subarachnoid blood with CT imaging. Lumbar puncture should be employed only after it has been determined, by noninvasive techniques, that no intracranial mass exists that could result in worsening of the patient's neurologic status subsequent to spinal fluid withdrawal.

Angiography remains without peer in the diagnosis of intracranial vascular lesions, specifically aneurysms or arteriovenous malformations. The presence of subarachnoid hemorrhage may be suspected on CT examination, but precise definition of the vascular tree depends on high-resolution cerebral angiography. The future may see MRI play an increasingly important role in the definition of intracranial vascular lesions, with the advent of computer-assisted three-dimensional image reconstruction, but at this time it is still limited in practical applicability.

Echoencephalography may provide a reasonable substitute where rapid CT or MRI is not available. This system allows assessment of the position of midline diencephalic structures and can yield valuable information with reference to the existence of a supratentorial mass. In experienced hands, this method may also allow crude evaluation of the ventricular system, thereby predicting the presence of hydrocephalus. However, the presence of a posterior fossa mass may be unappreciated, emphasizing the need for the greater precision offered by CT or MRI.

EVALUATION AND MANAGEMENT OF THE PATIENT WITH A DEPRESSED LEVEL OF CONSCIOUSNESS

Patients with a marked depression in the level of consciousness can be readily placed into two general categories: those harboring an intracranial mass lesion and those in whom depression is secondary to metabolic derangement. The clinician must establish, as readily as possible, the existence of an intracranial mass lesion, whether this be supra- or infratentorial, since surgical excision of this mass provides the sole modality for resolution of the CNS disorder. Such efforts consequently take on great urgency. The availability of diagnostic equipment will determine the rapidity with which the diagnostic dilemma will be resolved. While preparations are being made for such investigations, however, simultaneous actions can be taken to evaluate and treat disorders arising extrinsic to the CNS that may exert profound influence upon neural function.

Table 20-1 provides a detailed assessment of systemic as well as localized extraneural parameters that may cause profound neuroglic dysfunction even though the sources lie external to the CNS [12]. Review of these related disorders reveals a number of pertinent laboratory assessments that may be immediately undertaken during the evaluation of the comatose patient. Appropriate blood samples should be procured early in the evaluation of such patients. Once cardiopulmonary parameters appear stable, sufficient blood should be obtained to enable assessment of various metabolic parameters. These should include an immediate arterial sample to evaluate arterial blood gases, as well as serum samples for glucose, calcium, hepatic enzymes, renal substrates, electrolytes, and a toxicology screen that includes hypnotics, sedatives, and common narcotics, as well as alcohol. Institution of therapy need not await any of these values, but baseline assessment is imperative in order to plan a long-term therapeutic regimen. Once the blood for baseline laboratory studies has been procured, it is reasonable to administer 30 to 50 cc of a 50% dextrose solution intravenously over a period of several minutes. Although hypoglycemia is a relatively uncommon source of coma, this administration of glucose carries little risk and may be of great impact in restoring neural function.

Once it has been clearly ascertained that systemic and cerebral perfusion, oxygenation, and substrate availability in the form of glucose are adequate and that no intracranial mass threatens catastrophic distortion of brain substance, one can proceed to explore the numerous causes of depressed consciousness indicated in Table 20-1. Many of these will require gradual correction, with gradual restoration of neural function paralleling improvement in the underlying metabolic disorder. If intracranial pres-

Table 20-1. Metabolic causes of stupor and coma

I. Stupor or coma arising from intrinsic diseases of the neurons or neuroglial cells (primary metabolic encephalopathy)
    A. Gray matter diseases
        1. Jakob-Creutzfeldt disease
        2. Pick's disease
        3. Alzheimer's disease and senile dementia
        4. Huntington's chorea
        5. Progressive myoclonic epilepsy
        6. Lipid storage diseases
    B. White matter diseases
        1. Schilder's disease
        2. Marchiafava-Bignami disease
        3. The leukodystrophies
II. Stupor or coma arising from diseases extrinsic to neurons and glia (secondary metabolic encephalopathy)
    A. Deprivation of oxygen, substrate, or metabolic cofactors
        1. Hypoxia (interference with oxygen supply to the entire brain—CBF normal)
            a. Decreased oxygen tension and content of blood
                (1) Pulmonary disease
                (2) Alveolar hypoventilation
                (3) Decreased atmospheric oxyten tension
            b. Decreased oxygen content of blood—normal tension
                (1) Anemia
                (2) Carbon monoxide poisoning
                (3) Methemoglobinemia
        2. Ischemia (diffuse or widespread multifocal interference with blood supply to brain)
            a. Decreased CBF resulting from decreased cardiac output
                (1) Stokes-Adams; cardiac arrest; cardiac arrhythmias
                (2) Myocardial infarction
                (3) Congestive heart failure
                (4) Aortic stenosis
                (5) Pulmonary infarction
            b. Decreased CBF resulting from decreased peripheral resistance in systemic circulation
                (1) Syncope; orthostatic, vasovagal
                (2) Carotid sinus hypersensitivity
                (3) Low blood volume
            c. Decreased CBF due to generalized or multifocal increased vascular resistance
                (1) Hypertensive encephalopathy
                (2) Hyperventilation syndrome
                (3) Hyperviscosity (polycythemia, cryoglobulinemia or macroglobulinemia, sickle cell anemia)
            d. Decreased CBF due to widespread small vessel occlusions
                (1) Disseminated intravascular coagulation
                (2) Systemic lupus erythematosus
                (3) Subacute bacterial endocarditis
                (4) Fat embolism
                (5) Cerebral malaria
                (6) Cardiopulmonary bypass
        3. Hypoglycemia
            a. Resulting from exogenous insulin
            b. Spontaneous (endogenous insulin, liver disease, etc.)

Table 20-1 (continued)

    4. Cofactor deficiency
      a. Thiamine (Wernicke's encephalopathy)
      b. Niacin
      c. Pyridoxine
      d. Cyanocobalamin
B. Diseases of organs other than brain
    1. Diseases of nonendocrine organs
      a. Liver (hepatic coma)
      b. Kidney (uremic coma)
      c. Lung (CO_2 narcosis)
    2. Hyperfunction and/or hypofunction of endocrine organs
      a. Pituitary
      b. Thyroid (myxedema-thyrotoxicosis)
      c. Parathyroid (hypoparathyroidism and hyperparathyroidism)
      d. Adrenal (Addison's diease, Cushing's disease,
        pheochromocytoma)
      e. Pancreas
    3. Other systemic diseases
      a. Cancer (remote effects)
      b. Porphyria
C. Exogenous poisons
    1. Sedative drugs
      a. Barbiturates
      b. Nonbarbiturate hypnotics
      c. Tranquilizers
      d. Bromides
      e. Ethanol
      f. Anticholinergics
      g. Opiates
    2. Acid poisons or poisons with acidic breakdown products
      a. Paraldehyde
      b. Methyl alcohol
      c. Ethylene glycol
      d. Ammonium chloride
    3. Enzyme inhibitors
      a. Heavy metals
      b. Organic phosphates
      c. Cyanide
      d. Salicylates
D. Abnormalities of ionic or acid-base environment of CNS
    1. Water and sodium (hypernatremia and hyponatremia)
    2. Acidosis (metabolic and respiratory)
    3. Alkalosis (metabolic and respiratory)
    4. Potassium (hyperkalemia and hypokalemia)
    5. Magnesium (hypermagnesemia and hypomagnesemia)
    6. Calcium (hypercalcemia and hypocalcemia)
E. Diseases producing toxins or enzyme inhibition in CNS
    1. Meningitis
    2. Encephalitis
    3. Subarachnoid hemorrhage
F. Disordered temperature regulation
    1. Hypothermia
    2. Heat stroke

CBF = cerebral blood flow; CNS = central nervous system.

sure is elevated, with its potential for compromise of adequate cerebral perfusion, one must turn to the management of persistent intracranial hypertension.

PERSISTENT INTRACRANIAL HYPERTENSION: EVALUATION AND MANAGEMENT

Intracranial pressure above 15 mm Hg indicates an elevation above normal. Transient increases in intracranial pressure do not pose a significant hazard to the patient. However, repeated episodes of intracranial hypertension, as well as persistent increases in intracranial pressure, may well contribute to depressed cerebral metabolic activity in association with impaired cerebral blood flow. Increased intracranial pressure in and of itself may not be an ominous sign in a cerebrum that is otherwise metabolically functioning well. However, in a brain impaired by toxic, metabolic, or traumatic insult, such intracranial hypertension may have disastrous consequences. The need for measures to alter intracranial pressure will depend, of course, on accurate measurement and recording of intracranial pressure, followed by measurements to ascertain whether the measures instituted to alter intracranial dynamics have been effective.

When considering the genesis of increased intracranial pressure, it is convenient to think of three separate but interdependent components within the intracranial cavity—the vascular, cerebrospinal fluid, and cerebral parenchymal components. Although each of these obviously affects the others in the interplay that underlies intracranial physical dynamics, one may think of them as individual or independent when attempting to describe a program of therapy designed to decrease intracranial pressure.

Parenchymal causes of increased intracranial pressure relate to swelling of brain substance itself, generally referred to as cerebral edema, or to compression of such substance by extrinsic or intrinsic masses, comprising primarily tumors, abscesses, and hematomas. Without question, any mass lesion demands surgical excision as the effective treatment of increased intracranial pressure. However, diffuse swelling of the brain without focal mass effect provides the setting most desirable for institution of medical management. Brain swelling may be subdivided into two histopathologic entities, cytotoxic edema and vasogenic edema. Cytotoxic edema refers to cellular swelling with resultant increase in intracellular volume and decrease in the extracellular compartment. This form of edema relates primarily to ischemic and metabolic disturbances of cerebral parenchyma, at least in their initial phases. Correction of the underlying mechanism (such as improvement in cerebral oxygenation) will inhibit potential extension to unaffected areas but will not necessarily reverse the pathologic process that has already taken place. Attack upon this form of cerebral edema has limited potential at the present time. If the blood-brain barrier has been spared by the underlying process, then the use of hyperosmotic agents may be effective in reducing cytoplasmic swelling. The generation of serum hyperosmolarity will result in extraction of both extracellular and intracellular fluid, because of the osmotic gradient between CNS and serum. This can readily be accomplished by the administration of mannitol, 1/4 to 1/2 gm per kilogram of body weight, in a rapid bolus. This agent may be utilized for repeated administrations in such a relatively low concentration, but higher doses of mannitol may well result in severe hyperosmolarity, renal failure, and metabolic acidosis.

Vasogenic edema, on the other hand, results from a loss of the integrity of the blood-brain barrier, with a resultant increase in the extracellular space of brain secondary to leakage of osmotic particles from the intravascular compartment into the extracellular space. This form of cerebral edema may respond to high-potency glucocorticoids, which presumably act by helping to maintain the integrity of the blood-brain barrier. For short-term therapy, in the event that pressures are dangerously high, the use of hyperosmotic agents as described above may also help to reduce the extracellular component of the brain.

Intracranial hypertension may develop as a consequence of expansion of CSF, owing either to increased production or to decreased absorption. The latter mechanism is by far more frequently responsible for accumulation of excess volumes of CSF. The only entity that has been associated with increased production of CSF is the choroid plexus papilloma. This tumor obviously represents a cerebral mass lesion whose treatment is managed by surgical excision. Obstruction of CSF pathways, on the other hand, may produce two different syndromes. The first is dilatation of the cerebral ventricular system (hydrocephalus), which may occur as a consequence of accumulation of excess volumes of CSF. Evidence indicates that obstruction of CSF pathways is also the most frequent underlying cause of the development of the second syndrome, known as benign increased intracranial pressure, or pseudotumor cerebri. In this situation the ventricular system is generally normal if not actually reduced in size, but the increase in intracranial pressure can result in retinal ischemia and blindness, demanding prompt and vigorous treatment.

Reduction in intracranial pressure related to aberrant CSF dynamics may be accomplished by the use of a number of pharmacologic agents that have been shown to decrease CSF production. By establishing an osmotic gradient between CSF and serum, mannitol will decrease the production of CSF, as well decrease the volume of the CSF compartment by causing water shift from CSF to serum. This mechanism is, of course, a transient event that does not lend itself well to therapeutic efforts of even intermediate duration. Several additional pharmacologic agents are available, however, to assist in the reduction of CSF production. Acetazolamide (Diamox), a carbonic anhydrase inhibitor, will reduce the CSF production by approximately 50 percent. In addition, the loop diuretics furosemide and ethacrynic acid have both been found to reduce CSF production significantly. In a superb article, Pollay [13] reviews the numerous pharmacologic agents that have been found to reduce CSF production. Reduction of CSF production, however, will have a short-lived effect, since if the defect resides at the absorptive end of the spectrum, pressure may continue to rise as long as any CSF is produced in the face of impaired absorption.

Restoration of normal absorption relies on surgical intervention. In the presence of a noncommunicating hydrocephalus (obstruction at one or more of the ventricular foramina), relief can be provided only by CSF diversion directly from the ventricular system. This can be accomplished on a temporary basis by the use of an external ventriculostomy system or may be established permanently with the insertion of a ventricular-jugular or ventricular-peritoneal shunt. If the ventricular system freely communicates with the subarachnoid space, particularly the lumbar subarachnoid space, several additional options are available. Repeated lumbar punctures may be effective in transiently resolving intracranial hypertension due to a temporary process interfering with transmigration of CSF from the subarachnoid space to the venous dural sinuses. CSF is produced at a rate of approximately 500 ml per day, so that removal of 20 to 30 ml of CSF is compensated within approximately an hour following removal of this fluid. The effect of the lumbar puncture is dramatic in creating a fistulous communication between the subarachnoid space and the epidural space. This fistulous communication may be enhanced by nursing the patient in a head-up position, so as to maximize the hydrostatic gradient between the cranial cavity and the site of the lumbar puncture. Such a position obviously enhances venous return from the head as well as drainage of CSF; these effects, either alone or in combination, may suffice for the temporary amelioration of increased intracranial pressure. One may then increase the temporary drainage of CSF by inserting a lumbar subarachnoid catheter percutaneously through a Touhey needle and allowing constant drainage into an appropriate vehicle. This system permits meticulous control over the amount of drainage but has the liability of potential infection ascending through the externalized catheter; a significant risk of infection would arise if such a drainage system were allowed to remain in place for more than 5 days. If prolonged diversion of CSF appears necessary for patient management, insertion of a lumboperitoneal shunt or ventricular shunt, as described above, would be appropriate to maximize the benefits of CSF diversion yet minimize the opportunity for secondary infection.

Finally, one must consider the influence of the intracranial vascular compartment upon intracranial physical parameters. The process of cerebral autoregulation assures relative constancy of cerebral blood flow under varying states of cerebral metabolic activity and systemic arterial pressure variations. This mechanism is dependent on the reactivity of cerebral resistance vessels, comprising primarily the small arterioles and capillaries. If such vessels undergo vasoparalysis, vascular volume will be increased, and this may, in turn, be reflected in an increase in intracranial pressure. Usually, one would not find an increase in intracranial pressure, since an equivalent volume of CSF would be displaced from the intracranial compartment. However, if such compensation is lost, intracranial pressure will rise. One encounters this constellation of events in malignant systemic arterial hypertension, which breaks through the capacity of autoregulation to maintain a constant blood flow, and therein blood volume.

At the other end of this spectrum, one must be acutely aware of the adequacy of venous drainage. Significant impedance to venous drainage will result in expansion in the venous compartment, then will be reflected back through the vascular compartment, resulting in overall increase in intravascular volume as well as slowing of cerebral blood flow. One may look at any or all of these mechanisms in an effort to alleviate increased intracranial pressure related to vascular components.

In the absence of arterial hypotension, patients should always be nursed with the head elevated, so as to enhance venous drainage to the heart and minimize the potential for impaired venous drainage. If systemic arterial hypertension is a significant problem (mean arterial pressure of greater than 140 mm Hg), efforts directed primarily at altering cerebral vascular reactivity will be fruitless, since autoregulatory phenomena presumably have been lost. In such circumstances, it is imperative to restore normal systemic arterial pressure if the reflected intracranial pressure is to be lowered. However, too rapid a decrease of systemic arterial pressure may result in a marked depression of cerebral perfusion. As mentioned above, a cerebral perfusion pressure of 75 mm Hg is found under conditions of normal systemic arterial pressure. In lowering systemic arterial pressure, one must be careful not to generate significant cerebral ischemia by lowering systemic arterial pressure without a concomitant fall in intracranial pressure. Intracranial pressure may remain elevated because of secondary cerebral edema processes that require time to abate. In addition, some of the agents used to reduce systemic arterial pressure may significantly affect autoregulatory processes and potentially contribute to sustained intracranial hypertension. In severe cases, one ideally should monitor both systemic arterial pressure and intracranial pressure while maintaining adequate cerebral perfusion.

Cerebral autoregulation may be divided into two distinct parts—namely, pressure autoregulation and metabolic autoregulation. Metabolic autoregulation relates to the alteration in carbon dioxide content and hydrogen ion content surrounding the cerebral vasculature. Even in the absence of pressure autoregulation, it may be possible to reduce intracranial pressure and cerebral blood flow by employing hyperventilation techniques. The optimal situation appears to derive from a $PaCO_2$ of approximately 25 to 30 mm Hg, which will maximize the vasoconstrictive effects of hypocarbia without potential superimposed ischemia from excessive vasoconstriction.

Each of these parameters may play an important role in the generation of significant intracranial hypertension. Efforts to control intracranial hypertension should be directed at mechanisms that will reduce parenchymal swelling, decrease cerebral extracellular fluid, decrease CSF production, enhance CSF drainage, and assure an appropriate cerebral blood flow pattern without excessive intracranial cerebrovascular volume.

MANAGEMENT OF ACUTE SPINAL CORD INJURIES
Once the physical examination relevant to the spinal cord injury has been performed, appropriate radiographic studies should be made promptly to support the clinical impression and appropriate management should be instituted. Transportation of the patient with spinal cord injury must be carefully addressed by the attending physician. The area of concern should be immobilized and alignment maintained during any transportation—this, of course, applies to transportation from the site of the accident as

well as transportation within the medical facility during the course of diagnostic evaluation. If the patient has an adequate airway, a soft collar may be gently applied without any manipulation of the neck, so as to hold the head in alignment if the neck is an area of concern. Under all circumstances, transportation should be on a rigid board or firm stretcher, to avoid any undue manipulation. X-ray films should be secured in the anteroposterior and lateral projections, while extreme caution is exercised in manipulation of the patient. If satisfactory simple x-ray films show no evidence of bony disruption, but evidence of spinal cord dysfunction is found on clinical examination, the patient should be managed as a spinal cord injury without overt subluxation but with the assumption that covert vertebral instability may exist. Radiographic evidence should be sought for paravertebral soft tissue swelling, an index of spinal trauma. These patients should be nursed, under close supervision, in a facility clearly geared for monitoring neurologic function. We have adopted the policy of nursing these patients in regular hospital beds with "logrolling" manipulation of the patient, so as to maintain alignment of the vertebral column. We have found that the use of metal frames for turning patients results in more complications and difficulties than does the use of regular beds.

Once alignment has been determined to be satisfactory in the nondisplaced vertebral column, CT of the suspected area should be secured to provide evidence of any nonvisualized trauma that might result in instability of the spine. Any lack of integrity of the bony vertebral column should be considered an index of instability and should be treated acutely as such. We do *not* advise the implementation of flexion-extension views in the acute phase in an effort to assess stability of any area of the spine. Our experience has been that CT provides a valuable index of the integrity of the spinal canal. Once the acute phase has resolved (4–5 days), flexion-extension views under medical supervision may be obtained if the patient possesses an intact sensorium.

If plain x-ray films indicate subluxation or dislocation of vertebral elements, efforts should be directed at early reduction of the malaligned vertebral components. Several factors come into consideration with respect to the urgency of such maneuvers. In the cervical spine, such efforts should be undertaken initially by the use of traction provided by insertion of skeletal tongs. Weights may be appropriately applied under x-ray guidance in an effort to reduce the unaligned cervical spine. Although weights up to 85 lb have been applied for cervical traction, one must be acutely aware of the potential for distraction of the spine as well as the spinal cord with the application of greater than 35 lb for injuries involving the lower cervical spine. Lesions involving the upper cervical spine may lend themselves to distraction even with significantly less weight; a rough guide suggests 5 lb of weight for each level starting at C_1. Radiographic confirmation of spine position should be obtained with each addition of weight. Traction devices are, in general, totally ineffective in reducing dislocated fractures involving the thoracolumbar spine. Such reduction may be accomplished by postural influences while the patient is lying in bed or by attempts at open reduction. Considerations for emergency reduction vary with the clinical specialist involved and extend beyond the scope of this discussion, but clearly, acute operative reduction of the spine is rarely necessary in the care of spinal cord injuries.

Several specific parameters are of great import with respect to acute intervention in spinal cord injuries.

Careful attention must be paid to bladder function in the patient with a spinal cord lesion. This will almost always require an indwelling catheter during the acute phases. The patient's control of bladder function will ultimately direct the necessary long-term management of the bladder, but overdistention of the urinary bladder is to be avoided, since it can lead to major loss of muscle tone, which will prevent significant bladder recovery. Cervical and high thoracic cord injuries will, in addition, result in significant compromise to pulmonary function, because of loss of intercostal innervation. One of the severe early consequences of such an injury is the development of hypoxemia, which must be carefully monitored. Therefore, early and repeated evaluation of arterial blood gases is mandatory, along with twice-daily assessment of vital capacity by respirometer. If evidence of pulmonary insufficiency develops, nasotracheal intubation should be instituted before the potential for hypoxemic CNS deterioration ensues.

Attention must be carefully directed at repeated evaluation of cardiovascular parameters, particularly in cervical spine injuries. Interruption of the descending sympathetic system in cervical and upper thoracic spine injuries engenders a situation that promotes vascular pooling in the extremities, with subsequent development of hypotension. Should this occur, vasopressors must be utilized to combat hypotension, along with volume expanders for the patient who has been in bed for some time. The development of a bradycardia, presumably due to unopposed vagal impulses influencing the cardiac mechanism, must also be carefully observed; bradycardia with pulses in the 30s may result in significant organ ischemia. This should be treated with atropine to combat the vagal influences and may require repeated administration.

Minimization of skin breakdown can be accomplished by periodic "logrolling" of the patient and nursing on the so-called egg crate mattress. The potential for development of a decubitus ulcer must be continuously recognized, and one must strive to avoid compression at any given site that shows evidence of skin breakdown. Finally, careful attention must be paid to the potential development of thrombophlebitis in chronically bedridden patients without adequate muscle tone. Monitoring of the deep venous system using radio-labeled fibrinogen may detect the early development of deep vein thrombosis. Evidence exists that minidoses of heparin (5000 units subcutaneously) administered every 12 hours may minimize the potential for such development, and the use of inflatable stockings or pneumatic calf-compression devices may further reduce the chance for development of this potentially lethal situation.

TREATMENT OF STATUS EPILEPTICUS

Status epilepticus may be defined as repeated seizure activity without the regaining of consciousness between attacks. One may also consider prolonged, continuous seizure activity in the absence of loss of consciousness as representative of status epilepticus, with particular reference to petit mal epilepsy, myoclonic epilepsy, and epilepsy partialis continua. The last group of disorders, however, does not present so urgent a problem, since the potential for cardiorespiratory compromise is not so great. The prime intent, therefore, of treatment of status epilepticus is to prevent the development of hypoxemia, with its attendant multiple organ system disruption; in this regard, it should be considered a medical emergency, with a current mortality of up to 12 percent.

Approximately 75 percent of patients with generalized status epilepticus will respond within several hours to a variety of pharmacologic regimens employed to abort the seizure activity. However, as many as 25 percent may require up to 3 or 4 days to respond to any of the regimens. Under such circumstances, the patient may well experience the superimposition of iatrogenic or acquired complications in addition to the underlying disorder. Such problems relate specifically to the development of respiratory depression, cardiac arrest, hypotension, prolonged coma, and aspiration pneumonia.

In the approach to the management of a patient with status epilepticus, it is imperative initially to define the patient's vital signs, as well as to ascertain that an adequate airway exists. Attempts at insertion of devices such as tongue blades or bite blocks to protect the tongue have frequently resulted in tooth fractures, aspiration, and other problems, so these are generally discouraged. Blood samples should immediately be secured for toxicologic screen, including barbiturates, narcotics, phenothiazines, alcohol, and phenytoin. If possible, establish an intravenous line using 5% dextrose in water and administer 50 ml of 50% glucose rapidly, along with 100 mg of thiamine. If it is necessary to maintain blood pressure, any of the appropriate pressor agents may be utilized; a central venous pressure line or Swan-Ganz catheter may prove invaluable under such circumstances. Fluid balance should be carefully observed, along with evaluation of serum electrolytes.

To suppress seizure activity rapidly, the benzodiazepine lorazepam (Librium) is the current pharmacologic agent of choice. It should be administered intravenously in doses of 1 to 2 mg over a period of several minutes, to a total dosage of 8 mg in adults. Its activity is related to suppression of the spread of electrical activity on the cerebral cortex. This agent is extremely effective in the *short-term* control of seizures. The advantage of this agent over diazepam (Valium) is less respiratory suppression and hypotension associated with intravenous administration and a longer duration of action. The most common adverse side effect reported with its usage has been significant sedation. The drug is effective in controlling ongoing seizure activity in approximately 75 percent of cases of primary generalized tonic-clonic epilepsy; in cases of partial status the response rate is much lower, as with other anticonvulsants. Care must still be taken to observe the patient's airway with intravenous use of this agent; significant respiratory depression is possible, requiring assisted ventilation. The greatest liability of the use of this agent is that it is effective in the short term only and thus requires concurrent administration with another prophylactic agent [such as phenytoin (Dilantin) or phenobarbital], if the patient has not already been loaded with such. If lorazepam is unavailable, the next agent of choice would be intravenous diazepam administered in doses up to 10 mg over a period of 3 minutes, recognizing the significant potential for respiratory depression.

The administration of intravenous phenytoin must be carefully monitored with an electrocardiogram (ECG), since it may result in the generation of severe cardiac arrhythmias. Phenytoin may be administered in doses of up to 800 to 1000 mg intravenously, at a rate not to exceed 50 mg per minute, in association with constant monitoring by ECG. This regimen, in combination with the initial lorazepam, should be effective in establishing long-term control as well as cessation of status epilepticus. Once the intravenous phenytoin has been administered, one may resort to daily maintenance doses of 300 to 400 mg per day in divided doses, either orally or intravenously. Serum phenytoin levels should be secured to determine the adequacy of maintenance therapy.

An appropriate alternative to phenytoin may be the administration of phenobarbital to gain control of recurrent seizures. Phenobarbital can be administered intravenously at a rate of 200 mg per 20 minutes, to reach a total dose of 600 to 800 mg. As with Valium or lorazepam, one must be aware of the potential for respiratory depression and a prolongation of coma due to an accumulative effect of this long-acting barbiturate. Therefore, one must be prepared to offer ventilatory as well as cardiovascular support to such patients.

Another alternative, particularly in patients suffering from prolonged seizure activity secondary to alcoholic withdrawal, is the use of paraldehyde. Paraldehyde cannot be sterilized and therefore can only be administered by selected routes. One may administer 6 to 8 ml by the rectum or 4 to 6 ml intramuscularly. A 4% solution of paraldehyde may be administered intravenously, up to a total of 8 ml. However, this must be carefully titrated because of the potential development of pulmonary edema with such administration.

Finally, if the above potential regimens should be unsuccessful over a period of 12 to 24 hours, one should consider employing a general anesthetic. This should be done only in the attendance of an anesthesiologist and will require intubation and adequate ventilation. Penthrane administration to a level of stage III anesthesia appears to be the preferred choice of general anesthetic for uncontrolled status epilepticus, regulated by a competent anesthetist.

ACUTE CEREBRAL TRAUMA

The circumstances under which cerebral injuries occur are extremely variable and unpredictable. This section will review those elements of a strategic system that may prove useful in the intensive care setting. The basic objectives can be stated as follows: (1) to provide a milieu that will maximize recovery of cerebral tissue, (2) to recognize or prevent those intra- and/or extracranial complications demanding urgent therapeutic intervention, and (3) to establish a system of priorities for diagnosis and therapy in the best interest of the patient commensurate with the resources available.

The reaction of brain to injury is a dynamic process and, to some degree, follows a predictable pattern of recovery. A departure from this pattern usually provides the first clue to a potential complication. Recognition of ominous clues requires a standard of reference, composed for the most part of the basic neurologic examination. In a setting in which only casual observations have been made and recorded, the most important guideline in the management of the patient with cerebral trauma is frequently lost. Careful consideration of the essentials of the neurologic examination relevant to the trauma may avoid an unrecognized catastrophic sequence.

Appraisal of the state of consciousness is the single most important component of this examination, since a normal state of cognitive function requires a higher level of integrated performance of neuronal pathways than does any other mode of behavior. In a patient with acute posttraumatic encephalopathy, minor fluctuations in the state of consciousness will be observed from examination to examination. Ordinarily, insignificant or minor changes in the factors that alter cerebral metabolism—such as intracranial pressure, cerebral blood flow, or metabolic derangements—may produce some minute-to-minute changes in the conscious state that can be equally perplexing to the experienced and the inexperienced observer. However, the overall trend toward consciousness or unconsciousness appears to be the most critical factor.

One can therefore appreciate the need for explicit details during the course of observation. Terms such as *comatose* have variable meanings to different examiners; therefore, a clear statement of the precise level of consciousness and response to external stimuli is imperative. The only way to avoid misinterpretation of observations is to be certain that all of the evaluation parameters—including assessment of level of consciousness, degree of orientation, specific response patterns, and response to external stimuli—are consistently employed and recorded. Here again, the Glasgow Coma Score can be helpful not only in grading the severity of the cerebral trauma, but also in prognosticating recovery in the patient suffering head trauma.

Funduscopic examination at the outset is generally unremarkable but provides a baseline for evidence of the evolution of intracranial hypertension. One should *never* utilize mydriatic agents in an effort to visualize the fundus of a patient with a suspected intracranial mass. The importance of the pupillomotor reflex, on the other hand, cannot be overemphasized. In the unresponsive patient, the direct and consensual response of the pupil should be carefully recorded. Loss of either aspect of this response may be a moderately early index of progressive dysfunction of the visual or oculomotor apparatus, particularly in herniation syndromes. Evaluation of facial symmetry is another aspect of the neurologic examination that can be made in almost all patients except those with facial trauma extensive enough to produce soft tissue distortion by swelling. If a patient is unresponsive to pain, the symmetry of the grimace may be a useful indication of the integrity of the corticobulbar tract.

In most instances of cerebral injury resulting is posttraumatic encephalopathy of sufficient magnitude to alter the conscious state, detailed sensory testing is not helpful in evaluating the progress of the encephalopathy, but it is helpful in ascertaining whether an obvious motor deficit is of cerebral, spinal, or peripheral origin. The response to a gross painful stimulus will help to identify an afferent defect due to a peripheral nerve, plexus, or root injury. Fine sensory evaluation is not of major consequence in the patient with a cerebral injury.

The extent of information obtainable from assessing the motor system depends, of course, upon the state of consciousness. Active motor resistance testing depends upon the patient's ability to understand and willingness to carry out simple commands. In the alert patient without overt motor deficit, one may document with great precision the status of the neuromuscular system. The difficulty arises in the patient who is unresponsive to verbal stimuli. In such a patient, in addition to observing the response to painful stimuli, one must always assess the amount and nature of muscular resistance to passive movement—a process that can be deferred only in the presence of an extremity fracture. The solitary flaccid extremity offering no resistance to passive manipulation should alert the examiner to a lesion involving peripheral nerve or lower motor neuron, whereas a flaccid quadriplegia arouses suspicion of associated spinal cord injury. Although seen in terminal stages, this finding would be unusual as a consequence of head injury. Spasticity—increased resistance to passive motion of the joint at the very onset of the movement pattern—is an expression of exaggerated tendon stretch reflex. Spasticity is a reliable index of disturbance of the corticospinal system, which may occur at any point from the pyramidal cell in the cortex to the lower motor neuron. Babinski's sign also indicates a disturbance in the pyramidal system, and a change from a normal flexor pattern to the abnormal extensor pattern in Babinski's reflex may be of major significance in following the patient with head trauma.

Decerebrate rigidity does not actually describe rigidity, but rather a posture in which the trunk and extremities reflect an exaggerated spasticity in the antigravity (extensor) muscle groups. This posture represents a profound disturbance of conduction in the corticospinal (motor) pathways—the lesion occurring between the red and vestibular nuclei in the brain stem and resulting in uninhibited vestibulospinal reflexes. It may occur as a result of generalized increase in intracranial pressure, compression distortion of the brain stem from direct injury, or a marked shift of the neuraxis by a mass above or below the tentorium. Although this is a serious or grave sign, it is by no means an irreversible situation.

Frequent measurements of the vital signs (blood pressure, pulse, and respiration) provide a highly useful series of observations. The incidence of Cushing's phenomenon (increase in systolic and pulse pressures, slowing of pulse rate) is surprisingly low in supratentorial expanding mass lesions, but its occurrence may point to a possible posterior fossa lesion. Theoretically, a gradual fall and deepening of the respiratory pattern should be the earliest change in vital sign functions, but there certainly is no consistent pattern.

As indicated earlier, the reaction of the brain and, therefore, the clinical behavior of the patient to cerebral injury is not entirely predictable. The primary problem facing the clinician, therefore, is to recognize the remedial intra- and extracranial complications associated with cerebral injury. The classic, typical findings in extradural or subdural hematomas are rarer in practice than are the atypical or partial syndromes.

CLOSED HEAD INJURIES

Closed intracranial injuries are usually categorized as either concussion or contusion. Classical clinical and electrophysiologic criteria may be used to describe these; but absolute correlation of these criteria in a human subject is rare, and they offer the clinician little help in any given case of posttraumatic encephalopathy. Immediate posttraumatic encephalopathy can be diagnosed according to the following criteria: group I, patients rendered unconscious or sustaining a loss of neurologic function for relatively brief periods of time who, upon gaining consciousness, demonstrate no neurologic or behavioral deficits; and group II, patients rendered unconscious for a more prolonged period who demonstrate neurologic or behavioral deficits at the time of evaluation.

Group I patients meet, for the most part, the clinical definition of concussion. When this is the only medical problem, there is little active treatment that the physician need offer other than a period of observation in or near a facility that can provide the diagnostic and therapeutic help to manage potential complications. Assuming that ideal circumstances prevail, how long should the patient be kept in hospital for observation? Almost 100 percent of acute catastrophic intracranial hemorrhagic complications in this group of patients occur within the first 72 hours; 24 hours will cover most instances. Hospitalization is unnecessary if the patient is asymptomatic at the time of the evaluation. Cerebral edema is virtually nonexistent, at least in a clinically significant form, in group I patients (concussion). Therefore, a patient in this category who has an alteration in the state of consciousness, complains of increasing headache, or has discernible progressive neurologic deficit should be considered to have an intracranial hemorrhage until that diagnosis is excluded.

The foregoing discussion refers only to early management. Chronic subdural hematomas may develop and become evident several weeks or months following injury, along with the more insidious complication of posttraumatic hydrocephalus. Therefore, all of these patients should be seen as outpatients regularly for a minimum of 6 weeks.

Patients in group II (cerebral contusion) are obviously more severely injured and require hospitalization. The number of variables that affect the cerebral function and alter behavior is greatly increased in group II patients, and therefore, the number of dilemmas in management is correspondingly increased. Many of the patients who appear to be in group II at the time of the initial evaluation fall rapidly into group I when the effects of alcohol or other intoxicants have subsided; they can safely be discharged after 24 hours. A toxicology screen is obviously of paramount importance in all patients suspected of head injury, who must be managed in the same way as patients in group I until they are clearly out of danger.

Those showing evidence of progressive neurologic deficit documented along previously described lines demand more definitive diagnostic tests.

In addition to the initial forces of acceleration or deceleration that disrupt the structure and function of brain tissue, the brain itself exerts adverse effects in reacting to the initial injury. This process is commonly ascribed to cerebral edema, but although there is little doubt that edema contributes to cerebral swelling, it is only one component of what is quite likely to be a constellation of complex phenomena only partially understood. The process seems to be most severe between 24 and 48 hours after the injury; thereafter, it gradually subsides. The onset may be as early as 6 to 12 hours following injury. This period overlaps the expected time of onset of the surgically remediable hemorrhagic complications of cerebral injury. Time of onset of the decline in performance of the patient's cerebral function therefore provides little help in distinguishing between the two processes. This leads to the question of whether there is a particular pattern of neurologic dysfunction that characterizes one or both of these processes. The answer is clearly no.

Intra-axial cerebral swelling and extra-axial compression by extradural or subdural hemorrhage are frequently concomitant and interrelated. Clinical records too frequently refer only to the presence or absence of localized findings. Their absence, however, is not a reliable diagnostic sign in the evaluation of a potential expanding intracranial mass lesion. The hallmark of any expanding intracranial mass remains the progressive decline in level of consciousness. Thus, documentation of increasing neurologic deficit, in any sphere, should summon further diagnosis and therapy from attending personnel.

DIAGNOSTIC TOOLS

At the point in time when investigation beyond direct bedside observations is required, the clinician's course of action will be greatly influenced by the availability and reliability of diagnostic tools in the institution.

Plain Film Radiography

Conventional radiography of the skull will show the presence or absence of a fracture and provide some indication of whether there is a shift of the brain by the position of the pineal gland when it is calcified. The distribution, presence, or absence of fractures provides little help in diagnosing an intracranial hematoma, although it may be useful in lateralizing extradural hemorrhage. The most significant value of the plain skull radiograph in the assessment of the patient with head trauma is in identifying a depressed skull fracture that cannot be appreciated on clinical examination and in finding of incidental intracranial abnormalities that may have contributed to the original trauma.

Electroencephalography

Electroencephalography (EEG) is rarely helpful in the acute trauma setting.

Lumbar Puncture

Lumbar puncture is much the same as EEG in assessing the patient with posttraumatic encephalopathy. It provides an indication of intracranial pressure, but the clinical findings are of far greater consequence. The presence or absence of bloody cerebrospinal fluid also does not help in the clinician's decision-making process. As previously discussed, it can be argued that the lumbar puncture is contraindicated in the evaluation of an acute posttraumatic encephalopathy, since the release of even a small amount of fluid from the lumbar subarachnoid space may enhance an already existent hemispheric shift, due to an intra- or extra-axial hemispheric clot. Therefore, its most useful role is in the evaluation of *coma of unknown etiology.*

CT Scanning

Present-day CT equipment provides a rapid, extremely accurate, noninvasive means of defining intracranial pathology. Intracerebral hematomas and significant cerebral distortions can be readily perceived. In addition, a remarkably high percentage of extra-axial clots, both epidural and subdural, can be discerned. Acute epidural or subdural hematomas, however, may be missed, because of their isodense character relative to adjacent bone; one must understand this potential for a false-negative evaluation with smaller hematomas. One additional limiting factor is the risk of movement in the agitated patient, creating the need for general anesthesia in some patients, an undesirable situation in terms of patient management.

MRI

Magnetic resonance imaging provides superior intracranial resolution, allowing visualization of pathology often not discernible by other modalities. The information obtained by MRI often complements CT; for this reason, MRI and CT should not be considered equivalent. In general, intracranial lesions are visualized with great accuracy with the newer-generation scanners; if there are instances where CT is preferable, it would be in the delineation of an acute intracranial hemorrhagic event, as acute hemorrhage is often isointense with parenchyma within the first few days following the ictus on MRI and may be overlooked. For this reason, in addition to the superior bone resolution CT offers, CT is the modality of choice in the acute trauma setting.

Cerebral Angiography

Cerebral angiography has largely been replaced by CT or MRI scanning when these latter techniques are available within a given institution. However, angiography remains one of the best diagnostic studies in the acute setting for consistent establishment of suspected vascular injuries, especially in instances of penetrating cranial or neck trauma. Brachial, carotid, or transfemoral catheter angiography may be employed, depending upon the available facilities. If CT or MRI is not readily available, early appropriate angiography may certainly prove to be lifesaving in the demonstration of cerebral distortion from intracranial hemorrhage.

EARLY MANAGEMENT

Standard principles of homeostatic support apply to all patients with head injury as well as injuries elsewhere. Assessment of the cardiopulmonary system assumes priority in all circumstances. Airway patency must be uncompromised; endotracheal or nasotracheal intubation should be instituted when deemed advisable. When possible, a set of arterial blood gases should be obtained early, to corroborate the clinical impression of pulmonary function. In addition, cardiovascular stability should be secured. Once adequate systemic perfusion is assured, a good intravenous system is in place, and drainage of both gastric and urinary system is operant where deemed advisable, the physician may turn to assessment and initial management of CNS trauma.

Transport of patients with cerebral injuries should be accomplished with the head elevated 30 degrees above the heart, in order to maximize the venous drainage from the intracranial cavity. This, of course, must be compatible with a stable cardiovascular system, which must assume priority. The initial evaluation also must yield no evidence of vertebral instability; if there should be any question about a potential associated spinal injury, adequate measures to maintain spinal stability must be instituted at the time of initial transport. The physician must always be concerned with the real potential for cervical spine injury in association with cranial trauma. A good rule is to assume that any trauma severe enough to render a patient unconscious, even momentarily, should be considered severe enough to involve transmission of the axial loading force of the blow to the cervical spine, with possible disruption of the vertebral spinal axis.

Between 2 and 5 percent of patients with closed cerebral trauma will develop a focal or generalized seizure. This raises the question of prophylactic anticonvulsants in closed head trauma cases. In cases of discernible contusion or other intracranial hemorrhage on initial CT scanning, anticonvulsants (usually phenytoin, to avoid the confounding depressant effects of phenobarbital) are routinely administered. In the patient with no radiographically identifiable pathology, we believe that the potential for drug reaction outweighs the benefits derived and consequently withhold anticonvulsants until the clinical course (a focal or generalized seizure) indicates their need. Should a seizure intervene, however, vigorous efforts must be made to attain therapeutic levels of anticonvulsants, to avoid the potential complications of status epilepticus.

THE CURRENT STATUS OF CEREBRAL PROTECTION

Although the concept of protection of the neuronal pool following trauma or stroke is not unique to the modern era of medicine, the current century has been unique in its interest in the development of a pharmacologic panacea for the mitigation of stroke. Previous dogma had stated the inevitable irreversibility of neuronal damage following 4 to 8 minutes of complete anoxia; there now exists evidence from several models that neurons may sustain up to 60 minutes of ischemic anoxia without suffering irreversible injury and retain their ability to maintain cellular integrity as well as generate action potentials. Thus, the limits of cell viability must be redefined.

Perhaps more important, however, is the potential for *reversibility* of neuronal ischemic malfunction, utilizing treatments initiated before or after the ischemic insult.

The common pathophysiologic denominators of head trauma, stroke, increased intracranial pressure, and cardiopulmonary arrest are *ischemia* and *hypoxia*. Indeed, in the vast majority of cerebral insults, ischemia is the offender. Ischemia has been classically subdivided into focal and global subtypes; this differentiation is more than merely arbitrary, in that (1) experimental evidence indicates different pathophysiologic cellular events following focal or global ischemia, (2) focal ischemia allows the potential for collateral flow, and (3) experimentally proven therapies differ.

Glucose is the well-recognized preferential neuronal energy source. It is oxidized via the Embden-Myerhoff pathway to pyruvate, which is further oxidized via the tricarboxylic acid cycle, producing ATP from oxidative phosphorylation. In the absence of oxygen delivery or blood flow to cerebral tissue, oxidative phosphorylation ceases in approximately 15 seconds. Anaerobic metabolism quickly ensues, with the production of lactate from pyruvate, and a significant decrease in intra- and extracellular pH. The lactic acidosis and depletion of ATP stores trigger many catabolic cellular processes that culminate in the ultimate death of the ischemic neuron. Failure of ATP-dependent sodium-potassium pumps cause ion fluxes, depolarization of membrane potentials, and an increase in intracellular calcium. The functional result of increased calcium levels is platelet aggregation, vasoconstriction, and uncoupled oxidative phosphorylation, all of which ultimately further exacerbate tissue ischemia.

The several potential areas of therapeutic intervention in this catabolic sequence are perhaps best considered by their mode of action.

Methods of Decreasing Metabolic Demand

Therapy may directed toward decreasing the metabolic activity of the neuron, thereby improving the supply-demand mismatch under conditions of ischemia or hypoxia. Hypothermia is the archetypical method of decreasing the metabolic demand of the cell. It has long been suspected clinically, and has been supported by anecdotal case reports, that hypothermia increases neuronal resistance to hypoxic insults. By lowering of the core temperature from 37 to 22°C, the cerebral metabolic rate of oxygen consumption ($CMRO_2$) decreases linearly to 25 percent of normal. Hypothermia has long been a useful adjunct in cardiac surgery. Difficulties in applicability of hypothermia have been its limiting side effects—most notably, cardiac depression, pulmonary infections, and gastric ulceration. Prolonged hypothermia indeed may be detrimental, in light of increased viscosity of blood at lower temperatures and attendant sludging of flow. In the face of these omnipresent limiting features, a moderate hypothermia is advocated, with core temperature being lowered to no less than 32 to 33°C. Experimental evidence suggests that this degree of hypothermia has minimal myocardial depression while offering substantial decreases in $CMRO_2$. Perhaps more importantly, any hyperthermia often associated with head trauma or seizure activity should be aggressively managed; at these core temperatures, each degree of temperature elevation is associated with a concomitant rise of 9 to 10 percent in cerebral metabolic rate. Thermolytic agents, cooling blankets, or ice packs should be utilized in this setting to evoke a rapid normalization in temperature.

Barbiturates exhibit a dose-dependent diminution of $CMRO_2$ (up to 50%) until electrical silence of the cerebrum ensues. Additional doses after electroencephalographic silence is achieved offer no further effect; housekeeping cell functions are not affected. In addition to this major protective mechanism, barbiturates also exhibit lysosomal membrane stabilization, decrease cerebral edema formation, and scavenge free radicals, all of which processes have been implicated in continued catabolic effects following ischemia. Barbiturates also decrease flow in the nonischemic brain and thus may actually improve flow under conditions of *focal* ischemia by producing a "reverse-steal" phenomenon. The efficacy of barbiturate protection in focal ischemia is well documented both in pretreatment and early posttreatment (within 60 minutes of the insult) experimental models of middle cerebral artery occlusion. However, their efficacy following conditions of *global* ischemia is controversial; different animal experimental paradigms have offered opposing results; at this time the routine use of barbiturates following cardiac arrest or other conditions of complete anoxia or ischemia has shown no consistent clinical benefit. This is an important consideration in view of the deleterious side effects of most barbiturates—cardioplegic effects that are dose-dependent and require initiation of pressor support in a significant number of patients receiving burst-suppressive doses, the increased risk of infection attributable to their use, and depression of mental status that obscures neurologic evaluation. The efficacy of these agents in severe head trauma is also controversial; studies have failed to demonstrate unequivocally improved outcome following their use. Recent randomized trials have demonstrated improvement of ICP control [5] yet failed to show improvement in outcome [17]. Questionable benefits and severe potential side effects preclude their use in the majority of trauma cases. Clinical trials are presently underway to determine potential subgroups in which use of these agents may be of benefit.

Certain inhalational anesthetic agents similarly reduce neuronal metabolic demand. Isoflurane and etomidate both decrease $CMRO_2$ in a dose-related fashion. As with barbiturates, their primary metabolic depressant effect preferentially alters synaptic activity; metabolism maintaining cellular integrity is unaffected. In contrast to barbiturates, however, these inhalational agents exhibit no significant cardioplegic side effects. Etomidate offers the additional benefit of decreasing intracranial pressure in head trauma; this is related to its vasoconstrictive properties, which could potentiate ischemia in the face of a normal intracranial pressure.

Recently there has been enthusiasm regarding the potential clinical use of antagonists of excitatory neurotransmitters. A decrease in seizure activity should intuitively decrease the metabolic demand of the ischemic neuron, and this concept has been extended in attempts to suppress general cortical activity by utilizing antagonists of putative excitatory amino acid cerebral neurotransmitters. 2-amino-7-phosphoheptanoic acid, an antagonist of N-methyl-D-aspartate, has recently been demonstrated to decrease ischemic damage [14]. Future clinical use of these and other similar agents demands further research.

Methods of Increasing Supply

In the ischemic brain, autoregulation may be lost and cerebral blood flow may therefore become dependent on mean arterial pressure (MAP). In consideration of this, in the absence of elevated intracranial pressure it seems intuitively reasonable that elevation of MAP should enhance perfusion of the ischemic region. The administration of colloid or crystalloid infusions also produces a significant hemodilution effect that enhances microcirculatory flow. The combination of hypertension and hemodilution has been demonstrated to improve or reverse ischemic neurologic deficit in up to 70 percent of patients suffering from subarachnoid hemorrhage-induced vasospasm [2]. Moreover, clinical trials in ischemic stroke have offered promising results with the use of hemodilution. This should be utilized, however, with the caveat that the presence of hemorrhagic stroke, suspected increase in ICP following head trauma, or large infarction would be contraindications to the use of hypertensive therapy. There is also the potential for detrimental effects with the use of hypertensive therapy in the face of a disrupted blood-brain barrier; extravasation of osmotically active serum components may exacerbate tissue edema and contribute to increasing intracranial pressure [15].

Rheologically, microcirculatory flow is enhanced with a moderate reduction of hematocrit to a level of 30 to 35 percent. This level strikes a balance between a decrease in blood viscosity and the maintenance of sufficient oxygen-carrying capacity of the blood. Often this may be achieved with colloid and/or crystalloid infusion in the stroke patient; if this strategy is insufficient, phlebotomy may be necessary to reach this end.

The use of antiplatelet agents or anticoagulants such as heparin or coumadin following focal ischemia is controversial. The rationale for the use of these agents is that during ischemia, elevated intracellular calcium, with subsequent liberation of leukotrienes and thromboxane, enhances thrombogenesis and increases particulate flow. Although these agents have been used with much success during vascular surgical procedures and in patients with known sources of emboli (e.g., cardiac sources or carotid ulceration), at present there have been insufficient studies to demonstrate unequivocal benefits to the routine use of these agents in focal ischemia. Similarly, in head trauma the use of anticoagulants or antiplatelet agents has yet to be defined; it is likely that the increased risk of hemorrhagic complications in these patients will preclude their use.

During conditions of ischemia, thromboxane (TXA_2) is preferentially synthesized, producing an overall increase in platelet aggregation and vasoconstriction. The use of prostacyclin (PGI_2), the naturally occurring vasodilating prostaglandin, has been proposed as a nonspecific vasodilator in this circumstance. When administered concurrently with a cyclooxygenase inhibitor, it has been purported to be more efficacious in pro-

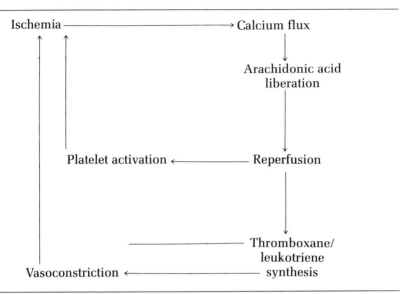

Fig. 20-2. Current hypothetical interrelated events in reperfusion following ischemia. (Adapted from White, Winegar, et al. [18].)

moting vasodilatation while actively preventing thromboxane synthesis. Indomethacin in combination with PGI_2 has been documented to decrease focal cerebral ischemia [1].

Recent interest in calcium ion activity relates to the fact that Ca^{++} shifts are central in the production of leukotrienes, prostantoids, and oxidative free radicals and are implicated heavily in the postischemic hypoperfusion syndrome [18]. All of these factors interrelate and contribute to neuronal injury (Fig. 20-2). Calcium-entry blockers (CEB), while decreasing ionic shifts, are purported to mitigate against this catabolic cascade. The use of CEB is potentially applicable in focal as well as global ischemia. Pretreatment with CEB has been reported to provide protection from global cerebral ischemia, both in short term (24 hours after aortic arch occlusion in dogs) and in the longer follow-up term in primates. At present, there is an ongoing trial of lidoflazine administration following human cardiac arrest. The use of calcium-channel blockers in SAH-induced vasospasm has evoked great enthusiasm; recent work studying nimodipine, a potent voltage-dependent calcium-channel blocker, has demonstrated reversal of neurologic deficit [18] and reversal of angiographic vasospasm [4] following its use. Recently, nicardipine, a cerebrospecific congener that is administrable intravenously, has been developed; a multicenter trial is presently underway to determine its efficacy.

The above potential advantages notwithstanding, in general all CEBs carry risk of hypotension and negative cardiac inotropic effects, which may limit their use in some clinical circumstances.

Membrane Stabilization

Membrane integrity is central to maintaining the homeostatic metabolic milieu necessary for normal neuronal function. Following ischemia, two basic membrane-associated factors are responsible for damage: the ion flux that results from the drop in pH and membrane depolarization (K^+ and Ca^{++} flux) and the direct lipid peroxidation of membranes from free radicals liberated in the calcium-dependent activation of phospholipases.

High-potency glucocorticoids have long been utilized prior to neurosurgical procedures, in the belief that they mitigate against edema and provide neuronal protection at a time of anticipated neuronal insult. Experimentally, they stabilize membranes and decrease arachidonic acid release following ischemia. Their protective effect is probably multifactorial; they increase blood flow to injured CNS tissue and enhance Na-K ATPase activity (presumably by decreasing lipid peroxidation), thus decreasing ion flux. Intrinsic antioxidant properties of glucocorticoids also function in free-radical scavenging (see following section). One proviso in their use, however, is potentiation of hyperglycemia with their administration, often at a time in which the patient is already hyperglycemic following the stress of trauma or stroke. Clinical trials have failed to demonstrate a consistent favorable effect on outcome following head trauma. In potential subsets of patients (most notably, younger patients) with severe head trauma, the use of high doses of methylprednisolone *may* improve outcome [7]. At the present time, however, the deleterious catabolic side effects (in addition to the increased risk of infection and gastrointestinal blood loss associated with their use) outweigh their proven benefit in the majority of head injured patients. Dosage and potential subgroups in which their use may be of benefit await definition.

Phenytoin, in addition to its anticonvulsant properties, has been demonstrated to reduce membrane-associated ion flux during both hypoxia and normoxia. It has no significant effect on $CMRO_2$ and produces an overall decrease in cerebral blood flow. Phenytoin has been shown to decrease K^+ concentration in CSF following global ischemia; this most certainly reflects an attenuated liberation of potassium from intracellular sites following ischemia. The mechanism of this is uncertain but may be enhanced Na-K pump activity or a direct membrane stabilizing effect. Immediate postischemic administration has decreased the neuropathologic changes associated with neuronal anoxia. Maximal benefits are gleaned from anticonvulsant dosages; larger doses produce attendant toxic side effects and provide no further ischemic protection.

Free-Radical Scavengers

As alluded to previously, free radicals have been implicated in the postischemic dissolution of membranes, especially under conditions of reperfusion, and are likely also involved in the formation of postischemic edema [9]. Several agents have free-radical–scavenging properties. Agents that are reported to readily quench this reactive species (e.g., barbiturates) have, as aforementioned, been demonstrated to reduce deficit after focal ischemia. Other naturally occurring antioxidants, such as vitamins C and

E (α-tocopherol), have been demonstrated to decrease cerebral lipid per-oxidation [6]. Mannitol, in addition to its primary rheologic effects, is pos-tulated to possess some free-radical–scavenging ability. The well-known scavenger superoxide dismutase, although experimentally promising, has not yet been demonstrated to be of advantage clinically.

Substrate Manipulation

Subsequent to the onset of ischemia, there is a rapid depletion of intracel-lular glucose stores and intracellular pH, as well as a preferential shift of metabolism to anaerobic mode, with production of lactate from pyruvate. Under conditions of *incomplete* ischemia, with continued delivery of glu-cose to the neuron, lactate production proceeds with further reduction in intracellular pH, thus increasing cellular toxicity and exacerbating the neu-rologic deficit. In this instance, as Hoff [9] appropriately described, "a little blood flow is worse than no flow at all, if followed by reperfusion." Ex-perimental work has correlated the degree of hyperglycemia with neuronal damage in incomplete ischemia. Thus, rapid establishment of *normogly-cemia* following the ischemic insult or trauma is advocated; one must, at the same time, be cognizant of the well-recognized detrimental effects of hypoglycemia.

The natural extension of this concept has been to identify alternative neuronal energy substrates that are metabolized to nontoxic products, in an attempt to circumvent this detrimental anaerobic glucose metabolism. Such substrates as γ-hydroxybutyrate and 1,3-butanediol are readily util-ized as energy substitutes in the hypoglycemic state and are catabolized into nontoxic metabolites. Both of these agents have been demonstrated experimentally to prolong hypoxic survival in the mice model. The pre-dominant limiting factor with the use of γ-hydroxybutyrate is the major reduction in CBF and cardiac output in clinical use. The clinical use of these agents in cerebral ischemia has yet to be defined.

With the continued acquisition of knowledge of the complex cellular events consequent to ischemia, our definition of the limits of neuronal viability will undoubtedly be expanded. While the above discussion alluded to many at-present experimental modalities of cerebral protection, we remain optimistic that clinical benefit will be substantiated in many instances.

THE CLINICAL DIAGNOSIS OF BRAIN DEATH

Implicit in the discussion in the care of the critically ill neurosurgical pa-tient is the recognition of hopeless loss of cerebral function, with subse-quent inability to sustain internal homeostatic function. Since the late 1950s neurologists and neurosurgeons have been interested in the defini-tion of strict criteria that substantiate the diagnosis of brain death. Mollaret and Goulon [11] in 1959 originally described a condition in which no dis-cernible neurologic function was present yet cardiovascular parameters could be maintained by artificial measures (aptly phrased *Le coma de-passe*). There is now verwhelming evidence that this state is a self-limited process that will culrⁱ nate in cardiopulmonary arrest within a few days in the majority of cases. Recent advancements in surgical transplantation emphasize the need for precise and relatively expedient determination of this state, as donor organ status is a major determinant in the success of organ transplantation. It should be stated at the outset that no single set of rigid and absolute criteria has been defined; and perhaps more important, the different criteria proposed all basically share common themes: that there be extensive cerebral and brain stem dysfunction resulting from known structural or metabolic disease that would ostensibly preclude recovery, that such a state be irreversible, and that there be no physical evidence of depressant drug, poison, or hypothermia that could mimic such a state [12].

Several sets of criteria have been published as guidelines for the determination of cerebral death; Table 20-2 outlines one of the more commonly utilized schemes, proposed by the Ad Hoc Committee of Harvard Medical School [3]. The fundamental criterion is the presence of an unresponsive coma, with no evidence of response to external stimuli of any modality, such as an auditory or noxious cutaneous stimulus. The presence of apnea indicates severe dysfunction of the lower medullary respiratory centers and is tested by a period of trial following disconnection from assisted ventilation. One must be certain that, as often is the case in the neurosurgical patient who is being treated with hyperventilation, sufficient time is spent off assisted ventilation to allow hypercarbia to develop to adequately stimulate respiratory centers (usually several minutes). Profound hypoxia may be avoided in this circumstance by ventilating the patient with 100 percent oxygen prior to apnea testing. No spontaneous respirations after several minutes off of the ventilator is a strong indicator of medullary damage incompatible with life. One absolute criterion in the determination of brain death is the persistent absence of brain stem reflexes, such as pupillary, corneal, vestibulo-ocular, and tracheal reflexes. Pupillary reactivity may be rapidly assessed; nonreactive pupils (either dilated or midposition) in the absence of known ocular disease or mydriatic agent use are important inclusionary criteria. Vestibulo-ocular reflex testing should be performed; the integrity of this mechanism may also be determined by the instillation of cold water in the external ear canal to test caloric reflexes, as previously described. One potential pitfall is the presence of foreign body in the external canal, superimposed labyrinthine disease, or previous exposure to ototoxic agents (e.g., aminoglycosides), which could produce false-negative results. Absent spinal reflexes as required by the Harvard Criteria are *not* universally accepted in the diagnosis of irrecoverable cerebral death. Primitive spinal reflexes, as in the form of stretch reflex, may persist despite a low medullary transection in man. For this reason, opposing schools have deleted this requisite in the determination of brain death.

Laboratory tests should include thorough urine and blood toxicology screening, as reported cases of sedative or hypnotic overdoses have eradicated all clinical signs of brain stem function with subsequent full recovery.

Ancillary examinations in the form of EEG may be of service in the establishment of cerebral death. Electrical cerebral silence (ECS) is estab-

Table 20-2. Summary of Harvard criteria for brain death [3]

1. Unresponsive coma to all stimuli
2. Apnea
3. Absence of cephalic reflexes
4. Absence of spinal reflexes
5. Electrocerebral silence (ECS)
6. Persistance of the above conditions for at least 24 hours
7. Absence of drug intoxication or hypothermia

lished by the continuous monitoring of EEG for a period of 30 minutes with no evidence of electrical activity exceeding 2 microvolts (the expected background interference level). The Harvard Criteria necessitate 24 hours of ECS in addition to the aforementioned clinical requirements; however, evidence suggests that sustained ECS in the nature of 2 sequential studies at least 6 hours apart provides strong collaborative evidence for clinical brain death, and for this reason the extended period is probably superfluous. Cerebral blood flow studies, such as standard cerebral angiography or technetium-99m isotope angiography may be helpful in the rapid determination of absent intracranial blood flow in circumstances of massive intracranial hypertension. In addition to ECS, this offers objective and reproducible evidence of irreversible cerebral death and may be useful in situations in which expeditious determination of this condition could benefit potential organ donor recipients.

CONCLUSION

In summary, several factors repeatedly appear in the consideration of the assessment and management of patients with acute cranial trauma. First, a precise, recorded neurologic examination should be made as soon as feasible—essentially, as soon as cardiopulmonary systems have been stabilized. Once this has been done and appropriate diagnostic studies have been secured, repeated evaluation of these basic parameters provides a detailed analysis of any changes in trend that will determine appropriate modifications of therapy. Finally, one must adhere closely to the tenet of introducing some change of therapy, whether medical or surgical, in the face of an increasing neurologic deficit.

REFERENCES

1. Awad, I., Little, J. R., et al. Modification of focal cerebral ischemia by prostacyclin and indomethacin. *J. Neurosurg.* 58:714, 1983.
2. Awad, I., Carter, L., et al. Clinical vasospasm after SAH: Response to hypervolemic hemodilution and arterial hypertension. *Stroke* 18:365, 1987.
3. Beecher, H. K. A definition of irreversible coma: Report of the Ad Hoc Committee of the Harvard Medical School to examine the definition of brain death. J.A.M.A. 205.⌐5, 1968.
4. Boker, D., Solymosi, L., and Wassman, H. Immediate postangiographic intra-

carotid treatment of cerebral vasospasm after subarachnoid hemorrhage with nimodipine. *Neurochirugia* 28:118, 1985.

5. Eisenberg, H. M., Frankowski, R. F., Contant, C. F., et al. High dose barbiturate control of elevated intracranial pressure in patients with severe head injury. *J. Neurosurg.* 69:15, 1988.

6. Flamm, E. S., Demopuolos, H. B., and Seligman, M. L. Free radicals in cerebral ischemia. *Stroke* 9:445, 1978.

7. Giannotta, S. L., Weiss M. H., Apuzzo, M. L. J., and Martin, E. High dose glucocorticoids in the management of severe head injury. *Neurosurgery* 15:497, 1984.

8. Hoff, J. T. Editorial Comment. *J. Trauma* 23:794, 1983.

9. Hoff, J. T. Cerebral protection. *J. Neurosurg.* 65:579, 1986.

10. Koos, W. T., Perneczy, A., et al. Nimodipine treatment of ischemic neurological deficits due to cerebral vasospasm after subarachnoid hemorrhage: Clinical results of a multicenter study. *Neurochirugia* 28:114, 1985.

11. Mollaret, G. F., and Goulon, M. Le coma depasse. *Rev. Neurol.* 101:3, 1959.

12. Plum, F., and Posner, J. (eds.). *The Diagnosis of Stupor and Coma* (3rd ed.) (Contemporary Neurology Series, No. 19). Philadelphia: F. A. Davis, 1980.

13. Pollay, M. Formation of cerebral spinal fluid. *J. Neurosurg.* 42:665, 1975.

14. Simon, R. P., Swan J. H., et al. Blockade of N-methyl-D-aspartate receptors may protect against ischemic damage in the brain. *Science* 226:850, 1984.

15. Symon, L., Branston, N. M., et al. Autoregulation in acute focal ischemia. *Stroke* 7:547, 1976.

16. Teasedale, G., and Jennett, B. Assessment of coma and impaired consciousness: A practical scale. *Lancet* 2:81, 1974.

17. Ward J. D., et al. Failure of prophylactic barbiturate coma in the treatment of severe head injury. *J. Neurosurg.* 62:383, 1985.

18. White, B. C., Winegar, C. D., et al. Calcium blockers in cerebral resuscitation. *J. Trauma* 23:788, 1983.

Renal Dysfunction

W. Scott McDougal

The kidneys play a major role in maintaining the appropriate extracellular fluid (ECF) volume and its proper electrolyte composition. Unfortunately, malfunction of this organ system is not uncommon in the critically ill. It is clear that renal dysfunction in these patients leads to a marked increase in mortality and morbidity. Oftentimes, major malfunctions can only be treated by supportive measures; therefore, the emphasis must be placed on early recognition of impending dysfunction, so that preventive measures may be instituted before the dysfunction becomes inevitable. There is considerable evidence to indicate that abnormalities, if corrected early, will result in rapid return of renal function, whereas delays will result in a markedly increased incidence of immediately irreversible abnormal renal function. Patients who develop renal failure must then be supported by dialysis until the kidney slowly regains function. Initial signs of renal dysfunction often involve abnormalities of urine flow. Note, however, that acute renal failure not infrequently occurs despite normal urine flow. This is particularly true for traumatized patients who are resuscitated shortly after the injury. The sine qua non of renal dysfunction is an elevated plasma creatinine concentration.

Abnormalities of urine flow include too little (oliguria) or too much (polyuria). Oliguria is generally defined as a urine flow of less than 400 to 500 ml/day, or less than 20 ml/hr. Polyuria may be defined as urine excretion exceeding 2400 ml/day, or 100 ml/hr. If urine output falls outside 20 to 100 ml/hr, the cause of the abnormality must be identified and corrective measures taken.

In this chapter, the pathophysiology and clinical management of each major category of oliguria and polyuria are discussed. An understanding of the pathophysiologic events leading to oliguria and polyuria forms the basis for correct interpretation of clinical and laboratory observations and for proper therapy.

OLIGURIA

The differential diagnosis of acute oliguria falls into three general pathophysiologic categories: acute postrenal failure, acute prerenal failure, and acute renal failure (ARF). *Acute postrenal failure* is due to obstruction or extravasation of urinary outflow from the urethra, bladder, ureters, or renal pelvis. *Acute prerenal failure* is functional renal insufficiency due to a deficient plasma volume, a deficient cardiac output, or an excessive nitrogen load. *Acute renal failure* is failure of the kidney itself to function. These entities will be discussed in the following section. (*Note:* Hyperkalemia, the most urgent disorder that accompanies any form of oliguria, must be recognized and treated early.)

Acute Postrenal Failure

Acute postrenal failure is defined as obstruction or extravasation of urinary outflow from the urethra, bladder, ureters, or kidneys.

Obstruction of urine flow initially causes an increase in hydrostatic pressure in the urinary tract proximal to the obstructing lesion. Increased intratubular hydrostatic pressure is short-lived and a consequence of outflow obstruction opposed by the hydrostatic pressure within the glomerulus. Subsequently, preglomerular vasoconstriction mediated by angiotensin II results in a fall in glomerular hydrostatic pressure, resulting in a decrease in glomerular filtration rate (GFR). Glomerular filtration rate, however, does not cease, even though the obstruction to urine flow may be complete. The tubular fluid that is filtered is reabsorbed by the tubules and the peripelvic lymphatic and venous vessels. A small amount of filtrate may be extravasated around the renal fornices and absorbed in the perirenal tissue. On occasion, striking peripelvic extravasation of urine can be demonstrated by intravenous pyelography during acute urinary obstruction.

Morphologic and functional damage to the renal parenchyma may occur. The extent of the damage is correlated with the degree and duration of obstruction, the level of the urinary tract where the obstruction occurs (the more proximal the obstruction, the greater the destruction of renal parenchyma per unit period of time), the compliance of the collecting system, the nutritional status of the patient, the degree to which renal blood flow is compromised by preexisting disease, the presence and virulence of associated pyelonephritis, and the previous state of renal function [14].

A triphasic response occurs following obstruction of urinary outflow. Initially, there is an increase in renal blood flow that lasts for approximately 2 to 4 hours and may be mediated by the vasodilator prostaglandins. Subsequently, there is a fall in renal blood flow that is associated with an increase in intratubular pressure, thought to be a consequence of efferent arteriolar vasoconstriction. This vasoconstriction results in an increased hydrostatic pressure gradient within the glomerular capillary, thus resulting in transmittal of increased pressure to the tubular lumen. This phase lasts for approximately 24 to 48 hours. Finally, under the influence of angiotensin II there is afferent arteriolar vasoconstriction that reduces intratubular pressure due to a decreased hydrostatic pressure gradient found within the glomerulus. These forces result in a reduction in glomerular filtration rate, which persists. The persistent afferent arteriolar vasoconstriction and reduction in glomerular filtration rate is maintained throughout the period of obstruction by the renin-angiotensin (RA) system.

Renin is found in the secretory granules of the juxtaglomerular cells of the juxtaglomerular apparatus [38]. Renin is released in the inactive form and is acted upon by a serum protease that converts it to the active form. Renin acts upon renin substrate, which is a globulin produced by the liver, to produce the decapeptide angiotensin I, which has little vasoactive properties until converting enzyme splits off the octapeptide angiotensin II, the most powerful pressor agent known. Within the kidney, angiotensin II causes constriction of the afferent and possibly efferent arterioles [81], a reduction in glomerular capillary hydrostatic pressure, and a fall in GFR.

The release of renin can be stimulated by (1) low pulse pressure in the afferent arteriole [102], (2) sympathoadrenergic stimuli [81], (3) prostaglandins, (4) calcium, and (5) reabsorbable sodium at the macula densa in the early distal tubule [101]. The action of the prostaglandins and the concentration of sodium in the first portion of the distal tubule may be the stimulus for the release of renin involved in obstruction. Micropuncture experiments 15 hours after the release of bilateral ureteral obstruction showed the Na^+ concentration in the early distal tubule to be twice as high as control values, demonstrating impaired net Na^+ transport in the proximal tubule and loop of Henle. The increased Na^+ delivery to the macula densa triggers the local RA system to lower GFR.

The renin-angiotensin system may not be solely responsible for the reduction in renal blood flow, and hence GFR, in postrenal failure. Accumulating evidence indicates that the prostaglandins and thromboxane may also participate in the mediation of this response. A relative absence of the vasodilator prostaglandins may result in unopposed renal vasoconstriction, resulting in a reduction in renal blood flow and thereby a diminished GFR. Although initially there was some evidence indicating that the vasoconstrictor thromboxane A_2 may play some role, recent findings cast some doubt on any role for thromboxane A_2 in altering renal blood flow in obstructive uropathy [15].

Etiology

The main causes of obstructive uropathy may be grouped under congenital, neoplastic, infectious, traumatic, and other acquired abnormalities. Prostatic enlargement, urethral transection, and strictures are among the common urethral causes of acute postrenal failure. In the bladder, urinary retention may occur for a variety of neurogenic reasons. Ureteral stones or tumor, inadvertently placed pelvic sutures or other ureteral injuries, retroperitoneal fibrosis, or retroperitoneal, bladder, or pelvic malignancies may cause outflow obstruction of the ureters. The ureteropelvic junction may be obstructed by congenital bands, aberrant vessels, neoplasms, infection, strictures, or stones. The differential diagnostic possibilities of acute postrenal failure are many; the foregoing examples are not exhaustive. Most commonly, however, acute postrenal failure is due to problems in the urethra or bladder, since bilateral involvement of both ureters or both kidneys is unusual, provided the patient has two kidneys.

Clinical and Laboratory Observations

Frequently, the patient with acute postrenal obstruction or extravasation of urine flow is anuric, in contrast with other acute oliguric states. A past history of hesitancy, weak urinary stream, frequency, nocturia, suprapubic pain, or renal colic may precede the acute illness and provide an etiologic clue. A history of recent trauma to the pelvis, back, or abdomen raises suspicion of urinary extravasation.

Physical examination of the patient may reveal the presence of tender kidneys, abdominal or pelvic masses, trauma, a distended bladder, or urethral blood.

A urinalysis may show occult or gross hematuria, and serum blood urea nitrogen (BUN) and creatinine indicate the degree of renal impairment and serve as a baseline to measure therapeutic progress. Renal function studies demonstrate impaired renal concentrating ability and impaired renal Na^+ conservation similar to that seen with acute intrinsic renal failure (Table 21-1).

Management

Catheter drainage of the urinary bladder frequently offers immediate relief of acute postrenal obstruction while narrowing the diagnostic possibilities to the urinary bladder or urethra. (*Note:* One must be certain that the catheter is properly placed and draining freely.) If there is acute postrenal obstruction higher in the urinary tract, a computerized abdominal scan or ultrasonography may be helpful. Ultrasonography has come to play an important role in the diagnosis of acute renal failure. It can be performed at the patient's bedside and therefore is ideally suited for the critically ill patient. The sonographic length of the kidney is calculated and compared to the measured x-ray height of L-2. The normal ratio of normally functioning kidneys is 3.58 ± 0.38. Ratios greater than two standard deviations from normal are considered enlarged and therefore likely to be obstructed. The ultrasonogram also directly visualizes the hydronephrotic system in patients suffering from postrenal failure [89]. However, one must remember that intrarenal pelves do not dilate significantly during acute obstruction, and therefore the patient may have complete ureteral obstruction without evidence of calyceal dilatation on either computerized tomography (CT) or renal ultrasound. In trauma patients, who may undergo surgical exploration for urinary tract injury, it is essential to know that the patient's other kidney is present and functioning. Valuable diagnostic information may be obtained by careful catheterization of the ureters and retrograde pyelography. Ureteral catheters may be left in place for a short time to relieve ureteral obstruction until definitive treatment is undertaken; sterile technique is essential. (*Note:* Any modality that introduces infection may initiate pyelonephritis and increase renal parenchymal damage. Frequent urine cultures are advised to identify pathogens and their antibiotic sensitivities, so that specific antibiotic treatment may be started early.)

Table 21-1. Laboratory distinction between acute postrenal, acute prerenal, and acute renal failure

Laboratory determination	Optimal renal function	Acute postrenal failure	Acute prerenal failure	Acute renal failure (ARF)
Plasma urea-creatinine concentration ratio	10 : 1	~10 : 1	>10 : 1	~10 : 1
Urine				
Sodium concentration (mEq/L)	15–40	>40	<20	>30
Potassium concentration (mEq/L)	15–40	Variable	Variable	Variable
Osmolality (mOsm/kg H_2O)	400–600	<400	>400	<400
Specific gravity	~1.010	~1.010	>1.020	~1.010
Volume (ml/day)	500–2400	<500	<500	Variable
Urine sediment	0–1 RBC 0–1 WBC Occasional hyaline cast No cellular casts	Look for RBCs, WBCs, malignant cells, crystals	Occasional hyaline cast	Tubular epithelial cells and casts, RBCs, free hemoglobin or myoglobin
Urine-plasma concentration ratios				
Urea	20 : 1	<8 : 1	>10 : 1	<4 : 1
Osmolality*	1.5 : 1–2 : 1	<1 : 1	>1.5 : 1	<1.1 : 1

RBC = red blood cells; WBC = white blood cells.

*The single most reliable observation that confirms the diagnosis of oliguric ARF is a urine-plasma osmotic concentration ratio <1.1

Two types of ureteral catheters may be placed. An external catheter may be placed to the renal pelvis; it is brought out through the urethra and fixed to a Foley catheter. This system allows irrigation of the catheter with ease and is ideal for acute management of obstruction due to bleeding disorders. The second type of ureteral catheter utilized is the double-J stent. This is an internal catheter that is placed from renal pelvis to bladder and is ideally suited for lesions that compress the ureter, thus causing obstruction, but do not involve the interior of the collecting system. The advantage of the double-J system is that it is internal and it does not require a Foley catheter to keep it in place, thus reducing the chances of infection to the upper urinary tract. Its disadvantage is that it does not allow for easy access to the renal pelvis or for irrigating the renal pelvis.

Definitive therapy of postrenal obstruction is directed to the site of obstruction. Immediate surgical procedures for decompression include suprapubic cystostomy, cutaneous ureterostomy, and nephrostomy. Urinary extravasation is relatively harmless for the first 24 to 36 hours. However, evidence of a preexisting urinary tract infection, especially with coliform or *Proteus* organisms, is cause for urgent concern; extravasation under these circumstances requires prompt drainage [71]. The early use of broad-spectrum prophylactic antibiotics in urinary extravasation is advisable, to avoid the development of infection in undrained hematomas.

Early relief of postrenal obstruction will avert permanent renal damage, provided infection has been avoided. A dramatic postobstructive diuresis may follow the release of postrenal obstruction within 2 to 24 hours. Impaired renal Na^+ transport throughout the nephron accounts for the massive loss of salt and water despite a low GFR. Preexisting volume overload and elevated BUN may also contribute to the diuresis. Management of postobstructive diuresis requires precise replacement of fluid and electrolyte losses, simultaneously avoiding sustained overhydration on the one hand and hypovolemia on the other.

Finally, a percutaneous nephrostomy can be placed under ultrasonographic guidance directly into the renal collecting system from the skin. This method of urinary diversion is ideal in the patient in whom cystoscopy is not possible or in whom the obstruction of the ureter cannot be negotiated by a ureteral catheter.

Acute Prerenal Failure

The most common cause of oliguria in critically ill patients is acute prerenal failure. Prerenal failure is defined as functional renal insufficiency [77] due to a deficient plasma volume, a deficient cardiac output, or an excessive nitrogen load. In acute prerenal failure the kidney itself is normal; it functions to excrete nitrogenous waste products in an economically small volume of urinary water.

Physiology of Extracellular Fluid Volume Regulation

It is especially important to understand the physiology of ECF volume regulation, in order to distinguish clinical and laboratory findings of functional renal insufficiency from failure of the kidney itself to function (ARF).

The physiology of ECF volume regulation is conveniently divided into systemic mechanisms and renal mechanisms. These mechanisms will be discussed briefly and correlated with clinical events and appropriate patient management.

SYSTEMIC MECHANISMS. Extracellular fluid volume regulation, reviewed comprehensively by Gauer et al. [33] and Share and Claybaugh [95], is determined by autoregulation, baroreceptors, volume receptors, and osmotic receptors.

Autoregulation. A modest fall in blood pressure does not directly lower renal blood flow (RBF) or GFR. Within a range of 30 mm Hg above or below normal systolic blood pressure, the renal vascular resistance changes directly with blood pressure, so that RBF and GFR are held nearly constant. This phenomenon is called autoregulation. The mechanism by which autoregulation of RBF is achieved is not clear, but it may be due to stretch receptors in the afferent arteriole that reflexly contract with a distending pressure and reflexly relax with a falling pressure [87]. An excessive fall in systemic blood pressure to 60 mm Hg or less cannot be compensated by renal autoregulation, and a fall in RBF, GFR, and urine output occurs. This is a coarse regulatory mechanism seen in shock.

Baroreceptors. Nevertheless, renal function can be altered by subtle changes in systemic blood pressure through neurohumoral pathways. A slight fall in arterial blood pressure will decrease vagal afferent impulses from the aortic arch and carotid sinus baroreceptors, to allow hypothalamic release of antidiuretic hormone (ADH), increased sympathoadrenergic activity, and increased renin-angiotensin-aldosterone (RAA) activity through sympathetic efferent nerve pathways. These mechanisms act on the kidney to conserve salt and water, thus restoring circulating plasma volume.

Volume receptors. Renal function can also be altered by a 10 percent loss of blood volume; such a loss is insufficient to alter systemic blood pressure. Volume receptors of the low-pressure system in both atria sense a 3-cm water pressure change. A fall in atrial pressure reduces vagal afferent impulses from the subendocardial stretch receptors, to allow hypothalamic centers to release ADH from the posterior pituitary. An excellent review of nonosmolar factors affecting renal water excretion has been published by Schrier and Berl [93].

Osmotic receptors. A loss of water in excess of salt causes plasma osmolality to increase. In 1946, Verney [105] first demonstrated the existence of intracranial receptors sensitive to plasma osmotic pressure in unanesthetized dogs undergoing a water diuresis. An injection of hypertonic sodium chloride or dextrose solution into an externalized carotid artery led to prompt interruption of water diuresis. Hypophysectomy blocked, and injections of ADH mimicked, the response to the hypertonic injections. Thus, intracranial osmotic receptors affect the diuresis through modulation of ADH and its release.

It is apparent that both osmolar and nonosmolar factors regulate ADH release. Arndt [3] studied the competition between osmotic and volume stimuli near threshold for control of ADH secretion. A 6 percent blood volume loss abolished a diuresis that followed an intracarotid injection of distilled water. When blood was retransfused, the water diuresis resumed. Thus, ECF volume stimuli supersede osmotic stimuli in modulating ADH release.

RENAL MECHANISMS. Renal salt and water excretion are modified by four general mechanisms: changes in GFR, RAA activity, atrial natriuretic factor, and ADH secretion.

Glomerular filtration rate. A fall in GFR reduces renal salt and water losses. It occurs in response to systemic hypotension outside the range where autoregulation of RBF and GFR can compensate. Glomerular filtration rate also falls in response to a net decrease in opposing hydrostatic and osmotic forces across the glomerular capillary wall, as predicted by Starling's hypothesis. Afferent arteriolar vasoconstriction in response to sympathoadrenergic stimuli or to angiotensin II also reduces GFR.

Renin-angiotensin-aldosterone system. The RAA system, previously described, plays a major role in both normal and pathophysiologic renal function. It is necessary to point out here that angiotensin II is a potent stimulus for aldosterone secretion by the adrenal cortex. Aldosterone restores ECF volume by increasing Na^+ resorption in the distal nephron. Other factors that also stimulate aldosterone secretion include elevated plasma K^+ concentration, adrenocorticotropic hormone (ACTH), and hemodynamic stimuli [54]. In addition to this mechanism, angiotensin causes efferent arteriole vasoconstriction, which attempts to maintain intraglomerular hydrostatic pressure and filtration rate in the face of falling afferent arteriolar pressures.

Atrial natriuretic factor. Atrial natriuretic factor is a 28-amino-acid polypeptide secreted by the atrium under the influence of increased atrial pressure. An atrial natriuretic factor results in a Na^+ and water diuresis and is a potent vasodilator. Its function becomes important in situations of volume overload and serves to return Na^+ and water balance to normal under these conditions.

Antidiuretic hormone. ADH permits the kidney to retain water by increasing the water permeability of the collecting-duct epithelium. The osmotic pressure driving force that causes the resorption of water from the collecting-duct lumen into the medullary tissue is established by active Na^+ or Cl^- transport in the thick ascending limb of the loop of Henle. Medullary hypertonicity is maintained by the countercurrent arrangement of the loops of Henle, vasa recta, and collecting ducts within the renal medulla.

The major solutes contributing to medullary hypertonicity are Na^+, Cl^-, and urea. The presence of concentrated urea in the renal medulla serves two related functions: (1) urea contributes to the osmotic pressure driving force to remove water from the collecting duct lumen, and (2) equilibration of urea concentration across the collecting-duct epithelium allows the generation of high urea urinary concentrations. The renal medulla, therefore, achieves the excretion of nitrogenous waste products in an economically small volume of water.

PLASMA UREA-CREATININE CONCENTRATION RATIO. Plasma urea concentration is elevated during extreme oliguria. Increased urea production due to deamination of protein for gluconeogenesis to satisfy hypermetabolic demands in a severely ill patient is partially responsible for the elevated plasma urea concentration. Elevated plasma urea concentration also occurs because of decreased glomerular filtration and increased back-diffusion of urea in prerenal failure.

In a physiologically normal kidney, a portion of filtered urea, which circulates within the medulla, diffuses back into the general circulation from the vasa recta and distal tubules [73], contributing to the elevated plasma urea concentration. The plasma urea-creatinine concentration ratio usually exceeds 10 : 1 in acute prerenal failure. In acute intrinsic renal failure, the medullary concentrating mechanism does not function, and the fraction of filtered water excreted is high. Since the renal handling of urea is dependent on the tubular water resorption, the fraction of filtered urea excreted should be high in ARF; less back-diffusion of filtered urea is expected. The plasma urea-creatinine concentration ratio is about 10 : 1 in ARF, since a failure of filtration alone is largely responsible for the failure of excretion of these two substances.

Etiology
The patient's history may reveal the cause of plasma volume deficiency. Deficits in plasma volume are commonly due to hemorrhage; acute gastrointestinal losses; excessive insensible losses; inadequate fluid intake; and large third-space losses, such as in pancreatitis, burns, or bowel obstruction.

Clinical and Laboratory Observations
Physical examination of a patient with acute prerenal failure may reveal signs of hypovolemia, including a rapid pulse, decreased skin turgor, and dry mucous membranes. A measure of central venous pressure (CVP), provided there is no myocardial disease, is low—usually 1 to 2 cm H_2O. Examination of the urine in functional renal insufficiency reveals the kidney is performing in a physiologically normal manner (see Table 21-1): the urine is concentrated with (1) a specific gravity above 1.020, (2) a urine osmolality of 400 to 1200 mOsm/kg H_2O, and (3) a urine-plasma (U/P) osmotic concentration ratio of at least 1.5. The kidney excretes its nitrogenous waste product urea in high concentrations, often exceeding 1000 mg/100 ml [48]; the U/P urea concentration ratio exceeds 10 [83]. Renal Na^+ conservation is efficient; the urine Na^+ concentration is less than 20 mEq/liter, and the urine Na^+ loss is negligible. Plasma urea and creatinine concentrations are elevated due to hemoconcentration and a diminished GFR, but the ratio of plasma urea to creatinine concentrations is greater than 10 : 1 in prerenal azotemia, because of back-diffusion of urea from

the vasa recta and distal tubules into the general circulation without a proportionate amount of reabsorption of creatinine.

Management
When the present illness and physical findings are consistent with plasma volume depletion, rapid expansion of plasma volume may confirm the diagnosis of prerenal failure while laboratory studies are pending. The type of intravenous fluid given depends on the type of fluid loss incurred. Isotonic losses should be replaced initially with normal saline or Ringer's lactate. Hypertonic dehydration is corrected with 0.45% saline. Whole-blood losses are initially replaced with crystalloid and/or volume expanders until blood is available. In the first hour or two, 500 to 1000 ml or more of fluids is infused rapidly (10–15 ml/kg/hr), to reexpand plasma volume and reestablish urine flow. Thereafter, full correction of fluid and electrolyte aberrations is best carried out at a more cautious rate.

A dilemma in managing oliguric postoperative patients often arises in deciding whether or not to give additional fluids. After extensive surgery or trauma, patients in ideal fluid balance gain 1 to 2 kg because of third-space sequestration of fluid and because of normal posttraumatic renal salt and water retention. CVP is not an entirely reliable guide in fluid balance. Usually, the need to give more fluids can be determined by clinical evaluation of the patient. Peripheral or presacral edema is a good sign that the circulating plasma volume compartment is saturated. Pulmonary auscultation and serial chest x-ray studies may reveal early signs of left heart failure that warn against further fluid administration. If uncertainty exists, a Swan-Ganz catheter should be inserted to measure pulmonary wedge pressure, which in turn reflects left atrial pressure. If the pulmonary wedge pressure is less than 15 mm Hg, further fluid may be infused safely.

Patients with heart disease may be oliguric from a low cardiac output. In these patients, the physical findings of congestive heart failure (CHF) and an elevated CVP (>15 cm H_2O) are usually detectable. Improved cardiac output is first obtained by fluid restriction, diuretics, oxygen, and positive-pressure breathing. These patients are best monitored with a Swan-Ganz catheter, allowing for measurement of pulmonary wedge pressure, pulmonary artery pressure, and cardiac output. If CHF persists after these measures, ionotrophic drugs may be given, and the blood-drug concentrations should be monitored by laboratory analysis. The acute use of these drugs in CHF caused by overhydration is unnecessary, and toxic effects of the drugs may be harmful.

When correction of plasma volume deficits and cardiac output fails to restore normal urinary flow and there is no evidence of an excessive exogenous nitrogen load, the ominous diagnosis of acute renal failure must be suspected.

Acute Renal Failure
A serious cause of oliguria is acute renal failure (ARF), or intrinsic failure of the kidney itself to function. However, with the advent of rapid resuscitation and early evacuation of traumatized patients, posttraumatic acute

Table 21-2. Etiology of acute intrinsic renal failure

Occlusion of renal arteries or renal veins

Arteriolar damage
  Malignant hypertension
  Polyarteritis
  Hypersensitivity angiitis

Disseminated intravascular coagulation (DIC)

Glomerulonephritis
  Lupus erythematosus
  Poststreptococcal glomerulonephritis
  Other

Parenchymal damage
  Acute interstitial nephritis
  Acute pyelonephritis
  Papillary necrosis
    Diabetes mellitus
    Nephrosclerosis
    Sickle-cell anemia
    Certain analgesics
  Cortical necrosis
  End-stage renal disease

Hepatorenal syndrome

Vasomotor nephropathy
  Shock
  Sepsis
  Transfusion reactions
  Crush injury
  Poisons
  Drugs (e.g., gentamicin, kanamycin, cephaloridine, methicillin,
    methoxyflurane)
  Idiopathic

renal failure is more often nonoliguric than oliguric. A list of causes of ARF is presented in Table 21-2.

The most common form of ARF encountered in the critically ill is the type that follows shock, sepsis, transfusion reactions, and so on. The term *vasomotor nephropathy* was first used for this syndrome in the early part of the century. Changing concepts of the pathophysiology of this entity are reflected in the changing nomenclature: lower nephron nephrosis, crush kidney, and acute tubular necrosis [11]. Recent studies have shown the primary abnormality to be a failure of glomerular filtration; the term *vasomotor nephropathy* has been reintroduced and has the advantage of conveying specific meaning [77]. Nevertheless, in this discussion, we will conform with current usage and retain the more general term *ARF* to refer to the kind of renal failure that follows shock, sepsis, and so on.

The usual course of ARF is one of transient oliguria lasting 8 to 16 days, with a mean duration of 11 days. The oliguric phase is followed by polyuria and a gradual return to near-normal renal function.

The mortality associated with ARF is high. In Vietnam, the U.S. Army reported a 63 to 69 percent mortality; sepsis was the single complication most responsible for death. Associated upper gastrointestinal bleeding carries an 80 percent mortality; jaundice carries 90 percent mortality [59, 60]. The range of published mortality rates for ARF in civilian surgical patients is 35 to 71 percent [16].

Pathophysiology

Four mechanisms have been proposed to account for the basic physiology of ARF: (1) renal vasoconstriction, (2) tubular obstruction, (3) back-leakage of filtrate, and (4) decreased ultrafiltration coefficient [65]. Renal vasoconstriction results in a reduction in total renal blood flow, with a shift of blood away from the cortex toward the medulla. Total renal blood flow is reduced; however, the blood flow to the cortex is reduced out of proportion to that of the medulla. Since 80 percent of the functional glomeruli are in the cortex, a shift away from these glomeruli results in a significant reduction in GFR [43]. Much circumstantial evidence implicates the RA system in the initiating phase of ARF, but the specific events that induce and prolong the filtration failure are not yet understood. ARF can be almost totally prevented in experimental animals by chronic saline loading [99], by pretreatment with mannitol and saline [107], or by the converting enzyme blocker captopril. The mechanism involved may be the depletion of renin stores prior to the renal insult and the prevention of the activity of renin-angiotensin on the renal vasculature. Tubular obstruction may also occur as a result of either swelling of tubular epithelial cells due to ischemia or the direct affect of tubular toxins such as heavy metals, intravenous contrast agents, myoglobin, glycols, halogens, and nephrotoxic drugs. As the tubules swell, they occlude the tubular lumen, which results in a blockage of the flow of filtrate. Tubules may also have increased permeability in some situations due to an ischemic event. The increased tubule permeability results in the back-leakage of filtrate from the tubule lumen into the interstitium. Thus, even though filtrate may arrive in Bowman's space, it leaks out of the tubule, reducing renal clearance.

The fourth mechanism that may play a role in the pathogenesis of acute intrarenal failure is decreased ultrafiltration coefficient. This occurs as the glomerular basement membrane becomes less permeable due to either protein or immunoglobins deposited upon it and/or a change in the charge of the membrane. The former mechanism impedes filtration by physically reducing its permeability, whereas the latter electrostatically decreases its permeability. Currently, tubular permeability, intratubular obstruction, decreased ultrafiltration coefficient, and redistribution of renal blood flow are all thought to contribute to some degree. The magnitude of the effect of each is dependent upon the etiology of the inciting cause [98].

Ischemic Acute Renal Failure

Alterations in renal perfusion brought about during transplantation or during procedures that result in acute occlusion of renal blood flow—such as abdominal aortic aneurysmectomy, renal artery surgery, and shock—all result in a very specific type of ARF that has been the subject of intense investigative effort recently. Since this type of renal failure is not uncommon to the critical care setting, it is important to understand in some detail the pathophysiology of the injury, so that its treatment and prevention can better be understood.

CELL BIOLOGY OF ISCHEMIC RENAL INJURY. The initiating event that leads to cell destruction is an increase in cell membrane permeability with a reduction in membrane electrical potential [96]. This results in an influx of calcium into the cell. Increased levels of intracellular calcium are thought to cause cell injury and contribute to cellular death [31]. Calcium enters injured cells through voltage- or receptor-dependent channels in exchange for the intracellular cations Na^+ and H^+ and nonspecifically through increased membrane permeability [6, 13, 32, 42]. With acute ischemic injury, an increase in intracellular calcium can be noted as early as 10 minutes following the event [76]. Once calcium begins entering the cell, it rapidly accumulates over a very short period of time. Normally, calcium is located within one of three pools within the cell. Ten to 20 percent is bound to the plasma membrane, approximately 60 to 70 percent is sequestered in intracellular organelles, and 10 to 20 percent is free within the cytosol [44]. It is the free calcium that is biologically active. Ischemia may also result in redistribution of intracellular calcium pools, with an increase in the cytosol of the free (biologically active) form. The increased calcium manifests its toxic effects on the cell by altering mitochondrial respiratory function, thereby reducing the rate of adenosine triphosphate (ATP) generation, and by stimulating calcium-dependent ATPase, which further depletes an already energy-deficient cell of high-energy phosphate stores. The impaired energy production and energy depletion reduce the ability of the active transport process to extrude the increased amounts of calcium from within the cell. The increased membrane permeability also makes it difficult to effectively extrude calcium from the cell. The increased permeability is due, at least in part, to the action of phospholipases on the membrane. Calcium activates the phospholipases [20], in addition to altering the membrane enzymes [22]. Calmodulin, which is a calcium regulatory protein present in most cells, is also important in controlling phospholipase activity [26] and may be altered during ischemia. Calcium increases cytosolic free fatty acids, which act as detergents and interfere with intracellular processes. It also alters cytoskeletal organelles with destruction of actin [110] and microtubular filaments [85].

Ischemia also results in the generation of free radicals. Free radicals and calcium work in concert to destroy lipids and thereby destroy the membrane. Free radicals may activate or inhibit enzymes, and they also alter cell function by reacting with intracellular molecules [78]. Free radicals are generated under conditions of normal respiration by the oxidation of NADPH to NADP. Two oxygen free radicals plus a hydrogen ion yields hydrogen peroxide. Hydrogen peroxide plus an oxygen free radical in the presence of iron yields a hydroxy free radical [17]. The free radicals produced under circumstances of normal respiration may damage the cell;

however, their concentration is kept at a minimum by the naturally occurring free-radical scavenger glutathione and by the enzyme glutathione peroxidase. In the presence of a limited oxygen supply, however, the mitochondria are required to increase their workload, and the production of free radicals markedly increases. Free radicals induce lipid peroxidation and in the presence of calcium, cause mitochondrial dysfunction [4, 78]. Another mechanism of free-radical generation occurs when high-energy phosphates (ATP) are degraded to adenosine monophosphates and subsequently to hypoxanthine. In the presence of ischemia, regeneration of ATP is limited and hypoxanthine accumulates. During reperfusion or when oxygen is supplied, hypoxanthine is converted to xanthine by xanthine oxidase, which results in the generation of an oxygen free radical. Thus, restoration of blood flow may be injurious, in that it increases the production of free radicals just as the limitation of blood flow in ischemia results in an increased production of free radicals—the latter through the mitochondrial respiratory mechanism and the former through degradation of high-energy compounds.

The cellular events that follow ischemic injury may be summarized as follows. Ischemia results in an influx of calcium into the cell, with activation of phospholipases that degrade the lipid bilayer of the cell membrane and further increase its permeability. Continued action of the phospholipases results in membrane disruption. Also, toxic lipid by-products from membrane degradation potentiate further membrane destruction. As intracellular calcium increases and defuses into the mitochondria, there is a disruption of mitochondrial respiration, a lack of energy production, and increased free-radical production—all of which combine to further destroy the membrane. Calcium, in conjunction with free radicals, injures mitochondria and reduces cellular respiration [4, 92]. Not only may the membrane be destroyed by these mechanisms during the ischemic event, but its destruction may also be enhanced when the ischemia is corrected and reperfusion established. This occurs as ATP is reduced to adenosine monophosphate, which then degrades to hypoxanthine during the ischemic episode. Hypoxanthine accumulates when the cell is reoxygenated and xanthine oxidase is stimulated to convert hypoxanthine to xanthine. This produces an oxygen free radical that attacks the membrane and destroys its structure.

HORMONAL ALTERATIONS DURING RENAL ISCHEMIA. The renin-angiotensin system is activated during renal ischemia and plays a significant role in altering both blood flow and the cellular response. This response has already been described (see preceding section). The eicosanoids, which are products of arachidonic acid metabolism, are significantly involved in renal ischemia. There are three main groups of products of arachidonic acid metabolism. When arachidonic acid is acted upon by the enzyme cyclooxygenase, endoperoxides are produced. Most tissues are capable of producing the endoperoxides; however, the enzymes that further facilitate the production of specific prostaglandins are unique to particular tissues. Within the kidney, the endoperoxides may be converted to prostacyclin

(PGI$_2$), PGE$_2$, PGF$_{2\alpha}$, or thromboxane A$_2$. PGI$_2$ and PGE$_2$ are vasodilators, whereas PGF$_{2\alpha}$ and thromboxane A$_2$ are vasoconstrictors. The renal medulla is the most active site of prostaglandin synthesis. The prostaglandins regulate renal blood flow and GFR, which they tend to maintain in the presence of vasoconstriction. They inhibit the action of ADH, decrease thick ascending-limb transport of Na$^+$ and Cl$^-$, interfere with urea reabsorption in the tubular epithelium, and also increase medullary blood flow. The prostaglandins most involved in these aspects of concentration and dilution are PGE$_2$ and PGF$_{2\alpha}$. They may also play a role in erythropoietin production [90].

The second group of products of arachidonic acid metabolism are the leukotrienes. These substances are formed when the enzyme lipoxygenase acts upon arachidonic acid to produce 5-HPETE. From this substance the leukotrienes are formed. The leukotrienes, although not indigenous to the kidney, are prominent within polymorphonuclear leukocytes. In many types of renal injury, polymorphonuclear leukocytes infiltrate into the interstitium. The leukotrienes are vasoconstrictors and increase membrane permeability. They are particularly active as chemotactic factors and when introduced into the kidney, reduce GFR [5, 88].

The third group of products of the eicosanoids are the hydroxy fatty acids, which are produced as a result of the enzyme lipoxygenase. These substances inhibit sodium transport [90].

These two hormonal systems, renin-angiotensin and the eicosanoids, work in concert—one affecting the other. Thus, when the juxtaglomerular cells produce renin, which subsequently generates angiotensin II, further output of renin is inhibited by the direct action of angiotensin II upon the juxtaglomerular cells. Angiotensin II results in vasoconstriction, and this, in addition to its direct action, activates phospholipase. Phospholipase activation results in an increased production of arachidonic acid, which results in an increase in the endoperoxides if cyclo-oxygenase is present. This results in an increased production of prostacyclin and PGE$_2$, which directly stimulate the juxtaglomerular cells to increase renin production. Thus, these hormones work in concert—one stimulating the other, and one performing the opposite action of the other. Under normal physiologic conditions, fine regulation of intrarenal blood flow and GFR is maintained by the appropriate production of these two hormonal products [90]. During ischemia, however, this balance is disrupted and their vasoconstrictive properties can be unopposed, thereby making the ischemia worse and prolonging its effect.

Clinical and Laboratory Observations

The diagnosis of ARF is suspected after other causes of oliguria have been eliminated or a rising creatinine is observed, i.e., urinary outflow obstruction, urinary extravasation, actions of drugs on inhibiting creatinine secretion, and functional renal insufficiency. Plasma volume, CVP, left atrial pressure, and cardiac output are restored to normal with no improvement in renal function in ARF.

Acute renal failure is manifested by oliguria or normal urine output, isosthenuria, and progressive uremia. Laboratory findings are presented in Table 21-1; the laboratory observations reflect severely abnormal renal function. The urine is dilute; the specific gravity is between 1.008 and 1.014, but the specific gravity may be misleadingly high due to the admixture of protein or sugar in the urine. The U/P osmotic concentration ratio is a more reliable index of renal concentrating ability; in ARF, it is less than 1.1. The failure to concentrate the urine is reflected by a low U/P urea concentration ratio. Renal handling of Na^+ is impaired; the urinary Na^+ concentration exceeds 30 to 40 mEq/liter. The urine sediment in ARF often contains tubular cells and casts.

Plasma creatinine concentration in ARF increases by 2 to 3 mg/d/day, and the BUN concentration increases by 25 to 35 mg/d/day. In some severe catabolic states the BUN may rise by 60 to 90 mg/d/day [100]. The ratio of plasma urea to plasma creatinine concentrations is equal to or less than 10 : 1.

Management

The treatment of ARF is not yet optimal, since there has been no major reduction in the 35 to 71 percent mortality rate in surgical patients. Although dialysis has reduced death from overhydration and hyperkalemia, sepsis and gastrointestinal hemorrhage remain difficult to control.

PREVENTION. Several factors are known to predispose patients to the development of ARF. These factors include (1) advanced age, (2) preexisting renal dysfunction, (3) recent exposure to aminoglycosides or other nephrotoxic agents, (4) volume depletion, (5) myoglobinuria, (6) hepatic insufficiency, and (7) unstable diabetic ketoacidosis [91]. It is critically important for all patients undergoing surgical procedures to be well hydrated preoperatively. In elective surgical procedures in which large third-space losses or hemorrhage are anticipated, overnight preoperative hydration is beneficial.

When the risk of inducing ARF is high under circumstances of renal artery cross-clamping or aneurysm repair, several manipulations are helpful in preserving renal function. Volume expansion prior to surgery with salt-containing solutions at least 12 hours prior to the procedure results in some depletion of renin reserves and thereby blunts the response of renin on the kidney. If the myocardial status can tolerate it, it is preferable several weeks prior to the procedure to place the patient on a high Na^+ diet, in an attempt to deplete the intrarenal renin reserves. In those patients who are hypertensive and who have no renal artery lesion, captopril may be a good choice for a preoperative antihypertensive. Captopril prevents the effects of renin on the kidney through its effect in blocking converting enzyme. It may also be an effective choice in some patients in whom prolonged renal ischemia is anticipated. Similarly, the use of allopurinol preoperatively, in an attempt to prevent the generation of free radicals during reperfusion by preventing the conversion of hypoxanthine to xanthine, may be considered when renal ischemia is anticipated to be over 70 minutes. Mannitol should also be given immediately before cross-clamping of the renal vessel. Barry et al. [7] reported a controlled study of 14 patients undergoing aneurys-mectomy of the abdominal aorta, in which mannitol reduced the expected fall in renal blood flow, GFR, and urine flow when given during the period of aortic clamping (20% mannitol given intravenously at 5.5 ml/min just before and during aortic clamping).

Intraoperatively, in those patients in whom the cross-clamp time will be less than 30 minutes, hypothermia is not required. In patients in whom the cross-clamp time exceeds 30 minutes, consideration should be given to cooling the kidney to a core temperature less than 20°C. Immediately fol-lowing renal ischemia or prior to its occurrence, there may be a place for the free-radical scavenger superoxide dismutase. Although currently not approved for general use, it is an effective means for preventing the dele-terious effects of free radicals and may be helpful in preventing the seque-lae of ischemic ARF.

In patients in whom ARF is discovered following the initiating event, early recognition and prompt treatment will lessen morbidity. Certain pa-tients with prerenal failure may remain oliguric despite correction of plasma volume deficits [61]. These patients are oliguric usually less than 50 hours; they have a U/P osmotic concentration ratio of 1.1 to 1.8, and they respond to intravenous mannitol (100 ml of a 20% solution infused over 10–20 minutes every 2–3 hours, to a maximum dose of 60 gm). In these circumstances, the action of mannitol is not clear. Either it may avert the development of ARF, or it may hasten the onset of diuresis following volume expansion. Mannitol has a vasodilatory effect on the renal vascu-lature; it serves as a free-radical scavenger; it also is an osmotic diuretic that may flush nephrons of cell debris and casts, although this effect is dubiously beneficial. Mannitol must be used with caution, to avoid precip-itation of congestive heart failure due to a shift of fluid into the circulating plasma volume compartment. Once the diagnosis of ARF is established by stringent laboratory criteria, mannitol is of no further value.

Low-dose dopamine (1 mg/kg/min) has been used in an attempt to pre-vent deterioration of renal function in ARF [36]. Dopamine has been shown to maintain renal blood flow, GFR, and urine output in the pro-drome of ARF. In established ARF, however, it has only been shown to improve urine flow; it does not alter the course of the disease. In some anecdotal case reports, the addition of furosemide may have altered the course of ARF. Furosemide has a theoretical advantage, in that it may re-duce transport work. However, it must be noted that it also potentiates nephrotoxic antibiotics, particularly the aminoglycosides [57, 58]. In estab-lished ARF, the roles of dopamine and furosemide appear to be in con-verting the oliguric renal failure patient to the nonoliguric state, so that fluid management and the administration of hyperalimentation solutions may be utilized during this period of critical illness. When these latter ef-fects of the drugs are separated from their direct effect on the kidney itself, it is unlikely that they have any effect in ameliorating ARF [40, 80]. It is our clinical impression, however, in dealing with a large group of septic burn patients, that in the prodrome of ARF, when renal cortical blood flow is shifting toward the medulla and urinary Na^+ concentration is inappropriately low in the volume-expanded patient, dopamine infusion may obviate or delay the onset of ARF until the sepsis can be corrected. This is a personal observation and is not founded in any prospective study.

Calcium-channel blockers such as verapamil impede calcium entry into the cell by interfering with the voltage-dependent calcium-channel transport mechanism. Verapamil also causes a profound vasodilation [45, 62] and solute excretion when infused into the renal artery [63, 106]. The vasodilatation is probably due to the ability of verapamil to block calcium entry into vascular smooth muscle during ischemia, as increased sarcoplasmic calcium has been shown to result in muscle spasm [104].

Whether or not calcium-channel blockers are beneficial in renal ischemia beyond their diuretic and vasodilatory effect is controversial. The data are conflicting, partially due to the fact that the effect of calcium-channel blockers has been studied in two different models of renal ischemia: the norepinephrine model and renal artery cross-clamp model. In the norepinephrine model, verapamil attenuates the fall in inulin clearance when administered before and after the insult in some studies [18] and only when administered before the insult in other studies [70]. In the renal artery cross-clamp model, some have reported an effect only if given prior to the insult [37], whereas others have noted no effect whatsoever [70]. These latter results were obtained in the isolated renal perfused model, in which changes in renal blood flow could be controlled [70].

Proponents of verapamil's effectiveness point out that renal blood flow can be maintained in the norepinephrine model of renal ischemia by secretin and acetylcholine without a protective effect, whereas verapamil gives protection, indicating that it does something in addition to maintaining renal blood flow. Secretin and acetylcholine, however, unlike verapamil, do not result in a solute diuresis. It may be the combination of increased renal blood flow and diuresis that confers the beneficial effect of calcium-channel blockers. Support for this theory comes from the fact that mannitol, which also improves renal blood flow and results in a solute diuresis, is as effective as verapamil in preserving renal function following renal ischemia [70]. Finally, Malis et al. have shown no protective effect histologically with verapamil in renal tubular cell brush borders [70]. In the norepinephrine model, however, some investigators have found that when verapamil is given prior to the insult, renal cortical mitochondrial respiration is maintained at normal levels and there is no intracellular accumulation of calcium when compared to controls. In summary, the protective effect of calcium-channel blockers in the renal artery cross-clamp model at present appears to be due to their ability to inhibit smooth-muscle vascular spasm and to establish a diuresis. The question of whether they play a role at the renal tubular level requires further investigation.

The generation of excess free radicals may occur during ARF if mitochondrial respiration is stimulated in the presence of decreased oxygen supply. In addition, reperfusion through the mechanism of conversion of hypoxanthine to xanthine may also produce free radicals. Allopurinol, which blocks hypoxanthine oxidation, has been shown to improve renal blood flow following renal ischemia [41]. It results in a decrease in peripheral resistance, which protects the kidney against renal failure. In a group of experiments in which plasma creatinine was followed over a period of days following renal ischemia, those animals who received allopurinol prior to the insult had a significant lesser rise in serum creatinine and a more rapid return to normal renal function than did those animals who did not receive the drug [78]. Although glutathione is a naturally occurring free-radical scavenger and glutathione peroxidase is effective in free-radical scavenging from induced lipid peroxidation, the quantities of these substances produced naturally are not sufficient to protect the patient in the face of excessive free-radical production. Several drugs have been introduced that are particularly effective as free-radical scavengers. Superoxide dismutase is specific for the oxygen free radical and dimethylthiourea nullifies the hydroxy free radical. Catalase, an enzyme that enhances the degradation of hydrogen peroxide to oxygen and water, has also been utilized but has not been found to be particularly effective in the kidney, because its large molecular size prevents it from being filtered. Dimethylthiourea, a hydroxy free-radial scavenger, when administered prior to the ischemic event, significantly diminishes the rise in plasma creatinine and results in a more rapid return in renal function. Superoxide dismutase appears to be the most effective drug of the free-radical scavengers in returning renal function to normal. When superoxide dismutase is given following an ischemic event, there is a 50 percent reduction in the rise of serum creatinine and a more rapid return of renal function than when the drug is not administered [78]. Of the drugs available, only superoxide dismutase is available at this time in a clinically limited way.

MYOGLOBIN NEPHROTOXICITY. Rhabdomyolysis has been reported to be the cause of ARF in approximately 5 percent of all patients. Prognosis for recovery is excellent, provided rhabdomyolysis is recognized promptly and therapy begun immediately. There are traumatic and nontraumatic causes of rhabdomyolysis. The former include crush injuries, electric burns, and surgery. Nontraumatic causes include increased muscle exertion, inflammatory muscle diseases, infection, toxic drugs, and metabolic abnormalities (particularly hypokalemia).

Following the precipitating event, the patient becomes acutely ill with fever, weakness, and pain. The urine is brownish and is dipstick-positive for heme. Since the molecular weight of myoglobin is much lower than that of hemoglobin, it is rapidly cleared from the serum. Thus a spun blood sample will reveal a clear serum—in contradistinction to hemolysis, in which the serum will be red due to retained hemoglobin. A high serum CPK level establishes the diagnosis. Serum potassium and phosphate are often elevated, and hyperuricemia may be severe. The mechanism(s) of this form of ARF is unclear, but it is probably due to a combination of events, including low flow, prolonged contact of the tubule lumen with myoglobin, and high uric acid concentration. Therapy is directed at establishing a diuresis either with a loop diuretic or by volume expansion with saline, combined with either mannitol or a loop diuretic. The diuresis dilutes the toxic myoglobin, removes it from the kidney, reduces the serum uric acid concentration, and modestly alkalinizes the urine. Alkalinization of the patient is advisable initially, since an acid medium promotes myoglobin disassociation into a ferrihemate and globin. It is the former that is toxic.

TREATMENT OF ESTABLISHED ACUTE RENAL FAILURE. Once a diagnosis of ARF is established, fluid intake is restricted to 400 ml/day plus the volume of other fluid losses. Body weight in an ARF patient in fluid balance will decline 500 gm/day due to protein catabolism. Sodium balance is maintained by quantitatively replacing losses. Frequent serum electrolytes are obtained to monitor Na^+ replacement and to detect hyperkalemia. The use of intravenous hyperalimentation solutions may obviate some of the weight loss and increase the rate of rise of BUN and creatinine. These solutions have been shown to reduce the morbidity of ARF, but they do not necessarily reduce its duration. If the patient is oliguric, dopamine and/or dopamine plus furosemide or furosemide alone may be utilized to convert the patient from an oliguric to a nonoliguric status. This is particularly helpful in the critically injured patient who is undergoing large fluid shifts and who, because of his hypermetabolic status, requires increased nutritional support. The ability to increase urine volume is critical, and these drugs may be helpful in allowing the physician to utilize other forms of treatment. It is unlikely, however, that the drugs in and of themselves will enhance the return of renal function. Perhaps an exception to this statement would be patients who are highly likely to develop acute renal failure, such as those who become septic and in whom the prodrome of ARF is recognized. In these circumstances the administration of dopamine may prevent the renal failure, or at least delay its onset. Finally, mannitol is useful in patients with myoglobin nephrotoxicity, because of its ability to flush the tubule of toxic myoglobin [28].

HYPERKALEMIA. Cardiac dysfunction occurs frequently with a serum K^+ concentration in excess of 8.0 mEq/liter; dysfunction is uncommon with a concentration of less than 7.0 mEq/liter. Cardiac manifestations of hyperkalemia include bradycardia, hypotension, and cardiac arrest from ventricular fibrillation or standstill. Hyperkalemia interferes with intra-atrial and intraventricular conduction. The sequential electrocardiogram (ECG) abnormalities of increasingly severe hyperkalemia are as follows: tall, peaked T waves, depressed S–T segments, decreased amplitude of R waves, a prolonged P–R interval, P waves that are diminished to absent, widening of the QRS complex, prolongation of the Q–T interval, and finally, a sine wave pattern. (Note: An initial ECG determines the severity of the hyperkalemia and the urgency of therapy while the return of laboratory serum electrolyte concentrations is awaited. The initial ECG serves as a baseline for further evaluation of therapy.)

Moderate hyperkalemia (6.0–7.0 mEq/liter) is treated by withholding K^+ administration in any form (it must be remembered that some antibiotics may contribute significant amounts of sodium or potassium) and by correcting existing metabolic or respiratory acidosis. Sodium polystyrene sulfonate (Kayexalate), a cation-exchange resin, is given either orally or as an enema; 15 to 60 gm is given in divided doses. Since Kayexalate may cause constipation, sorbitol is also administered. Although oral administration of cation exchange resins is more effective in lowering serum K^+ concentration, the rectal route is preferable in patients with alimentary tract dysfunction.

Severe hyperkalemia (>7.0 mEq/liter) should be rapidly controlled with intravenous sodium bicarbonate, and the myocardium can be protected temporarily by the administration of calcium gluconate or calcium chloride. Rarely, it may be necessary to give insulin and glucose (1 unit of regular insulin per 5 gm of glucose), but rebound hypoglycemia could prove fatal. Further control of hyperkalemia is achieved with Kayexalate followed by hemodialysis or peritoneal dialysis if necessary.

A Quinton-Scribner shunt [84] is placed early to control overhydration and hyperkalemic acidosis by hemodialysis when conservative measures are insufficient. Some nephrologists prefer to use percutaneous techniques to cannulate the femoral vessels for short-term dialysis [50]. Sheldon catheters may be placed in the femoral vessels by the Seldinger technique, or a MacIntosh double-lumen catheter may be inserted into the iliac vein through the saphenous vein. Other nephrologists prefer peritoneal dialysis. The choice of route must take into account the safety and comfort of the patient, the experience of the nephrologist, and the expected duration of renal failure.

OTHER THERAPEUTIC MEASURES. Once the diagnosis of ARF is established, the urinary catheter is removed, to eliminate a portal of entry for infection. Frequent cultures of sputum, urine, blood, and wounds are obtained. In the absence of specific infection, antibiotics are not recommended, but close observation for sepsis and early specific antibiotic treatment are required.

Ultrasonography of the kidneys (pyelographic visualization of the kidneys is usually not possible) should be obtained in an effort to determine whether or not prior renal disease is superimposed on the acute problem. Ultrasonography can determine renal size and thereby provide information about prior disease. Preexisting renal disease may be demonstrated by unilateral or bilateral small kidneys, which are indicative of vascular or infectious disease. An enlarged renal outline implies either acute renal vein thrombosis or infiltrative lesions, such as myeloma or lymphoma. Renal scans in suspected cases of bilateral renal artery thrombosis may indicate the need for arteriograms.

Since upper gastrointestinal hemorrhage may supervene, contributing to mortality, prophylactic antacid therapy should be used. Aluminum hydroxide is the most desirable antacid in ARF, since it helps to control the hyperphosphatemia of renal failure.

All diet and drug orders must be stopped, and a careful review of each order must be made in the light of absent renal function. The dosage of many therapeutic agents, including digitalis and antibiotics, may need to be adjusted [8, 86].

The timing and frequency of dialysis of patients with ARF are moot. Most centers regularly dialyze these patients three times a week as long as the BUN and serum creatinine concentrations continue to increase spontaneously. Kleinknecht and Ganeval [52] and Conger [23] report that preventive dialysis (to keep the BUN less than 70 mg/100 ml and the blood creatinine concentration less than 5 mg/100 ml) reduces mortality, bleeding episodes, and the incidence of major sepsis.

An important approach to improving the survival rate in ARF may lie in better nutritional management of these patients. Abel et al. [1] report with "improved survival in patients with ARF after they had been treated with intravenous essential L-amino acids and glucose." Perhaps combining better nutritional management with more-frequent dialyses will result in improved survival in this high-risk group of patients.

If renal function fails to improve spontaneously within 3 weeks, the diagnoses of renal infarction or acute cortical necrosis must be considered. Selective renal arteriograms may demonstrate obstruction of the renal artery and vein or may show loss of cortical blood flow. If a renal biopsy confirms the diagnosis, the patient should be placed on a chronic hemodialysis program. Renal transplantation may be considered if the patient is a suitable candidate.

Hepatorenal Syndrome

Hepatorenal syndrome (HRS) is a term that refers to the occurrence of ARF in patients with advanced liver disease. This variety of ARF deserves special comment. The renal failure is manifested by progressive azotemia, oliguria, a concentrated urine with a low urine Na^+ concentration, mild proteinuria, and occasionally, hyponatremia. The onset of renal failure in end-stage liver disease frequently marks the terminal stage of the patient's illness [79]. There is no satisfactory treatment for either the renal or the liver failure.

PATHOPHYSIOLOGY. The pathophysiology of HRS is not well understood, but the renal failure appears to be functional and is associated with abnormal renal blood flow. The morphology of kidneys from patients dying with HRS is often normal or shows only minimal changes. Epstein et al. [29] have demonstrated decreased renal blood flow, especially to the superficial cortex, using renal arteriography and xenon washout studies in these patients. Further evidence that the kidneys function normally when the liver malfunction is corrected comes from experiences in transplantation. Kidneys transplanted from a hepatorenal donor to noncirrhotic recipients function normally [53]. Conversely, recovery from HRS following successful liver transplantation has been reported [46].

The functional renal disturbance in HRS has been variously attributed to the following: (1) failure of the liver to detoxify a pressor substance, (2) release of a vasoactive hormone from the damaged liver, (3) abnormal function of the RA system, (4) a decrease in effective plasma volume associated with ascites and splanchnic pooling of blood, and (5) extrarenal diversion of blood through arteriovenous shunts. Clarification of the pathophysiology of the renal failure associated with advanced liver disease must await further studies.

CLINICAL AND LABORATORY OBSERVATIONS AND PATIENT MANAGEMENT. The hepatorenal syndrome usually develops with greatest frequency in patients with the most advanced liver disease; ascites and hepatic encephalopathy are frequently present. The onset of renal failure can be sudden and without apparent cause but is frequently associated with the use of diuretics, paracentesis, or surgical procedures.

There is no effective treatment for HRS, but the physician must always keep in mind that oliguria in a cirrhotic patient is not always due to the HRS and that other remediable causes, such as urinary obstruction or prerenal failure, may be involved. Therefore, the vigorous diagnostic efforts and treatment of acute oliguria described previously are required in these patients as well.

POLYURIA

The differential diagnosis of polyuria also falls into three general pathophysiologic categories: postrenal, prerenal, and intrinsic renal polyuria (Table 21-3). Postrenal polyuria is seen following the release of complete urinary obstruction or in the presence of chronic partial urinary occlusion. Prerenal polyuria is caused by insufficient circulating ADH and exogenous or endogenous diuretic agents. Renal polyuria is intrinsic renal impairment of the medullary concentrating mechanism due to anatomic disruption from disease, metabolic aberrations affecting ADH–collecting-duct interaction, or functional renal derangements.

To diagnose the type of polyuria and manage critically ill polyuric patients properly, it is essential to understand the normal physiology of the renal concentrating mechanism, since disturbances in this function ultimately result in polyuria.

Normal Renal Concentrating Mechanism

The bulk of the glomerular filtrate (60–70%) is resorbed isotonically from the proximal tubular lumen; 10 to 15 percent is resorbed from the loop of Henle and distal tubular lumen, and the remaining tubular fluid resorption is moderated in the medullary collecting duct by ADH.

Antidiuretic hormone is synthesized in the supraoptic nucleus of the hypothalamus and transported to the posterior pituitary, where it is stored. Release of the hormone occurs in response to increased plasma osmolality, decreased circulating blood volume, pain, stress, trauma, and anesthesia [35, 94]. Hypo-osmolar states, plasma volume expansion, and certain drugs (ethanol and nicotine) inhibit ADH release [51]. The hormone circulates to the kidney, where it binds to the collecting-duct cell membrane and activates adenyl cyclase, which facilitates the generation of adenosine $3' : 5' =$ cyclic monophosphate (cyclic AMP) from ATP. Cyclic AMP activates a protein kinase that is believed to increase water permeability in the collecting duct [39].

The driving force causing water to be resorbed from the medullary col-

Table 21-3. Differential diagnosis of polyuria

Postrenal polyuria
  In chronic, partial urinary obstruction
  Following release of complete urinary obstruction (postobstructive diuresis)
Prerenal polyuria
  Insufficient circulating antidiuretic hormone (ADH)
    Suppressed ADH release
      Iatrogenic expansion of extracellular fluid volume
      Compulsive water drinking
      Cerebral lesions causing thirst
    Defects in ADH synthesis (diabetes insipidus)
      Diabetes insipidus associated with tumor, trauma, infection, and
        granulomatous diseases
      Idiopathic diabetes insipidus
      Familial diabetes insipidus
Diuretic agents
  Inhibitors of renal tubular salt transport
    Diuresis following resolution of cardiac arrhythmias
    Addison's disease, Cushing's syndrome
    Nonosmotic pharmacologic agents
  Extrarenal osmotic diuretics
    Exogenous pharmacologic agents (e.g., mannitol)
    Endogenous diseases of metabolism (e.g., diabetes mellitus, excessive
      protein catabolism)
Renal polyuria (impaired renal concentrating mechanism)
  Anatomic disruption
    Sickle-cell anemia
    Pyelonephritis
    Polyarteritis nodosa
    Polycystic renal disease
    Medullary cystic disease
    Amyloidosis
    Myeloma
    Nephrocalcinosis
    Other
  Metabolic aberrations of ADH: collecting-duct interaction
    Hypercalcemia
    Potassium depletion
    Renal tubular acidosis
    Nephrogenic diabetes insipidus
    Other
  Functional renal derangements
    Acute renal failure, polyuric phase
    Posttransplantation acute renal failure
    Chronic renal failure
    Other

lecting-duct lumen is an osmotic pressure difference across the collecting-duct epithelium. Therefore, maintenance of medullary hypertonicity is essential for formation of concentrated urine. Conversely, should the medullary osmotic pressure gradient be dissipated, regardless of the circulating level of ADH, urinary concentration does not occur and polyuria results. Medullary hypertonicity is established by active transport of Cl^- or Na^+ by the thick ascending limb of the loop of Henle; it is maintained by the countercurrent flow arrangement of the loops of Henle, vasa recta, and collecting ducts. Medullary hypertonicity can be abolished by failure of ion transport mechanisms or by washout of medullary solute through rapid flow in either the vasa recta or tubules.

In each of the three broad categories of polyuria to be discussed, one or more elements of the normal renal concentrating mechanism is deranged.

Postrenal Polyuria

Postrenal polyuria occurs during partial chronic urinary obstruction [25] or following release of complete urinary occlusion (postobstructive diuresis) [108], provided that significant parenchymal damage has not occurred. Postrenal polyuria is characterized by excessive water, Na^+, and K^+ losses; decreased maximal tubular resorption of glucose; and decreased renal ability to acidify the urine [10, 27]. As much as 40 perent of filtered water, 30 percent of filtered Na^+, and 140 percent of filtered K^+ may be excreted in the urine [14, 103].

Pathophysiology

The mechanisms of postobstructive diuresis have been elucidated in experimental animal models [9, 66, 68, 109]. Postobstructive diuresis occurs despite a reduced glomerular filtration rate because of impaired nephron salt and water resorption. A brisk flow of tubular fluid ensues throughout the nephron, resulting in (1) a washout of the medullary osmotic gradient, (2) failure of the medullary concentrating mechanism, (3) an enhanced condition for K^+ secretion, and (4) increased urinary losses of water, Na^+, and K^+. There is a reduced glomerular filtration rate and renal blood flow due to the renin-angiotensin system that is unopposed by the vasodilator prostaglandins [64]; these mechanisms have been discussed in the section on postrenal failure. There is a nonspecific increase in tubule permeability [66, 68]. The permeability defect results in impaired hydrogen ion secretion and failure of the kidney to respond to salt-retaining hormones.

Other mechanisms have been proposed to explain the postobstructive diuresis. The roles of ECF volume expansion and solute retention during the period of urinary obstruction have been considered [30, 69, 74]. Extracellular fluid volume expansion and solute diuresis, when present, certainly enhance the diuresis, but the syndrome is seen in patients with volume contraction with normal urea loads to the kidney. Thus, both a physiologic diuresis and pathologic diuresis may occur following relief of urinary tract obstruction. The physiologic diuresis is due to ECF volume expansion and excess solute (urea), whereas the pathologic diuresis is fundamentally due to increased tubule permeability.

Clinical and Laboratory Observations and Patient Management
Clinically, postobstructive diuresis begins 2 to 24 hours after release of urinary obstruction. In these circumstances, the urine specific gravity is below 1.005, the U/P osmotic concentration ratio is less than 1.0, and the U/P urea concentration ratio is often less than 9 (Table 21-1). The urinary Na^+ concentration exceeds 50 mEq/liter, and the urinary K^+ concentration is over 20 mEq/liter.

The diuresis is self-limiting. Renal Na^+ and K^+ metabolism returns to normal in 48 to 72 hours, although the concentrating defect may persist for 1 to 2 weeks. On occasion, a spectacular diuresis of greater than 10 liters/day with excessive urinary Na^+ and K^+ losses may last for several weeks.

The diuresis is unresponsive to ADH, and the Na^+ transport defect is insensitive to mineralocorticoids. Excessive fluid replacement perpetuates the diuresis and increases urinary Na^+ losses. Generally, 5 gm/100 ml of dextrose in 0.45 gm/100 ml saline can be infused safely until laboratory measurements of urinary Na^+ and K^+ losses are available to guide replacement therapy. The intravenous infusion rate should be adjusted initially to match urine flow, provided the patient is not significantly overhydrated. After 24 hours, the intravenous fluid rate may be decreased cautiously, but ECF volume depletion and dehydration must be prevented. The clinical signs of ECF volume depletion are discussed in the section on clinical and laboratory observations of acute prerenal failure. Therapy to maintain homeostasis of the internal milieu must be continued until adequate renal function returns.

Clinically significant postobstructive diuresis is seen only when the total nephron mass has been obstructed: i.e., unilateral urinary obstruction causes inappropriate water, Na^+, and K^+ losses from that side, but their magnitude is such that routine fluid replacement is usually adequate to manage the patient properly [67].

Prerenal Polyuria
Prerenal polyuria is due to insufficient ADH or to exogenous or endogenous diuretic agents; the intrinsic integrity of the renal concentrating mechanism is maintained (Table 21-3). However, if prerenal polyuria is allowed to persist for prolonged periods, washout of the medullary osmotic pressure gradient occurs [2, 24], resulting in a superimposition of renal or prerenal polyuria.

Pathophysiology and Etiology of Insufficient Antidiuretic Hormone
Insufficient ADH activity results either from suppression of ADH release by normal physiologic mechanisms or through failure of ADH production. Physiologic suppression of ADH release is a consequence of ECF volume expansion or of a decrease in plasma osmolality. The more common causes of ECF volume expansion include overadministration of intravenous fluids, compulsive water drinking, and pathologic stimulation of the thirst center. Dilution of plasma osmolality occurs when salt and water losses are replaced with electrolyte-poor fluid. Absent or insufficient ADH pro-

duction occurs in diabetes insipidus (Table 21-3), which may be an inherited or acquired abnormality.

Clinical and Laboratory Observations and Patient Management

In the absence of ADH activity, laboratory findings reveal a low urinary specific gravity (<1.005), low urinary osmolality (<200 mOsm/kg H_2O), and a low urinary Na^+ concentration (<25 mEq/liter) [12, 21].

SUPPRESSED ADH RELEASE. Patients with physiologically suppressed ADH release respond to fluid restriction with a fall in urinary flow and a rise in urinary specific gravity and osmolality, provided the polyuric state has not washed out the medullary osmotic pressure gradient. When renal polyuria is superimposed on prerenal polyuria, the response to fluid restriction occurs slowly. In these circumstances, care must be taken to avoid ECF volume depletion and dehydration in the interim. Fluid restriction for several hours will lead to a stable urine osmolality above 250 mOsm/kg H_2O and will not respond to vasopressin administration [72].

DEFECTS IN AUTIDIURETIC HORMONE SYNTHESIS: DIABETES INSIPIDUS. Fluid restriction in patients with diabetes insipidus (Table 21-3) results in unabated renal water loss and progressive hypertonic dehydration. Diabetes insipidus is treated with exogenous vasopressin; several days may be required to reestablish the medullary osmotic pressure gradient before the effects of vasopressin are seen. In the interim, water restriction will cause the urine osmolality to stabilize between 60 and 200 mOsm/kg H_2O. In certain patients with low endogenous ADH production, chlorpropamide is beneficial, because it potentiates the action of ADH [56, 75]. In patients with no endogenous ADH, chlorpropamide is ineffective. Until the diuresis of diabetes insipidus is controlled, careful replacement of fluid and electrolytes is required.

Pathophysiology of Polyuria Due to Diuretic Agents

The polyuria produced by diuretic agents is caused basically by an increased osmotic content within the nephron, preventing water resorption. The diuretics either inhibit tubular salt transport or impose an extrarenal osmotic load.

INHIBITORS OF RENAL TUBULAR SALT TRANSPORT. Inhibition of Na^+ resorption may be due to nonosmotic pharmacologic agents [79], absence of salt-retaining hormones, renal disease, and cardiac arrhythmias. The solute diuresis that follows conversion of a cardiac arrhythmia—particularly paroxysmal atrial tachycardia—to a normal sinus rhythm appears to be due to inhibition of proximal tubular Na^+ resorption through unknown mechanisms [49]. Formerly, the etiology of the diuresis following correction of a cardiac arrhythmia was ascribed to physiologic suppression of ADH. However, since a solute rather than a water diuresis occurs, other etiologic mechanisms are being considered.

The failure of normal Na^+ resorption in these conditions results in a solute load to the collecting duct. The increased osmotic content of the collecting-duct fluid reduces the osmotic pressure difference between lumen and interstitium and, simultaneously, the driving force for water resorption. If the solute load is of sufficient quantity, polyuria results.

EXTRARENAL OSMOTIC DIURETICS. Osmotic diuresis is a frequent cause of polyuria in the critically ill. The osmotically active substance may be an exogenous pharmacologic agent (e.g., mannitol) or a product of an endogenous metabolic disease (e.g., glucose in diabetes mellitus).

The mechanism by which polyuria occurs with glomerular filtration of nonresorbable solute, such as mannitol, radiographic dyes, and excess urea or glucose, is as follows: The osmotic agent is filtered at the glomerulus in an isosmotic concentration to plasma. In the proximal tubule, Na^+ resorption into the intracellular space sets up an osmotic concentration gradient that leads to isotonic water resorption. However, the nonresorbable osmotic substance within the proximal tubular lumen initially increases in concentration and then balances the Na^+ osmotic concentration in the intracellular spaces. Further water resorption is inhibited. Net Na^+ transport is reduced, due to an increasing Na^+ concentration difference between the proximal tubular lumen and the intracellular spaces. Thus, decreased water resorption indirectly diminishes proximal tubular Na^+ resorption.

Similar inhibition of salt and water resorption in the distal nephron leads to a solute diuresis and dissipation of the medullary osmotic pressure gradient. Thus, even after the osmotic agent is removed, diuresis may continue because of loss of medullary tonicity. In addition to excessive Na^+ and water losses, increased excretion of K^+, Ca^+, phosphate, and magnesium may result in clinically significant deficiencies [34].

Renal Polyuria

Renal polyuria results from intrinsic impairment of the renal concentrating mechanism due to anatomic disruption from disease, metabolic aberrations affecting ADH–collecting-duct interaction, or functional renal derangements (Table 21-3).

Anatomic Disruption

A reduction in renal medullary tonicity due to sickle-cell anemia is representative of this group. Increased sickling of erythrocytes may occur in the renal medulla due to hypertonicity, decreased oxygen tension, and decreased pH. The abnormal sickle cell configuration retards blood flow in the medulla and reduces the amount of solute and water removed from the collecting duct [82]. Complete occlusion of the vasa recta with infarction of the papilla results in permanent alterations [97]. In children, and to a lesser degree in adults, fresh blood transfusions will correct this defect, demonstrating the reversibility of this disease process in its early stages [47]. Urine osmolality and specific gravity vary according to the degree of medullary vascular occlusion. Urinary Na^+ concentrations may be elevated to the levels as high as 60 mEq/liter [55]. Treatment is directed at replacing urinary salt and water losses. Exogenous vasopressin has been shown to be mildly effective in increasing urinary concentration.

Alterations that affect the collecting-duct structure (e.g., medullary cystic disease) or alter its permeability by surrounding it with impermeable protein deposits (e.g., amyloidosis [19]) may inhibit the concentrating mechanism sufficiently to produce polyuria.

Metabolic Aberration of ADH–Collecting Duct Interaction

Metabolic alterations in the renal concentrating mechanism are of particular interest, since they may coexist in the critically ill patient. Diagnostic evaluation of polyuric status requires careful evaluation of the serum chemistries and urine pH. Hypercalcemia, prolonged K^+ depletion, and renal tubular acidosis result in polyuria that is rapidly reversed when the primary disorder is corrected. Hypercalcemia initially interferes with the action of ADH on the collecting-duct epithelium; if it is corrected early, there is an immediate reversal of the concentrating defect. However, prolonged hypercalcemia with calcium deposition in the thick ascending limb of the loop of Henle, distal tubule, and collecting-duct epithelia may result in permanent loss of renal concentration ability.

The mechanism whereby hypokalemia exerts its effect in producing a diuresis is unclear; inhibition of the generation of adenyl cyclase, cyclic AMP, or protein kinase may be responsible. Hypokalemia may also directly inhibit the release of ADH from the posterior pituitary or stimulate hypothalamic thirst centers. Restoration of the K^+ levels in plasma corrects the renal concentrating mechanism [93].

Renal tubular acidosis results in hypokalemia; it is not known whether renal tubular acidosis interferes directly with the concentrating mechanism or whether its effect is mediated by reduced plasma K^+ concentrations. In either case, the renal concentrating mechanism is restored when acidosis and hypokalemia are corrected, provided nephrocalcinosis has not complicated the disease.

In nephrogenic diabetes insipidus, the collecting duct is insensitive to normal or elevated circulating levels of ADH. The urinary findings and response to fluid restriction are similar to those in diabetes insipidus; however, unlike the response in diabetes insipidus, urine osmolality is not affected by vasopressin administration.

Functional Renal Derangements

The pathophysiology of ARF has been discussed previously. In the diuretic phase of ARF, urine osmolality and specific gravity are low. The U/P osmotic concentration ratio is less than 1.1, the U/P urea concentration ratio is less than 4, and the urinary Na^+ concentration exceeds 30 mEq/liter. Sodium, fluid, and, rarely, K^+ losses can be excessive. During the diuretic phase of acute renal failure, urinary salt and water losses must be replaced carefully.

In summary, renal dysfunction often is manifested initially by oliguria or polyuria. Each of these two major categories may be subdivided into postrenal, prerenal, and intrinsic renal abnormalities. It is important to note that uremia may also occur despite normal urine flow; the sine qua non of renal dysfunction is an elevated plasma creatinine concentration. An understanding of the pathophysiology of acute uremia is essential for appropriate patient management.

REFERENCES

1. Abel, R. M., et al. Improved survival from acute renal failure after treatment with intravenous essential L-amino acids and glucose. *N. Engl. J. Med.* 288:695, 1973.

2. Andriole, V. T., and Epstein, F. H. Prevention of pyelonephritis by water diuresis: Evidence for the role of medullary hypertonicity in promoting renal infection. *J. Clin. Invest.* 44:73, 1965.

3. Arndt, J. O. Diuresis induced by water infusions into the carotid loop and its inhibition by small hemorrhage. *Pfluegers Arch.* 282:313, 1965.

4. Arnold, P. E., et al. In vitro versus in vivo mitochondrial calcium loading in ischemic acute renal failure. *Am. J. Physiol.* 248:F845, 1985.

5. Badr, K. F., et al. Renal and systemic hemodynamic responses to intravenous infusion of leukotriene C_4 in the rat. *Circ. Res.* 54:492, 1984.

6. Baker, P. F., et al. The influence of calcium on sodium efflux in squid axons. *J. Physiol.* (Lond.) 200:431, 1969.

7. Barry, K. E., et al. Mannitol infusion. II. The prevention of acute functional renal failure during resection of an aneurysm of the abdominal aorta. *N. Engl. J. Med.* 264:967, 1961.

8. Bennett, W. M., et al. A practical guide to drug usage in adult patients with impaired renal function. *J.A.M.A.* 214:1468, 1970.

9. Bercovitch, D. D., et al. The post-obstructive kidney. Observations on nephron function after relief of 24 hours of ureteral ligation in the dog. *J. Clin. Invest.* 50:1154, 1971.

10. Berlyne, G. M. Distal tubular function in chronic hydronephrosis. *Q. J. Med.* 30:339, 1961.

11. Berman, L. B. Vasomotor nephropathy. *J.A.M.A.* 231:1067, 1975.

12. Blom, P. S., et al. Sodium economy in the proximal and distal parts of the nephron studied in patients with diabetes insipidus. Their estimation under normal conditions and after salt restriction, chlorothiazide and a mercurial diuretic. *Acta Med. Scand.* 174:201, 1963.

13. Bolton, T. B. Mechanisms of action of transmitters and other substances on smooth muscle. *Physiol. Rev.* 59:606, 1979.

14. Bricker, N. S., et al. An abnormality in renal function resulting from urinary tract obstruction. *Am. J. Med.* 23:554, 1957.

15. Bricker, N. S., and Klahr, S. Obstructive Nephropathy. In M. B. Strauss and L. G. Welt (eds.), *Diseases of the Kidney.* Boston: Little, Brown, 1971. Pp. 997–1037.

16. Brown, C. B., et al. Establish Acute Renal Failure Following Surgical Operations. In E. A. Friedman and H. E. Eliahou (eds.), *Proceedings Acute Renal Failure Conference.* Washington, D.C.: DHEW Publication No. (NIH) 74-608, 1973. Pp. 187–201.

17. Bulkley, G. B. The role of oxygen free radicals in human disease processes. *Surgery* 94:407, 1983.

18. Burke, T. J., et al. Protective effect of intrarenal calcium membrane blockers before or after renal ischemia. Functional, morphological, and mitochondrial studies. *J. Clin. Invest.* 74:1830, 1984.

19. Carone, F. A., and Epstein, F. H. Nephrogenic diabetes insipidus caused by amyloid disease. *Am. J. Med.* 29:539, 1960.

20. Chien, K. R., et al. Accelerated phospholipid degradation and associated membrane dysfunction in irreversible, ischemic liver cell injury. *J. Biol. Chem.* 253:4809, 1978.
21. Coggins, C. H., and Leaf, A. Diabetes insipidus. *Am. J. Med.* 42:807, 1967.
22. Coleman, R. Membrane-bound enzymes and membrane ultra-structure. *Biochim. Biophys. Acta* 300:1, 1973.
23. Conger, J. D. A Controlled Evaluation of Daily Dialysis in Post-traumatic Acute Renal Failure. *Abstracts,* The American Society of Nephrology, Nov. 25–26, 1974. P. 18.
24. DeWardener, H. E., and Herxheimer, A. W. The effect of a high water intake on the kidney's ability to concentrate the urine in man. *J. Physiol.* (Lond.) 139:42, 1957.
25. Dorhout-Mees, E. J. Reversible water losing state, caused by incomplete ureteric obstruction. *Acta Med. Scand.* 168:193, 1960.
26. Dunn, M. J. Renal Prostaglandins. In M. J. Dunn (ed.), *Renal Endocrinology.* Baltimore: Williams & Wilkins, 1983. P. 4.
27. Eiseman, B., et al. Fluid and electrolyte changes following the relief of urinary obstruction. *J. Urol.* 74:222, 1955.
28. Eneas, J. F., Schoenfeld, P. Y., and Humphreys, M. H. The effect of infusion of mannitol-sodium bicarbonate on the clinical course of myoglobinuria. *Arch. Intern. Med.* 139:801, 1979.
29. Epstein, M., et al. Renal failure in the patient with cirrhosis. *Am. J. Med.* 49:175, 1970.
30. Falls, W. F., and Stacy, W. K. Postobstructive diuresis. Studies in a dialyzed patient with a solitary kidney. *Am. J. Med.* 54:404, 1973.
31. Farber, J. L. The role of calcium in cell death. *Life Sci.* 29:1289, 1981.
32. Fleckenstein, A. Specific pharmacology of calcium in myocardium, cardiac pacemakers, and vascular smooth muscle. *Annu. Rev. Pharmacol. Toxicol.* 17:149, 1977.
33. Gauer, O. H., et al. The regulation of extracellular fluid volume. *Annu. Rev. Physiol.* 32:547, 1970.
34. Gennari, F. J., and Kassirer, J. P. Osmotic diuresis. *N. Engl. J. Med.* 291:714, 1974.
35. Ginsburg, M. Production, Release, Transportation and Elimination of the Neurohypophyseal Hormones. In B. Berde (ed.), *Handbooks of Experimental Pharmacology.* Berlin: Springer, 1968. Pp. 286–371.
36. Goldberg, L. I. Dopamine—Clinical uses of an endogenous catecholamine. *N. Engl. J. Med.* 291:707, 1974.
37. Goldfarb, D., et al. Beneficial effect of verapamil in ischemic acute renal failure in the rat. *Proc. Exp. Dial. Med.* 172:389, 1983.
38. Goormaghtigh, N. Vascular and circulatory changes in renal cortex in the anuric crush-syndrome. *Proc. Soc. Exp. Biol. Med.* 59:303, 1945.
39. Handler, J. S., and Orloff, J. The Mechanism of Action of Antidiuretic Hormone. In J. Orloff, R. W. Berliner, and S. R. Geiger (eds.), *Handbook of Physiology.* Section 8, Renal Physiology. Washington, D.C.: American Physiological Society, 1973. Pp. 791–814.
40. Graziani, G., et al. Dopamine and furosemide in oliguric acute renal failure. *Nephron* 37:39, 1984.
41. Hansson, R., et al. Effect of xanthine oxidase inhibition on renal circulation after ischemia. *Transplant. Proc.* XIV:51, 1982.
42. Hinnen, R., Miyan.ito, H., and Racker, E. Ca^{2+} translocation in Ehrlich ascites tumor cells. *J. Membr. Biol.* 49:309, 1979.
43. Hollenberg, N. K., and Adams, D. F. Vascular Factors in the Pathogenesis of Acute Renal Failure in Man. In E. A. Friedman and H. E. Eliahou (eds.),

Proceedings Acute Renal Failure Conference. Washington, D.C.: DHEW Publication No. (NIH) 74-608, 1973. Pp. 209–229.

44. Humes, H. D. Role of calcium in pathogenesis of acute renal failure. *Am. J. Physiol.* 250:F579, 1986.
45. Ichikawa, I., Miele, J. F., and Brenner, B. M. Reversal of renal cortical actions of angiotensin II by verapamil and manganese. *Kidney Int.* 16:137, 1979.
46. Iwatsuki, S., et al. Recovery from "Hepatorenal syndrome" after orthotopic liver transplantation. *N. Engl. J. Med.* 289:1155, 1973.
47. Keifel, H. G., et al. Hyposthenuria in sickle cell anemia: A reversible renal defect. *J. Clin. Invest.* 35:998, 1956.
48. Kerr, D. N. S. Acute Renal Failure. In D. Black (ed.), *Renal Disease.* London: Blackwell, 1972. Pp. 447–452.
49. Kinney, M. J., et al. The polyuria of paroxysmal atrial tachycardia. *Circulation* 50:429, 1974.
50. Kjellstrand, C. M., et al. Technique of Hemodialysis. In J. S. Najarian and R. L. Simmons (eds.), *Transplantation.* Philadelphia: Lea & Febiger, 1972. Pp. 425–445.
51. Kleeman, C. R., et al. Studies on alcohol diuresis. II. The evaluation of ethyl alcohol as an inhibitor of the neurohypophysis. *J. Clin. Invest.* 34:448, 1955.
52. Kleinknecht, D., and Ganeval, D. Preventive Hemodialysis in Acute Renal Failure: Its Effect on Mortality and Morbidity. In E. A. Friedman and H. E. Eliahou (eds.), *Proceedings Acute Renal Failure Conference.* Washington, D.C.: DHEW Publication No. (NIH) 74-608, 1973. Pp. 165–184.
53. Koppel, M. H., et al. Transplantation of cadaveric kidneys from patients with hepatorenal syndrome: Evidence for the functional nature of renal failure in advanced liver disease. *N. Engl. J. Med.* 280:1367, 1969.
54. Laragh, J. H., and Sealey, J. E. The Renin-Angiotensin-Aldosterone Hormonal System and Regulation of Sodium, Potassium, and Blood Pressure Homeostasis. In J. Orloff, R. W. Berliner, and S. R. Geiger (eds.), *Handbook of Physiology.* Section 8, Renal Physiology. Washington, D.C.: American Physiological Society, 1973. Pp. 831–908.
55. Levitt, M. F., et al. The renal concentrating defect in sickle cell disease. *Am. J. Med.* 29:611, 1960.
56. Liberman, B., et al. Evidence for a role of antidiuretic hormone (ADH) in the antidiuretic action of chlorpropamide. *J. Clin. Endocrinol. Metab.* 36:894, 1973.
57. Linton, A. L. Acute renal failure. *Can. Med. Assoc. J.* 110:949, 1974.
58. Linton, A. L., et al. Protective Effect of Furosemide in Acute Tubular Necrosis and Acute Renal Failure. In E. A. Friedman and H. E. Eliahou (eds.), *Proceedings Acute Renal Failure Conference.* Washington, D.C.: DHEW Publication No. (NIH) 74-608, 1973. Pp. 71–87.
59. Lordon, R. E. Acute Renal Failure Following Battle Injury—Mortality, Complications, and Treatment. In E. A. Friedman and H. E. Eliahou (eds.), *Proceedings Acute Renal Failure Conference.* Washington, D.C.: DHEW Publication No. (NIH) 74-608, 1973. Pp. 109–123.
60. Lordon, R. E., and Burton, J. R. Post-traumatic renal failure in military personnel in Southeast Asia. *Am. J. Med.* 53:137, 1972.
61. Luke, R. G., et al. Factors determining response to mannitol in acute renal failure. *Am. J. Med. Sci.* 259:168, 1970.
62. MacLaughlin, M., ReMello Aries, M., and Malvic, G. Efeito do verapamil em differentes parametros da funcao renal. *Arq. Bras. Cardiol.* 32:335, 1979.
63. McCrorey, H. L., et al. Effect of Calcium Transport Inhibitors in Renal Hemodynamics and Electrolyte Excretion in the Dog. In B. Lichardus, R. W.

Schirer, and J. Ponce (eds.), *Hormonal Regulation of Sodium Excretion.* New York: Elsevier/North Holland, 1980. Pp. 113–120.

64. McDougal, W. S. Pharmacologic preservation of renal mass and function in obstructive uropathy. *J. Urol.* 128:418, 1982.

65. McDougal, W. S. The diagnosis, management and pathophysiology of acute renal failure in surgical patients. *A.U.A. Update Series* IV:7, 1985.

66. McDougal, W. S., Rhodes, R., and Persky, L. A histochemical and morphologic study of post-obstructive diuresis in the rat. *Invest. Urol.* 14:169, 1976.

67. McDougal, W. S., and Persky, L. Renal functional abnormalities in post-ureteral obstruction in man: A comparison of these defects to postobstructive diuresis. *J. Urol.* 113:601, 1975.

68. McDougal, W. S., and Wright, F. S. Defect in proximal and distal sodium transport in postobstructive diuresis. *Kidney Int.* 2:304, 1972.

69. Maher, J. F., et al. Osmotic diuresis due to retained urea after release of obstructive uropathy. *N. Engl. J. Med.* 268:1099, 1963.

70. Malis, C. D., et al. Effects of verapamil in models of ischemic acute renal failure in the rat. *Am. J. Physiol.* 245:F735, 1983.

71. Mitchell, J. P. Current concepts: Trauma to the urinary tract. *N. Engl. J. Med.* 288:90, 1973.

72. Moses, A. M., and Miller, M. Urine and plasma osmolality in differentiation of polyuric states. *Postgrad. Med.* 52:187, 1972.

73. Mudge, G. H., et al. Tubular Transport of Urea, Glucose, Phosphate, Uric Acid, Sulfate, and Thiosulfate. In J. Orloff, R. W. Berliner, and S. R. Geiger (eds.), *Handbook of Physiology.* Section 8, Renal Physiology. Washington, D.C.: American Physiological Society, 1973. Pp. 589–594.

74. Muldowney, F. P., et al. Sodium diuresis after relief of obstructive uropathy. *N. Engl. J. Med.* 274:1294, 1966.

75. Murase, T., and Yoshida, S. Mechanism of chlorpropamide action in patients with diabetes insipidus. *J. Clin. Endocrinol. Metab.* 36:174, 1973.

76. Nayler, W. G., Poole-Wilson, P. A., and Williams, A. Hypoxia and calcium. *J. Mol. Cell. Cardiol.* 11:683, 1979.

77. Oken, D. E. Nosologic considerations in the nomenclature of acute renal failure. *Nephron* 8:505, 1971.

78. Paller, M. S., Hoidal, J. R., and Ferris, T. F. Oxygen free radicals in ischemic acute renal failure in the rat. *J. Clin. Invest.* 74:1156, 1984.

79. Papper, S., and Vaamondo, C. A. The Kidney in Liver Disease. In M. B. Strauss and L. G. Welt (eds.), *Diseases of the Kidney.* Boston: Little, Brown, 1971. Pp. 1139–1154.

80. Parker, S., et al. Dopamine administration in oliguria and oliguric renal failure. *Crit. Care Med.* 9:630, 1981.

81. Peart, W. S. Renin-angiotensin system. *N. Engl. J. Med.* 292:302, 1975.

82. Perillie, P. E., and Epstein, F. H. Sickling phenomenon produced by hypertonic solutions: A possible explanation for the hyposthenuria of sicklemia. *J. Clin. Invest.* 42:570, 1963.

83. Perlmutter, M., et al. Urine-serum urea nitrogen ratios. *J.A.M.A.* 170:1533, 1959.

84. Quinton, W. E., et al. Eight months experience with Silastic-Teflon bypass cannulas. *Trans. Am. Soc. Artif. Intern. Organs* 8:236, 1962.

85. Redman, J. I., Binkley, B. K., and Means, A. R. Regulation of microfilaments and microtubules by calcium and cyclic AMP. *Adv. Cyclic Nucleotide Res.* 11:131, 1979.

86. Reindenberg, M. M. *Renal Function and Drug Action.* Philadelphia: Saunders, 1971.

87. Renkin, E. M., and Robinson, R. R. Glomerular filtration. *N. Engl. J. Med.* 290:785, 1974.

88. Rosenthal, A., and Pace-Asciak, C. R. Potent vasoconstriction of the isolated perfused rat kidney by leukotrienes C_4 and D_4. *Can. J. Physiol. Pharmacol.* 61:325, 1983.

89. Sanders, R. C., and Jeck, D. L. B-Scan ultrasound in the evaluation of renal failure. *Radiology* 119:199, 1976.

90. Schlondorff, D., and Ardaillou, R. Prostaglandins and other arachidonic acid metabolites in the kidney. *Kidney Int.* 29:108, 1986.

91. Schrier, R. W. Acute renal failure. *Kidney Int.* 15:205, 1979.

92. Schrier, R. W., et al. Protection of mitochondrial function by mannitol in ischemic acute renal failure. *Am. J. Physiol.* 247:F365, 1984.

93. Schrier, R. W., and Berl, T. Nonosmolar factors affecting renal water excretion. *N. Engl. J. Med.* 292:81 and 141, 1975.

94. Share, L. Vasopressin: Its bioassay and the physiological control of its release. *Am. J. Med.* 42:701, 1967.

95. Share, L., and Claybaugh, J. R. Regulation of body fluids. *Annu. Rev. Physiol.* 34:235, 1972.

96. Shires, G. T., et al. Alterations in cellular membrane function during hemorrhagic shock in primates. *Ann. Surg.* 176:288, 1972.

97. Statius von Eps, L. W., et al. Nature of concentrating defect in sickle-cell nephropathy. *Lancet* 1:450, 1970.

98. Stein, J. H., Lifschitz, M. D., and Barnes, L. D. Current concepts in the pathophysiology of acute renal failure. *Am. J. Physiol.* 234:F171, 1978.

99. Thiel, G., et al. Micropuncture studies of the basis for protection of renin depleted rates from glycerol induced acute renal failure. *Nephron* 7:67, 1970.

100. Thomson, G. E. Acute renal failure. *Med. Clin. North Am.* 57:1579, 1973.

101. Thurau, K. J., et al. Composition of tubular fluid in the macula densa segment as a factor regulating the function of the juxtaglomerular apparatus. *Circ. Res.* 20, 21 (Suppl. 2):79, 1967.

102. Vander, A. J. Control of renin release. *Physiol. Rev.* 47:359, 1967.

103. Vander, A. J., and Miller, R. Control of renin secretion in the anesthetized dog. *Am. J. Physiol.* 207:537, 1964.

104. Van Neuten, J. M., and Vanhoutte, P. M. Improvement of tissue perfusion with inhibitors of calcium ion influx. *Biochem. Pharmacol.* 29:479, 1980.

105. Verney, E. B. Absorption and excretion of water. *Lancet* 2:739, 781, 1946.

106. Wait, R. B., White, G., and Davis, J. H. Beneficial effects of verapamil on postischemic renal failure. *Surgery* 94:276, 1983.

107. Wilson, D. R., et al. Glycerol induced hemoglobinuric acute renal failure in the rat. *Nephron* 4:337, 1967.

108. Witte, M. H., et al. Massive polyuria and natriuresis following relief of urinary tract obstruction. *Am. J. Med.* 37:320, 1964.

109. Yarger, W. E., et al. A micropuncture study of post-obstructive diuresis in the rat. *J. Clin. Invest.* 51:625, 1972.

110. Yin, H. L., and Stossel, T. P. Control of cytoplasmic action gel-sol transformation by gelsalin, a calcium-dependent regulatory protein. *Nature* 281:583, 1979.

Endocrine Dysfunction and Emergencies in Critical Illness

John R. Corsetti
Gregory G. Stanford
Bart Chernow

Endocrine and metabolic emergencies are relatively rare yet dramatic, problems in critical care medicine [17]. The endocrine emergencies include myxedema coma, thyroid storm, adrenal insufficiency, and diabetes insipidus. These emergencies serve as the basis for discussion in this chapter. Other endocrine emergencies, including pheochromocytoma (see Chap. 16) and hyperosmolar coma (see Chap. 25) are reviewed elsewhere.

The initial step in any endocrine emergency is to move the patient to a special care unit, where appropriate management can be provided. Even though one is dealing with a biochemical problem, one must assure adequate oxygenation, ventilation, and tissue perfusion. Once this goal is achieved, the clinician must ensure that the evidence for the endocrine problem is verified, and then therapeutic action is taken.

Critical care practitioners see, and care for, many patients with endocrine disorders (e.g., hyperglycemia, mild diabetes insipidus, hyponatremia due to SIADH). Endocrine emergencies are merely exaggerated manifestations of the more common endocrinopathies.

MYXEDEMA COMA
Myxedema coma is characterized by altered mental status and is due to a deficit in circulating thyroid hormones. Establishing the diagnosis of myxedema coma is difficult, due to the rarity of the disease; however, early diagnosis is crucial, since rapid treatment is the key to survival. The disease classically affects elderly women in the winter months; however, it is being seen in younger people with increasing frequency, due to the widespread use of radioactive iodine (^{131}I) in the treatment of thyroid gland hyperactivity [80]. Most commonly, the disease develops in individuals with a long history of hypothyroidism; in fact, the presence of a scar on the neck may serve as an aid in diagnosis. Moreover, myxedema coma is almost

Supported in part by funds from the Henry K. Beecher Memorial Anaesthesia Research Laboratories.

always associated with a precipitating event that causes decompensation and often life-threatening illness in the hypothyroid patient.

Etiology

A deficiency of thyroid hormone causes defective thermogenesis. In the course of long-standing hypothyroidism, several physiologic adaptations occur in an effort to ensure the maintenance of body temperature. These efforts of heat conservation consist of peripheral vasoconstriction, bradycardia, decreased cardiac output, and a resultant decrease in blood volume (up to 1 liter) due to decreased circulating aldosterone concentrations [69]. These changes, along with manifestations that affect virtually every organ system, render the hypothyroid patient unable to maintain homeostasis when faced with any of a variety of precipitating stresses (Table 22-1). Hypothyroidism in patients with myxedema is most often due either to the loss of thyroid tissue (thyroprivic hypothyroidism) or to defective hormone biosynthesis (thyrotrophic hypothyroidism). Uncommonly (5%), the hormone deficiency is due to hypothalamic or pituitary disease (trophoprivic hypothyroidism).

Clinical and Laboratory Findings

The clinical manifestations of long-standing hypothyroidism are protean, affecting every organ system. Recognition of myxedema coma on physical examination is important because therapy is best started early, without waiting for the results of thyroid hormone determinations. The disease garners its name from the generalized edematous appearance of the patient. This edema is due to the accumulation of hyaluronic acid complexed with water in the dermis. Unlike the edema of congestive heart failure, it is nonpitting and especially noticeable periorbitally and on the dorsae of the hands and feet. Protein and fluid extravasation, as well as deranged lymph flow, have been documented [72]. In addition, the skin is dry and cool and often has a yellow hue, due to increased carotene levels. The hair is dry and brittle and has a tendency to fall out; classically, there is loss of the temporal side of the eyebrows. These changes tend to be much less pronounced when the hypothyroidism is due to pituitary deficiency rather than primary glandular failure.

The cardiovascular changes of myxedema are due both to efforts to ensure heat and to decreased sensitivity to adrenergic stimuli. There is reduced cardiac stroke volume, bradycardia, and reduced cardiac output. Also, there is an increased peripheral vascular resistance and a decreased blood volume. The state of generalized vasoconstriction causes decreased blood flow to vital organs and is the main reason vasopressors should be used only as a last resort in this illness. The heart is often enlarged and the heart sounds may be distant due to the presence of a pericardial effusion. The pericardial effusion of myxedema may rarely lead to tamponade and life-threatening hemodynamics [84]. There may be elevations of serum creatine phosphokinase (CPK) and lactate dehydrogenase (LDH) concentrations, with an increased cardiac isoenzyme that, together with the edematous appearance, may lead to the mistaken diagnosis of acute myocardial infarction.

Table 22-1. Common precipitants of myxedema coma

1. Infection
2. Hypothermia
3. Drugs: diuretics, digitalis, sedatives
4. Surgery or trauma
5. Cerebrovascular accident
6. Hypoglycemia
7. Hypovolemia/blood loss
8. Congestive heart failure

The respiratory changes in hypothyroidism are often implicated as one of the most important factors in the decompensation and development of coma. There is a state of hypoventilation, with hypercapnia and hypoxia in the presence of a decreased respiratory rate. In addition, there is a decreased diffusion capacity for carbon monoxide, as well as a decreased ventilatory response to hypercapnia [94]. There are several reasons for these pulmonary abnormalities. The chest wall may function abnormally secondary to myxedematous infiltrate of striated muscle [6]. Decreased amounts of pulmonary surfactant have been found in hypothyroid rats [77]. Anatomic changes such as macroglossia and oropharyngeal edema may cause airway obstruction, often exacerbated by the fact that many of these patients are obese. Also, these patients metabolize drugs at a much slower rate than do euthyroid people and so are very sensitive to the respiratory effects of sedatives, narcotics, and tranquilizers [57, 68]. Finally, there is evidence that these patients have a decreased central respiratory drive [57]. Patients in myxedema coma very often require endotracheal intubation and mechanical ventilation for respiratory support.

The gastrointestinal system is also affected with constipation, decreased peristalsis, decreased absorption, and paralytic ileus that may progress to "myxedema megacolon." The patients may have fecal impaction on presentation. Ascites is occasionally observed. Up to 50 percent of patients have achlorhydria, and 12 percent have pernicious anemia. The liver and pancreas are generally normal.

There is decreased renal blood flow and a decreased glomerular filtration rate in myxedematous patients [71]. Hyponatremia is often a feature and may be due to inappropriate antidiuretic hormone secretion [73] or to diminished delivery of filtrate to the distal nephron in this relatively volume-depleted state. Azotemia is not commonly seen in hypothyroidism; however, patients with myxedema coma often have marked prerenal azotemia or even acute renal failure. Much of the retained water is complexed with hyaluronic acid, which gives the myxedematous appearance. This excess water accounts for much of the weight gain seen in this illness. All these changes are reversed by thyroid hormone replacement therapy.

There is often a normochromic, normocytic anemia, due to decreased erythropoietin, as well as myxedematous involvement of the bone marrow. The white blood cell count may be decreased, and there may be defective ability to generate a leukocytosis in response to infection, often making the diagnosis of infection difficult. The physician should be alerted to the possibility of infection by a leftward shift in the differential white blood count [69].

Diagnosis

Myxedema coma should be suspected in any patient with a history of hypothyroidism who presents with an altered mental status. Definitive diagnosis can be established only by knowing the serum thyroxine (T_4), triiodothyronine (T_3) and thyroid-stimulating hormone (TSH) concentrations. It is recommended that presumptive therapy be started if the diagnosis of myxedema coma is suspected (before any thyroid hormone levels are determined), because the small risk of giving thyroid hormone to a euthyroid patient is far outweighed by the disastrous outcome that results from withholding thyroid hormone replacement therapy from a patient in myxedema coma.

To make a clinical diagnosis of myxedema coma, three elements should be present [69]. First, there must be altered mental status. Second, there should be evidence of disordered thermoregulation. Thyroxine stimulates thermogenesis by enhancing membrane sodium potassium adenosine triphosphate (ATP) and increasing amino acid and fatty acid turnover. The patient in myxedema coma typically has a reduced core body temperature. However, a normal body temperature in a patient with myxedema can occur in the possible presence of infection [81]. Third, there should be some evidence of a precipitating event (Table 22-1). A summary of the laboratory abnormalities found in patients with myxedema is contained in Table 22-2.

Therapy

The cornerstone of therapy for myxedema coma is early replacement of thyroid hormone, along with careful attention to cardiovascular and respiratory support.

Thyroid hormone replacement may be administered as T_4 or T_3 and may be administered orally, intramuscularly, or intravenously. Table 22-3 shows the currently available thyroid hormone preparations. The initial doses of thyroid hormone should be given intravenously, as gut absorption may be unpredictable. It is unclear whether the replacement hormone should be given as T_4 or T_3. There is evidence that in severe illness, the peripheral conversion of T_4 to T_3 is greatly reduced, and that reverse T_3 (rT_3), an inactive compound, is preferentially formed [20]. Some authors feel that rapid repletion of high doses of T_4 is the best therapy [37, 79]. Others feel the rapid repletion of body T_4 stores is too much of a stress on the cardiovascular system and that hormone replacement should be done more slowly [39]. Because injectable T_3 is not readily available, we agree with the recommendation of administering between 100 and 500 μg T_4 (the dosages shall be based upon cardiac function). However, if injectable T_3 were commonly available, we believe it would be the preferred medication [18].

Corticosteroid replacement therapy (hydrocortisone, 50–100 mg three times a day) [6] is routine in these patients and should be started at the

Table 22-2. A summary of the laboratory abnormalities found in patients with severe hypothyroidism and myxedema coma

Hyponatremia; hypoglycemia; elevated serum levels of triglycerides, LDL, uric acid, beta carotene, CPK, LDH; increased CSF protein

Normochromic normocytic anemia, normal to decreased WBC, normal platelet count, increased PTT

Arterial blood gases: decreased O_2, increased CO_2, decreased DLCO; diminished ventilatory response to hypercapnia

CXR: enlarged heart, pericardial effusion, pleural effusion

KUB: ileus, $+/-$ ascites.

EKG: sinus bradycardia, flattened T, low-voltage QRS changes consistent with pericardial effusion

Table 22-3. Commonly used thyroid hormone preparations

Preparation	Daily maintenance dose
Levothyroxine (T_4)	100–200 µg
Liothyronine (T_3)	25–75 µg
Liotrix ($T_4 : T_3 = 4 : 1$)	See package insert/PDR

same time that T_4 or T_3 therapy is begun. A 30-minute adrenocorticotropic hormone (ACTH) stimulation test should be performed before the hydrocortisone therapy is begun. Adrenal insufficiency may coexist with myxedema of central origin and may be precipitated by the rapid increase in metabolic rate that occurs with thyroxine therapy [61].

Attention should be directed to the respiratory and cardiovascular status of the patient with myxedema coma. Hypoxia and hypercapnia are often present, and concurrent pneumonia should always be suspected. The majority of these patients require expeditious intubation and mechanical ventilation. Endotracheal intubation may be difficult, due to airway obstruction from macroglossia and/or oropharyngeal edema; in this case, tracheostomy is indicated.

Hypotension and cardiovascular collapse are frequent problems in these patients. Due to their decreased blood volume, myxedematous patients are exquisitely sensitive to any perturbation in volume status, such as occult bleeding, sepsis, and vasodilation due to warming. Vasoconstrictive adrenergic agents are rarely indicated for blood pressure maintenance and should be avoided, since there is already volume depletion and compromised tissue perfusion due to the increased systemic vascular resistance and reduced cardiac responsiveness to adrenergic input.

A thorough search for a precipitant of metabolic decompensation should be undertaken. Temperature increases and leukocytosis are not reliable indices and their absence does not exclude infection.

Hypothermia should be corrected centrally rather than with warming blankets, since the peripheral vasodilation that may occur with peripheral warming may lead to circulatory collapse. Small amounts of hypertonic saline may be indicated to treat hyponatremia. This saline may be given with furosemide if there is danger of congestive heart failure from volume overload. Hemodynamic monitoring is helpful here.

EUTHYROID-SICK SYNDROME

The most common abnormality of thyroid function seen in critically ill patients is the euthyroid-sick syndrome, which results from the slowing of peripheral thyroid hormone metabolism. Critically ill patients have rapid changes in hormonal function with the onset of critical illness [16]. Thyroid function also changes rapidly in critically ill adults [96] and children [97]. Many of these patients have the euthyroid-sick syndrome. This syndrome is characterized by low serum T_4 and T_3 and increases in serum rT_3 [95]. The free fractions of T_4 and T_3 usually remain normal. This biochemical abnormality is due to the inhibition of thyroid hormone binding to protein and to diminished 5'-deiodinase activity (Fig. 22-1). This enzyme catalyzes the conversion of T_4 to the more active T_3 in organs such as the liver, kidney, and pituitary gland [19]. The other enzyme that acts on T_4 is 5-deiodinase. This enzyme converts T_4 to rT_3 and is not affected by critical illness. Therefore, T_4 is preferentially shunted to the rT_3 pathway in critical illness, due to the diminished activity of 5'-deiodinase. In addition, rT_3 is normally metabolized to 3,3-deiodothyronine by 5'-deiodinase; therefore, rT_3 accumulates due to an increased synthesis and decreased breakdown. These patients are clinically euthyroid and have normal serum thyrotropin (TSH) concentrations.

The euthyroid-sick syndrome appears to be an adaptive phenomenon in states of critical illness. The diminished T_3 production limits the utilization of protein and oxygen and decreases the metabolic demands on the heart [89]. Administration of thyroid hormone replacement may be deleterious in these patients and has been found to increase urinary nitrogen and 3-methyl-histidine excretion [12, 34]. It therefore becomes important to distinguish the euthyroid-sick syndrome, which does not require treatment, from hypothyroidism, which does require treatment. The serum TSH concentration is normally a sensitive indicator of hypothyroidism but can occasionally be misleading in critical illness. Serum TSH concentrations have not been found to be increased in response to decreases in circulating T_4 and T_3 in about 50 percent of patients with nonthyroidal illness [59]. A more reliable means of determining thyroid function in critical illness is to measure the free thyroxine index or perform a thyrotropin-releasing hormone (TRH) test, a simple bedside test in which 250 to 500 μg of TRH (available commercially as Relefact TRH) is administered intravenously. The TSH concentration is measured 15 to 30 minutes later. Serum TSH concentrations double or triple in response to TRH in patients with the euthyroid-sick syndrome, whereas the hypothyroid patient shows an exaggerated response of 6 to 8 times normal. In spite of the availability of new, highly sensitive TSH tests [27], evidence is accumulating that the TSH concentration may not be reliable in serious nonthyroidal illness [16, 85].

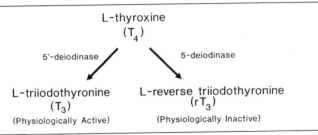

Fig. 22-1. In healthy individuals, the majority of T_4 is metabolized to T_3. However, in critical illness, T_4 is preferentially metabolized to the physiologically inactive rT_3, because of an inhibition of 5'-deiodinase.

The free thyroxine index is available and can be measured directly with an equilibrium dialysis method or approximated by multiplying the T_4 concentration by the T_3 resin uptake (T_3RU).

THYROID STORM
Thyroid storm is a life-threatening medical emergency in which prompt recognition and treatment are essential. Though there are no specific criteria for the diagnosis of thyroid storm, the condition is characterized by an accentuation of the usual signs and symptoms of thyrotoxicosis. The illness is most commonly seen in patients with a history of thyrotoxicosis.

Etiology
The causes of thyrotoxicosis are detailed in Table 22-4. Graves' disease, characterized by the presence of thyroid-stimulating immunoglobulin, is the most common form of thyrotoxicosis. Another cause of thyrotoxicosis is in toxic multinodular goiter, in which autonomously functioning areas of thyroid tissue secrete T_4 in the absence of an appropriate stimulus. Overproduction of TSH, usually by a pituitary adenoma, is an uncommon cause of thyrotoxicosis. These three conditions are similar in that they cause an enhanced uptake of radioactive iodine (RAIU) by the thyroid gland. Thyroiditis may cause a transient state of hyperthyroidism as T_4 leaks out from an immunologically damaged gland. Thyrotoxicosis due to overingestion of thyroid hormone and stroma ovarii, or ectopic thyroid tissue, may also be associated with a hyperthyroid state. These latter conditions do not represent true gland hyperfunction and are characterized by an abnormally low RAIU.

Thyroid storm is usually seen in patients under stress who have a long-standing history of thyrotoxicosis. Common precipitants include infection, surgery, trauma, psychologic stress, withdrawal from antithyroid drug treatment, treatment of poorly controlled thyrotoxicosis with radioiodine, diabetic ketoacidosis, and episodes of congestive heart failure. Thyrotoxicosis can also be induced in critically ill patients through the use of iodine-rich drugs, such as amiodarone, povidone-iodine, and radiographic contrast agents [50, 58, 76]. The incidence of thyroid crisis in patients admitted

Table 22-4. Causes of thyrotoxicosis

I. Conditions associated with gland hyperfunction
   1. Hypersecretion of TSH
   2. Graves' disease
   3. Trophoblastic tumor
   4. Hormone-producing adenoma
   5. Toxic multinodular goiter
II. Conditions not associated with gland hyperfunction
   1. Subacute thyroiditis
   2. Chronic thyroiditis with transient thyrotoxicosis
   3. Ectopic thyroid tissue (struma ovarii)

---

to the hospital for thyrotoxicosis was previously estimated at 5 to 10 percent [91]. Now, with β-blocker therapy, the frequency of thyroid storm is less than 0.5 percent. Even though thyroid storm is very rare in the United States, thyrotoxicosis is common. Patients who develop thyroid crisis generally have had symptoms of thyrotoxicosis for at least 2 months [91].

Thyroid storm or moderate thyrotoxic symptoms and signs may be observed postoperatively in patients undergoing subtotal thyroidectomy as therapy for hyperthyroidism. This unfortunate complication is essentially avoided by the preoperative administration of antithyroid medication and β-adrenergic receptor antagonists (β-blockers). Options for preoperative treatment of hyperthyroidism include antithyroid medications (propylthiouracil [PTU] or methimazole) in combination with iodine or lithium.

Some surgeons advocate the use of β-adrenergic blockers alone as preoperative therapy, citing reduced treatment time, fewer side effects, and faster relief of symptoms as advantages over the traditional use of PTU or methimazole preoperatively [45]. Other authors do not recommend using propranolol alone, especially in severely thyrotoxic patients requiring high doses of β-blocker to achieve acceptable heart rate control and relief of symptomatology. They note that although a mildly thyrotoxic patient may have a benign intra- and postoperative course when managed with propranolol alone, patients who are severely thyrotoxic, requiring supplemental β-blocker doses, have a higher heart rate during surgery and a more marked postoperative temperature rise, as well as a greater propensity to show signs of thyroid hormone excess (agitation, pyrexia, diaphoresis, tachycardia) [31, 51]. In summary, propranolol alone is safe and effective preoperative therapy for patients with relatively mild thyrotoxicosis whose symptoms are easily controlled with the drug. In more severe cases of thyrotoxicosis, it is prudent to use propylthiouracil or methimazole in combination with iodine or lithium to avoid adverse postoperative symptomatology.

Clinical and Laboratory Findings
Patients with thyroid storm present with the signs and symptoms of thyrotoxicosis. In addition, they commonly are febrile, due to the thermogenic properties of T_4, and have central nervous system alterations ranging from

agitation and confusion to lethargy, somnolence, and coma. Thyroid storm is a clinical diagnosis of a life-threatening illness due to the excess of thyroid hormone and cannot be differentiated from ordinary thyrotoxicosis by any laboratory criteria.

Symptoms include nervousness, heat intolerance, sweating, fatigue, palpitations, insomnia, irritability, emotional lability, shortness of breath, increased appetite or anorexia, nausea and vomiting, and an increased frequency of stools. Cardiovascular signs of thyrotoxicosis include tachycardia, loud S1 and S2, a systolic ejection murmur, and a hyperdynamic precordium. Pulmonary edema or even anasarca may be present if the patient has overt congestive heart failure. Nausea and vomiting with abdominal pain are not symptoms of thyrotoxicosis per se but may herald the onset of thyroid storm. The patient generally complains of severe muscle weakness, and muscular atrophy of the shoulder and pelvic girdle, as well as of the thighs, may be evident. There is shortening of the contraction and relaxation phases of the deep tendon reflexes. Males may exhibit gynecomastia, and females may have galactorrhea and oligo- or amenorrhea. Long-standing hyperthyroidism causes enhanced bone turnover with resorption exceeding formation, resulting in osteoporosis. In thyroid storm, the cardiovascular findings combine with fever and CNS signs to dominate the clinical picture. In addition, there should be a careful search for the signs and symptoms of a precipitating infection or illness.

The serum total T_4 concentration is not greater in thyroid storm than in patients with compensated thyrotoxicosis [2]. There is, however, a marked increase in the concentrations of free thyroxine, and a defect in binding to thyroxine binding globulin is postulated in thyroid storm [10]. Other than alterations in serum thyroid hormone values, there are few laboratory abnormalities characteristic of thyrotoxicosis. There may be hypercalcemia and hyperglycemia (due to the gluconeogenic and glycogenolytic effects of thyroid hormone). Thyrotoxicosis is a glucose-intolerant state with decreased glucagon suppression and impaired insulin response to hyperglycemia [46]. Some thyrotoxic patients develop a macrocytic, hypochromic anemia. A macrocytic anemia may be seen in patients with Graves' disease who also develop atrophic gastritis and pernicious anemia. An increase in the white blood cell count or a leftward shift in the differential should alert the physician to the possibility of infection. The serum cholesterol may be decreased, but circulating free fatty acid and triglyceride levels are increased. Serum alkaline phosphatase concentrations (from bone) are increased. Importantly, the electrocardiogram may show atrial fibrillation or flutter with a rapid ventricular response.

Diagnosis

The diagnosis of thyroid storm is best made on the basis of history of a precipitating event in the presence of a history and findings suggestive of hyperthyroidism. An early diagnosis permits therapy to commence at the earliest possible time, often before the results of any thyroid function tests are available. Laboratory tests demonstrate increases in RAIU, serum T_4 and T_3 [11], T_3RU, and free thyroxine index.

Therapy

Therapy for thyroid storm consists of general supportive measures in concert with definitive measures aimed at lowering the patient's metabolic rate. Hyperpyrexia should be treated with acetaminophen and cooling blankets as needed. Aspirin should be avoided, because it may cause an increased metabolic rate, possibly by displacing T_3 from binding globulin [47]. Congestive heart failure should be treated with diuretics and oxygen. Digitalis or calcium-channel blockers are indicated for the treatment of atrial fibrillation with a rapid ventricular response. Glucocorticoids are useful to prevent adrenal insufficiency; they also inhibit the peripheral conversion of T_4 to T_3. The usual glucocorticoid dose is 50 mg hydrocortisone intravenously every 8 hours (we recommend performance of an ACTH stimulation test prior to glucocorticoid administration). Of primary importance is to rapidly lower the serum T_4 and T_3 levels and to prevent the thyroid gland from releasing more hormone. This goal is best accomplished with PTU, which blocks synthesis of active hormone and inhibits peripheral T_4 to T_3 conversion. PTU is not available for intravenous use and must be administered orally or via a nasogastric tube if the patient is unable to swallow. PTU (250 mg) should be administered every 6 hours. Alternatively, methimazole can be used in dosages of 30 mg every 6 hours until the patient is euthyroid. The maintenance dose of methimazole is 10 to 30 mg a day. Unlike PTU, methimazole does not affect peripheral thyroid hormone conversion, and PTU is preferred in thyroid storm. Iodine can be administered as either iodine solution (Lugol's solution, 6 mg/drop) or potassium iodide solution (1 gm/ml). In thyrotoxic crisis, the dose of iodine used is either two drops of Lugol's solution or 50 to 100 mg of potassium iodide solution every 12 hours. Iodine should be given 1 to 2 hours after PTU or methimazole, to prevent iodine accumulation in the thyroid gland. Sodium iodide may also be given intravenously in doses of up to 1000 mg per day. β-adrenergic blockers are a mainstay of therapy. Propranolol can be administered intravenously at a rate of 1 mg/min up to a maximum of 5 mg. The dose should then be repeated in 4 to 6 hours. Oral maintenance dosages range from 20 to 200 mg every 6 hours in order to control symptoms. Subsequent dosing should be directed at maintaining a heart rate at 90 beats per minute or less. Propranolol, in addition to its cardiovascular actions, inhibits the peripheral conversion of T_4 to T_3. Other beneficial effects are improved carbohydrate tolerance and reduced negative nitrogen balance. Under this regimen, serum T_3 generally returns to normal in 24 to 48 hours. Iodine should then be withdrawn from the regimen and definitive therapy for hyperthyroidism instituted.

ADRENAL INSUFFICIENCY

Adrenocortical insufficiency is classified as primary or secondary. Primary failure is due to adrenal glandular disease (from autoimmune disease, infections, hemorrhage, or, rarely, metastasis). Secondary adrenal failure is due to hypothalamic-pituitary disease or to suppression of the hypothalamic-pituitary adrenal axis by exogenous corticosteroid therapy. The syndrome of adrenal insufficiency may develop insidiously or may have a sudden onset, depending on the etiology. Whatever the cause, early diagnosis and therapy are critical to the survival of the patient.

Etiology

The leading cause of primary adrenocortical insufficiency is now autoimmune-mediated atrophy of the adrenal glands. In a 1974 report concerning 108 patients with adrenal insufficiency, 66 percent were classified as idiopathic (autoimmune disease) and 17 percent were due to tuberculosis [67]. There is strong evidence that the idiopathic destruction of the gland is an immunologically mediated process. In one series, 73 percent of women and 50 percent of men with primary adrenocortical insufficiency had circulating antibodies to adrenocortical tissue [40]. In addition, there is a high prevalence of antibodies to other endocrine glands (islet cells of the pancreas, thyroid, parathyroid) in these patients [40]. Patients with tuberculous-induced adrenal insufficiency do not have these circulating antibodies.

Tuberculous infection of the adrenal gland was at one time the dominant cause of adrenocortical insufficiency, responsible for 80 percent of cases in one series [28]. It is now a much less common cause of the disease. Other infectious causes include histoplasmosis [24], blastomycosis [29], and coccidiomycosis [33].

Carcinomatous infiltration of the gland, although relatively common, rarely causes functional failure [14]. Only 20 percent of functional gland mass is required for normal plasma cortisol levels and responsiveness to exogenous ACTH. The most common primary sites of tumors metastatic to the adrenal glands are the lung and breast [14].

Impairment of vascular supply to the gland can also precipitate adrenal crisis. This problem may occur as a result of vasculitis and adrenal vein thrombosis [42]. Glandular hemorrhage may also be part of the sepsis syndrome or a result of trauma, or it may occur with large burns [48]. Hemorrhage of the adrenal glands is particularly associated with meningococcal sepsis. Another recognized cause of impaired vascular supply is the heparin-induced thrombotic thrombocytopenic syndrome [3]. The cause of this syndrome is postulated to be paradoxical adrenal vein thrombosis with resultant gland infarction. Rare causes of primary adrenal insufficiency include acquired immunodeficiency syndrome [87], amyloidosis [54], and the use of medications such as ketoconazole [74] and etomidate [49, 90].

Secondary adrenal insufficiency is due either to chronic gland suppression from endogenously produced or exogenously administered corticosteroids or to hypothalamic-pituitary lesions (neoplasms, infection, trauma, sarcoidosis). The most common cause of secondary adrenal insufficiency today is chronic adrenal suppression from the use of corticosteroids in the treatment of some other disease process. There is much variability in the duration of steroid therapy, which causes adrenal suppression and insufficiency. Adrenal insufficiency has been reported following discontinuation of glucocorticoids given for as short a time as 2 weeks [83].

Pathophysiology

The syndrome of adrenal insufficiency is characterized by disturbances in a number of organ systems. Failure to produce the mineralocorticoid aldosterone leads to sodium wasting as the ability of the distal nephron to retain sodium chloride is greatly diminished. Potassium excretion likewise fails, and hyperkalemia results; however, total body stores of potassium are generally decreased in this disease, due to vomiting and diarrhea. So while the initial therapy may be directed at reversing hyperkalemia, total body stores of potassium may eventually need to be repleted. The inability to retain sodium leads to a state of intravascular volume depletion and hypotension. The hyponatremia is worsened by the release of vasopressin by the pituitary in response to hypotension, causing further free-water retention [8]. Renal blood flow is compromised, reducing distal delivery of filtrate and further impairing the diluting ability of the kidney.

Clinical and Laboratory Findings

Weakness, fatigability, weight loss, anorexia, hypotension, and hyperpigmentation are seen in virtually all patients with adrenal insufficiency. The hyperpigmentation is most pronounced in skin creases, on extensor surfaces, and on old scars. Nausea and vomiting are seen in about one-half of patients.

All of the signs and symptoms of adrenal insufficiency take time to develop, and their absence may lead the clinician away from the correct diagnosis. One situation in which adrenal insufficiency is particularly difficult to diagnose is in the postoperative patient. Abdominal pain, hypotension, fever, tachycardia, volume depletion, nausea and vomiting, and delirium are all signs and symptoms of adrenal insufficiency; however, in the early postoperative period, they are often ascribed to other, more frequent, causes. In one series of patients who developed adrenal insufficiency after coronary artery bypass procedures, symptoms of adrenal insufficiency began 4 to 10 days postoperatively, but the diagnosis of adrenal insufficiency was made, on average, on postoperative day 19 [1]. Postoperative adrenal insufficiency may occur in patients with Addison's disease who are on inadequate corticosteroid doses considering the stress of surgery, or it may occur de novo due to adrenal hemorrhage as a complication of surgery or sepsis [38].

Although spontaneous adrenal hemorrhage may occur in any patient, it is more likely to occur in those patients subjected to the greatest stresses [41]. The etiology of adrenal hemorrhage is not known, but it may be produced experimentally with large doses of endotoxin or ACTH [53]. The diagnosis of adrenal insufficiency should at least be considered in postoperative patients with acute decompensation when other causes are not evident. The diagnosis is supported by fever, leukocytosis, increased BUN, hyperkalemia, and hyponatremia. An eosinophil count of greater than $500/mm^3$ is considered highly suggestive of adrenal insufficiency in the acutely ill patient [30].

Diagnosis

The diagnosis of adrenal insufficiency is very often a difficult one to establish, especially in the absence of some cardinal features, such as hyperpigmentation. Unfortunately, the proper diagnosis is often made at autopsy. The patient with adrenal insufficiency is characteristically acutely ill, has poorly responsive hypotension, and develops an evolving shock syndrome [52]. The symptoms [2] and electrolyte abnormalities [21] both take 2 to 3 days to evolve after adrenal failure. If the diagnosis is entertained, the clinician should become especially aware of such points as a history of tuberculosis, prior use of corticosteroids, use of anticoagulants, history of other autoimmune disorders, presence of widely metastatic cancer, history of pituitary or hypothalamic disease, or bacterial sepsis, especially meningococcal sepsis [66]. One study demonstrated that 20 percent of patients with sepsis had an impaired adrenal response to infection, as well as a subnormal response to endogenous ACTH stimulation [82].

Therapy

Treatment of the patient in Addisonian crisis has three principal objectives: (1) repletion of glucocorticoids, (2) repletion of sodium and water deficits, and (3) correction of hypoglycemia.

Addisonian crisis is a life-threatening syndrome, and treatment with high-dose intravenous glucocorticoids must be instituted as soon as the diagnosis is suspected. A rapid ACTH stimulation test may be performed if there is doubt regarding the proper diagnosis, and in this case initial glucocorticoid therapy should consist of dexamethasone instead of hydrocortisone hemisuccinate. Initially, hydrocortisone hemisuccinate, 100 to 200 mg, should be administered intravenously as a slow bolus. Volume resuscitation should begin immediately in the form of isotonic normal saline (0.9%) containing 50 g (5%) dextrose. The first liter should be given over 30 minutes, and then at 1 liter per hour until the patient is clinically euvolemic. Central venous monitoring is generally not necessary. Vasopressors may be required to sustain adequate blood pressure in the initial stages of therapy. If hypotension exists initially, vasopressor agents such as norepinephrine should be avoided, as tissue perfusion is already compromised, and inotropes such as dobutamine should be used instead. Hydrocortisone (50–100 mg every 6 hours) should be administered intravenously for the first 24 hours of treatment. Patients should not be allowed oral intake for at least 10 to 12 hours, to avoid potential vomiting and aspiration. Glucocorticoid therapy may be switched to oral supplementation on day 2 if the patient is well stabilized. Hydrocortisone (20 mg every 8 hours) should be given and then tapered at a rate of 10 to 15 mg/day until maintenance dosage (20 to 30 mg/day) is reached. Glucocorticoid doses in this range have enough mineralocorticoid activity to obviate the need for supplementation. Fludrocortisone (Florinef), 0.1 to 0.2 mg orally, may be required in primary adrenal failure when more mineralocorticoid activity is necessary [36].

Hyperkalemia is rarely in excess of 7 mEq/liter and usually responds rapidly to glucocorticoid replacement, glucose administration, and rehydration. Because these patients have deficient total body stores of potassium, supplementation (20 to 40 mEq) may be necessary after the first several hours of treatment. In addition to these therapeutic measures, a careful search for a precipitant of adrenal insufficiency should be made. This search includes a careful history and physical examination along with blood, urine, and sputum cultures and a chest radiograph. After all appropriate cultures are performed, it is wise to institute empirical broad-spectrum antibiotic coverage. Doses of glucocorticoid in excess of those outlined above may be required when adrenal crisis is precipitated by trauma or infection.

DIABETES INSIPIDUS

Diabetes insipidus (DI) is characterized by the inability to generate a concentrated urine and conserve solute-free water in the face of appropriate stimuli. This disease is due either to a failure of the pituitary gland to secrete adequate amounts of antidiuretic hormone (termed *central diabetes insipidus*) or to a lack of renal tubular responsiveness, either congenital or acquired, to the antidiuretic actions of antidiuretic hormone (termed *nephrogenic diabetes insipidus*). The cardinal features of the disease are polyuria, polydipsia, intense thirst, and a tendency toward hyperosmolar plasma [64].

Etiology
The most common causes of central diabetes insipidus are the following.

1. *Neoplastic or infiltrating lesions of the hypothalamus or pituitary,* such as craniopharyngioma, pituitary adenoma, metastatic lesions, sarcoidosis, histiocytosis, leukemia, and lymphoma. The presence of diabetes insipidus is the single most important feature in differentiating a metastatic pituitary lesion from a benign pituitary adenoma [55]. In one series, 14 percent of patients with diabetes insipidus had cancer metastatic to the pituitary gland [43]. Lung and breast cancers are the most common origins for metastases to the pituitary gland [44, 55, 75, 88].

2. *Head trauma,* usually severe enough to cause skull or facial fracture [7, 35] may cause DI, although cases of DI have been reported from minor head trauma [43]. The pathophysiology is thought to be shearing trauma to the pituitary stalk. The time of onset of posttraumatic diabetes insipidus is variable, but it generally becomes manifest 5 to 10 days after trauma [75].

3. *After surgery on the pituitary or hypothalamus.* Postoperative diabetes insipidus is more common in posteriorly located pituitary adenomas [4].

4. *Idiopathic diabetes insipidus.* One must be careful to exclude occult cancer in patients in whom a diagnosis of idiopathic diabetes insipidus is suggested. Apparently normal head CT scans should be followed up carefully to identify possible expanding pituitary lesions [26].

5. *Nephrogenic DI,* either congenital or acquired.

Pathophysiology

The defect in central diabetes insipidus may exist in (a) the osmoreceptors, (b) the cells of the synaptic or paraventricular nuclei or their axons, (c) the posterior pituitary storage site, or (d) the site of ADH action on the renal collecting tubule. Diabetes insipidus after surgery or trauma is presumably due to hemorrhage, trauma, or edema in the area of the neurohypophysis. Patients undergoing ablative pituitary surgery classically exhibit a triphasic vasopressin response [55] in the immediate postoperative period, initially exhibiting polyuria with a fall in urine osmolality and rise in urine volume. This phase is followed by 5 to 7 days of decreased urine output and a rise in urine osmolality. This so-called interphase is presumably due to vasopressin leak from damaged and degenerating neurons. The final stage is characterized by frank diabetes insipidus with a loss of concentrating ability. This sequence is important for the critical care specialist, because hypotonic fluids started during the initial polyuric phase may lead to water overload and cerebral edema if continued into the interphase period.

Simple removal of the posterior pituitary does not necessarily cause diabetes insipidus [13]. Rather, injury to the supraopticohypophyseal tract must be sufficiently high in the pituitary stalk to cause retrograde degeneration of the supraoptic and paraventricular nucleus neurons [32]. In patients undergoing surgery in the area of the hypothalamus or pituitary, it is always important to closely monitor urine output and the serum sodium postoperatively.

Clinical and Laboratory Findings

The classical clinical picture includes polyuria, intense thirst for cold fluids, and nocturia. Patients with complete loss of ADH secretion may urinate every 30 minutes and have a total daily urinary volume up to 18 liters, equal to the total filtrate reaching the collecting ducts. Those with partial ability to synthesize and secrete vasopressin may lose lesser amounts of fluid. If denied access to water, the patient may rapidly develop striking symptomatology, including stupor, lethargy, and coma.

Laboratory studies in patients with diabetes insipidus show persistently hypotonic urine, with urinary osmolality less than 200 mOsm/liter, serum hypernatremia, and normal glomerular filtration rate. Urine specific gravity is generally less than 1.005. Urine osmolality is not necessarily below that of plasma. In mild cases, the urine osmolality may be 300 to 600 mOsm/liter, and the disease manifests itself only when the patient is denied access to water. Under those circumstances, the inability to concentrate urine beyond a certain level causes excessive free-water loss, plasma hypertonicity, and thirst. DI is important to recognize in the unconscious postcraniotomy patient, since hypertonicity can develop rapidly when water is lost in excess of solute. Isotonic saline administration in large volumes is particularly dangerous unless adequate volumes of solute free water are also administered.

Diagnosis

The diagnosis of diabetes insipidus is made by establishing that the kidney is unable to produce a maximally concentrated urine in the presence of the osmotic stimuli of either dehydration or hypertonic saline infusion. The easiest and safest test to use is the dehydration test. Radioimmunoassay of plasma ADH is available but is seldom necessary to establish a diagnosis.

A water deprivation test can be used to confirm the diagnosis of diabetes insipidus. The principle of this test is to create an osmotic stimulus for the patient to maximally concentrate urine and to then assess the effect of exogenous ADH on the urine osmolality. The test can distinguish among normals, those with partial central DI, those with severe central DI, and those with nephrogenic DI.

1. The patient is denied access to all fluids until the urine osmolality reaches a steady state (<30 mOsm/kg increase for 3 consecutive hours). Fluid restriction should begin at 4:00 to 5:00 A.M. for severely polyuric patients (>10 liters/day), in order that they may be suppressed during the entire test. For mildly polyuric patients (2 to 6 liters/day), fluid restriction should begin at 6:00 P.M. on the previous day. Patients with severe polyuria will take 3 to 6 hours to achieve a constant urine osmolality, whereas those with mild polyuria may take up to 18 hours [60].

2. After the urinary osmolality stabilizes, the patient is administered vasopressin, either 5 units of aqueous vasopressin, 1 μg desmopressin subcutaneously, or 10 μg desmopressin intranasally. A urine specimen should be collected immediately before vasopressin administration.

3. Urine is collected every 15 minutes for the next hour, and osmolality determined.

Vasopressin increases the permeability of the collecting tubules to water, allowing the flow of water down the osmotic gradient between the lumen and the medullary interstitium. The ability to concentrate urine, therefore, is dependent both on the medullary interstitial tonicity and on the presence of vasopressin. The medullary tonicity is affected by previous water diuresis [9] and illnesses such as pyelonephritis, so it is not relevant to define an absolute minimum value for normal maximal concentrating ability. One study showed a maximal urine osmolality in randomly selected hospital patients of 764 and a value of 1067 in normal volunteers [62].

Patients with severe central diabetes insipidus are unable to concentrate their urine above plasma osmolality when challenged by dehydration. Furthermore, they demonstrate a greater than 50 percent increase in urine osmolality when administered exogenous ADH [9]. Patients with partial diabetes insipidus are able to produce urine that is hyperosmolar relative to plasma, but when given exogenous ADH, they show a greater than 10 percent rise in urinary osmolality [9]. This finding implies that the endogenous levels of vasopressin are insufficient to maximally stimulate the collecting tubules to reabsorb water. If patients with partial diabetes insipidus are dehydrated for longer periods of time, they eventually show a paradoxical fall in urine osmolality, implying exhaustion of a limited vasopressin reserve. Normal patients and patients with primary polydipsia are able

Table 22-5. Currently available vasopressin preparations

Preparation	Route	Dose
Aqueous vasopressin	Subcutaneous, intramuscular Intranasal	5–10 units bid or tid Individualized
Vasopressin tannate in oil	Intramuscular	0.3–1 ml (48–96 hr duration)
Lysine vasopressin	Intranasal	1–2 sprays each nostril qid
Desmopressin (dDAVP)	Intranasal Subcutaneous, intravenous	5–10 μg bid 1–2 μg bid

to concentrate their urine beyond plasma levels and do not increase their urine osmolality more than 10 percent with exogenous ADH. Patients with nephrogenic DI or polyuria from potassium depletion show little rise in plasma osmolality with dehydration and do not respond to exogenous ADH.

The diagnosis of polyuria in the critically ill patient is frequently encountered. Essentially, the physician must distinguish between excessive water intake (primary polydipsia, central thirst center disorders), central diabetes insipidus, nephrogenic diabetes insipidus (congenital, lithium, hypokalemia, hypercalcemia, chronic renal disease), and osmotic diuresis (glycosuria, mannitol, diuretics). Patients with primary polydipsia have a urinary concentrating defect due to a diluted medullary interstitium caused by long-standing polyuria. They can be distinguished from those with diabetes insipidus by the dehydration test. Urine should be examined for the presence of glucose, and a history of mannitol or other diuretic use should be elicited. The causes of renal resistance to vasopressin—particularly hypokalemia, hypercalcemia, drug use, and renal disease—should be sought.

Therapy

The primary goals in the treatment of diabetes insipidus are to decrease urine output and to restore plasma hypertonicity. Those patients with urine output of less than 5 liters/day may not require any specific therapy. A list of the currently available vasopressin preparations is provided in Table 22-5.

Desmopressin (1-deamino,8-D-arginine vasopressin [dDAVP]) may be administered intravenously, intranasally, or subcutaneously [78]. It is similar in structure to vasopressin; the modifications result in a molecule with a high antidiuretic-to-pressor potency (2000 : 1) and an increased duration of action (12 to 24 hours) compared with arginine vasopressin [22]. Because of its long duration of action, its availability as an intranasal spray, its paucity of side effects, and its potent antidiuretic activity, dDAVP has become the drug of choice for neurogenic diabetes insipidus. The intranasal dose of dDVAP is 5 to 10 μg twice a day. It can also be given intravenously or subcutaneously in doses of 1 to 2 μg twice a day. One should establish a dose by first determining the minimum dose that controls nocturia. The same or slightly higher dose can be used to control daytime polyuria [22]. Rarely, patients may exhibit tolerance to the drug [22].

Aqueous vasopressin is useful for the acute management of postoperative neurosurgical or trauma patients because of its short half-life. One should be careful not to administer vasopressin during the interphase period.

dDVAP also temporarily increases factor VIII:C and vonWillebrand factor and is useful in augmenting hemostasis [5, 54, 75]. It should not be used in patients with factor VIII:C activities less than 5 percent, patients with factor IX deficiency, or patients with type IIB vonWillebrand's disease [56]. The dosage used is 0.3 μg/kg in 50 ml of normal saline infused intravenously over 15 to 30 minutes. This dosage can be used daily, but administration more often than every 2 to 3 days diminishes the response.

Other drugs useful in the management of diabetes insipidus include chlorpropamide, clofibrate, carbamazepine, and thiazides. Chlorpropamide acts by potentiating the effect of ADH at the renal tubule [65]. It is useful in patients with some ability to produce ADH. Doses of 250 to 750 mg/day are usually sufficient to effect antidiuresis in 50 to 80 percent of patients. Clofibrate, given in doses of 400 to 600 mg/day, stimulates ADH release and produces an antidiuresis [63]. The combination of clofibrate and chlorpropamide is also effective [92]. Thiazide diuretics are also useful in both central and nephrogenic diabetes. They paradoxically reduce polyuria by producing a state of relative volume depletion, reducing GFR. Proximal solute reabsorption is increased and the delivery of filtrate to the diluting segment is reduced, interfering with the ability of the kidney to generate a dilute urine. The usual dose is 50 to 100 mg hydrochlorothiazide daily [23]. It is effective only in conjunction with salt restriction.

SYNDROME OF INAPPROPRIATE ADH SECRETION (SIADH)

The normal physiologic response to hyponatremia and increased arterial volume is the suppression of ADH secretion. When this system becomes deranged, the syndrome of inappropriate ADH secretion (SIADH) develops. It is characterized by hyponatremia, hypoosmolality, and increased intravascular volume. SIADH is most often associated with certain carcinomas, especially lung and pancreatic tumors. It can also develop after head trauma; with central nervous system disorders; in certain pulmonary diseases, such as tuberculosis; and in glucocorticoid deficiency. Drug-induced SIADH can occur after the administration of vincristine, chlorpropamide, cyclophosphamide, barbiturates, opiates, and indomethacin [70].

The diagnosis is based on the demonstration of inappropriately high urine concentration in relation to serum osmolality. The diagnostic criteria are hyponatremia, lower serum osmolality, urine osmolality less than maximally dilute with a urine sodium concentration greater than 20, no volume depletion, and normal renal, adrenal, and thyroid function [15]. The treatment of SIADH is water restriction. Other effective treatment modalities are furosemide [25], lithium [93], and phenytoin [86]. Demeclocycline decreases the renal response to ADH and is effective in dosages of 300 mg every 6 hours [25].

SUMMARY

Endocrine problems are common in critical care medicine but are rarely fatal if recognized and treated promptly. Critical care physicians should maintain a high index of suspicion, especially in those patients who do not have a clear etiology for their cardiovascular or metabolic abnormalities. It is not uncommon for subclinical disease to become manifest during the stress of a serious illness, and therefore, endocrine function should be aggressively evaluated in all cases of complicated critical illness.

REFERENCES

1. Alford, W., Mihalevich, J., Glassford, D., and Thomas, C. Acute adrenal insufficiency following cardiac surgical procedures. *J. Thorac. Cardiovasc. Surg.* 78:489, 1979.
2. Amador, E. Adrenal hemorrhage during anticoagulant therapy. *Ann. Intern. Med.* 63:559, 1965.
3. Anduson, K., Kuharjda, F., and Bell, W. Diagnosis and treatment of anticoagulant-related adrenal hemorrhage. *Am. J. Hematol.* 11:379, 1981.
4. Balestrieri, F., Chernow, B., and Rainey, T. G. Post-craniotomy diabetes insipidus—Who's at risk? *Crit. Care Med.* 10:108, 1982.
5. Bichet, D. G., Razi, M., Lonergan, M., Arthus, M. F., Papukna, V., Kortas, C., and Barjon, J. N. Hemodynamic and coagulation responses to 1-desamino (8-D-arginine) vasopressin in patients with congenital nephrogenic diabetes insipidus. *N. Engl. J. Med.* 381:881, 1988.
6. Blum, M. Myxedema coma. *Am. J. Med. Sci.* 264:432, 1972.
7. Bowerman, J., and Heslop, I. Diabetes insipidus associated with maxillofacial injury. *Br. J. Oral Surg.* 8:197, 1971.
8. Boykin, T., DeTorrente, A., Erickson, A., Robertson, G., and Shrier, R. Role of plasma vasopressin in impaired water excretion of glucocorticoid deficiency. *J. Clin. Invest.* 62:738, 1978.
9. Bray, G. Freezing point depression of rat kidney slices during water diuresis and antidiuresis. *Am. J. Physiol.* 199:915, 1960.
10. Brooks, M., and Waldstein, S. Free thyroxine concentrations in thyroid storm. *Ann. Intern. Med.* 93:694, 1980.
11. Brooks, M., Waldstein, S., Bronsky, D., and Sterling, K. Serum triiodothyronine concentration in thyroid storm. *J. Clin. Endocrinol. Metab.* 40:339, 1975.
12. Burman, K. D., Wartofsky, L., Dinterman, R. F., et al. The effect of T_3 and reverse T_3 administration on muscle protein catabolism during fasting as measured by 3-methyl-histidine excretion. *Metabolism* 28:805, 1979.
13. Camus, J., and Roussy, G. Experimental researches on the pituitary body. *Endocrinology* 4:507, 1920.
14. Cedermark, B., and Sjoberg, H. The clinical significance of metastases to the adrenal glands. *Surg. Gynecol. Obstet.* 152:607, 1981.
15. Chernow, B. Hormonal and Metabolic Considerations in Critical Care Medicine. In W. C. Shoemaker, W. L. Thompson, and P. R. Holbrook (eds.), *Textbook of Critical Care*. Philadelphia: Saunders, 1984. Pp. 646–664.
16. Chernow, B., Alexander, H. R., Thompson, W. R., Cook, D., Beardsley, D., Fink, M. P., Smallridge, R. C., and Fletcher, J. R. Hormonal responses to graded surgical stress. *Arch. Intern. Med.* 147:1273, 1987.
17. Chernow, B., and Anderson, D. M. Endocrine responses to critical illness. *Semin. Respir. Med.* 7:1, 1985.

18. Chernow, B., Burman K. D., Johnson, D., O'Brian, J. T., Wartofsky, L., and Georges, L. P. T_3 may be a better agent than T_4 in the critically ill hypothyroid patient: Evaluation of transport across the blood-brain barrier in a primate model. *Crit. Care Med.* 11:99, 1983.

19. Chopra, I. An assessment of daily production and significance of thyroidal secretion of 3,3′,5′-triiodothyronine (reverse T_3) in man. *J. Clin. Invest.* 58:32, 1976.

20. Chopra, I., Chopra, U., Smith, S., Rega, M., and Solomon, D. Reciprocal changes in serum concentrations of 3,3,′5′-triiodothyronine (reverse T_3) and 3,3′,5 triiodothyronine (T_3) in systemic illness. *J. Clin. Endocrinol. Metab.* 41:1043, 1975.

21. Clark, O. Postoperative adrenal hemorrhage. *Ann. Surg.* 182:124, 1975.

22. Cobb, W., Spare, S., and Reichlin, S. Neurogenic diabetes insipidus: Management with dDAVP (1-desamino-8-D-arginine vasopressin). *Ann. Intern. Med.* 88:183, 1978.

23. Crawford, J., and Kennedy, G. Clinical results of treatment of diabetes insipidus with drugs of the chlorothiazide series. *N. Engl. J. Med.* 262:737, 1960.

24. Crispell, K., Parson, W., Hamlin, J., et al. Addison's disease associated with histoplasmosis. *Am. J. Med.* 20:23, 1956.

25. Decaux, G., Waterlot, Y. Ganette, F., et al. Treatment of the syndrome of inappropriate secretion of antidiuretic hormone with furosemide. *N. Engl. J. Med.* 304:329, 1981.

26. Dietemann, J., Banneville, J., and Hirsch, E., et al. The need for repeated CT examinations in hypothalamic-pituitary pathology. *J. Neuroradiol.* 12:113, 1985.

27. Dubuis, J. M., and Burger, A. G. Thyroid-stimulating hormone measurements by immunoradiometric assay in severely ill patients. *Lancet* 2:1036, 1986.

28. Dunlop, D. Eighty-six cases of Addison's disease. *Br. J. Med.* 2:887, 1963.

29. Eberle, D., Evans, R., and Johnson, R. Disseminated North American blastomycosis occurrence with clinical manifestations of adrenal insufficiency. *J.A.M.A.* 238:2629, 1977.

30. Faloon, W., Reynolds, R., Beebe, R. The use of the direct eosinophil count in the diagnosis and treatment of Waterhouse-Friederichsen syndrome. *N. Engl. J. Med.* 242:441, 1950.

31. Feely, J., Crooks, J., Forrest A., Hamilton, W., and Gunn, A. Propranolol in the surgical treatment of hyperthyroidism, including severely thyrotoxic patients. *Br. J. Surg.* 68:865, 1981.

32. Fisher, C., Ingram, W., and Ranson, S. Relation of hypothalamico-hypophysio system to diabetes insipidus. *Arch. Neurol. Psychiat.* 34:124, 1935.

33. Forbes, W., and Beiterbreutje, A. Coccidiomycosis: A study of 95 cases of the disseminated type with special reference to the pathogenesis of the disease. *Military Surg.* 99:553, 1946.

34. Gardner, D. F., Kaplan, M. M., Stanley, C. S., et al. The effect of triiodothyronine replacement on the metabolic and pituitary responses to starvation. *N. Engl. J. Med.* 300:579, 1979.

35. Goldman, K., and Jacobs, A. Anterior and posterior pituitary failure after head injury. *Br. Med. J.* 2:1924, 1960.

36. Graber, A., Ney, R., Nicholson, W., et al. Natural history of pituitary adrenal recovery following long term suppression with corticosteroids. *J. Clin. Endocrinol. Metab.* 25:11, 1965.

37. Holvey, D., Goodner, C., Nicoloff, J., and Dowling, J. Treatment of myxedema coma with intravenous thyroxine. *Arch. Intern. Med.* 113:89, 1964.

38. Hubay, C., Weckesser, E., and Levy, R. Occult adrenal insufficiency in surgical patients. *Ann. Surg.* 181:325, 1975.

39. Hylander, B., and Rosenqvist, U. Treatment of myxedema coma—Factors associated with fatal outcome. *Acta Endocrinol.* 108:65, 1985.
40. Irvine, W. Autoimmunity in endocrine disease. *Proc. R. Soc. Med.* 67:548, 1974.
41. Jagatic, J., and Rubnitz, M. Massive bilateral adrenal bleeding: Five-year review of cases. *Ill. Med. J.* 2:68, 1942.
42. Kaufman, G. Adrenal cortical necrosis. An autopsy study. *Arch. Pathol.* 97:395, 1974.
43. Kern, K., and Meislin, H. Diabetes insipidus: Occurrence after minor head trauma. *J. Trauma* 24:69, 1984.
44. Kimmel, D., and O'Neill, B. Systemic cancer presenting as diabetes insipidus. *Cancer* 52:2355, 1983.
45. Kovacs, K. Metastatic cancer of the pituitary gland. *Oncology* 27:533, 1973.
46. Lam, K. S. L., Yeung, R. T. T., Ho, P. W. M., and Lam, S. K. Glucose intolerance in thyrotoxicosis: Roles of insulin, glucagon and somatostatin. *Acta Endocrinol.* 114:228, 1987.
47. Larsen, P. Salicylate-induced increases in free triidothyronine in human serum. *J. Clin. Invest.* 51:1125, 1972.
48. Lead article: Adrenal hemorrhage and apoplexy. *Lancet* 2:295, 1976.
49. Ledingham, I. Mc. A., and Watt, I. Influence of sedation on mortality in critically ill multiple trauma patients. *Lancet* 1:1270, 1983.
50. Leger, A. F., Massin, J. P., Laurent, M. F., Vincens, M., Auriol, M., Helal, O. B., Chomette, G., and Savoie, J. C. Iodine-induced thyrotoxicosis: Analysis of eighty-five consecutive cases. *Eur. J. Clin. Invest.* 14:449, 1984.
51. Lennquist, S., Jortso, E., Anderberg, B., and Smeds, S. Beta blockers compared with antithyroid drugs as preoperative treatment in hyperthyroidism: Drug tolerance, complications and postoperative thyroid function. *Surgery* 98:1141, 1985.
52. Leshin, M. Acute adrenal insufficiency: Recognition, management and prevention. *Urol. Clin. North Am.* 9:229, 1982.
53. Levin, J., and Cluff, L. Endotoxemia and adrenal hemorrhage: A mechanism for the Waterhouse-Friderichsen syndrome. *J. Exp. Med.* 121:247, 1965.
54. Liddle, G. Pathogenesis of glucocorticoid disorders. *Am. J. Med.* 53:638, 1972.
55. Lipsett, M., Maclean, J., West, C., et al. An analysis of the polyuria induced by hypophysectomy in man. *J. Clin. Endocrinol. Metab.* 16:183, 1956.
56. Mannucci, P. M., Cancaini, M. T., Rota, L., and Donovan, B. S. Response of factor VIII/von Willebrand factor to dDAVP in healthy subjects and patients with haemophilia A and von Willebrand's disease. *Br. J Haematol.* 47:283, 1981.
57. Massumi, R., Winnacker, J. Severe depression of the respiratory center in myxedema. *Am. J. Med.* 36:876, 1964.
58. Martino, E., Aghini-Lombardi, F. Mariotti, S., Bartalena, L., Braverman, L., and Pinchera, A. Amiodarone: A common source of iodine-induced thyrotoxicosis. *Horm. Res.* 26:158, 1987.
59. Maturo, S. J., Rosenbaum, R. L., Pan, C., et al. Variable thyrotropin response to thyrotropin-releasing hormone after small decreases in plasma free thyroid hormone concentrations in patients with nonthyroidal disease. *J. Clin. Invest.* 66:451, 1980.
60. Max, M., Deck, D., and Rottenberg, D. Pituitary metastasis: Incidence in cancer patients and clinical differentiation from pituitary adenoma. *Neurology* (*NY*) 31:998, 1981.
61. McCullock, W., Price, P., Hinds, C., and Wass, J. Effects of low dose oral triiodothyronine in myxedema coma. *Int. Care Med.* 11:259, 1985.

62. Miller, M., Dalakos, T., Moses, A., Fellerman, H., and Streeten, D. Recognition of partial defects in antidiuretic hormone secretion. *Ann. Intern. Med.* 73:721, 1970.

63. Moses A., Howanitz, J., van Gemert, M., and Miller, M. Clofibrate-induced antidiuresis. *J. Clin. Invest.* 52:533, 1973.

64. Moses, A., Frontiers of Hormone Research. In P. Czunichow and A. Robinson (eds.), *Diabetes Insipidus in Man*, Vol. 13. Basel, Kayer, 1985.

65. Moses, A., Numann, P., and Miller, M. Mechanism for chlorpropamide-induced antidiuresis in man: Evidence for release of ADH and enhancement of peripheral action. *Metabolism* 22:59, 1973.

66. Migeon, C., Kenny, F., Hung, W., and Voorhess, M. Study of adrenal function in children with meningitis. *Pediatrics* 40:163, 1967.

67. Nerup, J. Addison's disease—clinical studies: A report of 108 cases. *Acta Endocrinol.* 76:127, 1974.

68. Nichel, S., and Frame, B. Nervous and muscular system in myxedema. *J. Chronic Dis.* 14:570, 1961.

69. Nicoloff, J. Myxedema coma and thyroid storm. *Med. Clin. North Am.* Sept. 1985.

70. Oh, M. S., and Carroll, H. J. Electrolyte and acid-base disorders. In B. Chernow (ed.), *The Pharmacologic Approach to the Critically Ill Patient.* Baltimore: Williams and Wilkins, 1987. Pp. 803–817.

71. Papper, S., and Lancestremere, R. Certain aspects of renal function in myxedema. *J. Chronic Dis.* 14:495, 1961.

72. Parimy, H., Hansen, J., Nielsen, S., Rossing, N., Munck, O., and Lassen, N. Mechanism of edema formation in myxedema—increased protein extravasation and relatively slow lymphatic drainage. *N. Engl. J. Med.* 301:460, 1979.

73. Pettinger, W., Talner, L., and Ferris, T. Inappropriate secretion of antidiuretic hormone due to myxedema. *N. Engl. J. Med.* 272:362, 1965.

74. Pont, A., Williams, P., Loose, D., Feldman, D., Reitz, R., Bochra, C., and Stevens, D. Ketoconazole blocks adrenal steroid biosynthesis. *Ann. Intern. Med.* 97:370, 1982.

75. Porter, R., and Miller, R. Diabetes insipidus following closed-head injury. *J. Neurol. Neurosurg. Psychiat.* 11:258, 1948.

76. Rajatanavin, R., Safran, M., Stoller, W. A., and Mordes, J. P. Five patients with iodine-induced hyperthyroidism. *Am. J. Med.* 77:378, 1984.

77. Redding, R., Douglas, W., and Stein, M. Thyroid hormone influence upon lung surfactant metabolism. *Science* 175:994, 1972.

78. Richardson, D. W., and Robinson, A. G. Desmopressin. *Ann. Intern. Med.* 103:228, 1985.

79. Ridgway, E., McCammon, J., Benotti, J., and Maloof, F. Acute metabolic responses in myxedema to large doses of intravenous L-thyroxine. *Ann. Intern. Med.* 77:549, 1972.

80. Senior, R., and Birge, S. The recognition and management of myxedema coma. *J.A.M.A.* 217:61, 1971.

81. Senior, R., Birge, S., Wessler, S., and Anoli, L. The recognition and management of myxedema coma. *J.A.M.A.* 217:61, 1971.

82. Sibbald, W., Short, A., Cohen, M., and Wilson, R. Variations in adrenocortical responsiveness during severe bacterial infections. *Ann. Surg.* 186:29, 1977.

83. Slaney, G., and Brooke, B. Postoperative collapse due to adrenal insufficiency following cortisone therapy. *Lancet* 1:1167, 1957.

84. Smolar, E., Rubin, J., Avramides, A., and Carter, A. Cardiac tamponade in primary myxedema and review of the literature. *Am. J. Med. Sci.* 272:345, 1976.

85. Spencer, C., Elgen, A., Shen, D., Duda, M., Quails, S., Weiss, S., and Nicoloff, J. Specificity of sensitive assays of thyrotropin (TSH) used to screen for thyroid disease in hospitalized patients. *Clin. Chem.* 33:1391, 1987.
86. Tanay, A., Yust, I., Peresecenschi, G., et al. Long-term treatment of the syndrome of inappropriate antidiuretic hormone secretion with phenytoin. *Ann. Intern. Med.* 90:50, 1978.
87. Tapper, M., Rotterdam, H., Lerner, C., Al'Khafaji, K., and Seitzman, P. Adrenal necrosis in the acquired immunodeficiency syndrome. *Ann. Intern. Med.* 100:239, 1984.
88. Teears, R., and Silverman, E. Clinicopathologic review of 88 cases of carcinoma metastatic to the pituitary gland. *Cancer* 36:216, 1975.
89. Utiger, R. D. Decreased extrathyroidal triiodothyronine production in nonthyroidal illness: Benefit or harm? *Am. J. Med.* 69:807, 1980.
90. Wagner, R. L., White, P. F., Kan, P. B., et al. Inhibition of adrenal steroidogenesis by the anesthetic etomidate. *N. Engl. J. Med.* 103:1415, 1984.
91. Waldstein, S., Slodki, S., Kaganiec, G., and Bronsky, D. A clinical study of thyroid storm. *Ann. Intern. Med.* 52:626, 1960.
92. Weitzman, R., and Kleeman, C. The clinical physiology of water metabolism. Part II: Renal mechanisms for urinary concentration; diabetes insipidus. *West. J. Med.* 131:486, 1979.
93. White, M. G., and Fetner, C. D. Treatment of the syndrome of inappropriate secretion of antidiuretic hormone with lithium carbonate. *N. Engl. J. Med.* 292:390, 1975.
94. Wilson, W., and Bedell, G. The pulmonary abnormalities in myxedema. *J. Clin. Invest.* 39:42, 1960.
95. Woeber, K. A., and Maddux, B. A. Thyroid hormone binding in nonthyroidal illness. *Metabolism* 30:412, 1981.
96. Zaloga, G. P., Chernow, B., Smallridge, R. C., Zajtchuk, R., Hall-Boyer, K., Hargraves, R., Lake, C. R., and Burman, K. D. A longitudinal evaluation of thyroid function in critically ill surgical patients. *Ann. Surg.* 201:456, 1985.
97. Zucker, A., Chernow, B., Fields, A. I., Hung, W., and Burman, K. D. Thyroid function in critically ill children. *J. Pediatr.* 107:552, 1985.

Fluid and Electrolyte Management

Robert J. Freeark
Robert C. Morris

DEFINITION OF THE PROBLEM

Management of the fluid and electrolyte requirements of the critically ill is an exercise in optimizing physiologic function [2]. Fluid and electrolyte therapy requires knowledge of the normal physiology of water and the serum electrolyte constituents. In addition, certain organ systems are of paramount importance—in particular, the kidney, which plays a central role in water and sodium conservation through several mechanisms, including the effects of antidiuretic hormone, the effects of the renin-angiotensin axis, and the effects of aldosterone.

Potassium and acid-base balance are also influenced by renal function and the effects of drug therapy, particularly diuretics.

Extrinsic to organ systems function, problems in fluid and electrolyte therapy may arise as a consequence of the therapies involved in the management of the ill or injured. One example is the use of mannitol for the patient with a closed head injury. If not carefully observed, alterations in tonicity, as well as an alteration in volume status, may occur, further complicating the management of the head-injured patient.

Less-emphasized but important constituents may be altered because of dietary restrictions imposed by illness or injury. This leads to abnormalities secondary to deficits in calcium, phosphorus, and magnesium.

A detailed discussion of cardiac physiology as it pertains to cardiac filling pressures and volume status is beyond the scope of this discussion, but the determination of adequate volume status is sometimes inaccurate using standard bedside indices of heart rate, blood pressure, and urine output.

Normal physiology as it pertains to water and electrolyte distribution will be discussed briefly, and discussion of pathophysiologic events will be presented in terms of changes in volume, concentration, and composition.

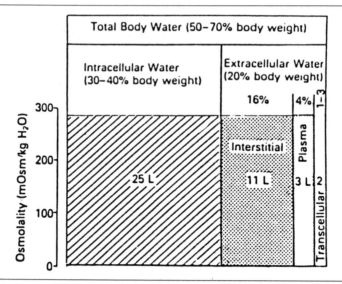

Fig. 23-1. Approximate sizes of major body fluid compartments, expressed as both percentage body weight and in mean absolute values. (From H. Valtin, *Renal Function: Mechanisms Preserving Fluid and Solute Balance in Health.* [2nd ed.] Boston: Little, Brown, 1983. P. 24.)

THE ANATOMY OF BODY FLUIDS

Body Water

Total body water (TBW) is distributed between two major compartments: those of intracellular fluid (ICF) and extracellular fluid (ECF). The ECF is further distributed between plasma and the interstitial fluid. (So-called transcellular fluid—gastrointestinal, cerebrospinal fluid, etc.—is not important in fluid balance except where sequestration of fluid may be excessive.)

The relative proportions of TBW, ICF, and ECF are as follows: total body water is approximately 60 percent (50–70%) of body weight, and of that, two-thirds is distributed in the ICF and one-third in the ECF [26] (see Fig. 23-1).

Concentration and Composition of Fluid Compartments

The composition of the various fluid compartments is illustrated in Table 23-1 and graphically depicted in Figure 23-2. In Table 23-1, total amounts are listed, and in Figure 23-2, the various concentrations of constituents in mEq/liter H_2O are depicted.

The osmolality (a function of the number of particles in solution) is essentially equal in all compartments, so there is no net water movement between compartments in the steady state. In the ECF, since Na^+ is the cation of the greatest concentration, it contributes most to the osmolality, as illustrated by the calculation

$$Osm = 2(Na^+) + 1/2.8(BUN) + 1/18(glucose)$$

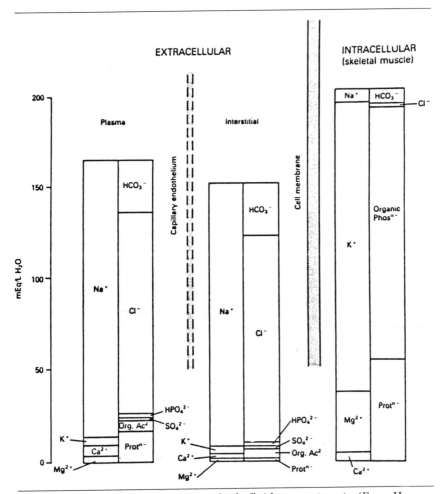

Fig. 23-2. Solute constituents of major body fluid compartments. (From H. Valtin, *Renal Function: Mechanisms Preserving Fluid and Solute Balance in Health.* [2nd ed.] Boston: Little, Brown, 1983. P. 28.)

Because the cell membrane and vascular endothelium are semipermeable to constituents such as proteins and there are active mechanisms to maintain the intracellular electrolyte composition, there is an unequal distribution of diffusible substances between the ICF and the ECF and between plasma and interstitial fluid, respectively. Because plasma proteins are not freely diffusible to the interstitium, they serve to retain water in the vascular space. This creates a small hydrostatic pressure difference. Oncotic pressure is the difference in osmotic pressure between two compartments accounted for by differing concentrations of proteins in the two compartments [7].

Where this fact may be of some importance is in the observation that in some disease states, hypoproteinemia may contribute to a loss of oncotic

Table 23-1. Composition of 70-kg man

Component	Extracellular		Intracellular	Bone	Total
	Plasma	Interstitial fluid			
Body water (kg or liter)	3.5	10	33	3.5	50
% body water	7	20	66	7	100
% body weight	5	15	50	5	71
mOsm/liter	290	290	290		
Na^+ (mEq)	500 (10%)	1,400 (30%)	600 (15%)	2,000 (45%)	4,500 (100%)
K^+ (mEq)	15 (<1%)	40 (1%)	3,300 (94%)	145 (4%)	3,500 (100%)
Ca^{++} (mEq)	18 (<1%)	50 (<1%)	100 (<1%)	59,900 (99%)	60,000 (100%)
Mg^{++} (mEq)	7 (<1%)	20 (<1%)	1,073 (50%)	1,000 (48%)	2,100 (100%)
Cl^- (mEq)	350 (15%)	1,000 (45%)	350 (15%)	500 (25%)	2,200 (100%)
$H_2PO_4^-$ and $HPO_4^=$ (mM)*	4 (<1%)	12 (<1%)	2,800 (14%)	17,000 (85%)	20,000 (100%)

*Because of different valence states, mass is expressed as millimoles (mM).

pressure in plasma that may favor fluid losses to the interstitial space, contributing to edema formation.

Implications for Fluid Therapy

As the foregoing discussion indicates, alterations in body fluid can occur as a result of volume changes and compositional changes. Volume changes in general are the result of the excess administration or loss of isotonic fluid and are confined to the ECF, whereas concentration changes in general are the result of the loss or gain of water or Na^+, respectively, and result in water movement between ICF and ECF.

Composition changes reflect excesses or losses in constituents such as K^+, Mg^{++}, and Ca^{++} and may lead to cellular dysfunction.

ALTERATIONS IN VOLUME STATUS

The least complicated changes in volume status are those that result from a gain or loss of isotonic fluid. Because there are no concentration changes, there is no water movement between the ICF and ECF compartments.

Volume deficits may be the result of protracted emesis, diarrhea, or translocation of plasma volume into the so-called third space, as is frequently seen in the postoperative patient. In these patients, volume deficits are best replaced with isotonic fluids, since isotonic fluids are lost. How rapidly deficits are replaced will depend upon the severity as assessed by vital signs. Occasionally, as alluded to earlier, invasive monitoring may be required to assess cardiac performance and adequacy of cardiac filling.

There are several methods of replacing deficits and carrying out maintenance fluid therapy. In general, these methods are based on body surface area or body weight determinations, or on estimates of measured (sensible) or unmeasured (insensible) losses (see Table 23-2).

A useful method of estimating fluid requirements is to do so using body weight. This calculation is based on the fact that a certain amount of water is required for metabolic needs, and that metabolic activity is proportional to body weight. Approximately 1 ml of water is required for each kilocalorie generated, and the number of kilocalories required has been computed as related to body weight. This calculation takes into account basal metabolic rate, in addition to providing some additional calories to allow for expenditures during normal activities [16]. The formula is as follows:

100 ml/kg for first 10 kg

50 ml/kg for second 10 kg

20 ml/kg for remaining body weight

For a 70-kg man, accordingly, this daily fluid is 2500 ml. The composition of the replacement fluid for maintenance requirements is generally hypocaloric and hypotonic. In general, the kidney can regulate sodium excretion, but because of obligatory loss, potassium must be supplemented, usually in the form of potassium chloride.

Sodium usually is administered in the form of 0.45% NaCl solutions, which give approximately 9 gm of sodium chloride daily.

Table 23-2. Sensible/insensible water loss

Route	Volume (cc/day)
Sensible	
Urine	800–1500
Stool	0–250
Sweat	0
Insensible	
Lungs/skin	600

Potassium is provided by giving 0.5 to 1.0 mEq K^+/kg body weight per day as potassium chloride.

Volume deficits can be replaced by giving an estimated amount or if losses are known, a measured amount. One method of administering deficit volume in the postoperative patient is to give additional volume based on a quadrant scheme of the abdomen [10]. Each quadrant accounts for additional volume to be given as one-fourth of calculated maintenance based on the involvement of that portion of the abdomen.

Regardless of the method used to calculate fluid requirements, therapy should be based on adequacy of tissue perfusion and cardiac function as assessed by blood pressure, urine output, heart rate, and normal acid-base status.

In the chronically ill patient, fluid replacement therapy may be complicated by the effects of malnutrition and hypoproteinemia. Whether colloid-containing solutions (albumin, dextran, hydroxyethyl starch) should be used to supplement or replace electrolyte-containing solutions is a controversial issue in fluid replacement therapy [16].

ALTERATIONS IN CONCENTRATION AND TONICITY

Alterations in the concentration of solutes generally are related to the ratio of solutes to water. Because the sodium ion is the predominant cation in the ECF, changes in sodium concentration reflect TBW gain or deficit. Less important are the contributions of urea and glucose, as they represent only a small portion of osmotically active particles under normal conditions. However, urea and glucose can be important in conditions such as renal failure with severe azotemia and hyperglycemia, especially when associated with diabetic ketoacidosis and nonketotic coma.

The mechanisms of Na^+ and water balance involve a number of organ systems and depend on intact renal function (salt and water handling), hypothalamic function [antidiuretic hormone (ADH) secretion, osmoregulation, and thirst], and adrenal function (aldosterone), in addition to the effects of drugs that may sensitize the kidney to ADH or stimulate the release of ADH. A number of disease states (e.g., neoplasms, pulmonary infections, central nervous system infections), trauma, stress, and metabolic disorders may contribute to ADH release by nonosmotic mechanisms [20].

Serum osmolality is normally in the range 285 to 290 mOsm/kg water. In the evaluation of patients in whom disorders of concentration are sus-

Table 23-3. Osmolar gap (measured-calculated)
of greater than 10 mOsm/kg H_2O

I. Decreased serum water
   Hyperlipidemia
   Hyperproteinemia
II. Low-molecular-weight substances
   Mannitol
   Ethanol
   Methanol
   Ethylene glycol

---

pected, determination of osmolar "gap" leads to consideration of certain diagnoses, including decreased serum water content, as might be seen in lipid disorders, or the addition of low molecular weight substances, as might be seen in ingestion of ethylene glycol (Table 23-3) [13]. Use of the calculated osmolality may give some idea of the magnitude of water excess or water loss.

Tonicity

Tonicity is a measure of water movement across a semipermeable membrane. Because sodium ion is an impermeable solute, an accumulation of extracellular sodium will cause water movement from ICF to ECF. Urea is freely permeable to cell membranes and will increase osmolality but will not affect tonicity, so no water movement occurs between ICF and ECF on the basis of urea accumulation alone.

As tonicity takes into account only the effects of sodium and glucose, it is calculated as follows [9]:

$$\text{Tonicity} = 2(Na^+) + (\text{glucose}/18)$$

Tonicity, then, as measured in mOsm/liter of water, is slightly less than osmolality, as the effects of freely permeable substances such as urea do not affect water movement from the intracellular to the extracellular compartment.

Hypertonic syndromes seen in the intensive care setting are those related to water loss in excess of sodium loss, solute increase in excess of water gain, or solute increase in the face of water losses [12].

One clinical situation in which one sees these syndromes is in the patient who is administered mannitol for the treatment of increased intracranial pressure. The end point of therapy is to increase tonicity to cause cellular dehydration.

Mannitol also causes an osmotic diuresis with ECF volume contraction that may manifest itself, depending on water movement from the ICF. Treatment of this condition involves replacement of the free-water deficit in addition to replacement of losses (volume deficit) due to the diuretic effect. An estimation of the water deficit can be obtained from the relationship [8]

Deficit = 0.6(kg body wgt) × [1 − (140/measured sodium)]

The calculation of pure water deficit is based on several assumptions. There is an increase in impermeable solute in the ECF, which causes water movement from the ICF in order to restore tonicity between the ECF and ICF. Total body solute remains constant, and therefore hypertonicity is proportional to water loss.

$$(TBW \times posm)_i = (TBW \times posm)_f$$

where TBW = total body water, posm = plasma osmolality, and the subscripts denote initial and final conditions, respectively.

$$
\begin{aligned}
\text{Water deficit} &= TBW_i - TBW_f \\
&= TBW_i [1 - (p_i osm/p_f osm)]
\end{aligned}
$$

Serum sodium may be substituted, since in the absence of solute change, sodium is the major determinate of osmolality in plasma [13].

Example
In a 70-kg man with a serum sodium of 155 mEq/liter, a 4-liter water deficit is calculated.

Replacement should be guided by the degree of dehydration and patient response.

A second clinical scenario in which hypertonicity develops is that of hyperglycemia [9]. The setting is the administration of an acute glucose load without glucose utilization. Depending on the level of glucose elevation, pseudohyponatremia may be seen because of water shift (1.5 mEq/liter decrease for every 100 mg% increase). More often, one sees a diuresis because of the osmotic effects of glucose, ECF volume contraction, azotemia, and ketosis in those patients with absolute insulin deficiency with the aggravating consequences of metabolic acidosis and a further contribution to hyperosmolality by ketoacids.

In using serum sodium to assess for dehydration, a "corrected" serum sodium allows for better estimation of the water deficit. Treatment involves replacement of the volume deficit with isotonic solutions; correction of hyperglycemia, which may or may not require insulin; and then replacement of the water deficit lost as a result of hypertonicity [9].

A third clinical scenario in which hypertonicity may be seen is diabetes insipidus associated with head trauma or in the postoperative period following pituitary or hypothalamic surgery. Use of low-dose vasopressin administered intravenously has been described [3,19]. The dose described has been in the range of 1 IU/hour. This regimen can be used to control ongoing losses while replacing the water deficit.

In summary, the treatment of hypertonicity should replace deficits, match ongoing losses, and decrease those ongoing losses. This involves obtaining some estimate of the "pure" water deficit and treating the underlying disease processes.

Table 23-4. Causes of hyponatremia

↑ *ECF*
CHF
Liver failure
Nephrotic syndrome
↓ *ECF*
Diuretics
Vomiting
Adrenal insufficiency
Normal ECF
SIADH
Postoperative states

Adapted from N.F. Rossi and P. Cadnapapornehai, Disordered water metabolism: Hyponatremia. *Crit. Care Clin.* 5:759, 1987. With permission.

Hyponatremia ($Na^+ < 134$ mEq/liter) may occur in a number of clinical settings [22]. Generally, the cause of hyponatremia is the combined consequence of excessive water intake and impaired water excretion (Table 23-4).

In the disease states of congestive heart failure, liver failure, and renal failure (nephrotic syndrome) ECF volume is increased. There is decreased water excretion on the basis of the effects of a decrease in glomerular filtration rate and neurohumoral factors on tubular function leading to increased water absorption. Vasopressin is increased on the basis of nonosmotic stimulation and leads to further water absorption by its effect on the distal tubule.

Where ECF volume is decreased, as in mineralocorticoid deficiency or vomiting, salt wasting occurs (renal or extrarenal) with volume contraction; nonosmotic stimulation of vasopressin occurs; and water excretion is limited in the face of continued sodium and electrolyte loss. The water retention is inadequate to correct ECF volume deficit, because it is predominantly distributed to ICF [14].

Where ECF volume is normal, as in the syndrome of inappropriate ADH secretion (SIADH), the increased activity of vasopressin is operative. As the patient continues to receive water or hypotonic replacement fluids, hyponatremia results (see Table 23-4).

Assessment of the patient with hyponatremia first involves a determination of osmolality. Hyponatremia with normal osmolality occurs in the states of hyperlipidemia or hyperproteinemia. Hyponatremia associated with increased osmolality may occur with hyperglycemia, because of water shift secondary to the change in tonicity caused by glucose.

The next assessment is of volume status, which proceeds with a history and physical examination. Signs of orthostasis, the presence of edema, and jugular venous distention are sought. Additionally, ECF fluid volume in hyponatremia may be more accurately determined with a measure of urine Na^+ [4]. In patients found to be responsive to saline loading (ECF contracted), the urine Na^+ averaged 18 mEq/liter; in those nonresponsive to saline infusion, urine Na^+ averaged 72 mEq/liter [4].

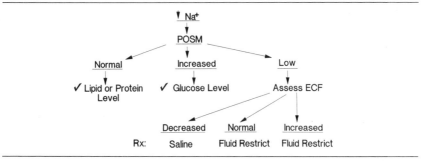

Fig. 23-3. Treatment scheme for hyponatremia. (Adapted from N.F. Rossi, Disordered water metabolism: Hyponatremia. *Crit. Care Clin.* 5:772, 1987.)

After determination of volume status and osmolality, treatment of those patients with hypotonic hyponatremia who have expanded or normal ECF volume involves fluid restriction. Patients who are hypovolemic should be treated with normal saline [22] (Fig. 23-3). There is some controversy over how rapidly one should correct hyponatremia [25]. With severe hyponatremia (Na$^+$ < 110 mEq/liter), symptoms primarily related to neurologic dysfunction are commonly seen, but these may also be related to the rate of change in the sodium concentration.

In patients who are symptomatic, and particularly in those with SIADH, one regimen recommended is to induce diuresis with furosemide, measure urinary electrolyte losses, and replace the losses with hypertonic saline (3% or 5% sodium chloride) and supplemental potassium chloride [15,22]. Use of demeclocycline may have some benefit in chronic SIADH. This antagonist of vasopressin on the kidney is reversible but requires 5 to 7 days to take effect and is not useful in acute situations.

In all forms of hyponatremia, the end point of therapy is restoration of serum Na$^+$ to normal levels. How rapidly this is accomplished will depend on the severity of symptoms manifested.

ALTERATIONS IN POTASSIUM HOMEOSTASIS

Potassium homeostasis is controlled by a number of extrarenal mechanisms. It is influenced by certain drugs used and disease states seen in the critical care setting (Table 23-5).

Briefly, potassium is the most abundant intracellular cation, with a concentration in the range of 150 to 160 mEq/liter. ECF concentration is in the range of 3.5 to 5.5 mEq/liter. Only a small proportion of total body potassium resides in the ECF (70 mEq, or 2% of the 3500 mEq of total body potassium) [5].

The significance of this is that the resting membrane potential of excitable cells depends primarily on the concentration gradient of potassium ion across the cell membrane. Small changes in serum K$^+$ have significant effects on the ratio of extracellular to intracellular K$^+$, leading to membrane depolarization with hyperkalemia and to hyperpolarization with hypokalemia. The clinical consequences of abnormal potassium levels in-

Table 23-5. Drug therapies affecting potassium balance

↑ *Intake*
KCl Supplements
Antibiotics
↑ *Output*
Diuretics
↓ *Output*
K^+-sparing agents
Nonsteroidal anti-inflammatory agents
Angiotensin converting-enzyme inhibitors
Distribution (ICF → ECF)
Digitalis toxicity
Hypertonic solutions

Table 23-6. Manifestations of abnormal K^+

	Hyperkalemia	Hypokalemia
Cardiac	Arrhythmias	Arrhythmias (digoxin toxicity)
Neuromuscular	Paresthesia	Paresthesia
	Weakness	Weakness
	Paralysis	Paralysis
Metabolic	—	Alkalosis
		Glucose intolerance
		Nitrogen wasting

Adapted from L.S. Weisburg, H. M. Szerlip, and M. Cox, Disorders of potassium homeostasis in critically ill patients. *Crit. Care Clin.* 5:834, 1987.

volve cardiac and skeletal muscle function [28], although metabolic derangements may also occur with extremes in potassium concentration (Table 23-6).

The factors that influence potassium homeostasis affect mechanisms controlling internal potassium balance (the distribution between ICF and ECF), external potassium balance (intake and excretion), or both [5]. In patients, the categories of interventions or processes that affect the above mechanisms include the use of certain drugs, acid-base disorders, hypomagnesemia, and renal insufficiency [28].

Hyperkalemia is commonly seen in association with renal failure when the glomerular filtration rate (GFR) has decreased to low levels, with an additional potassium load presented to the kidney either by exogenous administration or cellular necrosis. Drugs contribute to hyperkalemia by increasing input (KCl supplements and antibiotics such as carbencillin and potassium penicillin). Drugs that affect potassium excretion by lowering aldosterone levels include potassium-sparing diuretics, angiotensin converting-enzyme inhibitors, and nonsteroidal anti-inflammatory agents.

Drugs that affect the distribution of K^+ between ICF and ECF include digitalis derivative overdose, by inhibition of sodium-potassium adenosine triphosphatase (ATPase), and hypertonic solutions, presumably due to water shift with accompanying potassium ion or membrane alterations with potassium leak due to hypertonicity. In certain denervation syndromes, succinylcholine has been documented to cause hyperkalemia because of increased membrane sensitivity and marked release of intracellular amounts. Diuretic use leads to hypokalemia because of increased potassium losses in the urine [21].

Acute metabolic mineral acidosis consistently predisposes to hyperkalemia, and chronic metabolic alkalosis leads to hypokalemia because of obligatory potassium wasting. Replacement with potassium chloride effectively treats both the alkalosis and the hypokalemia.

Hypomagnesemia can cause refractory hypokalemia by renal wasting. Improvement may not occur until magnesium stores are replenished.

Because both hyperkalemic and hypokalemic states can be life-threatening, knowledge of the proper therapy of both conditions is important. Hyperkalemia can be treated by intravenous calcium infusions (10–20 ml of 10% solution as chloride or glugonate), glucose/insulin infusion (500 ml of 10% dextrose with 10–20 units regular insulin); administration of sodium bicarbonate (50–100 mEq), administration of kayexalate enterally or by enema (25–50 gm in 70% sorbital), or dialysis [28]. As all of these methods act by different mechanisms, they may be used in combination to achieve early onset and prolonged duration of effect.

The treatment of mild hypokalemia can usually be accomplished by oral KCl supplements. Severe hypokalemia (<2 mEq/liter), if symptomatic, requires emergent therapy. Even if severe hypokalemia is not symptomatic, it still requires urgent therapy. Low serum potassium always indicates a total body potassium deficit [27].

The administration of 20 mEq KCl in 100 ml saline over 1 hour with subsequent frequent checks of serum potassium provides a safe regimen and will guide the need for further supplementation.

ALTERATIONS IN MAGNESIUM, CALCIUM, AND INORGANIC PHOSPHATE HOMEOSTASES

Less often realized is the clinical importance of the roles of magnesium, calcium, and phosphate. In each of the constituents, the kidney and the gut are the key organ systems that regulate intake and excretion. The more common clinical problems are discussed below.

Magnesium

Magnesium is essential for many bodily functions (and for a number of enzyme systems)—including maintenance of calcium homeostasis and metabolism of fat, glucose, and protein—for a number of enzyme systems [17]. Because magnesium also serves to stabilize excitable membranes, magnesium deficiency has important consequences [11]. Magnesium homeostasis is normally regulated by the kidney and is largely independent of parathyroid hormone (PTH) and vitamin D, although absorption may be influenced by these hormones.

Hypermagnesemia is rarely seen except in situations of excess administration of antacids in patients with renal insufficiency. Hypermagnesemia

Table 23-7. Hypomagnesemia

Causes
  NPO
  Malabsorption
  Diarrhea
  Diuretic use: furosemide
  Antibiotic use: amphotericin B, gentamicin
Consequences
  Neuromuscular irritability
  Arrhythmia
  Hypocalcemia

---

can lead to neuromuscular and cardiac dysfunction, the most life-threatening of these conditions being muscle paralysis with apnea and heart block with asystole. These effects can be antagonized by calcium administration. Serum levels can be decreased by saline diuresis with furosemide or by dialysis in patients with oliguric renal failure.

Hypomagnesemia is more common in the critically ill population. Among its multiple causes are decreasing dietary intake and a host of conditions that enhance losses, including diuretic use, antibiotic use, diarrhea, and malabsorption. The clinical consequences of magnesium deficiency are tetany, weakness, and cardiac arrhythmias. Parathyroid gland suppression leads to hypocalcemia, with an additional effect of decreased sensitivity of PTH on bone (Table 23-7).

Treatment of mild deficiency can be accomplished by diet or oral supplements. Parenteral preparations are recommended for symptomatic hypomagnesemia and levels below 1.1 mEq/liter (1 mg%). A suggested regimen for replacement is administration of 600 mg of elemental Mg^{++} (6 gm of $MgSO_4$) initially over 3 hours and 900 mg of elemental Mg^{++} over the next 24 hours. Subsequent requirements are determined by measurement of levels. Losses should be replenished over 5 to 7 days [17].

Calcium

Calcium homeostasis is maintained by the combined effects of PTH and vitamin D metabolites on the gut, bone mass, and kidney and by the effects of PTH-independent mechanisms on renal function.

The physiologically active form of calcium is the ionized portion, which makes up approximately 50 percent of circulating calcium [29]. Measurement of ionized calcium is necessary to evaluate changes in the active fraction, because total serum calcium will vary with the level of serum albumin and ionized calcium will vary with acid-base status.

The causes of hypocalcemia include hypomagnesemia, vitamin D deficiency, renal insufficiency, alkalosis, sepsis, and hyperphosphatemia [6]. The clinical manifestations include neuromuscular irritability (tetany and seizures), cardiac arrhythmias, and hypotension (Table 23-8). Treatment of hypocalcemia acutely can be accomplished by giving calcium as a bolus injection (100–200 mg elemental calcium over 10 minutes, with a maintenance infusion of 1–2 mg/kg/hr elemental calcium) [29]. Magnesium and

Table 23-8. Hypocalcemia

Causes
↓ Mg^{++}
Vitamin D deficiency
Renal failure—chronic
Alkalosis
Consequences
Neuromuscular irritability: tetany
Seizures

phosphorus levels should be monitored to avoid hypophosphatemia or the administration of large doses of calcium in the presence of hyperphosphatemia. Correction of magnesium deficits will aid in the correction of calcium by restoring the normal mechanism of calcium homeostasis.

Hypercalcemia is caused by a number of disease processes, including hyperparathyroidism, malignancy, thyrotoxicosis, and certain granulomatous disorders [1]. Treatment regimens differ, depending on severity.

Saline diuresis, either with furosemide [18] or without diuretics, has been found to be effective. When diuretics are used, water and electrolyte losses must be monitored and replaced as necessary. Calcitonin has also been used in the management of patients in the acute setting [23]. After initial management, the underlying cause should be treated.

Phosphate

Phosphate homeostasis, like that of calcium, is modulated by the effects of PTH and vitamin D on the gut and kidney. Hyperphosphatemia results from increased intake or decreased excretion. The most common cause is decreased excretion due to renal failure [24]. Treatment involves decreasing gut absorption by phosphate binders (aluminum salts).

Hyposphatemia (see Table 23-9) is more common in the clinical setting and results from dietary restriction associated with alcoholism and starvation, alkalosis, and glucose loading, as occurs with hyperalimentation and the recovery phase of ketoacidosis [6].

Reported complications associated with hypophosphatemia include muscle weakness and rhabdomyolysis, hemolysis, and red cell dysfunction in oxygen release (↓ 2,3-DPG). Phagocytic cell function may be decreased, and neurologic abnormalities (seizures, paresthesias, coma) may occur. A suggested mechanism of these abnormalities involves a decrease in the cellular levels of phosphorus-containing metabolites and membrane phospholipids.

For the treatment of severe hypophosphatemia (<1 mg/dl), parenteral therapy is recommended. An initial dose of 2.5 mg/kg body weight (0.08 mM/kg) is administered for states that are uncomplicated and acute. For symptomatic patients, 5 mg/kg is administered. Lower doses are recommended for patients who are hypercalcemic. Doses are given over a 6-hour period, and serum levels are monitored. Subsequent doses are determined by serum levels and patient status. As the serum rises to above 1 mg/dl, replacement should be given orally, as tolerated by the patient.

Table 23-9. Hypophosphatemia

Causes
NPO
Alkalosis
Glucose loading
Consequences
Phagocytic cell dysfunction
Red cell dysfunction
Rhabdomyolysis
Seizures
Coma

SUMMARY

Fluid and electrolyte therapy in critically ill patients requires some knowledge of the normal physiologic mechanisms of homeostasis and of the disease states that alter those mechanisms. In all of the alterations discussed, multiple etiologies are often causative, and the syndromes can often occur simultaneously.

Anticipation and possible prevention of those disorders may be realized more easily than treatment of those conditions and their complications.

REFERENCES

1. Agus, Z. S., and Goldfarb, S. Clinical disorders of calcium and phosphate. *Med. Clin. North Am.* 65:385, 1981.
2. Berk, J. L., and Sampliner, J. E. (eds.). *Handbook of Critical Care* (2nd ed.). Boston: Little, Brown, 1982. Chapter 15.
3. Chanson, P., Jedynak, C. P., Dabrowski, G., Rohan, J. E., Bouchama, A., Rohan-Chabot, P., and Loirat, P. Ultralow doses of vasopressin in the management of diabetes insipidus. *Crit. Care Med.* 15:44–46, 1987.
4. Chung, H., Kluge, R., Schrier, R. W., and Anderson, R. J. Clinical assessment of extracellular fluid deficit in hyponatremia. *Am. J. Med.* 83:905, 1987.
5. Cox, M. Potassium homeostasis. Medical Clinics of North America, 65:363, 1981.
6. Desai, T. K., Carlson, R. W., and Geheb, M. A. Hypocalcemia and hypophosphatemia in acutely ill patients. *Crit. Care Clin.* 5:927, 1987.
7. Falk, J. L., Rackow, E. C., and Weil, M. H. Colloid and crystalloid fluid resuscitation. *Acute Care* 10:59, 1983/84.
8. Feig, P. U., and McCurdy, D. K. The hypertonic state. *N. Engl. J. Med.* 297:1444, 1977.
9. Feig, P. U. Hypernatremia and hypertonic syndromes. *Med. Clin. North Am.* 65:271, 1981.
10. Filston, H. C., Edwards, C. H., Chitwood, W. R., Larson, R. M., Marsicano, T. H., and Hill, R. C. Estimation of postoperative fluid requirements in infants and children. *Ann. Surg.* 196:76, 1982.
11. Flink, E. B. Magnesium deficiency, etiology and clinical spectrum. *Acta Med. Scand.* Suppl. 647, p. 125, 1981.
12. Geheb, M. A. Clinical approach to the hyperosmolar patient. *Crit. Care Clin.* 5:797, 1987.
13. Gennari, F. J. Serum osmolality uses and limitations. *N. Engl. J. Med.* 310:102, 1984.

14. Goldberg M. Hyponatremia. *Med. Clin. North Am.* 65:257, 1981.
15. Hantman, D., Rossier, B., Zohlman, R., and Schrier, R. Rapid correction of hyponatremia in the syndrome of inappropriate secretion of antidiuretic hormone. *Ann. Intern. Med.* 78:870, 1973.
16. Holliday, M. A., and Segar, W. E. The maintenance need for water in parenteral fluid therapy. *Pediatrics* 19:823, 1954.
17. Lee, C., and Zaloga, G. P. Magnesium metabolism. *Semin. Resp. Med.* 7:75, 1985.
18. Lenz, R. D., Brown, D. M., and Kjellstrand, C. M. Treatment of severe hypophosphatemia. *Ann. Intern. Med.* 89:941, 1978.
19. Levitt, M. A., Fleischer, A. S., and Meislin, H. W. Acute post-traumatic diabetes insipidus: Treatment with continuous intravenous vasopressin. *J. Trauma* 24:532, 1984.
20. Narins, R. G., Jones, E. R., Stom, M. C., Rudnick, M. R., and Bastl, C. P. Diagnostic strategies in disorders of fluid, electrolyte and acid base homeostasis. *Am. J. Med.* 72:496, 1982.
21. Ponce, S. P., Jennings, A. E., Madias, N. E., Harrington, J. T. Drug induced hyperkalemia. *Medicine* 64:357, 1985.
22. Rossi, N. F., and Cadnapaphornehai, P. Disordered water metabolism: Hyponatremia. *Crit. Care Clin.* 5:759, 1987.
23. Silva, O. L. and Becker, K. L. Salmon calcitonin in the treatment of hypercalcemia. *Arch. Intern. Med.* 132:337, 1973.
24. Slatopolsky, E., Rutherford, W. E., Rosenbaum, R., Martin, K., and Hruska, K. Hyperphosphatemia. *Clin. Nephrol.* 7:138, 1977.
25. Sterns, R. H. Severe symptomatic hyponatremia: Treatment and outcome. *Ann. Intern. Med.* 107:656, 1987.
26. Valtin, H. *Renal Function: Mechanisms Preserving Fluid and Solute Balance in Health* (2nd ed.). Boston: Little, Brown, 1982. Chapter 2.
27. Valtin, H. *Renal Dysfunction: Mechanisms Involved in Fluid and Solute Imbalance.* Boston: Little, Brown, 1979. Chapter 4.
28. Weisburg, L. S., Szerlip, H. M., and Cox, M. Disorders of potassium homeostasis in critically ill patients. *Crit. Care Clin.* 5:834, 1987.
29. Zaloga, G. P., and Chernow, B. Hypocalcemia in critical illness. *J.A.M.A.* 256:1924, 1986.

Acid-Base Disturbances

Paul M. Starker
Charles Weissman

The maintenance of acid-base homeostasis requires the integration of a number of physiologic mechanisms, including cellular and extracellular buffering and the compensatory actions of the lungs and kidneys. Critically ill patients frequently develop disorders in acid-base balance, and the interpretation and treatment of these problems is based on a firm understanding of the basic principles of acid-base physiology. This chapter will first address the basic concepts and terminology of acid-base therapy and then discuss the major alterations associated with the disease state.

CONCEPTS AND TERMS

An acid is an organic or inorganic compound that can dissociate and release a proton, and a base is a compound that can accept a proton.

The reaction indicated below shows the dissociation of an acid into a hydrogen ion (proton) and its associated base.

$$HA \rightarrow H^+ + A^-$$

It is important to appreciate that the tendency of the acid to donate a hydrogen ion is counterbalanced by an opposing tendency toward accepting a proton. A better way to show the reaction is as follows:

$$HA \rightleftarrows H^+ + A^-$$

At equilibrium, every acid in solution dissociates to a greater or lesser degree. A fully dissociated acid will be able to donate more protons and is thus considered to be strong, whereas a weak acid's conjugate base shows a greater affinity for protons, thus limiting dissociation.

The term *pH* represents the concentration of free hydrogen ion in solution; the pH value is inversely proportional to the concentration of hydrogen ions in the solution. The addition of a strong acid to water will obviously lower pH, but the presence of buffers will modify these changes.

561

Buffering is critical in the physiology and pathophysiology of acid-base, but the precise chemical mechanisms need not concern us here. Rather, it is far more valuable to look at the effect of body buffers and how these systems operate in conjunction with the kidney and lung to maintain the pH of extracellular fluid at 7.4.

Body Buffers

In vivo pH is held in the normal range primarily by maintaining plasma concentration of two substances: HCO_3^- at 24 mM/liter and CO_2 near 1.2 mM/liter. This represents the normal 20 : 1 ratio of HCO_3^-/CO_2. Although it might be arbitrary to focus on the concentrations of HCO_3^- and CO_2 when many other buffer pairs are present in plasma, the important point is that the organism exercises acid-base homeostasis by controlling arterial carbon dioxide tension ($PaCO_2$) and HCO_3^- levels.

There are two principal reasons for the primacy of HCO_3^- among the buffers of extracellular fluid (ECF)—one physiochemical, one physiologic. First, because of the open-ended system resulting from pulmonary control of $PaCO_2$, plus the evolutionary selection of 7.4 as the pH of ECF, the HCO_3^- and CO_2 buffer system accommodates more nonvolatile acid accumulating in ECF and yields more protons to added base than all the other buffers present collectively. This is true even in whole blood, despite the contribution of hemoglobin. As indicated, the second reason for the importance of HCO_3^- among the extracellular buffers is physiologic. Fluctuation of plasma HCO_3^- is the principal normal stabilizer of plasma pH as the acid-base load varies, because the change in plasma HCO_3^- affects urine pH in such a way that a steady state of zero acid-base balance normally is always approximated.

Several other nonvolatile buffers require consideration. Ammonia (NH_4^+ and NH_3) is of great importance in the urine but of less importance in the ECF, because ammonia is in low concentration there. On the other hand, circulating protein, the principal plasma buffer, and inorganic phosphates are important in plasma, and hemoglobin in both its oxygenated and deoxygenated forms is the primary whole-blood buffering agent.

Returning to consideration of the plasma bicarbonate buffer system: the 20 : 1 ratio of HCO_3^- to H_2CO_3 points up the quantitative relationship between the concentrations of the dissociated and nondissociated constituents of a buffer pair. This can be expressed by an equation that sets forth the relationship between hydrogen ion concentration (H^+) and the ratio of the constituents of the bicarbonate (HCO_3^-)–carbonic acid (H_2CO_3) buffer system.

$$(H^+) = K \frac{(H_2CO_3)}{(HCO_3^-)}$$

K represents the equilibrium constant for this system. Since pH [$-\log (H+)$] is used clinically instead of (H^+), the equation is rewritten

$$pH = pK + \log\frac{(HCO_3^-)}{(H_2CO_3)}$$

In this form it is the familiar Henderson-Hasselbach equation. This expression is applicable to the plasma bicarbonate system and is fundamental to any quantitative treatment of acid-base balance.

Role of the Kidney

The role of the kidney in acid-base homeostasis is to rid the body of any additional acid load. In order to add net acid to the urine, the kidney must reabsorb all the filtered HCO_3^- prior to secreting additional H^+ into the urine. The same cellular mechanism is involved in both. Every time a proton is added to the urine and trapped by a urinary buffer (HCO_3^-, NH_3, or $HPO_4^=$), an HCO_3^- molecule is released into the blood. In the proximal tubule, H^+ is titrated with HCO_3^- and forms H_2O and CO_2. When all the HCO_3^- is removed, the H^+ is trapped in the lumen of the tubule and excreted. The presence of urinary buffers (NH_3 and $HPO_2^=$) is crucial, because once the urinary pH drops below 4.5, protons will leak back into the tubular cells. These buffers thus allow a great increase in total acid excretion before luminal pH declines to a minimum value. Therefore, urine pH is not an indication of the total amount of acid excreted by the kidney. If the urinary concentration of buffer is high, the amount of acid excreted will be great prior to a fall in urinary pH and will be the ultimate limitation of excretion.

Role of the Lung

The muscles of respiration are innervated by lower motor-neurons that are controlled by the respiratory center lying in the brain stem. Any alteration in the chemical composition of the blood will immediately influence respiration through stimulation of the respiratory center.

Normally, the $PaCO_2$ is held at a value of 40 mm Hg. This implies a balance between CO_2 production and alveolar ventilation. If either one of these factors varies, the balance will be disrupted, and stimulation of the respiratory center to compensate will occur. Carbon dioxide production is often increased in the critically ill patient, due to hypermetabolism. However, this CO_2 load generally is easily handled by the lungs. Unfortunately, in the ICU alveolar hypoventilation is often a problem, and the excretion of this excess CO_2 can become a problem. This particular problem will be reviewed in greater detail during the discussion of respiratory acidosis.

Interpretation of Clinical Disorders of Acid-Base Balance

Before discussing particular disorders of acid-base balance, the concepts of compensation and steady state must be considered. Compensation for acid-base abnormalities is accomplished by rapid pulmonary mechanisms and slower renal mechanisms. Thus, the final blood pH is determined not only by the primary acid-base abnormality, but also by its compensatory process. Primary respiratory abnormalities are compensated for by alterations in HCO_3^- reabsorption by the kidney, and compensation for metabolic derangements occur by alteration in the handling of CO_2 by the lungs.

Several points about these compensatory mechanisms must be stressed. First, no compensating organ will overcompensate for an acid-base abnormality. Since the act of compensation is stimulated by a change in pH, correction of the pH will remove the stimulus and turn off the compensatory mechanisms. Second, compensatory changes require normal function of the compensatory organ. Obviously, if the lungs or kidneys are not functioning normally, they cannot perform their compensatory role. Third, the act of compensation causes its own abnormalities in either $PaCO_2$ or serum HCO_3^- levels. Therefore, correction of the primary acid-base problem may leave a different acid-base problem induced by the compensatory mechanism. This point leads to the consideration of the concept of steady state.

In managing patients with acid-base abnormalities, one must consider whether the patient is in steady-state conditions. If not, it is critical to determine the direction and rate of change in the patient's pH. For instance, a patient who develops acute respiratory acidosis from hypoventilation can be treated in the early phase with hyperventilation. However, if time has passed and renal compensatory mechanisms place the patient into a steady state, hyperventilation will induce a metabolic alkalosis. Thus, the proper management of an acid-base disorder must take into consideration whether the patient is in a steady state.

ALKALOSIS

Respiratory Alkalosis

Respiratory alkalosis is caused by hyperventilation inducing a decrease in $PaCO_2$ levels. Most acutely ill patients will exhibit some degree of hyperventilation, which is extremely common in states of early sepsis and peritonitis, as well as in early stages of acute respiratory failure.

A marked degree of alkalosis is undesirable and should be aggressively treated. Alkalosis makes patients more prone to arrhythmias. Also, cerebral blood flow decreases with progressive hypocapnia and with alkalosis as well. Treatment is directed at reversing the cause of the hyperventilation. Often, all that is necessary is supplemental oxygen to relieve concurrent hypoxemia. If the patient is on mechanical support the initial therapy is to decrease the amount of minute ventilation by decreasing respiratory frequency. Occasionally, it may be necessary to increase the dead space in the system. Acidifying agents are not required in the treatment of respiratory alkalosis.

Metabolic Alkalosis

Metabolic alkalosis can be induced by a number of factors, many of which are often present in the intensive care unit (ICU) setting. These factors include diuretic use, loss of gastric juice, hypovolemia, resuscitation with sodium bicarbonate solutions, and steroid use. Precipitating events that lead to metabolic alkalosis can be divided into those of base gain and those of acid loss.

Loss of acid through vomiting or nasogastric suction is a potential source of large net acid loss. Often, there is associated potassium depletion that may further exacerbate alkalosis. In addition to the loss of these ions, hypovolemia may also be present—a situation that causes aldosterone levels to rise. This causes H^+ secretion into the urine to increase and increases

Table 24-1. Urinary chloride in metabolic alkalosis

Chloride-responsive	Chloride-resistant
UCL < 15 mEq/liter	UCL > 15 mEq/liter
Vomiting—nasogastric suction	Diuretics
Posthypercapnia	Severe potassium depletion
Postdiuretic	Alkali loading
Nonreabsorbable anion	Bartter's syndrome, primary aldosteronism

the ability of the kidney to reabsorb $HCO_3{}^-$, further aggravating the alkalemic state.

States of chronic diuretic use induce hypovolemia and therefore stimulate increased aldosterone levels. The losses of sodium chloride and potassium induced by the diuretics can lead to a state of profound alkalosis.

Metabolic alkalosis can also be induced by a gain in base. Most commonly, this gain is associated with infusion of sodium bicarbonate during resuscitation. However, the administration or presence of endogenous anions that can be converted to bicarbonate can also result in alkalosis. Citrate from the rapid transfusion of large amounts of blood or lactate in a patient recovering from lactic acidosis are converted to $HCO_3{}^-$ and in large enough quantities can cause a significant alkalosis. Calculation of the urinary chloride concentration will help distinguish "chloride-responsive" from "chloride-resistant" causes of metabolic alkalosis (Table 24-1).

Chloride-responsive alkalosis can be treated by replacement with sodium chloride and potassium chloride. Total body potassium deficits may be as large as 300 to 500 mEq. In general, these deficits should be replaced slowly over time, to allow the relatively low serum concentrations of potassium to equilibrate with the extravascular space. If rapid replacement is necessary, rates of up to 20 mEq/hr can be given intravenously. In conjunction with such rapid infusion, serum levels must be closely followed and the cardiogram must be monitored for evidence of hyperkalemia. Replacement therapy with sodium and potassium chloride will improve volume status as well as potassium depletion and reverse the renal stimulus for proximal tubular reabsorption of $HCO_3{}^-$. In patients in whom cardiac failure or cirrhosis has caused a reduction in the effective circulatory volume with total body fluid overload, the use of a carbonic anhydrase inhibitor such as acetazolamide (250–500 mg/day) may be required. This agent will inhibit proximal reabsorption of $HCO_3{}^-$ and thus will return bicarbonate levels toward normal.

Chloride-resistant alkalosis suggests a state of volume expansion and reduced chloride reabsorption. Chloride replacement is obviously ineffective in these cases. Simple maneuvers such as discontinuing thiazide or loop diuretics, increasing potassium replacement, or reducing alkali intake will reverse the alkalosis in cases in which these etiologies can be established. In patients with hyperaldosteronism, aldosterone antagonists (spironolactone) or distally acting potassium-sparing diuretics (triamterene, amiloride) will be of value. Surgery to remove an adrenal tumor may be the ultimate therapy for these patients.

Finally, if severe alkalosis persists and is othewise irreversible, an infusion of either dilute HCl (0.1 N) or arginine monohydrochloride may be necessary. In order to infuse hydrochloric acid, 100 ml of one normal hydrochloric acid is added to 1 liter of saline or dextrose. This volume is infused into a central vein over 6 to 24 hours, during which time measurements of pH, PCO_2, and serum electrolytes are made every 4 hours.

ACIDOSIS

Respiratory Acidosis

Respiratory acidosis is caused by the retention of CO_2, leading to an increase in the PCO_2. This is due to an imbalance in the production of CO_2 and its elimination through alveolar ventilation. The production of CO_2 is increased in hypermetabolic states. The increase in CO_2 stimulates the respiratory center to increase ventilation. If there is depression of the respiratory center (e.g., by sedatives and hypnotics), acidosis will develop. Disorders in alveolar ventilation can also lead to respiratory acidosis. Diseases that cause mechanical chest-wall dysfunction as well as direct pulmonary processes—such as asthma, emphysema, or ventilation perfusion abnormalities caused by pulmonary emboli—will all lead to respiratory acidosis.

The treatment of respiratory acidosis centers around the improvement in the excretion of CO_2. This entails the improvement in alveolar ventilation and minute ventilation. Some techniques may entail withdrawal of respiratory depressant medications, such as sedatives, or alternatively, administration of sedation if pain is limiting chest wall motion. Stabilization of flail chest, improvement of a partially obstructed airway, and bronchodilators may also be indicated, depending on the underlying cause of the CO_2 retention. Ultimately, these patients may require support with mechanical ventilation. Hypoventilation can be easily corrected by this method. The hypoxemia associated with the acute respiratory distress syndrome commonly seen in the ICU is not often associated with hypercapnia, due to the high diffusibility of carbon dioxide.

Metabolic Acidosis

Metabolic acidosis results from either an accumulation of acid or a loss of base. The clinical picture is characterized by decreases in blood pH and plasma HCO_3^-.

The acidosis produced by acid gain can be divided into those cases in which acid production results from spontaneous alterations in metabolic processes and those that develop because of the effects of an ingested toxin. These forms of metabolic acidosis introduce an unmeasured anion into the plasma, thus increasing the anion gap. In other forms of metabolic acidosis the initiating event is loss of HCO_3^- or addition of an acid whose anion is chloride. These disorders are called hyperchloremic or non–anion gap acidoses (Table 24-2).

Table 24-2. Metabolic acidosis

Anion gap	Non–anion gap
Lactic acidosis	Gastrointestinal loss of HCO_3^-
Renal failure	Renal loss of HCO_3^-
Ketoacidosis	Addition of acid containing Cl
Ingestion of toxins	Dilutional acidosis

Anion Gap

The anion gap is estimated by the equation $Na - (Cl + HCO_3)$, with a normal value being between 8 and 12 mEq/liter. The term *anion gap* is obviously a misnomer, since the concentration of cations must equal the concentration of anions. An alternative term, *unmeasured anion*, is also somewhat misleading, because the concentration of unmeasured anion is about 23, not 12, mEq/liter. This is because there is about 11 mEq/liter of unmeasured cation. The concept of anion gap may be better understood through the following statement. Since total serum cation is equal to sodium (Na) and unmeasured cation (UC), and total serum anion is equal to chloride (Cl) and bicarbonate (HCO_3) and unmeasured anion (UA), the following equation is true.

$$Na + UC = Cl + HCO_3 + UA$$

Therefore,

$$Na - (Cl + HCO_3) = UA - UC$$

Since

$$Na - (Cl + HCO_3) = \text{anion gap}$$

then

$$UA - UC = \text{anion gap}$$

Normal concentrations of unmeasured anions and cations are listed in Table 24-3.

INCREASED ANION GAP. The anion gap can be increased by one of three mechanisms: a decrease in unmeasured cation, an increase in unmeasured anion, or a laboratory error involving the measurement of Na, Cl, or HCO_3.

An increase in anion gap due to a decrease in unmeasured cations is rarely seen clinically. Increased anion gap is most often associated with an increase in unmeasured anions. This may be due to an accumulation of organic acids, as in lactic acidosis or ketoacidosis, or of inorganic acids such as sulfate or phosphate, as in uremic acidosis. Exogenous anions,

Table 24-3. Normal concentrations of unmeasured anions and cations

Unmeasured cations (mEq/liter)		Unmeasured anions (mEq/liter)	
K	4.5	Protein	15
Ca	5.0	PO$_4$	2
Mg	1.5	SO$_4$	1
		Organic acids	5
Totals	11		23

such as formate and salicylate, can accumulate in association with ingestion of toxins and cause an increased anion gap.

An increase in the anion gap due to laboratory error can be seen with falsely increased serum sodium or falsely decreased serum chloride or bicarbonate.

Metabolic Acidosis Associated with an Increased Anion Gap

LACTIC ACIDOSIS. Lactic acidosis is probably the most common form of metabolic acidosis encountered in clinical medicine. Lactic acid is the end product of anaerobic glucose metabolism and is normally converted by the liver back to glucose or oxidized to CO_2 and H_2O.

Lactic acidosis occurs when the rate of lactic acid production exceeds the rate of its metabolism. The result is the accumulation of lactate anion and hence a high anion gap. The most common cause of severe lactic acidosis, especially in an ICU, is circulatory failure and shock. Severe lactic acidosis indicates tissue hypoxia, increased anaerobic metabolism, and insufficient hepatic utilization of lactate. Treatment centers around reestablishing blood pressure and cardiac output to allow hepatic metabolism to convert the lactate to bicarbonate. If acidosis is severe, immediate compensation can be accomplished by inducing a respiratory alkalosis via hyperventilation and the judicious infusion of bicarbonate-containing solutions. Overzealous treatment may lead to a metabolic alkalosis following resuscitation.

RENAL FAILURE. In acute renal failure the glomerular filtration rate (GFR) and urine output are reduced. This limits the opportunity to add H$^+$ to the urine. The anions that accompany the acidosis (sulfate, phosphate, or organic acids) are not filtered and remain in the ECF, thus contributing to the increased anion gap.

In chronic renal failure, as the number of functioning nephrons is reduced, the ability to generate ammonia also is reduced. The tubules can no longer generate enough NH$_3$ to buffer the H$^+$, and urinary pH drops to 4.5 and no more H$^+$ can be added to the urine. An anion gap will not develop until the GFR drops below 10 ml/min, at which point an anion gap will form.

KETOACIDOSIS. Diabetic ketoacidosis is a classic example of organic acidosis. With impaired glucose utilization, incomplete oxidation of lipids leads to the increased production of β-hydroxybutyrate, acetoacetate, and acetone. The H^+ load is buffered by HCO_3^-, leading to an anion gap. When insulin is administered and glucose is once again utilized adequately, the oxidation of lipids and production of organic acids and ketones decreases. Bicarbonate therapy is rarely needed.

INGESTION OF TOXINS. Toxins such as ethylene glycol, methanol, paraldehyde, and salicylate can cause severe anion gap acidosis.

Ethylene glycol metabolism leads to toxic metabolites such as glycolic, lactic, and oxalic acids. Renal precipitation of the oxalate leads to acute tubular necrosis. Therapy includes hemodialysis, administration of ethanol to inhibit metabolism of the toxin, and hydration to promote oxalate excretion. Recent evidence also points to 4-methylpyrazole as an antidote.

Methanol is metabolized to formaldehyde and formic acid, which interfere with oxidative metabolism and cause acidosis. Bicarbonate and ethanol are the mainstays of treatment, along with hydration, hemodialysis, and diuresis.

Salicylate ingestion is associated with a mixed acid-base disorder characterized by metabolic acidosis and respiratory alkalosis. Treatment centers around diuresis to promote excretion of salicylate. Alkalinization of the urine aids in this therapy.

Metabolic Acidosis Not Associated with an Increased Anion Gap

GASTROINTESTINAL LOSSES OF HCO_3^-. Diarrhea, biliary fistula, pancreatic fistula, and small bowel fistula all cause loss of fluid with bicarbonate concentrations greatly in excess of serum levels. Many patients in a surgical ICU will experience these ongoing losses and will develop a hyperchloremic acidosis. Therapy is centered around replacement of volume and ions that are lost—i.e., bicarbonate.

RENAL LOSSES OF HCO_3^-. Renal loss of bicarbonate is known as renal tubular acidosis (RTA). In one type of RTA, urinary pH is high in mild or severe acidosis. Bicarbonate levels in the urine are less than 3 percent of the filtered load, and supplemental HCO_3^- required to normalize serum pH is only 1 to 3 mEq/kg/day. A second type of RTA is characterized by a high urinary pH that will decrease as the acidosis becomes severe. There is a marked loss of HCO_3^- in the urine, and large amounts of HCO_3^- (5–20 mEq/kg/day) are required to maintain homeostasis. The third and final type of RTA is characterized by low urinary pH and small amounts of bicarbonate loss in the urine. The problem is inability to excrete NH_4^+. The need for exogenous HCO_3^- is small, and the use of exogenous mineralocorticoids may be helpful.

ADDITION OF CHLORIDE-CONTAINING ACIDS. Acids such as HCl, lysine HCl, or arginine HCl can produce non–anion gap acidosis if infused or ingested in significant amounts. Amino acids conjugated with Cl^- and delivered in a TPN solution can also lead to a hyperchloremic acidosis. Therapy centers around decreasing the chloride load; this can be accomplished by conjugating cations with acetate, which will be metabolized to bicarbonate.

DILUTIONAL ACIDOSIS. Large gains of isotonic fluid cause a dilution of the available HCO_3^- and in the face of a stable PCO_2 lead to a metabolic acidosis. The acidosis is only present after extremely large volumes have been delivered, and even then is of a mild degree.

MIXED ACID-BASE DISTURBANCES
Hemorrhagic, cardiogenic, and septic shock produce complex abnormalities of acid-base regulation, usually associated with hypoxia, increased ventilation, and hypocapnia. Alkalemia is often seen in the early stages, and acidemia may become predominant later on. In addition, some degree of lactic acidosis is generally present. Such patients are commonly found in the ICU population.

The complexity of these states, as well as poorly defined alterations involving the metabolism of heart, lung, brain, kidney, and peripheral tissues, produces acid-base disturbances that are often mixtures of the four basic abnormalities described above. Clinically, it is common to see simultaneous respiratory and metabolic derangements. It is essential for the clinician not only to look at the arterial blood gases and associated derived acid-base values, but also to evaluate the clinical setting carefully. Losses of acid or alkali are usually recognized, whereas gains related to therapy frequently receive less attention or are overlooked completely. Resolution of many complex acid-base problems depends on taking into account not only the underlying disease process, but also its treatment. This is especially true in the ICU, where critical illness and vigorous therapy exist in combination.

As a general principle, compensatory mechanisms are incomplete, so that despite compensation, the abnormal pH remains abnormal and in the direction of the primary disturbance. In other words, if a patient loses HCO_3^- from a pancreatic fistula, pH and total serum CO_2 will decrease. The resulting metabolic acidosis will stimulate the respiratory center, and hyperventilation will reduce $PaCO_2$. Respiratory alkalosis thus compensates for the previously uncompensated metabolic acidosis, and pH tends to return toward normal. However, the pH would still remain below the normal value of 7.4, indicating that the primary disturbance is acidosis rather than alkalosis.

"Overcompensation" is possible under certain special circumstances that should be mentioned here. In patients with chronic respiratory alkalosis with maximal compensation, abrupt correction of the hypocapnia will lead to acidosis. Overcompensation occurs because the rate of renal adjustment lags behind the respiratory correction. Similarly, overcompensation can develop in patients with long-standing CO_2 retention (respiratory acidosis) and maximal compensation if their hypercapnia is abruptly corrected. Once again, this is related to the time required for renal adjustments, which lag behind the rapid respiratory correction. Awareness of overcompensation is important in the ICU, because mechanical ventilation provides the means for abruptly changing body CO_2 stores. As is the case in many other ICU problems, acid-base management requires not only careful consideration of the patient's underlying disease, but also serial observations that make it possible to interpret evolving patterns that would otherwise be extremely confusing when considered in isolation.

SELECTED READINGS

Appel, G. B., and Chase, H. S., Jr. Diagnosis and Treatment of Acid-Base Disorders. In J. Askanazi, C. Weissman, and P. M. Starker (eds.), *Fluid and Electrolyte Management in Critical Care*. Boston: Butterworth, 1986. Pp. 145–170.

Astrup, P. K., et al. Acid-base metabolism: A new approach. *Lancet* 1:1035, 1960.

Baud, F. J., Galliot, M., Astier, A., et al. Treatment of ethylene glycol poisoning with intravenous 4-methylpyrazole. *N. Engl. J. Med.* 319:97, 1988.

Black, R. M. Metabolic Acid-Base Disturbances. In J. M. Rippe, R. S. Irwin, J. S. Alpert, and J. E. Dalen (eds.), *Intensive Care Medicine*. Boston: Little, Brown, 1985.

Davenport, H. W. *The ABC of Acid-Base Chemistry* (4th ed.). Chicago: University of Chicago Press, 1958.

Filly, G. F. *Acid-Base and Blood Gas Regulation: For Medical Students Before and After Graduation*. Philadelphia: Lea & Febiger, 1971.

Gamble, J. L., Jr. *Regulation of the Acidity of the Extracellular Fluids: Teaching Syllabus*. Baltimore: Johns Hopkins University Press, 1966.

Heird, W. C., et al. Metabolic acidosis resulting from intravenous alimentation mixtures containing synthetic amino acids. *N. Engl. J. Med.* 287:943, 1972.

Hills, A. G. *Acid-Base Balance*. Baltimore: Williams & Wilkins, 1973.

OH, M. S., and Carroll, H. J. The anion gap. *N. Engl. J. Med.* 297:814, 1977.

Siggaard-Anderson, O., et al. Micro method for determination of pH, carbon dioxide tension, base excess and standard bicarbonate in capillary blood. *Scand. J. Clin. Lab. Invest.* 12:172, 1960.

Siggaard-Anderson, O. Titratable acid or base of body fluids. *Ann. N.Y. Acad. Sci.* 133:41, 1966.

Singer, R. B., and Hastings, A. B. Improved clinical method for estimation of disturbances of acid-base balance of human blood. *Medicine* 27:223, 1948.

Van Slyke, D. D., and Cullen, G. E. Studies of acidosis. I. Bicarbonate concentration of blood plasma; its significance, and its determination as measure of acidosis. *J. Biol. Chem.* 30:289, 1917.

Winters, R. W., et al. *Acid-Base Physiology in Medicine*. London, Ont.: Talbot, 1967.

Nutritional Management

Daniel W. Benson
Josef E. Fischer

Nutritional support has become an integral part of care of the critically ill patient. Since the pioneering work of Rhoads and Dudrick in parenteral nutrition and of Randall and Levenson in the area of predigested and elemental diets, continued expansion in our understanding of the complex interrelationships of nutrient delivery and metabolism have transformed nutritional support from a supportive therapy to, in some cases, a therapeutic one.

As the field of nutritional support has evolved, certain fundamental principles of nutritional management have undergone revision. Whereas 5 to 10 years ago the principle was "more is better," with patients commonly receiving 3500 to 4000 calories/day, now the mean caloric supplementation is closer to 2000 to 2500 calories/day. The overzealous administration of calories is now recognized to contribute to the deleterious side effects of excessive CO_2 production, hyperglycemia, pulmonary edema, worsening of preexisting congestive heart failure, hepatic steatosis, and perhaps an increased incidence of non–catheter-related infection. Another principle regarding the institution of nutritional support that has needed tempering is, "If you think of it, you probably should do it." This point of view is based on the fact that it is easier to prevent the complications of starvation than to treat them once they have occurred. This type of thinking has fostered practices such as preoperative parenteral nutrition to "beef up" patients showing anywhere from mild to moderate signs of malnutrition. There is now evidence that in the mild to moderately malnourished patient, this practice may not result in a net benefit, as any decrease in complications in the mild to moderately malnourished group is offset by an increase in non–catheter-related infections. However, in the severely malnourished group, the decrease in operative complications makes preoperative nutritional supplementation worthwhile [10]. Increases in infection have also been demonstrated in two series in which the early institution of parenteral nutrition in patients with acute pancreatitis resulted in a higher incidence of catheter sepsis [23, 36]. A final principle that has been revived rather than revised is, "If the gut works, use it." We are becoming increasingly aware of the importance in maintaining the structural and functional integrity of the gastrointestinal tract. Also, it is being increasingly demonstrated that the gut works more often than heretofore has been supposed, provided that one makes a sustained attempt to use it.

In order to gain a proper perspective of the role of nutritional management in critical care, several statements about the gravity of the problem are in order. An estimated 25 to 60 percent of hospitalized patients are reported to suffer from protein/calorie malnutrition. During the course of any illness a loss in lean muscle mass of 10 percent is felt to be significant, a loss of 20 percent is considered critical or premorbid, and a loss of 30 percent or more is regarded as lethal. In addition to skeletal muscle catabolized for gluconeogenesis and energy, a significant additional source of protein is the rapidly turning over and more recently synthesized protein from metabolically active tissue—namely, the liver enzymatic proteins, renal tubular enzymes, and gastrointestinal mucosa. This type of "autocannibalization" serves as a form of "internal nutritional support," providing the patient with the energy (glucose, free fatty acids, and proteins) necessary for host defense and tissue repair. Although this response may be adaptive in cases of mild trauma and infection or the early stages of sepsis, in prolonged starvation and sepsis it becomes maladaptive, resulting in the failure of individual or multiple organ systems that often determines the final outcome.

The goals of nutritional management, therefore, are (1) to identify patients at nutritional risk early in their course, so that further nutritional deterioration can be prevented; (2) to maintain lean body mass and provide the necessary energy and nutrients to sustain physiologic systems; (3) to select the nutritional formulations and methods of administration appropriate to the patient's condition or disease; and (4) continual reassessment of the patient, including adequacy of the nutritional regimen, the patient's response to that regimen, and the changing requirements as the patient goes through the phases of hypermetabolism, stabilization or recovery, and finally, repletion.

GENERAL INDICATIONS

If neither significant economic costs nor complications were factors in nutritional support, all patients who were unable to take adequate nutrients for any length of time would be candidates for such therapy. Since cost and complications must be considered, guidelines for the timing and method of nutritional support must be established.

Time

The length of time an individual can withstand inadequate nutritional intake depends on age, previous state of health, previous state of nutrition, degree of trauma, and presence of sepsis. The effect of age is demonstrated in the following guidelines. An adult with previously normal nutrition who is in a moderately catabolic state generally will tolerate up to 14 days of starvation without demonstrating a measurable defect. This holds true up to age 60. For patients 60 to 70 years old, tolerance falls to 10 days of starvation; and for those over 70 years of age, it drops to 7 days.

Parenteral Nutrition

In general, patients without a functional gastrointestinal tract or who are about to undergo some form of therapy that will prevent them from taking adequate intake for the reasonable future are candidates for parenteral nutrition. The indications can be further divided into primary therapy, supportive therapy, and investigational. Primary therapy includes those diseases in which nutritional support has been shown to affect the disease process or improve the outcome—enterocutaneous fistula, short-bowel syndrome, acute tubular necrosis, major burns, and acute or chronic hepatic insufficiency. Supportive therapy includes conditions for which a positive effect on disease outcome has not been clearly established—gastrointestinal toxicity from chemotherapy or radiation therapy, preoperative total parenteral nutrition, cardiac cachexia, pancreatitis, large wounds losing nitrogen, prolonged ileus, stomal dysfunction, and prolonged ventilatory support. Areas currently under investigation are the treatment of sepsis and the treatment of cancer.

In addition to these general guidelines, the use of parenteral nutrition will vary from institution to institution and will reflect both the current status of the procedure's safety in a given institution and the understanding and acceptance of this mode of therapy by the staff. It is a truism that in an institution with a low rate of complications, a wider range of indications is used. Conversely, in institutions in which the administration of parenteral nutrition by a central route is accompanied by a high rate of complications, this treatment modality will be reserved for only the most seriously ill. In our institution, parenteral nutrition generally is instituted within 5 to 7 days in any seriously injured patient who is unable to resume an enteral diet, and immediately following stabilization if it is clear that eating will not resume for a period of time.

Enteral Nutrition

Patients with a functioning small-bowel tract who cannot take food by mouth and/or cannot meet nutritional requirements are candidates for special supplements and/or tube feedings. These indications include the inability or lack of desire to take adequate oral intake; neurologic or physiologic disorders; oropharyngeal/esophageal lesions or trauma; burns; and select gastrointestinal disorders, including the use of needle or tube catheter jejunostomy following upper gastrointestinal surgery, mild flare-ups of inflammatory bowel disease, pancreatitis, and the adaptation period in short-bowel syndrome.

NUTRITIONAL NEEDS

Normal Adult Needs

It is appropriate at this point to review the normal nutritional needs of adult patients. This is perhaps artificial, since most of what is known in nutrition has been derived from normal human volunteers or patients in a comparatively steady state. Thus, all of our "ideal" amino acid criteria, for example, are derived either from the ideal composition of a protein, such as egg albumin, thought to be of high biologic value, or from the safe requirements of amino acids, such as those proposed by Rose, that, again, have been based on investigations in well patients in the steady state.

Normal nutritional needs include a basal caloric expenditure rate of 1800 to 2000 calories/day, or, more accurately, not more than 35 kcal/kg. This basal expenditure does not increase significantly following minor sugery or after minor trauma. In the typical diet, approximately 40 to 50 percent of calories are derived from carbohydrates, 10 to 20 percent from protein, and 40 percent from fat. Under normal conditions, the body can oxidize glucose at a rate of 2 to 4 mg/kg/min, with a minimum of 100 to 150 gm of carbohydrate per day necessary to achieve a protein-sparing and anti-ketogenic effect. The normal protein requirement is about 10 gm of nitrogen in approximately 60 to 70 gm of protein, or 0.8 gm/kg/day of protein. The figure of 40 percent fat far exceeds normal needs, with only 4 to 6 percent dietary fat required to prevent essential fatty acid deficiency.

Nutritional Needs Following Injury (Patterns)

Following massive injury with or without sepsis, the energy consumption pattern changes, so that an increased fraction of the caloric needs is derived from protein. During stress the maximal oxidation rate of glucose increases only slightly, to 3 to 5 mg/kg/min. In contrast, protein requirements increase significantly, with some recommending 1.2 to 1.5 gm/kg/day.

The altered substrate utilization is largely due to the glucose intolerance that develops during sepsis or major trauma. The causes of this glucose intolerance are multifactorial and include elevated levels of the catabolic hormones, a high glucagon-insulin ratio, and the inability of tissues, especially the liver, to take up glucose. The latter phenomenon has been termed *insulin resistance*. Various mechanisms for this insulin resistance have been postulated, including a receptor defect and post-receptor defects. Postreceptor alterations in glucose metabolism may be in the steps that involve glucose uptake (transport and phosphorylation), glycogenolysis (phosphorylase), glycolysis (phosphofructokinase), or oxidation (pyruvate dehydrogenase). In the absence of exogenous glucose, as in starvation, the muscle and brain, among other tissues, will use either glucose derived from gluconeogenesis—derived in turn from muscle breakdown and proteolysis—or ketone bodies derived from free fatty acids generated from lipolysis. In addition, the muscle, at least, will utilize branched-chain amino acids, valine, leucine, and isoleucine for energy. These substances, which also serve as sources of alanine for the glucose-alanine cycle (and thus gluconeogenesis), are unique in that they may be oxidized for energy directly, without the intervention of glucose. This unique property makes them more valuable in trauma and sepsis.

In sepsis and severe trauma, glucose intolerance, decreased ability of the liver to manufacture ketone bodies, and perhaps impaired utilization of fatty acids all conspire to increase the energy demands and increase the breakdown of lean body mass to provide the caloric supply for vital-organ function.

Numerous direct effects of injury or of major surgery increase caloric needs. These include fever; tissue damage; blood, plasma, and protein loss; plasma exudation by damaged capillaries into the surrounding tissues; and the metabolic requirements for clearance of the damaged tissues. The plasma lost at injury is often not replaced, and increased synthesis of albumin and other protein by the liver is an additional metabolic drain in the early postinjury period. Additional metabolic requirements may be secondary to the increased work of breathing and respiratory function. Fever remains the most significant factor in the increase in caloric needs. It is estimated that each degree of fever brings about a 10 to 13 percent increase in oxygen consumption. The caloric equivalent of a 10 to 13 percent increase in oxygen consumption has not been demonstrated exactly, but one may calculate approximately 500 to 1000 calories for each degree (Fahrenheit) of fever. This may not take into account the increased loss of water vapor with the diaphoresis and tachypnea that occurs with fever.

EFFECTS OF STARVATION

The nonspecific deleterious effects of starvation include wound disruption, poor healing, and decreased anastomotic strength; lack of mobility leads to an increased tendency to phlebitis and skin breakdown, with formation of decubiti (also aided and abetted by poor skin nutrition). There are nonspecific effects on the central nervous system as well. Patients become less alert. They sleep more, cooperate in their care to a lesser extent, and have a decreased ability to clear secretions. It is not established whether these central nervous system effects are mediated by the lack of caloric intake for the brain and resulting decreased brain function or by other nonspecific toxic factors, including the accumulation of products from the breakdown of muscle. It is known that some of the transmitter functions of the central nervous system are influenced by the concentration of certain amino acids in the serum and that these amino acids compete at the blood-brain barrier for entry into the brain and in turn determine the neurotransmitter profile of the brain. In liver disease and perhaps renal disease, amino acid imbalances may contribute to the decreased alertness. It is therefore possible that some of the effects of starvation on the central nervous system may be mediated to the brain by the known alterations in plasma amino acid patterns.

As starvation goes on and muscle is utilized for gluconeogenesis, the patient may ultimately reach a point at which so many intercostal and upper abdominal muscles are compromised that insufficient muscle mass remains to perform the work of breathing. This is one common reason for the inability to wean patients who have been on the respirator for a prolonged period. The intercostal muscles of such patients may have been so wasted away by starvation that even if they are repleted and hyperalimented, respiratory failure due to loss of muscle mass may become almost irreversible, since the muscles are unable to hypertrophy with respiratory work. In addition, there are data that clearly relate nonspecific host resistance to deficits in protein and perhaps the essential amino acids. Since death from sepsis is common in starvation, loss of host resistance probably plays a greater role than we have heretofore been made aware.

Starvation in the presence of sepsis may contribute to multiple organ systems failure, such as the liver and kidneys. It has been previously noted that rapidly-turning-over proteins may be used for gluconeogenesis under certain circumstances and that these proteins include the newly synthesized enzymatic elements of both liver and kidney. To be sure, most instances of inexplicable hepatic and renal failure in patients who are overwhelmingly ill reflect generalized organ failure and the inability of the organism to provide homeostasis. It is possible, however, that a significant contribution to hepatic and renal failure may be the cannibalization of useful functional elements for gluconeogenesis.

NUTRITIONAL ASSESSMENT
The basic objectives of nutritional assessment are to identify the patient at high risk nutritionally and to provide optimal nutritional support throughout the hospitalization, thereby preventing hospital-onset of malnutrition. Efforts to develop a formula to predict patients at risk or to develop use of other sophisticated measurements have proven to be no better than the clinical observations ("global assessment") of an experienced physician [12].

The major parameters used in nutrition assessment are the patient's history, the physical examination, anthropometrics, and laboratory data. Important aspects of history include medical and surgical conditions that impair ingestion, digestion, or absorption of food; usual dietary habits; and food allergies. During the physical examination, one should look for evidence of overall protein-calorie malnutrition or other deficiencies, such as essential fatty acid deficiency; anemia; and vitamin and/or trace element deficiency. A practical and immediately useful measurement of anthropometrics is determination of height and weight. This should be compared to the patient's usual body weight (UBW) rather than a calculated ideal body weight (IBW) or one determined from life insurance tables. Weight gain or loss from UBW can have important clinical implications. Other measures of anthropometrics, such as skinfold thickness and midarm circumference, have proven to be of less value. Finally, one should assess laboratory data indicative of electrolyte balance; renal, hepatic, bone, hematopoetic, and pulmonary function; visceral and somatic protein status; and fat tolerance. The proteins most often evaluated in assessing visceral protein status are serum albumin, transferrin, thyroxine-binding prealbumin, and retinol-binding protein. It is important to remember, however, that these values can be affected by factors other than nutritional status, particularly the state of hydration. Somatic protein status can be measured by determining nitrogen balance. This can be calculated by the equation

$$N \text{ balance} = N \text{ intake} - N \text{ excretion}$$

$$= \frac{\text{protein intake}}{6.25} - (24\text{-hr UUN} + 4)$$

where N = nitrogen and UUN = urinary urea nitrogen.

This equation is accurate so long as the urine remains the major source of nitrogen loss—i.e., in the absence of diarrhea or weeping wounds. Its use is also limited in nitrogen retention diseases such as renal or hepatic failure. The figure of 6.25 gm of protein per gram of nitrogen is not accurate when modified (i.e., high branched-chain) amino acid solutions are used, in which case there are approximately 7 gm of protein per gram of nitrogen.

Somatic protein status can also be qualitatively assessed by estimating protein breakdown and turnover. This is accomplished by measuring the urinary excretion of 3-methylhistidine (3-MH), a minor amino acid derived largely from actin and myosin that is neither metabolized nor reutilized following release during proteolysis. It is not entirely clear what urinary 3-MH measures, but it probably reflects not only muscle lean body mass, but also a small, rapidly-turning-over protein pool derived from the gut. Therefore, 3-MH will measure a derivative of lean body mass and cannot be taken as a measurement of total skeletal muscle turnover.

Determination of Needs

Based on the nutritional assessment of the past and current nutritional status of the patient, a projection of nutrient needs can be made based on basal metabolic needs and additional requirements related to activity, stress factors, and thermal regulation. As a rule of thumb, in the absence of severe sepsis, trauma, or major burn, 30 to 35 kcal/kg body weight/day is probably adequate. Equations are available that allow for greater individualization, including age, sex, height, and weight of the patient, as well as the activity and stress level. The Harris-Benedict equation [26] and Calvin Long's activity and stress factors [31] are usually used for this purpose:

Harris-Benedict—Basal Energy Expenditure (BEE)

$$BEE = 66.5 + 13.7W + 5.0H - 6.8A \text{ (male)}$$

$$BEE = 65.5 + 9.6W + 1.7H - 4.7A \text{ (female)}$$

where W = weight (kg), H = height (cm), and A = age.

Calvin Long—Activity Factor

1. Calculate the increased energy expenditure imposed by activity
   a. BEE × activity factor = REE
      (1) Confined to bed—1.2
      (2) Out of bed—1.3
2. Calculate the increased energy expenditure imposed by injury
   a. BEE × activity × injury factor = total estimation of energy requirements (TEE)
      (1) Minor operation—1.2
      (2) Skeletal trauma—1.35
      (3) Major sepsis—1.6
      (4) Severe thermal burn—2.10

These factors probably overestimate caloric needs.

Finally, indirect calorimetry can be used to calculate energy expenditure by the measurement of respiratory gas exchange. The actual measurements made during indirect calorimetry are $\dot{V}O_2$ (oxygen consumption), $\dot{V}CO_2$ (CO_2 production), and V_E (minute ventilation). From these variables the REE and respiratory quotient (RQ) can be calculated. This technique has become increasingly attractive in the critical care setting, as it is noninvasive, is portable, and can be used on spontaneously breathing or mechanically ventilated patients. Accurate measurement of REE and RQ is particularly helpful in the mechanically ventilated patient, both for the monitoring of nutritional support and to aid in weaning. In these patients it can be extremely difficult to estimate the various contributions of mechanical ventilation, immobilization, sedative drips, etc., in the final REE. In general, if the patient is properly at rest, indirect calorimetry usually underestimates the needs by 10 to 15 percent, because no allowance is made for activity. The figure derived should be increased by 10 to 15 percent to allow for caloric expenditure by activity.

It should be emphasized that the primary goal of nutritional therapy is to maintain lean body mass and support physiologic systems. This is not the time to try to "build up" patients nutritionally, which rarely happens under these circumstances.

METHODS OF NUTRITIONAL SUPPORT
Nutritional support can be administered by the parenteral route, via peripheral or central veins, or by the enteral route, using the stomach or small bowel as the entry point. Although the two methods are equally effective in providing nutritional support, there are some important differences that clinicians should keep in mind when prescribing these therapies [5].

Parenteral nutrition alters the normal sequence by which nutrients are received, metabolized, and distributed to the body. The cost of this to the patient is a disruption of normal physiology and metabolism. Physiologic changes include an altered body composition and an increased gut blood flow [41]. Metabolically, parenteral nutrition commonly leads to some degree of hepatic dysfunction, to changes in the levels of pancreatic and gastrointestinal hormones, and to the absence of direct enteral stimulation by nutrients that is required to maintain the structural and functional integrity of the gut [6, 13, 20, 29, 30]. For the critically ill patient, these physiologic and metabolic changes may lead to inappropriate and/or inefficient substrate utilization and a higher incidence of complications such as gastrointestinal bleeding and acalculous cholecystitis.

Another important function of the gut that becomes compromised in the absence of enteral nutrition is its role as an immune organ. The gut can be an important portal of entry for infectious agents. Bacterial translocation refers to the passage of viable bacteria from the gastrointestinal tract through the epithelial mucosa into the mesenteric lymph nodes and then to other organs. Gastric acidity, mucus production, intact peristalsis, and the normal indigenous bacterial microflora protect the intestinal mucosa from bacterial translocation. These are frequently altered in the intensive care patient by antacids or H_2-blockers, broad-spectrum antibiotics, and disuse atrophy of the gut. In addition, secretory immunoglobulin A (IgA), a major component of this mucosal defense system, is decreased in parenterally fed patients, suggesting the presence of intraluminal nutrients are necessary for the maintenance of normal levels [2].

A brief statement as regards the cost, efficiency, and safety of parenteral and enteral nutrition is in order. Enteral nutrition is less expensive and generally has a wider range of applications, being suitable for acute care facilities, nursing homes, and home use. Furthermore, since the end point of nutritional therapy is usually tolerance of an enteral diet, enteral support is more expedient in meeting this goal.

Although it is often claimed that enteral nutrition is safer than parenteral nutrition, we have not found this to be the case. Both methods can be associated with serious technical, metabolic, and infectious complications. Mortality is more common with enteral feedings into the stomach and is usually due to vomiting and aspiration. However, studies have shown that morbidity and mortality can be reduced to acceptable levels by the institution of strict clinical protocols. Therefore, we feel that safety should not be a primary factor in choosing the method of therapy.

PARENTERAL NUTRITION
Parenteral nutrition can be given by either peripheral or central veins. Regardless of the route, the basic ingredients of the parenteral solution are the carbohydrate, amino acid, and fat components, along with appropriate amounts of electrolytes, vitamins, and trace elements. The parenteral formulary used at the University of Cincinnati is given in Table 25-1.

Caloric Source
In the United States, the only solutions available for use contain glucose as the principal caloric source. In other countries, fructose and polyhydrate alcohols are also available; the rationale for their use is to improve on the glucose intolerance present in posttraumatic patients, who may be more tolerant of fructose and alcohol in small amounts for the first 3 to 4 days following the injury. These advantages seem more apparent than real, since alcohols and fructose generate problems in turn, such as lack of physiologic control, difficulty in readily measuring blood excess of such carbohydrates, hepatic damage (in the case of xylitol), and lactic acidosis secondary to fructose. These must remain theoretic considerations, since it is unlikely that other carbohydrate sources will be commercially available in the future, and fructose, which is commercially available, has not proven popular.

Amino Acid Source
The protein component can be either a hydrolysate or a mixture of single amino acids of synthetic origin.

Hydrolysates
Discussion of hydrosalates is really of historical interest only. Hydrolysates were the first solutions in use, the protein source being the hydrolysate of either casein or fibrin. There appears to be a small but theoretic advantage

Table 25-1. Parenteral nutrition formulary currently in
use at the University of Cincinnati Medical Center

---

1. **Central formulation**

   Indications: Standard formulation used on most patients.

   Composition (each 1000 ml):

Amino acids	(4.25%)	42.5 gm	Nitrogen 6.5 gm/liter
Balanced			

Dextrose	(25%)	250 gm	Nonprotein calories 850 kcal
Total calories	1020 kcal	kcal/ml 1.02	kcal/nitrogen 131/1

Standard electrolytes (mEq/liter)	K	Na	Mg	Ca	P (mM)	Cl	Acetate
	13–40	20–52	8	4.7	14–17	10–27	45–81

2. **Modified substrate formulation**

   Indications: (a) Lowered dextrose formulation (D15%) designed to have fat
   emulsion administered as substitute for carbohydrate
   calories.

   (b) For patients with glucose intolerance.

   (c) For patients with evidence of carbohydrate overfeeding.

   Composition (each 1000 ml):

Amino acids	(4.25%)	42.5 gm	Nitrogen 6.5 gm/liter
Balanced			

Dextrose	(15%)	150 gm	Nonprotein calories 510 kcal
Total calories	680 kcal	kcal/ml 0.68	kcal/nitrogen 78/1

Standard electrolytes (mEq/liter)	K	Na	Mg	Ca	P (mM)	Cl	Acetate
	13–40	20–52	8	4.7	14–17	10–27	45–81

3. **Cardiac formulation**

   Indications: Concentrated formulation for reduced volume in patients with
   fluid intolerance.

   Composition (each 1000 ml):

Amino acids	(5%)	50 gm	Nitrogen 7.65 gm/liter
Balanced			

Dextrose	(35%)	350 gm	Nonprotein calories 1190 kcal
Total calories	1390 kcal	kcal/ml 1.39	kcal/nitrogen 156/1

Standard electrolytes (mEq/liter)	K	Na	Mg	Ca	P (mM)	Cl	Acetate
	0–50	5	8	0	5–12	1	44–84

4. **Renal formulation**

   Indications: Patients with acute tubular necrosis who can tolerate a modest
   fluid load and in whom it is felt dialysis can be delayed or
   prevented.

   Composition (each 750 ml):

Amino acids	(1.7%)	12.75 gm	Nitrogen 1.6 gm/750 ml
Essential L-amino acids (Nephramine)			

Dextrose	(46.6%)	350 gm	Nonprotein calories 1190 kcal
Total calories	1240 kcal	kcal/ml 1.65	kcal/nitrogen 744/1

Standard electrolytes (mEq/liter)	K	Na	Mg	Ca	P (mM)	Cl	Acetate
	0	1.2	0	0	0	0	0

5. **Hepatic formulation**

   Indications: (a) Patients with chronic liver disease intolerant to standard
   formulations.

   (b) Patients with a grade-II or greater encephalopathy.

Table 25-1 (continued)

Composition:
Amino acids   (4%)   40 gm   Nitrogen 6 gm/liter
35% branched-chain amino acids (Hepatamine)
Dextrose   (25%)   250 gm   Nonprotein calories 850 kcal
Total calories   1010 kcal   kcal/ml 1.01   kcal/nitrogen 142/1

Standard electrolytes (mEq/liter)	K	Na	Mg	Ca	P (mM)	Cl	Acetate
	12–40	5–50	8	4.7	5–14	13.5–46.5	31–58

6. **Stress formulation**

   Indications: Critically ill, hypermetabolic, traumatized, or septic patients in the immediate postinjury period.

Composition:
Amino acids   (5.2%)   52 gm   Nitrogen 7.3 gm/liter
45% branched-chain amino acids
Dextrose   (17.5%)   175 gm   Nonprotein calories 595 kcal
Total calories   803 kcal   kcal/ml   kcal/nitrogen 82/1
                     0.803

Standard electrolytes (mEq/liter)	K	Na	Mg	Ca	P (mM)	Cl	Acetate
	13–40	23–55	8	4.7	9–12	10–27	51–87

7. **Peripheral formulation**

   Indications: (a) Patients who have no central venous access or in whom central venous catheterization is contraindicated.

   (b) For 3 to 5 days of nutritional support in patients who may not be able to take an adequate oral intake.

Composition:
Amino acids   (3.5%)   35 gm   Nitrogen 5.5 gm/liter
  Balanced
Dextrose   (5%)   50 gm   Nonprotein calories 170 kcal
Total calories   310 kcal   kcal/ml 0.31   kcal/nitrogen 31/1

Standard electrolytes (mEq/liter)	K	Na	Mg	Ca	P (mM)	Cl	Acetate
	3–20	0–50	8	4.7	0–6	0–28	52–82

In addition, vitamins and trace elements are added to each of the formulations. The standard electrolyte concentrations can be altered as long as the maximal allowable concentration is not exceeded. Insulin may be added as required.

---

to casein, although fibrin gave excellent clinical results. The solution is generally used as a formulation of 30 gm protein to approximately 200 to 250 gm of glucose per liter. Only approximately 55 percent of the available nitrogen in casein hydrolysate, for example, is available as α-amino nitrogen. It is known that hydrolysis is not complete, and it is not known whether or not dipeptides and tripeptides can be efficiently utilized by the body. Thus, the wastage in this type of solution accounts for the small amount (approximately 2.2 gm of nitrogen per liter of solution) available to the patient for use in protein synthesis. In some situations (e.g., with burns), patients may be extremely septic and their catabolic rate, even in the presence of parenteral nutrition, may exceed this figure. In such patients, rather than promoting anabolism, this solution may merely maintain the body at a near steady state.

Table 25-2. Ingredients of the mixed amino acid solution (Freamine) currently in use at the University of Cincinnati Medical Center[a]

Ingredient	Amount
Protein equivalent (gm)	40
Nitrogen, utilizable (gm)	6.4
Nitrogen, total (gm)	6.4
Total calories	959
Potassium (mEq/liter)	40
Sodium (mEq/liter)	21
Chloride (mEq/liter)	8
Magnesium (mEq/liter)	8
Calcium (mEq/liter)	4.7
Phosphate (mM/liter)	13.4
Acetate (mEq/liter)	29
Insulin USP (units)	15[b]
Vitamins	B Group, C (A, D, E)

[a]There is a certain amount of variation in the ionic components that the pharmacy will mix at the physician's request. The pharmacy will prepare the following variations: low potassium, 0; additional sodium, 50 mEq/liter (total).
[b]Optional.

Synthetic Amino Acid Solutions

The theoretic advantages to a synthetic amino acid solution are that its composition is known exactly, there are no dipeptides or tripeptides, and the amino acid composition may be varied with different situations. It has been demonstrated in a few patients that the smaller amount of protein in a synthetic amino acid solution and its slower rate of infusion as compared with a hydrolysate may be successful in promoting positive nitrogen balance.

Theoretic objections to these solutions involve their amino acid composition. An amino acid imbalance appears to contribute to a metabolic acidosis, a problem that can be easily remedied by the administration of sodium as the acetate rather than as the chloride (Table 25-2). Hyperammonemia has been reported with Freamine, but this appears to be confined to neonates of low birth weight. No cases have been observed since the original report (R. Winters, personal communication). In our own studies, only slight increases in blood ammonia have been observed in large numbers of adults given Freamine.

Fat

The use of fat has undergone several phases of evolution. In the early stages of parenteral nutrition, fat was omitted, largely due to the lack of a safe fat emulsion. As the latter became available, the administration of fat was used to prevent essential fatty acid deficiency by giving 4 to 6 percent of daily caloric supply as fat. More recently, fat has been used as a major caloric source as well as a source of essential fatty acids. Under normal circumstances or in patients with only moderate stress, fat and carbohydrate are indistinguishable with respect to nitrogen balance, and 25 to 30 percent of nonprotein calories as fat seems optimal for hepatic protein synthesis. Most agree, however, that the dose of calories provided by fat emulsions should not exceed 60 percent of total nonprotein calories, since caloric doses of fat in excess of this amount may exceed the patient's metabolic capacity for safe removal and oxidation, as well as impair nitrogen balance.

An area of remaining controversy is the use of fat in sepsis. During sepsis, fat utilization becomes altered, with the impairment of fat oxidation comparatively early in sepsis, followed later by impaired fat clearance. For this reason we believe that in the severely stressed or septic patient, reliance should be placed primarily on glucose and amino acids and the usage of fat decreased to only 10 percent of needs.

Others have suggested that the type of fat used may strongly influence immunologic and inflammatory processes in the septic patient and have focused on the relationship between the fatty acids linoleic and linolenic acid, and prostaglandin (PG) metabolism [24]. Linoleic acid, a W6 fatty acid, is the precursor of arachidonic acid and its metabolites, PGE_2, PGI_2, and thromboxane A_2 of the cyclo-oxygenase pathway and of certain leukotrienes. These metabolites have potent biologic effects, including the regulation of vascular responses, platelet aggregation, thrombosis, and immunosuppression. Linolenic acid, a W3 fatty acid, is converted to eicosapentaenoic acid, the precursor to the triene E_3 prostaglandins. Eicosapentaenoic acid is an inhibitor of linoleic acid metabolism and suppresses leukotriene B_4, a potent chemotactic and aggregating factor of neutrophils. It has therefore been suggested that dietary enrichment with eicosapentaenoic acid may be beneficial, whereas the use of standard fat emulsions containing a high percentage of linoleic acid may be harmful. Studies are underway in patients to test the effects of substitution of W3 fatty acids on outcome in critically ill patients.

Peripheral Parenteral Nutrition

Peripheral parenteral nutrition is, as the name implies, the technique of supplying total intravenous nutrition through a peripheral vein using a fat emulsion as a principal source of calories, with some glucose and a nitrogen source. This method avoids the use of hypertonic carbohydrate and the central venous catheter, the principal source of complications from the central parenteral technique. The cornerstone of peripheral therapy is the use of approximately 500 ml of 10% fat emulsion with each liter of peripheral formulation, which typically contains 3 to 4% amino acids and 5% dextrose. This may be carried out sequentially over a 24-hour period, giving 5% glucose and 3 to 4% amino acids for a 16-hour period and fat emulsion over an 8-hour period. Alternatively, solutions may be administered in Y fashion, giving fat and carbohydrate simultaneously.

Limitations

There are several limitations to the use of the peripheral technique as total support.

This "lipid system" uses fat almost exclusively as the caloric source and is often unable to supply the full nutritional support needed in the severely stressed patient. The amount of fat that can be given is limited to approximately 2 gm/kg/24 hr. Although occasional investigators have exceeded this amount, the incidence of thrombocytopenia and fat embolism increases significantly above the level of 2 gm/kg. In addition, fat utilization may be impaired during severe stress or sepsis, as previously noted.

The amino acid solution, even if administered as 10% glucose, contains only 500 calories/liter, making it difficult to meet the needs of a patient with high caloric demands without the infusion of large volumes of solution. For patients in delicate fluid balance due to congestive heart failure (CHF), respiratory failure/acute respiratory distress syndrome (ARDS), hepatic failure/ascites, etc., this practice would clearly be injurious. Some authors have suggested the use of diuretics; however, it seems more logical to use a central technique, which can supply a greater number of calories in a smaller volume.

It is difficult to conceive of keeping peripheral intravenous lines in patients for a prolonged period of time—say, 6 to 8 weeks—without an extraordinary amount of attention to intravenous technique. Prolonged peripheral administration leads to loss of peripheral venipuncture sites in patients who are chronically ill, due to phlebitis and sclerosis. This may constitute a drawback, particularly if surgery is contemplated.

Nonetheless, the peripheral technique lends itself well to circumstances in which supplemental rather than total nutrition is desired and when the risks of central total parenteral nutrition are great. Alternatively, when the patient resumes oral intake and one is not certain that gastrointestinal function will return rapidly, it may serve as an intermediate technique. In our experience, it can rarely be successfully carried out for more than 10 days, owing to the loss of venous access.

Monitoring

Frequent monitoring is necessary in patients on peripheral parenteral nutrition. Monitoring should be done daily for the first 3 days and should include triglycerides and cholesterol, which may not be cleared initially. Frequent monitoring of blood sugar, electrolytes, calcium, phosphorus, and magnesium is also essential, although serious ionic deficiencies are less likely to occur than they are with central nutrition. Fat emulsions, however, will provide essential fatty acids—usually required after 1 week in patients totally maintained—and to a certain extent will decrease the need for phosphate replacement, since they contain phospholipids in abundance.

Protein Sparing

The infusion of amino acids has been advocated by some as a means of decreasing the catabolism of lean body mass with subsequent reliance on endogenous caloric sources (i.e., fat). This proposal has been entirely discredited, both from a theoretic point of view [25] and from the fact that most patients for whom the possibility of parenteral nutrition is entertained are so catabolic that exogenous calories are required. In addition, in the original studies carried out by Blackburn and coworkers, 90 gm of amino acids were compared with 70 gm of amino acids and glucose [4]. Other authorities have clearly shown that the provision of glucose is beneficial [25]. This technique deserves no place in the nutritional support of any patient, and particularly the sick patient.

Central Parenteral Nutrition

There is little question that provision of large amounts of calories and protein to seriously ill patients by central parenteral nutrition has already saved many lives. Unfortunately, the method is not free of complications, and as with most complex therapy, recognition of the pitfalls has come with experience. By far the most serious of these complications are septic ones, generally catheter-related. It appears that even with an extremely rigid protocol, such as that used in many institutions throughout the United States, a certain minimal level of septic complications appears to be unavoidable, at least with our present techniques. In our experience, catheter care is the most important of all factors involved in reducing the sepsis rate to 1 to 3 percent, or even lower—in our institution, the current catheter sepsis rate is 0.8 percent.

Limiting Factors

Several factors limit the amount of solution that can be administered to a given patient in 24 hours. Some of these factors are variable—the patient's age, metabolic status, and endocrine reserve. The practical limit in the administration of glucose readily metabolized in the normal adult is approximately 400 to 500 mg/day, above which metabolic problems occur at greatly increased frequency. Most solutions currently available utilize a 25% glucose caloric source; the limit of administration is therefore approximately 2 to 3 liters/24 hr.

The calorie-nitrogen ratio is a magic number unsupported by hard data. The calorie-nitrogen ratio for efficacy of nitrogen utilization falls between 125 and 200 nonprotein calories per gram of nitrogen; there is little evidence of which we are aware to suggest that any ratio higher than this offers any significant advantage. Most studies, including our own, have concluded that a calorie-nitrogen ratio of about 150 : 1 is appropriate [27].

PLACEMENT OF THE CATHETER IN INTRAVENOUS NUTRITION

Site

Only two sites are acceptable for prolonged intravenous nutrition—the subclavian and internal jugular veins, terminating in the superior vena cava. Other sites (i.e., femoral vein, saphenous vein, external jugular, and long arm lines) appear to be associated with too high an incidence of infection or thrombosis, or both. Of the two, the subclavian approach is preferable, although it is accompanied by a slightly higher incidence of technical complications in placement. These complications decrease with

Table 25-3. Subclavian intravenous catheter placement set in use
at the University of Cincinnati Medical Center

Quantity	Item*
2	3-ml disposable syringe with 22-gauge needle
1	3-0 silk with straight needle (put on 3 × 3 sponge)
1	5-ml vial of lidocaine
1	Kelly "Pean"
1	Thumb forceps 5½"
1	B&S scissors 5½"
3	Towel clips
1	Folded half-sheet
3	Flat towels
10	3 × 3 Topper sponges
1	Disposable precaution gown

*The instructions are as follows. Place in Ekco tray, wrap in two 25 × 25 autoclave papers, and label. After set is autoclaved, put in a 12 × 20 Tower bag with a #16 Intracath 8" #3112, Betadine ointment, two filter masks, two pairs of size-7½ gloves. Seal. Date 2 months ahead. Flush equipment with distilled water before sterilizing for removal of pyrogens.

experience, although even the most experienced personnel will occasionally cause a complication. The subclavian catheter is more easily cared for,
the occlusive dressing is more easily carried out, and it is also more comfortable for the patient.

In our institution catheter placement is made easier by the prepackaging
of kits for subclavian placement that include catheter, masks, gowns,
gloves, sterile towel, half-sheets for draping of the patient, and simple instruments, including a Kelly clamp, scissors, and forceps (Table 25-3).
These kits are available on all floors and on special hyperalimentation
carts placed at strategic locations throughout the hospital. In addition to
the kits, the carts contain intravenous and "prep" solutions. Orders are
available on each unit.

Procedures

As with all procedures, proper preparation is essential. The placement of
central venous catheters is an elective procedure. Before the attempted insertion, the patient should be well hydrated and should have adequate
platelets and normal coagulation studies. The actual procedure may be
performed in the patient's room with the patient in bed; mild sedation is
helpful. The area of catheter placement is shaved and prepared with a surgical "prep" solution, including acetone, iodine, and alcohol. In general, it
is preferable to prepare both the subclavian and the internal jugular sites.
Then, if one is not successful in passing a subclavian catheter, an internal
jugular placement may be attempted, and vice versa. A nurse experienced
in the technique should be present. Fewer technical errors and breaches
of technique will occur under these circumstances.

The patient is placed in bed with a towel roll between the shoulder
blades to throw the shoulders back and the head of the manubrium sterni

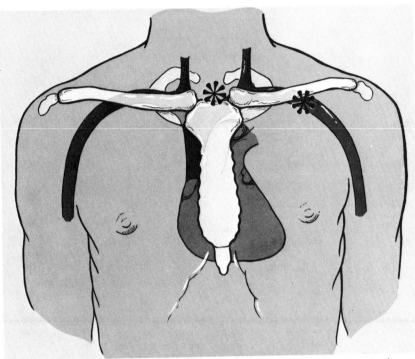

Fig. 25-1. Landmarks in placement of a subclavian catheter. Two principal landmarks are midpoint of clavicle, 1 cm below and 1 cm lateral to point at which clavicle bends, and a point 1 finger-breadth above manubrium sterni (toward which the needle should point).

forward; the arm is at the side. The subclavian vein is more easily approached in this fashion. The landmarks we use are approximately midway along the clavicle, 1 cm medial and 1 cm caudad to the bend. The point of the needle is directed toward 1 finger-breadth above the manubrium sterni (Fig. 25-1). In general, we prefer to locate the subclavian vein with a #22 needle in which the lidocaine has been placed in the skin and infiltrated around the periosteum. When the vein is located, the large-bore needle through which the catheter is passed will then be directed in a similar direction (toward the manubrium sterni). It is important not to direct the needle more than 10 or 15 degrees to the horizontal (Fig. 25-2). One must recall that the subclavian vein is the most anterior of all the structures in the thoracic inlet; all the structures that can be damaged, including the subclavian artery, the brachial plexus, and the apex of the lung, are posterior.

Once the needle is in place, the patient is asked to perform a Valsalva maneuver, and the catheter is passed through the open end of the needle. Alternatively, a Seldinger or guidewire technique can be used. This technique uses a smaller 18-gauge needle to enter the vein; in some cases, this may be preferable to the large 14-gauge needles used in the catheter-

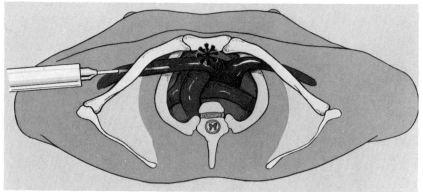

Fig. 25-2. Position of subclavian vein in reference to clavicle. Note that subclavian vein is uppermost structure in thoracic inlet. All the other structures, including subclavian artery, brachial plexus, and apex of lung, lie inferior and, to a certain extent, caudad. Needle is kept horizontal. If it is inserted at an angle of no greater than 10 or 15 degrees to the horizontal, complications will be avoided.

through-the-needle technique. To avoid placing the catheter in the internal jugular vein, the hub of the needle is directed cephalad. The catheter is then sutured into place, and an infusion of 5% D/W is started and continued until the catheter's position can be confirmed by a chest x-ray film; hypertonic solutions should not be administered before the x-ray is taken. A final 0.22-μ filter is inserted in the line. (This is optional; the additional manipulation may actually increase line sepsis rates.)

With respect to the internal jugular percutaneous puncture, one must remember that the internal jugular vein is anterior and lateral to the carotid artery. The landmark used here is a point 2 finger-breadths above the clavicle at the posterior border to the sternocleidomastoid border. The patient's neck is turned to the opposite side, and the arm is alongside the body. Again, the vein may be located with a #22 needle containing lidocaine, pointing toward the notch above the manubrium sterni. Here again, the catheter is sutured in place. It may be possible to pass the catheter subcutaneously under local anesthesia over the clavicle, so that the exit point is on the chest. This procedure gives the additional protection of the subcutaneous tunnel, which should theoretically decrease the incidence of sepsis; it is our belief that sepsis occurs by bacteria growing along the site of the venipuncture from the skin into the vein [3]. Also, dressing is easier in this position. Again, a chest x-ray is used to confirm the location of the catheter tip, which should be in the superior vena cava and not in the right atrium. Several cases of arrhythmia have been reported from placement of the catheter too close to the sinoatrial node.

Aftercare
The dressing is changed every 48 hours after the site has been cleansed with acetone iodine and alcohol solutions and an antifungal and a povi-

done ointment is applied. The position of the catheter when the dressing is done should be such that it is directed toward the nipple over the chest, and not over the arm, shoulder, or any other point.

GUIDELINES FOR PARENTERAL NUTRITION
General Guidelines
The most frequent metabolic complications in parenteral nutrition occur following too-rapid administration of hypertonic dextrose solutions when hyperalimentation is begun. Consequently, if the body is allowed time to equilibrate and if one allows an endogenous insulin response to build up, parenteral nutrition should be carried out safely and without hyperglycemia. The infusion is started at a rate of 40 ml/hr (assuming 25% dextrose as the caloric source). This is increased by increments of 20 ml/hr every day, until a target rate of infusion is reached. Insulin is added to the infusion in all patients over 30 years of age; this is our own preference and is not followed by many other investigators working in the area. Urine testing is carried out routinely, as shown in the printed orders (Fig. 25-3) that are with every patient's chart and are signed by the physician initiating the hyperalimentation. However, unless blood sugar is elevated, the presence of urinary glucose alone (at least within the first 48 hours) should not be used as an indication to administer insulin by test.

The ideal weight gain should be between ½ and 1 lb a day. A gain of over 1 lb almost certainly indicates fluid retention, signs of which in legs or sacrum will usually be detectable.

It is our custom never to use a pump in patients who are not in intensive care situations; we use a rate controller, as pumps generally tend to cause more problems than they solve. Of course, in cases in which fluid overload is critical, a pump is safe if supervised by a well-trained nurse, but such supervision rarely exists on a general hospital floor.

Ion Requirements
Ion requirements for patients on parenteral nutrition will vary from patient to patient, depending on previous body stores, renal function, and the primary disease for which the patient is being treated. Before initiating parenteral therapy, one should correct major fluid and electrolyte deficits. Although it is possible to add additional fluid and electrolytes to parenteral solutions to accomplish this, the early fluctuations in volume and electrolytes usually lead to frequent changes in formulation that result in excessive waste and increased cost. Furthermore, when there are ongoing losses of large amounts of fluid and electrolytes, as in small-bowel obstruction or high-output gastrointestinal fistulas, a separate intravenous infusion should be established to manage them.

It is possible, however, to suggest approximate requirements for the maintenance and/or repletion of lean body mass.

Potassium
Whole-body potassium stores are depleted in starved patients, potassium being the primary intracellular cation that tends to be lost in the urine as muscle is catabolized for gluconeogenesis. Thus, repletion of lean body

UMC-374
Revised 5/88

University of Cincinnati Hospital
Physician's Checklist/Order Sheet

All applicable orders have been checked. A line has been placed through orders that have been voided. ORDERS NOT CHECKED ARE NOT TO BE FOLLOWED. Orders have been modified according to the medical condition of the patient. These orders have been dated, timed and signed by a physician. As an order is filled, the individual doing so must date/time and initial in the space provided. Further orders will be added as needed.

PAGE __1__ OF __1__

ORDER NUMBER	√	PHYSICIAN'S STANDING ORDERS PARENTERAL NUTRITION	ORDER NOTED (DATE/TIME)	(INITIAL)
1.	√	Infuse only through a new subclavian or internal jugular or existing implanted catheter which terminates in superior vena cava or brachiocephalic vein.		
2.	√	STAT portable chest x-ray.		
3.	√	Initial and subsequent dressing by nurse (per Nursing Procedure).		
4.	√	Infuse D_5W at 40 ml/hr until TPN is available.		
5.	√	Administration via infusion device.		
6.	√	Catheter may be used only for TPN except by order of Nutritional Support physician.		
7.	√	Vital signs Q 6 hours.		
8.	√	Urine sugars Q 6 hours with Diastix.		
9.	√	Intake and Output Q 24 hours.		
10.	√	Weights Monday, Wednesday, and Friday.		
11.	√	Blood Work: MONDAY: Renal (4203), Bone (4041) & Hepatic (4162) Profiles. THURSDAY AND PRIOR TO STARTING PARENTERAL NUTRITION: Renal (4203), Bone (4041) & Hepatic (4162) Profiles, CBC (4032), Prothrombin Time (4204), Transferrin (4706), Prealbumin (4705), Retinol Binding Protein (4707), Magnesium (4229), Cholesterol & Triglyceride (4726), Amino Acid Profile (4265).		
12.	√	STAT blood glucose for 1/4% or greater glycosuria.		
13.	√	If parenteral nutrition solution is interrupted, infuse D_5W at the same rate until it is restarted.		
14.	√	Notify Nutritional Support for catheter removal and culture Mon.-Fri. 9:00 a.m.-4:00 p.m.		

White-Chart   Yellow-Kardex

Physician's signature _____

Date _____ Time _____

Developed by _____   Date _____

Fig. 25-3. Protocol for administration of parenteral nutrition at the University of Cincinnati Hospital.

mass is usually accompanied by a tremendous requirement for potassium—approximately 100 to 120 mEq/day. Its fate is varied; much enters intracellularly through repletion of protein and an anabolic state, some is lost in the urine, and some is lost in perspiration. Patients with compromised renal function will not tolerate 120 mEq of potassium, and a decreased dose is administered carefully. Potassium is generally determined twice weekly in patients who are stable and is administered as the chloride, phosphate, or acetate.

Magnesium

The requirements for magnesium appear to vary with calcium and phosphorus metabolism. In patients with a normal serum phosphorus and normal bony stores of calcium, approximately 8 to 16 mEq/day of magnesium is reasonable. Magnesium is useful as a cofactor, and much is taken up intracellularly. Again, patients whose renal function is impaired will have a lower requirement for magnesium than will patients with normal renal function. Magnesium is administered as the sulfate.

Phosphate

Hypophosphatemia is not a complication of hyperalimentation; it is a deficiency state, since most total parenteral nutrition (TPN) solutions do not contain adequate phosphate. Unfortunately, numerous cases of hypophosphatemic coma occurred prior to the realization that phosphate, which is present in normal diets, had been omitted. The requirement for phosphate is approximately 30 to 45 mM/24 hr; it is greater in very depleted patients. Much of this is utilized for membrane phospholipids, high-energy phosphate bonds, and perhaps some storage in the bone. Patients with renal impairment will excrete and require less phosphate than will those with normal renal function. Phosphate is generally administered as the sodium or potassium salt.

Calcium

The requirement for calcium is approximately 3 to 8 mEq/day but may in fact be much higher. It will be increased if the patient is allowed to become hypophosphatemic or hypomagnesemic. Serum levels, of course, do not reflect total body stores, since bone contains vast calcium stores; rather, they reflect the levels of magnesium and phosphate. Calcium is administered as the chloride or gluconate.

Sodium

One does not ordinarily think of sodium in terms of requirement. If sodium is not administered, urine excretion of water may be impaired, with resultant water retention and hyponatremia. It is currently our practice to administer approximately 70 to 100 mEq of sodium daily, even in patients in whom fluid retention is suspected and peripheral edema may be a problem. Paradoxically, the administration of sodium to these patients appears to enable them to excrete sodium along with water, and the incidence of peripheral edema and hyponatremia does not appear to be so high under these circumstances. Sodium may be administered in the form of chloride or as acetate, which will tend to counteract any metabolic acidosis in amino acid preparations.

Most patients on parenteral nutrition tend to become hypochloremic. Hypochloremia rarely becomes a problem. If there is a metabolic syndrome associated with hypochloremia, we have not recognized it. Approximately 50 to 100 mEq of chloride appears to be required. Its fate is uncertain; it may be stored in the bone or be lost in perspiration. Requirements for chloride will, of course, be increased if the patient has a large gastrostomy or nasogastric tube output; in this case, increased amounts of chloride may be given as potassium chloride or sodium chloride; both may be required.

Ionic Compatibilities

In most patients, it should not be necessary to administer extra intravenous fluids to manage metabolic problems. Additives are sufficiently varied to enable management with hyperalimentation solution alone. A list of compatibilities is shown in Table 25-4.

Trace Metals

Multiple trace-element solutions are now commercially available and are added daily to parenteral solutions. Trace elements participate in a variety of important metabolic functions, including protein and nucleic acid synthesis, membrane transport, mitochondrial function, nerve conduction, and muscle contraction. Essential trace elements for human existance are iodine (I), cobalt (Co), zinc (Zn), copper (Cu), chromium (Cr), and manganese (Mn). Other important trace elements are selenium (Se), molybdenum (Mb), vanadium (Va), nickel (Ni), and silicon (Si). Although not common today, some of the clinical syndromes associated with deficiencies of trace elements are as follows.

Zinc—acrodermatitis enteropathica, impaired wound healing
Copper—anemia, neutropenia
Chromium—hyperglycemia
Manganese—impaired growth, skeletal abnormalities, ataxia, convulsions
Selenium—muscle weakness, cardiomyopathy

Essential Fatty Acids

With the ready availability of safe fat emulsions, essential fatty acid deficiency should be a rarely seen deficiency. Essential fatty acid deficiency in patients receiving prolonged parenteral nutrition was recognized as long ago as 1929 [9]. At present, however, the early lesions are difficult to recognize, but essential fatty acid deficiency probably has serious implications for the patient on prolonged parenteral nutrition. In addition to the skin lesions and anemia associated with fatty acid deficiency, it is clear that wound healing is adversely affected.

Biochemical lesions suggesting essential fatty acid deficiency are manifested as a change in the ratio of unsaturated fatty acids and the appearance of eicosatrienoic acid in the serum, generally after 3 to 4 weeks without

Table 25-4. Allowable additive supplementation

Additives	Available products	Maximum allowable total per liter bottle
Calcium	*Calcium gluconate inj. Calcium chloride inj.	9 mEq
Magnesium	Magnesium sulfate	12 mEq
Phosphate	*Sodium phosphate inj. Potassium phosphate inj.	21 mM
Potassium	*Potassium chloride inj. Potassium acetate inj.	80 mEq
Sodium	*Sodium chloride inj. Sodium acetate inj.	Patient tolerance or need
Chloride	*Sodium chloride inj. Calcium chloride inj. Potassium chloride inj.	Limited by amount of cation
	HCl inj.	100 mEq
Acetate	*Sodium acetate inj. Potassium acetate inj.	Limited by amount of cation
Insulin	Regular insulin inj.	50 units

*With these electrolytes, unless otherwise specified on Physician's Order Form, additives supplemental to the established formulas will be added as the asterisked salt.

oral intake. Other biochemical lesions, such as failure of prostaglandin synthesis, manifested as decreased intraocular pressure, are present a week after fat-free parenteral nutrition [18]. At 4 weeks, skin lesions begin to appear. Anecdotal reports on some patients have indicated that wound healing appears to improve with correction of essential fatty acid deficiency.

Essential fatty acid deficiency can be prevented by the administration of fat emulsions as approximately 4 to 5 percent of the caloric requirement daily—i.e., about 200 ml of 10% fat emulsion in the average patient. As an alternative, 50 gm of corn or safflower oil given daily through a gastrostomy or jejunostomy tube should be sufficient to prevent fatty acid deficiency.

Vitamins

Although there are many data on the requirements for vitamins in normal patients, it is not clear whether these requirements are increased in patients who are stressed, injured, starved, or septic. There is some evidence that surgical patients require large amounts of vitamin C, and it is our practice to administer between 2 and 3 gm of vitamin C over 24 hours to such patients. A daily requirement for vitamin B appears to be easy to satisfy (see Table 25-5), and vitamin B toxicity has not been recognized. Clinical syndromes from overdosage with the fat-soluble of vitamins A and D have been recognized for some time in patients on prolonged parenteral nutrition. We have observed at least two cases of vitamin D toxicity and one

Table 25-5. Daily vitamin requirements[a]

Vitamin	Amount
Thiamine	5–10 mg
Riboflavin	4–5 mg
Niacin	8–20 mg
Pyridoxine	20 mg
Pantothenate	20 mg
Vitamin C	300–500 mg[b]
Vitamin A	2500–5000 IU
Vitamin D	400 IU
Vitamin E	10 IU

[a]This is one of several schemata for daily vitamin requirements. The exact requirements are not known, but this is a reasonable approximation.
[b]In injury and large wounds, up to 2 gm of ascorbic acid may be given. Evidence for efficacy is not well established.

case of vitamin A toxicity, the latter including eye and skin lesions and jaundice. With this in mind, our practice has been to give 5000 units of vitamin A and 500 units of vitamin D on a weekly basis. This has been sufficient to prevent the appearance of clinical deficiency of these vitamins, and toxicity has not been observed. There is less knowledge about vitamin E, and the existence of a clinical vitamin E deficiency state is controversial. It is therefore appropriate to administer small amounts of vitamin E, together with the other fat-soluble vitamins. Folate, vitamin B_{12}, and vitamin K apparently are not stable within the solution, and thus we do not add them, but administer them parenterally.

Monitoring

Monitoring of a patient with hyperalimentation depends on the patient's overall stability. In patients who are stable without massive fluid requirements or shifts, it is sufficient to monitor vital signs and urine glucose four times daily. Weights should be obtained approximately every other day. At the initiation of therapy, a complete battery of laboratory data is obtained, including the following profiles: renal (sodium, potassium, chloride, bicarbonate, blood urea nitrogen, creatinine, serum glucose); bone (calcium, phosphate), hepatic (albumin, total bilirubin, alkaline phosphatase, SGOT, SGPT), lipid profile (cholesterol, triglycerides), complete blood count, platelet count, prothrombin time, amino acid; and nutrition screen (transferrin, prealbumin, retinol-binding protein). Subsequently, the patient is monitored by twice-weekly labs. On Monday, renal, bone, and hepatic profiles are obtained, and on Thursday the complete initial battery of tests is repeated. Other aspects of monitoring are detailed in the Standard Order (Fig. 24-3) that is included in each patient's record. More-frequent determination of electrolytes and other parameters may be required by the patient's condition, especially if large amounts of fluid shifts occur or if gastrointestinal losses are high, as in patients with fistulas or high-gastrostomy drainage.

The adequacy of the nutritional regimen should be reassessed each week. We generally reserve nitrogen balance studies and the use of indirect calorimetry for the more complicated cases.

COMPLICATIONS OF PARENTERAL NUTRITION

Metabolic Complications

Significant metabolic complications are the result of deficiency states and disorders of glucose metabolism. Deficiency states include alterations in sodium, potassium, and more commonly, magnesium and phosphorus, which are present in the normal diet in large amounts but are not thought of as being specifically required. Thus, the administration of adequate amounts of magnesium and phosphorus is of greatest importance. The requirements for sodium, potassium, and chloride will depend on the basic disease for which the patient is being treated.

Disorders of glucose metabolism are one of the most dangerous complications of parenteral nutrition. Finally, a usually less serious but frequently discussed metabolic complication is hepatic dysfunction.

Hypomagnesemia

Hypomagnesemia may be suspected clinically by complaints of tingling in the extremities and around the mouth; agitation is also common. Serum magnesium will often be less than 0.6 mg/100 ml or undetectable. In patients with normal renal function, 8 to 16 mEq/day is generally required. However, during repletion states, and particularly in patients with liver disease or with profound diarrhea, this level may be exceeded. Magnesium can be replaced as the 10% sulfate in the solution or 50% sulfate in 2-ml intramuscular injections.

Hypophosphatemia

Hypophosphatemia coma was late in being recognized, merely because a clinical counterpart previously had not been seen often. It is not a complication of hyperalimentation per se, but rather a deficiency state secondary to inadequate intravenous administration of phosphate. It is estimated that 90 mEq of phosphate is required normally. During periods of repletion, this level may be exceeded. The symptomatology of hypophosphatemic coma is striking; having once observed it, one will not easily forget it. The earliest manifestations are lethargy and a slurring of speech; the patient complains of a "thick tongue." Thereafter, hypophosphatemia progresses to unconsciousness and coma. Anemia and abnormalities in phagocyte function and oxygen delivery have been attributed to hypophosphatemia.

Hyperglycemia

Hyperglycemia may be caused by too-rapid infusion of hypertonic dextrose solutions, by decreased insulin output secondary to diabetes or pancreatitis, or by the side effect of medications (steroids). Not uncommonly, however, the appearance of hyperglycemia in a previously stable patient who had not been spilling glucose signals the onset of sepsis; the latter will usually become apparent within 12 to 18 hours. The appearance of a 4+ glucose urine in a patient whose urine was previously negative should provoke an intensive search for sources of sepsis before it assumes overwhelming proportions. Prompt treatment will result in subsidence of the tendency toward hyperglycemia.

One stage beyond the development of hyperglycemia is the symptomatic hyperosmolar nonketotic state leading to coma. This clinical syndrome, comprising fever, osmotic diuresis, obtundation, and finally death, may be recognized by the presence of large quantities of glucose in the urine and the change in the mental status of the patient, without symptoms that would suggest acidosis. Ketone bodies are not present in the blood or urine, but the blood sugar will range from 400 to 1000 mg/100 ml. If this is not corrected, death follows rapidly. The serum sodium tends to be low if measured during the acute episode, but this is spuriously low secondary to hyperglycemia. With the correction of hyperglycemia, serum sodium will return to normal without the addition of exogenous sodium.

Therapy consists of prompt cessation of glucose infusion, administration of heroic quantities of insulin, and administration of large volumes of glucose-free solutions. Potassium is also required.

Hypoglycemia
Hypoglycemia is a rare occurrence that usually is the result of the sudden termination of a glucose infusion while still at a high rate. Parenteral infusions should usually be tapered, and this can be done over several days or several hours if necessary. If, for whatever reason, the infusion should be stopped while still at a high rate, hypoglycemia can be prevented by the peripheral infusion of D_5/W.

Hepatic Dysfunction
Some degree of hepatic dysfunction usually occurs in patients on parenteral nutrition following 1 to 3 weeks of therapy. Although poorly understood, it is usually a self-limited complication. It is manifested biochemically by elevations in alkaline phosphatase and the transaminases. In adult patients, significant elevations in serum bilirubin are almost never due to parenteral nutrition. Histologically, hepatic dysfunction appears as hepatic steatosis. Suggested causes include toxins (breakdown products of amino acids and bacterial endotoxins), deficiency states (essential fatty acid deficiency), excess carbohydrate administration, inappropriate proportion of nutrients, lack of enteral stimulation of the gut with altered levels of gut hormones, and abnormal portal ratios of insulin and glucagon. The keys to prevention are careful adjustments of nutritional support to meet needs, avoidance of deficiency states, and utilization of the gut whenever possible in order to maintain the structural and functional integrity of the gut.

Technical Complications
Complications secondary to catheter placement often occur with distressing frequency when hyperalimentation is initiated at a given institution. However, with increasing experience, the number of such complications should decrease. The most common complication in placement of internal jugular catheters is carotid artery cannulation or laceration, with second-

ary neck hematomas. Occasionally, respiratory obstruction may result, requiring urgent tracheostomy. Usually, however, an inadvertent carotid artery puncture will subside with pressure alone, except in patients with bleeding disorders.

Subclavian catheterization results in a much more interesting and varied group of complications. Technical complications may be largely avoided by keeping the needle near the horizontal plane, since the vein is most anterior. The most common complication by far is pneumothorax. Since many patients will be on the respirator when catheterized, it is our practice to take them off the respirator and hand-beathe them with a self-inflating bag—e.g., Ambu bag*—for the duration of the catheter insertion, since this will not hyperinflate the lungs to the same extent as the respirator does, and the apex of the lung remains posterior and inferior to the vein. Laceration of the subclavian artery for the most part is uncommon, and since the subclavian artery lies posterior to the subclavian vein, one will rarely strike it if the needle is kept at an angle no steeper than 15 degrees to the horizontal. Pressure above and below the clavicle will result in the cessation of hemorrhage. Another avoidable complication is administration of fluid intrathoracically, which occurs because x-ray confirmation of catheter position is imperfect. Infusion of hypertonic solutions will bring about a hydrothorax, recognizable by the development of pain, tachypnea, respiratory distress, and, often, shock. The chest film will confirm what has been detected by physical examination. This complication may be prevented by making certain before starting infusions that blood can be aspirated through the catheter.

Not all hydrothoraxes are secondary to catheter malposition. A rare and poorly understood complication is the development of "sympathetic effusion," in which the material infused does not enter the thoracic cavity, but a clear "sympathetic" exudate free of glucose is obtained. The reason for this complication is not known, although it may follow a mediastinal hematoma.

Many other mechanical complications have been described in the literature, covering virtually every situation imaginable, including arteriovenous fistula, thoracic duct fistula, bronchopleural cutaneous fistula, and superior vena cava bronchial fistula. Air embolism may be prevented at the time of insertion by having the patient perform a Valsalva maneuver as the catheter is passed. Some minimal technical complications appear to be unavoidable. Even physicians with extensive experience will occasionally cause a pneumothorax. However, the incidence can be decreased to an unavoidable minimum with experience.

Sepsis

The most dreaded complication of parenteral nutrition is the development of bacterial or fungal sepsis. It is generally agreed that adherence to strict catheter care protocols and the use of catheters that are reserved only for

---

*Air-Shields, Inc., Hatboro, PA.

parenteral nutrition have been responsible for the decline in catheter sepsis rates from 6 to 27 percent to the currently acceptable rates of 1 to 3 percent.

Catheter sepsis may originate from contaminated solutions, violations of the administration set, intraluminal migration of bacteria from the catheter hub, colonization of the skin adjacent to the insertion site, or hematogenous seeding of the catheter from blood-borne organisms from distant foci of infection. Based on epidemiologic studies at our institution, we believe that the skin site is the most frequent source of infection [3]. According to this theory, when a threshold number of organisms at the skin site (10^3 CFU) is exceeded, the fibrin sleeve that forms around the catheter becomes colonized, and catheter sepsis follows. The most commonly encountered bacterial pathogens are gram-positive cocci, *Staphylococcus epidermidis* and *Staphylococcus aureus,* and *Candida albicans* is the most common fungal pathogen. *S. aureus* and *C. albicans* appear to have an increased ability to colonize the fibrin sheath of central venous catheters through hematogenous seeding, whereas *S. epidermidis* is more likely to infect catheters via colonization of the skin site. For this reason, we feel that a positive blood culture for *S. aureus* or *C. albicans* requires the immediate removal of all central venous catheters.

The diagnosis and treatment of catheter-related sepsis can often be a troublesome issue. We define catheter sepsis as an episode of clinical sepsis in a patient with a central venous catheter who has no other apparent source of sepsis and whose symptoms and signs resolve with removal of the catheter. Clinical evidence of catheter-related sepsis may include fever (100.5°F PO or 101.5°F rectal), chills, leukocytosis, glucose intolerance, marked erythema or purulence of the catheter insertion site, worsening of the patient's condition, septic shock, or a previous positive blood culture. In the absence of other sources of infection, the immediate removal of the central venous catheter is clearly indicated and is usually all that is necessary for treatment. Another catheter is not placed for an additional 24 hours, to allow the septicemia to subside.

If *Candida* sepsis develops, however, it is absolutely necessary not to reinstate glucose infusions until serial blood cultures have been demonstrated to be free of *Candida* organisms. It has been our experience that not all patients with blood cultures positive for *Candida* need to be treated with amphotericin B if cultures revert to negative. However, even after catheter removal and negative blood cultures for several days, *Candida* may appear in the bloodstream when hyperalimentation is resumed. If this is the case, hyperalimentation must be stopped, and the possibility of alternative means of nutrition, such as fat infusion or tube feedings, must be entertained.

More controversial is what to do with the patient who does have a non-catheter source of infection and in whom catheter sepsis must be ruled out. Obviously, one would like to avoid the needless removal of sterile catheters. For these patients it is helpful to obtain confirmatory evidence of catheter sepsis, which may include positive cultures of the patient's blood or of the tip of the catheter, if it was removed. As an alternative, we have found semiquantitative cultures of the skin at the catheter insertion site helpful in avoiding unnecessary removal of sterile catheters from patients who are septic from a noncatheter source. In our experience, a sterile culture of the skin is 99 percent predictive of a sterile catheter, providing that neither *S. aureus* nor *C. albicans* has been cultured from the blood. Another alternative is the exchange of central venous catheters over a guidewire and culturing of the catheter tip. This may be of limited usefulness in patients who are at risk for repeated central venous cannulation or who have very limited intravenous access. If the results of the culture are positive, the newly exchanged catheter must be removed. It is important to stress that we feel this is a diagnostic and not a therapeutic maneuver, as some have advocated [7]. The site of the infection is the fibrin sheath, not the catheter. Therefore, it makes little sense to us to change the catheter, leaving the infected fibrin sheath in place.

A final controversial issue is the use of multilumen catheters. Some investigators have reported an acceptably low rate of catheter sepsis with these catheters, whereas others have reported higher rates of sepsis. It is our impression that the rate of catheter sepsis is increased with multilumen catheters. It remains our preference to use a single-lumen catheter whenever possible, even if it means placing a second intravenous catheter for administration of fluids, blood, or medications. In patients with limited access in whom we feel the use of a multilumen catheter is justified, we recommend changing the catheter every 3 days over a guidewire, with culture of the tip. If the culture is negative, the catheter can continue to be used; however, if it should return positive, it must be discontinued. We realize that there are those who disagree, but this is our practice.

Subclavian Thrombosis

The complication of subclavian thrombosis has been overlooked in the past. Although the incidence of clinically apparent thrombosis ranges from 2 to 5 percent, the actual occurrence of thrombosis as determined by studies utilizing venography is closer to 20 to 50 percent, with the majority being asymptomatic [8].

Postulated mechanisms include those related to the placement and maintenance of the catheter, to the composition of the catheter, and, finally, to the host. Catheter insertion by itself leads to intimal disruption of the vein and may instigate thrombus formation. With time, a fibrin sleeve usually forms on catheters and can also serve as the nidus for thrombus formation or a "sleeve thrombus." Other factors that may contribute include irritation of the acidic, hypertonic infusion and direct contact of the catheter along the vein (Fig. 25-4).

Composition of the catheter is another important determinant of thrombus formation. Polyvinylchloride appears to be the most thrombogenic, and silastic catheters the least. Finally, host factors related to blood stasis or hypercoaguability may contribute to venous thrombosis and include immobilization, congestive heart failure, sepsis, and malignancy.

In addition to the pain and swelling that may occur in the affected arm, subclavian vein thrombosis may be the source of sepsis (venous thrombophlebitis) and/or pulmonary emboli. If this is suspected, diagnosis is

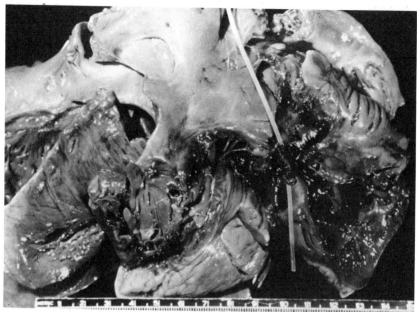

Fig. 25-4. Pathologic specimen depicting thrombosis of subclavian vein. Note that catheter extends through thrombus and that thrombus originates from subclavian vein wall in an area of impingement but not necessarily an area where hypertonic solution runs into vein wall. This suggests that subclavian vein thrombosis, an overlooked complication, occurs because of catheter reactivity rather than because of impingement of hypertonic solution against the vein.

made by upper extremity venography. Noninvasive techniques that have also proven to be useful are B-mode ultrasonography and phleborrheography.

Treatment involves immediate removal of the catheter, elevation of the extremity, and anticoagulation with heparin. If treatment is prompt, the arm swelling will usually decrease markedly, with minimal residual effect. A prominent venous pattern, however, will remain in the upper extremity and around the shoulder of the thrombosed subclavian vein. Occasionally, these will recanalize and allow the placement of another catheter. However, in our experience, this has almost never happened, and the affected side is lost for cannulation (Fig. 25-5).

Treatment of septic thrombophlebitis is more difficult and involves the removal of the catheter, use of antibiotics, and, potentially, removal of the infected vein.

SOLUTIONS FOR USE IN SPECIFIC ORGAN SYSTEM FAILURE
Renal Failure
Although the use of specific solutions for organ failure is still evolving, there has been sufficient experience with total parenteral nutrition in dif-

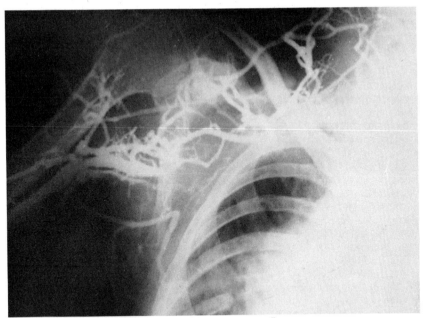

Fig. 25-5. Venogram of vessels in shoulder area following thrombosis of subclavian vein. Note that there is complete obliteration of subclavian vein, which is replaced by a number of smaller vessels, none of which is suitable for cannulation.

ferent disease states at our institution and others to suggest that specific diseases may require alterations in solution composition for greater efficacy. By far the largest amount of information available is on the administration of essential amino acids and hypertonic dextrose to patients in acute renal failure. This solution, with which extensive experience has been gathered, is an intravenous modification of the Giordanno diet. Giordanno [21] had shown that in patients with chronic renal failure, positive nitrogen balance can be achieved, with lowering of the blood urea nitrogen and improved patient well-being, provided that essential amino acids primarily are given and that the amount of nonessential amino acids is limited. Under such circumstances, urea nitrogen, previously thought to have been an end product in man, is split by gut bacteria to ammonia, reabsorbed, and made available for synthesis by transamination into nonessential amino acids. The combined essential and nonessential amino acids are then synthesized into protein, provided adequate energy is available. The entire process takes place at a lower protein intake than had been previously thought.

The first reports on the use of renal failure solution for patients who could not eat and required hyperalimentation were those by Wilmore and Dudrick [40] and Abel et al. [1]. In the study by Abel et al., the solution used consisted of essential amino acids and 47% dextrose (Table 25-6) and was used as primary therapy for patients with acute renal failure. It was

Table 25-6. Composition of 750-ml unit of Nephramine (renal failure solution) in use at the University of Cincinnati Medical Center*

Constituent	Amount
Essential amino acids	
L-Isoleucine	1.40 gm
L-Leucine	2.20
L-Lycine HCl	2.00
L-Methionine	2.20
L-Threonine	1.00
L-Tryptophan	0.50
L-Valine	1.63
Total	13.13 gm
Vitamin content	
Thiamine HCl (B$_1$)	25 mg
Riboflavin (as phosphate) (B$_2$)	5 mg
Pyridoxine HCl (B$_6$)	7.5 mg
Niacinamide	50 mg
Dexpanthenol	12.5 mg
Vitamin A	5000 USP units
Vitamin D (ergocalciferol)	500 USP units
Vitamin E (di-α-tocopheryl acetate)	2.5 IU
Ascorbic acid (vitamin C)	1.25 gm
Calories (47% dextrose)	1400
Total nitrogen	1.46 gm
α-Amino nitrogen	1.3 gm

*This intravenous modification of the Giordanno diet is well within the tolerance of most patients, even those with oliguric or anuric renal failure.

used both for the caloric-sparing effect of glucose—at which there are apparently two break points, 800 and 2200 calories, as was so well shown by Professor Henry Lee [28]—and for the Giordanno diet: that is, to lower BUN. Although the frequency of dialysis among the patients was not decreased, a somewhat unexpected but statistically significant increase in survival was observed, and renal failure was of shorter duration. Another beneficial effect was an improvement in the patients' ability to withstand complications. Although complications such as infection, gastrointestinal hemorrhage, and pneumonitis were not prevented, a higher survival rate followed if the complication occurred when the patient was receiving essential amino acids. A protective effect on uremic coma was observed as well.

Other trials of similar regimens have been unable to reproduce the same effects on recovery of acute renal failure, although the number of patients studied was much too small [14]. This led to the recommendation by some to use both essential and nonessential amino acids for patients with acute renal failure requiring TPN. However, this also has not been associated with consistent results related to the recovery of renal function after acute renal failure or to patient survival. A retrospective study by Freund and Fischer [19] concluded that treatment with essential and nonessential amino acids was associated with a decreased survival in comparison to a historical control group that received essential amino acids.

We continue to advocate the use of essential amino acids in 47% dextrose in all patients with acute tubular necrosis, either intravenously or as an elemental diet (AminAid*), which may be substituted for the intravenous form and which is discussed below. Since elemental diets must be started slowly, we generally start with intravenous infusion and gradually introduce the elemental diet if the patient's gastrointestinal tract is functioning.

The components of the solution are given in Table 25-6. Note that 47% dextrose is given in a small volume, so that even patients who are oliguric may receive a substantial number of calories. If there are gastrointestinal tract losses from a gastrostomy or nasogastric tube, an intake of 2250 calories is easily achieved. The solution is started at 30 ml/hr and increased 10 ml/hr each day until a rate of 70 ml/hr is reached. Since urinary glucose is notoriously unreliable in renal failure, the blood glucose should be checked at least daily when therapy is started. Insulin is added to the bottle as necessary, since hyperglycemia tends to develop in these patients, particularly if hepatic malfunction is present. It is not clear that a rate of greater than 70 ml/hr offers any significant advantage and the incidence of hyperglycemia increases markedly beyond this rate. Hypokalemia, hypomagnesemia, and hypophosphatemia occur regularly, and electrolytes should be checked every other day instead of twice weekly or every 5 days, as with the standard solutions.

Although the use of this solution may forestall the need for dialysis, a statistically significant effect on the incidence of dialysis has not been observed. If aggressive chronic dialysis is undertaken, both essential and nonessential amino acids will be lost, as we would suggest that patients be then changed to a solution containing both essential and nonessential amino acids. This will cause a marked increase in blood urea. This type of solution is suggested only for patients who are dialyzed every other day regardless of their symptoms or blood urea nitrogen. If a more flexible schedule of dialysis can be undertaken, we suggest that the patient be given only essential amino acids and hypertonic dextrose, in order to decrease the frequency of dialysis; dialysis in itself may be harmful, particularly in the elderly or in patients with unstable cardiovascular function. We have not observed more-frequent sepsis or metabolic complications in patients with renal failure who receive total parenteral nutrition, perhaps because of the importance of the essential amino acids in nonspecific host resistance.

Cardiac Failure

The patient with rheumatic heart disease, particularly with mitral stenosis and insufficiency, is often cachectic on the basis of long-standing anorexia and cardiac malfunction. If one adds cardiopulmonary bypass to an already nutritionally depleted patient, the complications most frequently seen (hepatic dysfunction, renal dysfunction, and respiratory insuffi-

*Kendall-McGaw Laboratories, Irvine, CA.

ciency) undoubtedly have a significant nutritional component. Preliminary hyperalimentation of patients undergoing cardiopulmonary bypass may be beneficial, although this remains to be verified in prospective fashion. For such patients, who frequently can tolerate only a limited fluid volume, a synthetic amino acid solution with 35% dextrose, known as Cardiac Hyperal for lack of a better name, is being utilized. This offers the advantage of a large number of calories in a small volume. Precautions in its administration are similar to those for the so-called renal failure solution. Infusion is started at 30 ml/hr and gradually increased by 10 ml/hr on a daily basis until the rate of 60 or 70 ml/hr is reached. If a patient can tolerate 1500 ml, it is doubtful that the hypertonic glucose solution is required; and since it is not known whether or not such hypertonic solutions are well tolerated indefinitely (for example, is the incidence of subclavian thrombosis higher?), it would seem reasonable to change to a 15 or 25% dextrose solution in patients who can tolerate the volume.

Monitoring is carried out every other day, as suggested with renal failure patients. The occurrence of hyperglycemia and other metabolic problems can be much more sudden in patients receiving 35% dextrose than in those receiving the 25% solution.

Hepatic Failure

The liver is the central metabolic organ of the body. Therefore, when it fails, multiple metabolic processes become deranged. The implications of this for the critically ill patient are obvious. Therapy for hepatic failure is geared toward the support of affected organ systems while allowing time for hepatic regeneration to occur. Of the known hepatotrophic factors, nutrition is the most easily manipulated, making the provision of adequate calories, protein, and micronutrients the cornerstone of the management of these patients. Implementation of this program becomes complicated, however, since both the provision of conventional nutrition or the restriction of protein because of encephalopathy may result in a worsening of hepatic function. The objective of nutritional management then is to administer nutrients in sufficient quantity and of appropriate quality to avoid intolerance.

To understand the basis for current nutritional management of hepatic failure, one must understand the basic metabolic alterations that occur and how they relate to hepatic encephalopathy. Common features of hepatic failure are accelerated catabolism and gluconeogenesis caused by elevated levels of circulating catabolic hormones, glucagon, epinephrine, and cortisol. This is brought about by the shunting of blood flow away from the liver and impaired hepatic degradation of amino acids and hormones. Peripheral insulin resistance develops that impairs glucose utilization and results in the rapid depletion of hepatic and skeletal muscle carbohydrate stores. The body responds by attempting to recruit alternate energy sources. In the normal fasting state, fat would be used; however, fat utilization also becomes impaired in hepatic failure.

The body then turns to protein by default, and alterations in amino acid metabolism are probably the most prominent biochemical changes in hepatic failure. The breakdown of skeletal muscle releases a variety of amino acids, with local utilization of branched-chain amino acids (BCAA) for energy and the accumulation of aromatic amino acids (AAA) because of the decreased ability of the failing liver to catabolize them. The end result is the distinct amino acid pattern that characterizes hepatic failure, with elevation of AAA, threonine, and methionine, and lowered levels of BCAA. The molar ratio of BCAA to AAA [(valine + leucine + isoleucine)/(phenylalanine + tyrosine)] begins to fall from 3.5, the usual value in the normal person. In hepatic failure, a molar ratio of 1.4 to 2.0 usually represents significant liver disease, and a ratio of 1.0 or less has correlated with the presence of hepatic encephalopathy. Other amino acid abnormalities include a decreased ability to convert phenylalanine to tyrosine.

The development of encephalopathy represents a serious complication of hepatic failure and serves as a useful end-point guideline during nutritional support. A detailed discussion of the theories on the etiology of hepatic encephalopathy is beyond the scope of this chapter; however, the amino acid/neurotransmitter theory as it relates to current nutritional therapy will be presented. According to this theory, developed by Fischer and Baldessarini to explain the neurologic and cardiovascular findings in cirrhotic patients with encephalopathy [16], BCAA and AAA share a common pathway across the blood-brain barrier and compete for transport into the cerebrospinal fluid. Because plasma BCAA levels are reduced, the AAA are transported in increased amounts and accumulate in the brain. These increased levels of AAA result in the formation of "false neurotransmitters" that compete with normal neurotransmitters for binding sites. Centrally, this process leads to the extrapyramidal symptoms of asterixis and disturbances of consciousness. Peripherally, the false neurotransmitters may play a role in the high cardiac output, low peripheral vascular resistance, and hepatorenal syndrome associated with liver failure [33].

Based on this information, it appeared logical that manipulation of both plasma and brain AAA levels could serve as treatment for encephalopathy [17]. In principle, this is accomplished by three mechanisms: (1) through decreased exogenous intake of AAA; (2) by establishing anabolism (positive nitrogen balance), which reduces AAA by incorporation into intracellular protein synthesis; and (3) by the administration of BCAA that may decrease skeletal muscle breakdown and thereby decrease the release of AAA, as well as decrease brain levels of AAA by increasing competition for transport. A specialized nutritional solution was developed with these goals in mind. Experimentally, this formula is known as F080; it is available commercially as Hepatamine.* The solution contains 35% BCAA, in contrast to the 14 to 25% BCAA of standard solutions; decreased concentrations of phenylalanine and methionine; and increased amounts of arginine and alanine.

Several large, properly randomized, prospective trials have compared BCAA therapy with standard forms of therapy [11, 15, 22, 32, 34, 37, 39]. The BCAA therapy has been shown to be effective in those studies that

---

*Kendall-McGaw Laboratories, Irvine, CA.

used hypertonic dextrose as a caloric source, whereas studies that used lipid emulsion as a major caloric source failed to demonstrate a benefit for the BCAA [32, 39].

In clinical practice, BCAA therapy is most beneficial in patients with chronic liver disease who become encephalopathic due to superimposed illness—"acute-on-chronic" disease. Nutritional therapy should be used in combination with standard forms of therapy: adequate oxygenation, careful fluid regulation, control of sepsis, control of gastrointestinal hemorrhage, use of nonabsorbable antibiotics such as neomycin, and the use of lactulose.

Following stabilization of hemodynamic, respiratory, and neurologic status, nutritional support should be instituted. Patients with grade-0 to -I encephalopathy can usually tolerate standard amino acid formulations without exacerbation of symptoms. Patients who do not tolerate this regimen or have grade-II or greater encephalopathy should be started on a formulation containing Hepatamine. Patients should be started on 0.75 gm/kg/day of amino acids and gradually advanced daily to achieve approximately 1.5 gm/kg/day of amino acids or as tolerated. Following the resolution of the acute illness and return of hepatic function, patients may be given a trial of a standard amino acid formula and, if there is no worsening of clinical status or amino acid pattern, remain with the standard solution until resumption of an oral diet.

ENTERAL NUTRITION

Enteral nutrition has come a long way since the administration of "nutrient enemas" to patients in need of nutritional support. A greater understanding of gastrointestinal physiology and the development of supporting technologies have helped to overcome many of the obstacles that plagued early efforts to use the gut.

Physiology

The relative roles of the stomach and small bowel as they relate to the delivery of enteral nutrition have been more clearly defined. The stomach initiates the digestive process but does not participate in nutrient absorption. Gastric acid secretion serves to sterilize gastric contents, thus preventing bacterial contamination of the gastrointestinal tract. A principal function of the stomach is to protect the gastrointestinal tract against an osmotic load. In the presence of hyperosmotic fluid, gastric motility is inhibited. Gastric secretion then dilutes the gastric contents until they are isoosmotic before allowing passage across the pylorus. The small intestine is less capable of diluting a hyperosmotic load, and this is why patients experience more difficulty when hyperosmolar tube feedings are instilled directly into the small bowel.

The small intestine, in addition to being the principal site of nutrient digestion and absorption, should be regarded as a metabolically active organ that both consumes nutrients and processes them before delivery to the liver via the portal circulation. Proteins are almost completely absorbed in the proximal jejunum, with dipeptides and tripeptides the preferred configuration. Carbohydrates are also absorbed high in the jejunum, with simple sugars the preferred form. Fats are the most difficult nutrients to absorb, requiring the proper release and mixing of bile and pancreatic enzymes. Long-chain fatty acids require micelle and chylomicron formation and must be transported through the lymphatic system, whereas short- and medium-chain fatty acids enter directly into the portal circulation. Calcium, iron, and other metals are absorbed in the duodenum. In addition to its absorptive functions, the small bowel serves important hormonal and immunologic functions that are only beginning to be fully appreciated.

Finally, enteral nutrition has benefited from an improved understanding of the pathophysiology of postoperative ileus. Although the stomach may have an ileus for 1 to 2 days and the colon one for 3 to 5 days postoperatively, the small intestinal absorption and motility may continue almost without interruption. This realization opened the way for immediate postoperative enteral feeding by needle catheter jejunostomy.

Formulas

Numerous enteral products are now available, and although this has broadened the applications of enteral nutrition, it has also caused some confusion. For simplicity, enteral products can be divided into the following categories: oral supplements, tube feedings, and modular components. Oral supplements are flavored products for oral consumption and are used in addition to other oral intake.

Tube feedings are generally unflavored products intended for delivery by tube. Enteral formulas for tube feedings differ in their nutritional completeness, viscosity, caloric density, lactose content, osmolality, and molecular form of the substrate. The most clinically important of these are the lactose content, the osmolality, and the molecular form of the substrate. A common difficulty in the seriously ill patient is acquired lactose deficiency, and therefore lactose-containing products may result in diarrhea. Osmolality of a solution is particularly important when feeding beyond the pylorus for reasons previously discussed. The molecular form of the substrate refers to the complexity of the carbohydrate, protein, and fat components. Each differs in its extent of hydrolysis, ranging from blenderized or partially hydrolyzed to the elemental, chemically defined formulas.

If possible, it is better to use the blenderized or partially hydrolyzed diets, as they have a lower osmolality, are less expensive, and are more balanced, having a better nitrogen-to-calorie ratio than many elemental diets. The use of elemental diets should be limited to patients with impaired absorption caused by a variety of factors, including the short-bowel syndrome, gastrointestinal fistulas, inflammatory bowel disease, or prolonged ileus. Finally, disease-specific enteral formulas are available for the treatment of renal failure, hepatic failure, and sepsis; these are similar in composition to their parenteral counterparts.

Modular components are sources of carbohydrates, protein, fat, vitamins, and minerals that can be added to existing formulations to increase caloric density, alter distribution of calories from carbohydrate, protein, and fat, or improve adequacy of the final composition.

The enteral formulary at the University of Cincinnati is given in Table 25-7.

Delivery Systems

Clinicians in the past were hampered by having to use stiff, large-bore nasogastric tubes that frequently caused an uncomfortable pharyngitis, otitis media, rhinitis, gastroesophageal reflux, impaired cough, and aspiration. The development of flexible, soft, small-bore feeding tubes has lowered the morbidity associated with enteral nutrition and made it more tolerable for the patient.

Another problem in the administration of enteral nutrition was the lack of a practical and safe means to regulate the infusion, resulting in the frequent bolus administration of tube feedings. This practice was often accompanied by bloating, cramping, and diarrhea. At present, however, infusion pumps have been specifically designed for enteral nutrition, making it safer, with less gastrointestinal intolerance, and more time-efficient.

Alternatives in Enteral Nutrition

Enteral nutrition can be provided orally, nasoenterically, or by tube enterostomy. Obviously, oral administration is the preferred route, but this is frequently not possible in the seriously ill patient.

If inadequate caloric intake occurs in a patient with intact gastrointestinal function, consideration should be given to nasogastric tube feedings. This method of nutritional support is normally well tolerated by patients for short periods of time (days to weeks). Tube feedings can be given nasogastrically or nasointestinally if gastric motility is impaired or if aspiration is a concern. Feeding tubes can be placed blindly or with fluoroscopic or endoscopic guidance. It is our practice to bridle feeding tubes around the nasal septum or palate when patients are uncooperative, due to altered mental status or there are other concerns about the tube becoming dislodged.

When enteral nutritional therapy is necessary for prolonged periods of time (weeks, months, years), consideration should be given to one of the tube enterostomies. The primary reason for this is increased patient comfort. Potential sites for tube enterostomies include the pharynx, esophagus, stomach, duodenum, and jejunum, although the stomach and jejunum are by far the most common [38].

Gastrostomy can be performed by an open technique or by the percutaneous endoscopic technique (PEG). Indications include esophageal obstruction, neurologic conditions associated with impaired swallowing, oropharyngeal trauma, and head and neck cancers. Contraindications include high gastrointestinal fistulas, disease of the gastric wall, and gastric outlet obstruction.

Jejunostomy is necessary when there is obstruction of the stomach, duodenum, and proximal jejunum. A frequently cited advantage of this method over gastrostomy is a decreased risk of reflux and aspiration. In experienced hands, the technique of needle catheter jejunostomy (NCJ) is a relatively fast, simple, and safe method of jejunostomy. Currently reported major complication rates are 2 to 3 percent. Indications for NCJ now include malnourished patients undergoing major upper gastrointestinal surgery for benign disease, malignancy, or trauma. Contraindications include local and systemic factors [35]. Local factors include Crohn's disease, extensive adhesions, radiation enteritis, and peritonitis. Systemic factors include ascites, immunosuppression, and coagulopathy.

General Guidelines

Enteral feedings are given either on an intermittent or continuous basis. The administration of intermittent tube feedings involves dividing the 24-hr volume of tube feeding into 4 to 6 feedings. The quantity to be delivered can then be allowed to flow into a feeding tube over 15 to 20 minutes via controlled gravity infusion or can be bolused by syringe infusion or rapid gravity infusion. The slower infusion rate is usually better tolerated.

Continuous tube feedings involve dividing the total dose by 24 hours to estimate an hourly rate, then infusing without interruption throughout the day, via gravity or by enteral pump. The pump is preferred for better regulation.

For intragastric feedings, the strength of a solution is increased first, then the rate. If a product is hyperosmolar at full strength, one should begin at a concentration that will be isoosmolar. If the product is isoosmolar at full strength, begin with full strength. Administration is usually begun at approximately 30 cc/hr. The strength is then increased in increments (1/2 strength to 3/4 strength to full strength) each 24 hours until the highest concentration required or tolerated is reached. Next, the rate is increased by increments of 20 ml/hr/day until the desired rate and concentration are achieved.

For the small-bowel feedings, the rate increases first, followed by the strength. Again, the tube feedings are begun at isoosmolar concentrations at approximately 30 cc/hr. The rate increases at increments of 20 ml/hr/day until the desired volume is achieved that, at full-strength concentration, will meet the patient's needs. Thereafter, increases in the strength in increments each 24 hours are made until the highest concentration required or tolerated is reached.

Monitoring

The protocol followed at the University of Cincinnati Hospital is given in Figure 25-6. A few points require emphasis. The use of pumps does not alleviate nurses of responsibility for checking patients frequently while on tube feedings. Patients should be positioned with the head of the bed elevated at 30 to 45 degrees. Strict intake-output monitoring should be done, especially the amount and frequency of diarrhea and aspirates. Urine glucose should be checked every 6 hours. Tube position should be checked every shift and prior to feeding or administering medications.

Complications

The complications of enteral therapy can be divided into gastrointestinal intolerance, mechanical complications, and metabolic complications. The

Table 25-7. Adult enteral formulary currently in use at the University of Cincinnati Hospital

	Vivonex TEN (Norwich Eaton)	Amin-Aid (Kendall-McGaw)	Hepatic-Acid II (Kendall-McGaw)	Isocal (Mead Johnson)	Magnacal (Biosearch)	Sustacal Liquid (Mead Johnson)	Ensure Plus (Ross)	C.I.B. (Carnation)
Kcal/ml	1	1.9	1	1	2	1	1.5	1
Protein, gm/liter (source)	38 (amino acids, 30% of total as branched-chain amino acids)	19 (crystalline essential amino acids)	44 (amino acids, 40% of total as branched-chain amino acids, low in aromatic amino acids)	34 (calcium + sodium caseinates, soy protein isolate)	70 (calcium + sodium caseinates)	60 (sodium + calcium caseinates, soy protein isolates)	55 (sodium + calcium caseinates, soy protein isolates)	58 (milk, soy protein, sodium caseinate)
Fat, gm/liter (source)	3 (safflower oil)	66 (partially hydrogenated soybean oil)	36 (soy oil, monodiglycerides)	44 (soy oil, MCT oil)	80 (soy oil)	23 (soy oil)	53 (corn oil)	31 (milk fat)
Carbohydrate, gm/liter	206 (maltodextrins and modified food starch)	330 (maltodextrin, sucrose)	169 (maltodextrins, sucrose)	133 (glucose)	250 (maltodextrin, sucrose)	138 (sucrose, corn syrup solids)	200 (corn syrup, sucrose)	135 (lactose, sucrose, corn syrup solids)
Lactose, gm/liter	0	0	0	0	0	0	0	100
Minerals (per liter)								
Calcium, mg	500		Negligible	630	1000	1000	634	1371
Phosphorus, mg	500		Negligible	530	1000	920	634	1105
mg	200		Negligible	210	400	380	317	459

Magnesium, mg	9		Negligible	9.5	18	17	14	18
Iron, mg	20		Negligible	23	43	40	46	42
Sodium, mEq	20		Negligible	34	32	53	49	72
Potassium, mEq	23		Negligible	30	27	44	45	147
Chloride, mEq	75		Negligible	79	150	140	105	16
Iodine, mcg	10		Negligible	11	30	14	23	2
Zinc, mg	1		Negligible	1	2	2	2	
Copper, mg	1	<15		2.6	5	3	2	
Manganese, mg								
Volume required to meet 100% RDA, ml	2,000	NA	NA	2000	1000	1100	2000	1373
Kcal/gm N₂	175/1	625/1	174/1	167/1	179/1	104/1	171/1	108/1
mOsm/kg H₂O	630	900	560	300	590	625	600	
Preparation	Powder	Powder	Powder	Ready to use	Ready to use	Ready to use	Ready to use	Powder
Comments	Supplement, tube feeding, enriched with branched-chain amino acids, absorbed in upper gut	Supplement, tube feeding, low electrolytes indicated for renal disease	Supplement, tube feeding, low electrolytes, indicated for liver disease, contains aspartame	Tube feeding	Supplement, tube feeding, high calorie, high protein	Supplement, high protein	Supplement	Palatable, easily available, inexpensive

UMC-396
Revised 5/88

University of Cincinnati Hospital
Physician's Checklist/Order Sheet

All applicable orders have been checked. A line has been placed
through orders that have been voided. ORDERS NOT CHECKED
ARE NOT TO BE FOLLOWED. Orders have been modified
according to the medical condition of the patient. These orders
have been dated, timed and signed by a physician. As an order is
filled, the individual doing so must date/time and initial in the
space provided. Further orders will be added as needed.

PAGE __1__ OF __1__

ORDER NUMBER	✓	PHYSICIAN'S STANDING ORDERS ADULT TUBE FEEDING	ORDER NOTED (DATE/TIME)	(INITIAL)
1.	✓	Small bore tube to be placed by certified physician.		
2.	✓	Chest/abdominal x-ray for position of feeding tube. Write		
		"for feeding tube placement" on requisition.		
3.	✓	Do not infuse formula until tip position is documented in		
		patient's chart.		
4.	✓	Elevate head of bed >30° during enteral feeding.		
5.	✓	Aspirate tube Q 4 hours for continuous feedings and prior		
		to each intermittent feeding with a 50 ml or larger syringe.		
		−If aspirate <150 ml return aspirate and continue feeding.		
		−If aspirate >150 ml hold aspirate and notify physician.		
6.	✓	Irrigate feeding tube Q 4 hours with 30 ml H_2O per nursing		
		procedure with a 50 ml or larger syringe.		
7.	✓	Administer continuous feeding via enteral pump.		
8.	✓	Vital signs Q 6 hours.		
9.	✓	Urine sugars Q 6 hours with Diastix.		
10.	✓	Intake and Output Q 24 hours.		
11.	✓	Do not let formula hang for longer than 8 hours.		
12.	✓	Change administration set Q 24 hours.		
13.	✓	Weights Monday, Wednesday, and Friday.		
14.	✓	Do not administer crushed medication via small bore		
		feeding tube.		
15.	✓	Irrigate tube before and after each medication.		
16.	✓	Blood work		
		Monday: Renal (4203)		
		Thursday: Renal (4203), Bone (4041), Hepatic (4162)		
		Profiles, CBC (4032), Prothrombin Time (4204),		
		Transferrin (4706), Prealbumin (4705), Retinol Binding		
		Protein (4707)		
17.	✓	STAT blood glucose for 1/4% or greater glycosuria.		

White-Chart   Yellow-Kardex

Physician's signature _____

Date _____ Time _____

Developed by _____   Date _____

Fig. 25-6. Protocol for adult tube feeding at the University of Cincinnati Hospital.

most frequently encountered complications are gastrointestinal problems, the most prevalent of which is diarrhea. The causes of diarrhea include gastric hypersecretion, lactose intolerance, concomitant drug therapy, altered stool flora, malabsorption, low serum albumin, and hyperosmolar formulas. Some of these can be easily avoided: for example, by the use of nonlactose-containing formulas and the careful titration of hyperosmolar formulas. For patients with a low serum albumin (<2.5), we have sometimes found it helpful to give a trial of albumin therapy to achieve a level ≥ 3.0). This is sometimes all that is needed to change the bowel from a secretory to an absorptive state.

Mechanical complications include luminal obstruction, gastric erosion, aspiration, tube displacement, and tube malpositioning. The latter complication is a particularly worrisome one, as pneumothorax resulting from attempted placement of these tubes has become an all-too-frequently reported occurrence. It is therefore imperative that the position of the tube be documented radiographically before the initiation of enteral therapy. In patients who are obtunded or mechanically ventilated, we recommend the use of fluoroscopy for placement of feeding tubes.

The metabolic complications are generally similar to those of parenteral nutrition. However, because of the gastrointestinal tract's buffering capacity, there is a greater margin of safety.

REFERENCES

1. Abel, R. M., Beck, C. H., Abbott, W. M., et al. Improved survival from acute renal failure after treatment with intravenous essential L-amino acids and glucose: Results of a prospective, double-blind study. *N. Engl. J. Med.* 288:695, 1973.
2. Alverdy, J., Chi, H. S., and Sheldon, G. E. The effect of parenteral nutrition on gastrointestinal immunity: The importance of enteral stimulation. *Ann. Surg.* 202:681, 1985.
3. Bjornson, H. S., Colley, R., Bower, R. H., et al. Association between microorganism growth at the catheter insertion site and colonization of the catheter in patients receiving total parenteral nutrition. *Surgery* 92:720, 1982.
4. Blackburn, G. L., Flatt, J. P., Clowes, G. H. A., et al. Protein sparing therapy during periods of starvation with sepsis or trauma. *Ann. Surg.* 177:588, 1973.
5. Bower, R. H., Talamini, M. A., Sax, H. C., et al. Postoperative enteral versus parenteral nutrition: A randomized controlled trial. *Arch. Surg.* 121:1040, 1986.
6. Bower, R. H. Hepatic complications of parenteral nutrition. *Semin. Liver Dis.* 3:216, 1983.
7. Bozzetti, F., Terno, G., Bonfanti, G., et al. Prevention and treatment of central venous catheter sepsis by exchange via guide wires. *Ann. Surg.* 198:48, 1983.
8. Bozzetti, F., Scarpa, D., Terno, G., et al. Subclavian venous thrombosis due to indwelling catheters: A prospective study on 52 patients. *J.P.E.N.* 7:560, 1983.
9. Burr, G. O., and Burr, M. M. A new deficiency disease produced by the rigid exclusion of fat from the diet. *J. Biol. Chem.* 82:345, 1929.
10. Buzby, G. P. Case for preoperative nutritional support. Presented at the American College of Surgeons 1988 Clinical Congress Postgraduate Course "Pre- and Postoperative Care: Metabolism and Nutrition," Chicago, October 25–28, 1988.

11. Cerra, F. B., Cheung, N. K., Fischer, J. E., et al. Disease-specific amino acid infusion (F080) in hepatic encephalopathy: A prospective, randomized, double-blind controlled trial. *J.P.E.N.* 9:288, 1985.
12. Detsky, A. S., McLaughlin, J. R., Baker, J. P., et al. What is subjective global assessment of nutritional status? *J.P.E.N.* 11:8, 1987.
13. Dupre, J., Curtis, J. D., Unger, R. H., et al. Effects of secretin, pancreozymin, or gastrin on the response of the endocrine pancreas to administration of glucose or arginine in man. *J. Clin. Invest.* 48:745, 1969.
14. Feinstein, E. F., Blumenkrantz, M. J., Healy, M., et al. Clinical and metabolic responses to parenteral nutrition in acute renal failure: A controlled double-blind study. *Medicine* 60:124, 1981.
15. Fiaccadori, F., Ghinelli, F., Pedretti G., et al. Branched chain amino acid enriched solutions in the treatment of hepatic encephalopathy: A controlled trial. In L. Capocaccia, J. E. Fischer, and F. Rossi-Fanelli (eds.), *Hepatic Encephalopathy in Chronic Liver Failure.* New York: Plenum Press, 1984. Pp. 323–333.
16. Fischer, J. E., and Baldessarini, R. J. False neurotransmitters and hepatic failure. *Lancet* 2:75, 1971.
17. Fischer, J. E., Rosen, H. M., Ebeid, A. M., et al. The effect of normalization of plasma amino acids on hepatic encephalopathy in man. *Surgery* 80:77, 1976.
18. Freund, H. R., Floman, N., Schwartz, B., and Fischer, J. E. Essential fatty acid deficiency in total parenteral nutrition. *Ann. Surg.* 190:139, 1979.
19. Freund, H., and Fischer, J. E. Comparative study of parenteral nutrition in renal failure using essential and nonessential amino acid containing solutions. *Surg. Gynecol. Obstet.* 151:652, 1980.
20. Gimmon, Z., Murphy, R. F., Chen, M., et al. The effect of parenteral and enteral nutrition on portal and systemic immunoreactivities of gastrin, glucagon, and vasoactive intestinal polypeptide (VIP). *Ann. Surg.* 196:571, 1982.
21. Giordanno, C. Use of exogenous and endogenous urea for protein synthesis in normal and uremic subjects. *J. Lab. Clin. Med.* 62:231, 1963.
22. Gluud, C., Dejgaard, A., Hardt, F., et al. Preliminary treatment results with balanced amino acid infusion to patients with hepatic encephalopathy. *Scand. J. Gastroenterol.* 18(suppl 86):19(abstract), 1983.
23. Goodgame, J. T., and Fischer, J. E. Parenteral nutrition in the treatment of acute pancreatitis: Effect on complications and mortality. *Ann. Surg.* 186:651, 1977.
24. Gottschlick, M. M., and Alexander, J. W. Fat kinetics and recommended dietary intake in burns. *J.P.E.N.* 11:80, 1987.
25. Greenberg, G. R., Marliss, E. B., Anderson, G. H., et al. Protein-sparing therapy in postoperative patients: Effects of added hypocaloric glucose or lipid. *N. Engl. J. Med.* 294:1411, 1976.
26. Harris, J. A., and Benedict, F. G. Biometric studies of basal metabolism in man. *Carnegie Institute of Washington Publication #279,* 1919.
27. Holter, A., and Fischer, J. E. The effects of perioperative hyperalimentation on complications in patients with carcinoma and weight loss. *J. Surg. Res.* 23:31, 1977.
28. Hyne, B. E. B., Fowell, E., and Lee, H. A. The effect of caloric intake on nitrogen balance in chronic renal failure. *Clin. Sci.* 43:679, 1972.
29. Johnson, L. R., Copeland, E. M., Dudrick, S. J., et al. Structural and hormonal alterations in the gastrointestinal tract of parenterally fed rats. *Gastroenterology* 68:1177, 1975.
30. Levine, G. M., Deken, J. J., Steiger, E., et al. Role of oral intake in maintenance of gut mass and disaccharide activity. *Gastroenterology* 67:979, 1974.

31. Long, C. L., Schaffel, N., Geiger, J. W., et al. Metabolic response to injury and illness: Estimation of energy and protein needs from indirect calorimetry and nitrogen balance. *J.P.E.N.* 3:452, 1979.

32. Michel, H., Pomier-Layrargues, G., Aubin, J. P., et al. Treatment of hepatic encephalopathy by infusion of a modified amino acid solution: Results of a controlled study in 47 cirrhotic patients. In L. Capocaccia, J. E. Fischer, and F. Rossi-Fanelli (eds.), *Hepatic Encephalopathy in Chronic Liver Failure.* New York: Plenum Press, 1984. Pp. 301–310.

33. Nespoli, A., Bevilcqua, G., Staudacher, G., et al. The role of false neurotransmitters in the pathogenesis of hepatic encephalopathy and hyperdynamic syndrome in cirrhosis. *Arch. Surg.* 116:1129, 1981.

34. Rossi-Fanelli, F., Riggio, O., Cangiano, C., et al. Branched chain amino acids vs. lactulose in the treatment of hepatic coma: A controlled study. *Dig. Dis. Sci.* 27:929, 1982.

35. Ryan, J. A., Jr., and Page, C. P. Intrajejunal feeding: Development and current status. *J.P.E.N.* 8:187, 1984.

36. Sax, H. C., Warner, B. W., Talamini, M. A., et al. Early total parenteral nutrition in acute pancreatitis: Lack of beneficial effect. *Am. J. Surg.* 153:117, 1987.

37. Strauss, E., Santos, W. R., DaSilva, E. C., et al. A randomized controlled clinical trial for the evaluation of the efficacy of an enriched branched chain amino acid solution compared to neomycin in hepatic encephalopathy. *Hepatology* 3:862 (abstract), 1983.

38. Torosian, M. H., and Rombeau, J. L. Feeding by tube enterostomy. *Surg. Gynecol. Obstet.* 150:918, 1980.

39. Wahren, J., Denis, J., Desurmont, P., et al. Is intravenous administration of branched chain amino acids effective in the treatment of hepatic encephalopathy? A multicenter study. *Hepatology* 3:475, 1983.

40. Wilmore, D. W., and Dudrick, S. J. Treatment of acute renal failure with intravenous essential L-amino acids. *Arch. Surg.* 99:669, 1969.

41. Yeung, C. K., Smith, R. C., and Hill, G. L. Effect of an elemental diet on body composition: A comparison with intravenous nutrition. *Gastroenterology* 77:652, 1979.

26

Sepsis Syndrome

Mitchell P. Fink

DEFINITION

Sepsis is an imprecise term denoting a variable constellation of nonspecific signs and symptoms (e.g., altered mental status, oliguria, jaundice) and laboratory abnormalities (e.g., leukocytosis hypoalbuminemia, azotemia) that are presumably caused by bloodstream invasion by microbes or microbial products. Pepe et al. [41] defined the sepsis syndrome as a "clinical picture of serious bacterial infection with a concurrent, deleterious systemic response." It is clear, however, that serious fungal and even viral infections can lead to clinical findings indicative of sepsis [15]. Indeed, it is increasingly apparent that a subset of critically ill patients manifest many of the features characteristic of the sepsis syndrome despite repeatedly negative blood cultures and no obvious focus of infection.

HEMODYNAMIC DERANGEMENTS

Systemic Hemodynamics

Systemic vascular resistance (SVR) is abnormally low in most septic patients [1,39]. Low SVR is so characteristic of the sepsis syndrome that this finding has been used as a diagnostic criterion in clinical research studies [34,41]. Cardiac output (CO) is usually well-preserved in sepsis. During periods of relative hemodynamic stability, CO is typically supranormal; this is the so-called hyperdynamic septic state. During episodes of systemic arterial hypotension ("septic shock"), CO often decreases into the normal range while SVR remains abnormally low [1].

Differentiating sepsis into early hyperdynamic and late hypodynamic phases is not a useful construct. Several studies have documented that CO remains normal or supranormal in most septic patients until just hours before death. Thus, subnormal CO is a preterminal event in a process that often lasts for days or even weeks. The low CO characteristic of many animal models of septic or endotoxic shock probably reflects inadequate maintenance of circulating volume: i.e., many of these models reflect the combined effects of hypovolemia superimposed upon the septic/endotoxic insult.

Myocardial Dysfunction

Although CO is well preserved in septic states, convincing data indicate that ventricular performance is impaired by serious systemic infection. These data come from both clinical and animal studies.

The most convincing evidence that myocardial dysfunction occurs in septic patients was provided by Parker and her colleagues from the National Institutes of Health [39]. These investigators used gated radionuclide ventriculography to assess left ventricular performance in 20 patients with at least one episode of profound hypotension, hyperthermia, and documented infection. Three of the patients had negative blood cultures (attributed to the administration of broad-spectrum antibiotics). Blood cultures in the remaining 17 patients were positive for gram-negative bacilli, gram-positive cocci or bacilli or *Candida albicans.* In this study, sepsis was associated with a marked decrease in left ventricular ejection fraction (EF). The alteration in EF was reversible; in survivors, EF typically returned to normal 7 to 10 days after the initial episode of septic shock. Analysis of the data indicated that decreased EF was not explainable by changes in a variety of factors (positive end-expiratory pressure, preload, afterload, and heart rate) known to affect this parameter. Therefore, the decrease in EF was almost certainly a manifestation of impaired systolic function. Despite the decrease in EF, stroke remained normal: i.e., left ventricular end-diastolic volume increased significantly. This acute, reversible dilation of the heart was apparently a compensatory response that allowed survivors to maintain a normal or even supranormal CO.

Using radionuclide cardiography to assess serial changes in left ventricular performance in a hyperdynamic canine peritonitis model, Natanson et al. [36] documented that EF is reversibly decreased in septic dogs, the decrement in EF being directly correlated with the magnitude of the septic challenge [37]. Furthermore, when 2-point Starling curves were constructed by rapidly infusing a large volume of crystalloid solution, these authors obtained additional evidence to support the idea that sepsis leads to profound (but reversible) myocardial depression.

Recently, Goldfarb and colleagues utilized a porcine endotoxemia model to study the effect of lipopolysaccharide (LPS; see below) on the end-systolic pressure-volume relationship. Originally described by Sugawa [49], the end-systolic pressure-volume relationship provides unambiguous information about the inotropic state of the ventricle. In both acute studies using anesthetized animals [21] and chronic studies using awake animals [29], Goldfarb and colleagues showed that administering LPS leads to marked depression of the inotropic state of the heart, even when CO is supranormal. These data, in addition to the results from the canine studies described above, are important because they indicate that the myocardial depression observed in patients is a manifestation of sepsis per se and is not a side effect of treatment with antibiotics, vasoactive drugs, or other agents.

The mechanisms responsible for sepsis- and LPS-induced ventricular dysfunction are poorly understood. One potential explanation that is almost certainly incorrect is that decreased cardiac performance in sepsis is due to myocardial ischemia secondary to coronary hypoperfusion. Both Cunnion et al. [13] and Dhainaut et al. [16] showed that coronary sinus blood flow is supranormal in septic patients without coronary artery disease. In addition, both groups showed that net myocardial lactate production does not occur in sepsis; rather, lactate uptake by the myocardium is significantly increased in septic patients as compared with nonseptic controls.

Another possible mechanism is that sepsis or endotoxicosis leads to the release of one or more circulating factors that depress myocardial performance. In 1966, Brand and Lefer discovered that the plasma of cats in hemorrhagic shock contains a "myocardial depressant factor" [8]. Wangensteen et al. subsequently showed that myocardial depressent factor is similarly released in experimental endotoxic shock [53]. In 1979, using a Langendorf rat heart preparation as a bioassay, Maksad et al. showed that plasma from septic (but not control) patients contains a myocardial depressant substance [32]. Recently, Parrillo et al. confirmed and extended these early observations in an elegant study that correlated results from an in vitro bioassay with clinical assessments of left ventricular performance [40]. Myocardial depressant substance, detected by its effect on the extent of shortening of an isolated, spontaneously beating newborn rat myocardial cell, was present in serum samples from patients with septic shock, but not serum specimens from normal laboratory personnel, people with decreased EF due to structural heart disease, critically ill nonseptic controls, or patients with septic shock during the preshock or recovery phases of their illness. Furthermore, within the group with septic shock, there was a significant (although relatively weak) correlation between the patient's acute phase EF (determined by radionuclide scan) and the percent decrease in myocardial cell shortening elicited by adding the patient's acute phase serum to the in vitro assay medium.

As yet, myocardial depressant factor has not been characterized at a molecular level. Preliminary data suggest that it is probably a protein (or glycoprotein) [23,40]. Based upon studies using animals, Greene and colleagues estimate a molecular weight of about 600 [23]. Parrillo et al. estimate a molecular weight of about 2000 [40].

Alterations in Regional Perfusion

Despite extensive interest in the hemodynamic derangements occurring in sepsis and septic shock, remarkably little is known about the effect of severe systemic infection on organ blood flow in humans. The paucity of good information in this area is a result of the difficulties inherent in the measurement of regional perfusion in patients. Methods useful in animal studies (e.g., electromagnetic or ultrasonic flow probes, radioactive microspheres) are generally not applicable in the clinical setting. Clearance methods are relatively noninvasive and can be used in humans to estimate "effective" perfusion of the kidney and liver. Typically, para-aminohippurate (or a closely related compound) is used to measure renal plasma flow, and indocyanine green dye is used to measure hepatic plasma flow.

Clearance methods, in order to be valid, require strict adherence to a rigorous set of rules [31]. First, there is an absolute requirement for near steady-state conditions during the clearance periods. This means that plasma levels of the indicator (i.e., para-aminohippurate or indocyanine green) must be stable _and_ the actual value of organ (i.e., kidney or liver) plasma flow must be constant over the clearance interval. Second, there is an absolute requirement for measurements of extraction across the organ of interest. Extraction efficiency can vary over a wide range (particularly in critically ill patients with varying degrees of organ failure who are receiving a wide range of potentially interfering pharmacologic agents). Third, when measuring renal plasma flow (or glomerular filtration rate), it is important that urine flow be relatively constant, to avoid large errors due to wash-out effects. In many published clinical studies using clearance methods to estimate kidney or liver perfusion in sepsis, one or more of these rules was not obeyed.

The best available data suggest that effective renal plasma flow increases in septic patients. In 1967, Gombos studied the renal effects of administering pyrogen to normal volunteers [22]. Pyrogen led to a biphasic renal response, characterized by early, transient vasoconstriction followed by sustained renal vasodilatation. During the second phase, renal plasma flow (corrected for extraction) increased 36 percent (average value for 10 subjects). Para-aminohippurate extraction decreased in all subjects. These data are remarkably similar to results obtained by Lucas et al., who, in a study of renal function in 11 septic patients, reported that average renal plasma flow (corrected for extraction) was 154 percent of normal and extraction efficiency was 46 percent of normal [30]. Whether renal blood flow is preserved in profoundly hypotensive patients with septic shock currently is not known, although very limited and preliminary data suggest that this is the case [9].

Three studies used indocyanine green dye clearance to estimate total liver (i.e., portral plus hepatic arterial) blood flow in septic patients [14,24,54]. Using previously published values for normal humans as the basis for comparison, these studies all suggest that hepatic blood flow is elevated in normotensive septic patients. Two of the studies, however, administered indocyanine green as a bolus [14,54]; this can lead to estimates of hepatic blood flow that are substantially different from the true value [14]. The study by Gump et al. [24] used a primed continuous infusion of green dye, but true steady-state conditions were not always achieved, and therefore the results from this study also may be invalid.

From the preceding, it should be apparent that current knowledge is limited regarding the effect of sepsis and septic shock on visceral blood flow in humans. For this reason, results obtained using clinically relevant animal models are pertinent. Findings from several such studies are summarized in Table 26-1. In models of compensated (i.e., normotensive and hyperdynamic) sepsis, perfusion is typically increased to the heart, intestine, and liver. Renal blood flow is generally well-preserved. Among

Table 26-1. Effect of sepsis or endotoxicosis on organ blood flow in several animal models

Species	Model	MAP[a]	CO[b]	Heart	Intestine	Liver	Kidney	Ref. no.
Monkey	IV LPS	→	↑	←	←	←	↑	55
Monkey	IV *E. coli*	→	←	←		→	→	12
Rat	Peritonitis	↑	←	←	←	←	↑	28
Rabbit	IP LPS	→	←	←	←	↑	↑	19
Pig	IV LPS	→	↑	↑	↑		→	10

[a]Mean arterial pressure.

[b]Cardiac output.

[c]Arrows indicate relative change from normal values: ↑ = increased; → = no change; ↓ = decreased.

models characterized by low SVR and profound hypotension, results are quite variable, presumably because of differences in species, degree and technique of resuscitation, anesthesia, and severity of the septic (or endotoxic) challenge. Despite the variability among results from these studies, it seems clear that perturbations in the distribution of blood flow in sepsis can lead to regional hypoperfusion, even when CO is within the normal range.

Oxygen Delivery and Uptake

In most tissues (the heart being a notable exception), perfusion is ordinarily greater than that necessary for adequate oxygen delivery ($\dot{D}O_2$). A corollary of this statement is that cellular oxygen consumption (uptake; $\dot{V}O_2$) is normally not limited or regulated by the availability of oxygen. When perfusion decreases (e.g., secondary to hemorrhage or heart failure), oxygen extraction increases, the oxygen content of postcapillary venous blood decreases, and the arteriovenous oxygen gradient widens. Thus, in most tissues, moderate decrements in perfusion affect $\dot{D}O_2$ but not $\dot{V}O_2$. Similarly, when metabolic demand increases without a commensurate increase in blood flow, oxygen extraction typically increases sufficiently so that $\dot{V}O_2$ rises appropriately. However, if flow falls by too great an extent and/or metabolic demand increases by too great an extent, then the reserve $\dot{D}O_2$ is exceeded and tissue ischemia results.

There is considerable interest in myocardial dysfunction and deranged distribution of CO in sepsis, because one or both of these phenomena could lead to global or regional inadequacies in $\dot{D}O_2$, particularly if metabolic demands are elevated. Indeed, there is accumulating evidence that systemic oxygen delivery ($\dot{D}O_2$) is insufficient to meet metabolic demands in certain subsets of septic patients, even when CO is normal or supranormal. Results from two of the studies that support this view will be summarized here.

Haupt et al. prospectively examined the effect of fluid loading in 20 septic patients [25]. Intravascular volume loading increased systemic $\dot{D}O_2$ in 14 patients, although the mean preresuscitation cardiac index (CI) in this subset was already high normal (3.59 liters/min/M²). In response to the increase in $\dot{D}O_2$ effected by the volume challenge, systemic $\dot{V}O_2$ increased in eight subjects and was unchanged in the other six. Of note, preresuscitation blood lactate levels were significantly higher in the former than in the latter subgroup. This key observation suggests that at least in some instances, lactic acidosis in sepsis is due to cellular anaerobic metabolism secondary to inadequate $\dot{D}O_2$, even when CO is normal or supranormal.

Bihari et al. measured systemic $\dot{D}O_2$ and $\dot{V}O_2$ in 27 critically ill people with acute respiratory failure secondary to proven or suspected sepsis [4]. The patients were evaluated before and during infusion of prostacyclin, a potent vasodilator (afterload-reducing agent). As expected, in both the 14 survivors and the 13 nonsurvivors, infusion of prostacyclin significantly increased $\dot{D}O_2$, although the mean preinfusion CI in both subgroups was in excess of 3.2 liter/min/M² (i.e., normal range). Despite the increase in $\dot{D}O_2$, however, $\dot{V}O_2$ increased only in a subgroup of patients who died of their illness. This finding suggests the presence of an oxygen debt due to inadequate perfusion in patients with ultimately fatal sepsis.

Clinical Implications

Despite a lack of understanding about the pathophysiology of sepsis and septic shock, it is reasonable to conclude the following: (1) myocardial performance is impaired in sepsis, even when CO is normal or supranormal; and (2) at least some septic patients manifest evidence of supply-dependent oxygen uptake, even when CO is normal or supranormal. If it is accepted that inadequate $\dot{V}O_2$ is bad for patients, then certain therapeutic guidelines seem reasonable.

First, it is imperative that septic patients be adequately resuscitated. Sepsis leads to marked alterations in capillary permeability; thus, inadequate resuscitation can result in superimposing the perfusion abnormalities associated with hypovolemia on those already present due to sepsis. Adequate maintenance of intravascular volume is especially important in sepsis, because adequate compensation for decreased myocardial performance apparently depends on diastolic ventricular dilatation (i.e., increased preload). Volume-loading septic patients is not without risk. A major concern, of course, is the possibility of worsening pulmonary edema (and hence impairing oxygenation) in patients with sepsis-related adult respiratory distress syndrome (ARDS). From a practical standpoint, fluid is infused until further increments in intravascular volume do not improve $\dot{D}O_2$ or until the pulmonary artery wedge pressure exceeds 15 to 18 mm Hg (in patients without preexisting heart disease treated with low or moderate levels of positive end-expiratory pressure [PEEP]). The choice of fluid (i.e., crystalloid or colloid) is less important than the volume of fluid administered, although it seems prudent to maintain an adequate circulating hemoglobin concentration (>10 gm/dl) by judicious transfusion of packed red blood cells.

Second, since myocardial performance is impaired in sepsis, it is logical to support CO using inotropic agents. Measuring a normal CO in an obviously septic patient does not ensure that $\dot{V}O_2$ is not supply-limited. Therefore, $\dot{D}O_2$ should be optimized (first with volume, then with inotropes and/or vasodilators) until there is no further improvement in $\dot{V}O_2$. At present, information is lacking regarding the relative merits of inotropic versus vasodilator therapy, although currently in our intensive care unit, we tend to choose the former approach, utilizing dobutamine as the inotropic agent of choice. Hemodynamic support for frankly hypotensive patients in septic shock is a more problematic issue. Some authorities advocate using a relatively pure inotropic agent (e.g., dobutamine), whereas others advocate using agents with both inotropic and peripheral vasoconstrictor properties (e.g., dopamine at higher doses, norepinephrine). Our first-line agent is dobutamine (5–20 µg/kg/min); however, in profoundly hypotensive patients (particularly those with known or presumed coronary artery occlusive disease), very low diastolic pressures may compromise coronary perfusion. Hence, in this population, norepinephrine (4–60 µg/min) is used in an effort to increase mean arterial pressure to greater than 60 mm Hg. However, as soon as feasible, we wean this agent and substitute dobutamine. Since some data suggest that adding "low-dose" dopamine to norepinephrine improves renal perfusion [45], dopamine is infused at 2 to 4 μg/kg/min when norepinephrine is used as a vasopressor.

ADJUVANT THERAPY
Introduction
Despite the complexity and seriousness of the problem, the basic management principles for sepsis and septic shock are straightforward. Above all, it is essential to institute early appropriate therapy for the primary problem. This implies administering intravenous antibiotics plus identifying and correcting surgical problems, if present. Initial antibiotic (including, in some instances, antifungal or antiviral) therapy is typically broad-spectrum, the antibiotic regimen subsequently being tailored as culture results become available. It is beyond the scope of the present discussion (see Chapter 27) to provide specific recommendations for antibiotic regimens and surgical procedures appropriate for different problems leading to sepsis. In addition to measures directed at the primary problem, current standard supportive therapy includes hemodynamic support (see above) and support for failing organs (e.g., PEEP and mechanical ventilation for ARDS).

Even with timely intervention and optimal supportive care, the mortality rate for septic shock remains very high. Therefore, there is intense interest in studies designed to evaluate adjunctive measures that might improve outcome. Some of these approaches are briefly reviewed below.

Steroids
Many studies (too numerous to cite here) using laboratory animals have demonstrated that steroids improve hemodynamic parameters and survival in experimental endotoxic and septic shock. Although pretreatment works far better than posttreatment in these laboratory models, even early intervention with steroids after a septic challenge clearly improved outcome in some studies. These data notwithstanding, the use of steroids as adjuvant therapy for septic patients was, until recently, very controversial. Although Schumer reported that high-dose steroid therapy significantly improves survival in septic shock [47], this study was criticized [46]. Furthermore, other data, notably those obtained by Sprung et al. [48], failed to support the idea that steroids are beneficial.

Currently, the controversy surrounding this issue seems to have been settled by the publication of results from two placebo-controlled, prospective, randomized trials of adjuvant therapy of the sepsis syndrome with methylprednisolone [5,52]. Although differing somewhat in design, both studies supported the conclusion that irrespective of clincial subset, pharmacologic doses of methylprednisolone do not improve survival in septic patients. Furthermore, there is evidence that in certain subsets of patients—i.e., patients with diminished renal function [5] or ARDS [6]—steroids significantly worsen outcome. Thus, steroids should not be utilized as adjuvant therapy for the sepsis syndrome (unless, of course, adrenal insufficiency is proven or suspected).

Naloxone

In a classic paper published in 1978, Holiday and Faden reported that naloxone, an opioid antagonist, reverses hypotension in a rat model of endotoxic shock [27]. Subsequent studies confirmed this observation and provided evidence that, at least in some experimental models, administering naloxone improves survival [43]. These data prompted a fruitful series of studies in numerous laboratories investigating the role of endogenous opioid peptides as mediators in endotoxic and septic shock.

Based on promising results from laboratory studies, there was considerable enthusiasm about using naloxone as a therapeutic adjuvant in the management of septic patients. This enthusiasm was fostered, in part, by Peters et al., who reported that naloxone (0.4–1.2 mg) increased blood pressure in 8 of 13 hypotensive septic patients [42]. Subsequently, however, other anecdotal clinical data were published that failed to support the idea that naloxone is beneficial in the management of septic shock in humans. Rock et al. studied the effect of graded bolus doses of naloxone (0.1–1.6 mg/kg) in 12 patients with septic shock and found that, by repeated measures analysis of variance, the drug had no effect on mean arterial pressure or any other hemodynamic variable [44]. Furthermore, four patients experienced major adverse reactions (severe hypotension, seizure, pulmonary edema) after receiving naloxone. Bonnet et al., in a series of seven patients, were similarly unable to detect any hemodynamic effects of naloxone in septic shock [7].

In addition to these discouraging results from clinical studies, there are data from animal experiments suggesting that naloxone therapy may not be salutory. For example, Fettman et al., using an unanesthetized porcine endotoxemia model, showed that naloxone significantly worsens survival and increases blood lactate levels [18]. Thus, at the present time, naloxone therapy cannot be advocated as an adjunctive therapy for septic shock in humans, although further studies using animal models may permit better delineation of the circumstances in which this agent is likely to be of benefit [35].

Cyclooxygenase Inhibitors

Cyclooxygenase-derived metabolites of arachidonic acid (i.e., thromboxane A_2 and prostaglandins) have been implicated as important mediators of many of the pathophysiologic events occurring in septic and endotoxic shock. The data supporting this view have been extensively reviewed elsewhere [20] but can be briefly summarized as follows: (1) cyclooxygenase inhibitors (e.g., ibuprofen and indomethacin) ameliorate hypotension and/or improve survival in many animal models of endotoxic and septic shock; (2) in endotoxin-challenged rats, survival is improved when eicosanoid biosynthesis is limited nonpharmacologically by dietary manipulations that induce a state of essential fatty acid deficiency; (3) inhibitors of thromboxane synthetase prevent the marked pulmonary hypertension that is characteristic of acute experimental endotoxicosis; (4) plasma levels of thromboxane B_2 (thromboxane A_2 metabolite) and 6-keto-$PGF_1\alpha$ (prostacyclin metabolite) are elevated in many animal models of septic or endotoxic shock and in many septic patients.

Despite these data, there is a paucity of information regarding the effect of cyclooxygenase inhibitors in humans. A "phase two" randomized prospective trial of adjuvant therapy with ibuprofen for the sepsis syndrome has been completed, but as of this writing, no results have been reported. Until these and other similar data become available, the role in the clincial management of sepsis for ibuprofen or other cyclooxygenase inhibitors remains unclear.

Antibodies Against Lipopolysaccharide

The outer cell wall of gram-negative bacteria is a trilaminer structure containing a mucopolysaccharide-peptidoglycan layer, a phospholipid-protein layer, and an (outermost) lipopolysaccharide (LPS) layer. Although the terms are commonly used interchangeably, endotoxin and LPS are not synonomous, since endotoxins contain protein in addition to LPS.

LPS is a complex molecule (depicted schematically in Fig. 26-1) with a wide variety of biologic effects. The biologic activity of LPS resides primarily in the lipid A portion of the molecule. LPS is unique for each strain of bacteria. Differences in the structure of the O-antigen polysaccharide chain are responsible for most of the variability in the structure of LPS among strains. In contrast, the structure of the core polysaccharide is conserved among species and strains of gram-negative organisms. Certain mutant strains of bacteria (e.g., the J5 variant of *Escherichia coli*) lack key enzymes and hence are unable to add sugar residues to the core region.

Because of the wide diversity of O-antigen determinants, adoptive anti-LPS immunotherapy is protective against the biologic effects of the immunizing strain of bacteria but is relatively ineffective against other organisms. Reasoning that antisera raised against the core determinants of LPS should have activity against most gram-negative organisms, Ziegler and coworkers immunized rabbits against the J5 mutant of *E. coli* and demonstrated that adoptive immunotherapy with rabbit anti-J5 antiserum markedly enhances survival in neutropenic rabbits infected with *E. coli, Klebsiella,* or *Pseudomonas* [56,57]. Based upon these results, these investigators initiated a clinical trial of anti-J5 antiserum for gram-negative septic shock in humans [58]. The antiserum was prepared in healthy human volunteers using a vaccine prepared from heat-killed J5 *E. coli.* Serum collected from the same donors prior to immunization was used for the control arm of the double-blind, prospective study. Overall, among 212 patients, treatment with a single dose of J5 antiserum decreased mortality from 39 to 22 percent (P = .011). Among patients in profound shock requiring pressors, adoptive immunotherapy decreased mortality from 77 to 44 percent (P = .003).

Despite these dramatic results, adoptive immunotherapy is not currently a component of standard therapy for sepsis and septic shock. Raising antiserum in human volunteers on a large scale is clearly impractical; furthermore, passively immunizing patients with antisera raised in humans carries an unacceptable risk of transmitting diseases (particularly hepatitis and acquired immunodeficiency syndrome). The recent development of technology that permits synthesis of monoclonal antibodies in large quan-

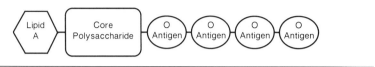

Fig. 26-1. Schematic diagram of the structure of lipopolysaccharide.

tities, however, offers the possibility that adoptive immunotherapy for septic shock may become a clinical reality in the near future. Along with approximately 20 other centers, we are currently entering patients into a randomized prospective trial of adjuvant therapy with a human anti-J5 monoclonal antibody. At least one other clinical study of adoptive immunotherapy for sepsis and septic shock is also in progress.

Interleukin 1 and Tumor Necrosis Factor

During the past several years, it has become increasingly apparent that several monokines are important pathophysiologic mediators in the sepsis syndrome. Monokines are peptide hormones that are synthesized by macrophages and other related cell types.

Interleukin 1 (IL1) is the name for two related peptides with a wide variety of biologic actions. The biology of IL1 was extensively reviewed recently by Dinarello [17]. IL1 is synthesized by numerous cell types, including mesangial cells, Langerhans cells in the skin, synovial fibroblasts, and monocytes. The synthesis and release of IL1 is stimulated by viable microorganisms as well as bacterial products (endotoxins and exotoxins). Many of the systemic actions of IL1 are prominent features of the sepsis syndrome, including fever, sleepiness, anorexia, increased synthesis of hepatic "acute phase proteins," neutrophilia, and lymphopenia. In addition, infusing rabbits with recombinant human IL1 elicits a hyperdynamic, vasodilated, shocklike state that is very similar to that observed in septic patients [38]. Taken together, these data suggest that IL1 is an important mediator in septic patients.

Tumor necrosis factor (TNF), also called cachectin, is another monokine that seems to be a key mediator in endotoxic and septic shock. The biologic actions of TNF were extensively reviewed by Beutler and Cerami [2]. In a landmark publication, these authors showed that passive immunization of mice with a rabbit polyclonal antiserum against murine-derived TNF protected against the lethal effect of intraperitoneally injected E. coli LPS [3]. Subsequently, this group showed that intravenously injecting rats with recombinant human TNF leads to systemic arterial hypotension, diffuse pulmonary injury, and ischemic hemorrhagic gastrointestinal tract lesions: i.e., recombinant human TNF elicits hemodynamic changes and tissue injury patterns in rats that are remarkably similar to those observed in response to LPS [50]. Further support for the notion that TNF is an important mediator in endotoxic shock derives from studies showing that plasma levels of this monokine increase in animals injected with viable bacteria [33]. Indeed, at least two groups have documented that plasma TNF levels are markedly increased in human volunteers injected with nanogram doses of LPS [26,33].

These data suggest that antibodies against TNF might have a therapeutic role in human sepsis. This idea is supported by data reported by Tracey et al. [51]. These authors showed that pretreating baboons with F(ab')₂ fragments of an anti–human TNF monoclonal antibody provides complete protection against the lethal effects of an intravenous infusion of viable *E. coli* bacteria. As yet, no data are available from animal studies indicating that delayed passive immunization against TNF improves outcome in shock states induced by injecting either purified LPS or viable bacteria, and, obviously, post- rather than pretreatment is the most probable scenario in the clinical setting. Thus, the future role for this form of adjunctive therapy is unclear at present; nevertheless, the concept is an exciting one that clearly warrants intense further investigation.

SUMMARY

Although sepsis and septic shock continue to carry a high risk of mortality, there have been substantial gains during this decade in our understanding of the pathophysiology of serious systemic infection. At present, optimal care in the intensive care unit consists of providing aggressive surgical debridement and drainage (where indicated), administering potent and appropriate antibiotics, and optimizing visceral oxygen delivery. It seems quite probable, however, that, before long, new adjunctive measures (e.g., cyclooxygenase inhibitors, monoclonal antibodies) will be a part of the armamentarium of practicing clinicians caring for septic patients.

REFERENCES

1. Abraham, E., Shoemaker, W. C., Bland, R. D., et al. Sequential cardiorespiratory patterns in septic shock. *Crit. Care Med.* 11:799, 1983.
2. Beutler, B., and Cerami, A. Cachectin: More than a tumor necrosis factor. *N. Engl. J. Med.* 316:379, 1987.
3. Beutler, B., Milsark, I. W., and Cerami, A. C. Passive immunization against cachectin/tumor necrosis factor protects mice from lethal effects of endotoxin. *Science* 229:869, 1985.
4. Bihari, D., Smithies, M., Gimson, A., et al. The effect of vasodilation with prostacyclin on oxygen delivery and uptake in critically ill patients. *N. Engl. J. Med.* 317:397, 1987.
5. Bone, R. C., Fisher, C. J., Jr., Clemmer, T. P., et al. A controlled clinical trial of high-dose methylprednisolone in the treatment of severe sepsis and septic shock. *N. Engl. J. Med.* 317:653, 1987.
6. Bone, R. C., Fisher, C. J., Jr., Clemmer, T. P., et al. Early methylprednisolone treatment for septic syndrome and the adult respiratory distress syndrome. *Chest* 92:1032, 1987.
7. Bonnet, F., Lhoste, B. F., Mankikian, L. H., et al. Naloxone therapy of human septic shock. *Crit. Care Med.* 13:972, 1985.
8. Brand, E. A., and Lefer, A. M. Myocardial depressant factor in plasma from cats in irreversible post-oligemic shock. *Proc. Soc. Exp. Biol. Med.* 122:200, 1966.
9. Brenner, M., Mallory, D. L., Schaer, G. L., et al. Renal blood flow in septic and critically ill patients. *Clin. Res.* 34:884A, 1986.

10. Breslow, M. J., Miller, C. F., Parker, S. D., et al. Effect of vasopressors on organ blood flow during endotoxin shock in pigs. *Am. J. Physiol.* 252:H291, 1987.

11. Burczynski, F. J., Pushka, K. L., Sitar, D. S., et al. Hepatic plasma flow: Accuracy of estimation from bolus injections of indocyanine-green. *Am. J. Physiol.* 252:H953, 1987.

12. Carroll, G. C., and Snyder, J. V. Hyperdynamic severe intravascular sepsis depends on fluid administration in cynomolgus monkey. *Am. J. Physiol.* 243:R131, 1982.

13. Cunnion, R. E., Schaer, G. L., Parker, M. M., et al. The coronary circulation in human spetic shock. *Circulation* 73:637, 1986.

14. Dahn, M. S., Lange, P., Lobdel, K., et al. Splanchnic and total body oxygen consumption differences in septic and injured patients. *Surgery* 101:69, 1987.

15. Deutschman, C. S., Konstantinides, F. N., Tsai, M., et al. Physiology and metabolism in isolated viral septicemia: Further evidence of an organism-independent host-dependent response. *Arch. Surg.* 122:21, 1987.

16. Dhainaut, J.-F., Huyghebaert, M.-F., Monsallier, J. F., et al. Coronary hemodynamics and myocardial metabolism of lactate, free fatty acids, glucose, and ketones in patients with septic shock. *Circulation* 75:533, 1987.

17. Dinarello, C. A. Biology of interleukin 1. *FASEB J.* 2:108, 1988.

18. Fettman, M. J., Hand, M. S., Chandrasena, L. G., et al. Naloxone therapy in awake endotoxemic yucatan minipigs. *J. Surg. Res.* 37:208, 1984.

19. Fink, M. P., Fiallo, V., Stein, K. L., et al. Systemic and regional hemodynamic changes after intraperitoneal endotoxin in rabbits: Development of a new model of the clinical syndrome of hyperdynamic sepsis. *Circ. Shock* 22:73, 1987.

20. Fink, M. P. Role of prostaglandins and related compounds in the pathophysiology of endotoxic and septic shock. *Semin. Resp. Med.* 7:17, 1985.

21. Goldfarb, R. D., Nightingale, L. M., Kish, P., et al. Left ventricular function during lethal and sublethal endotoxemia in swine. *Am. J. Physiol.* 251:H364, 1986.

22. Gombos, E. A., Lee, T. H., Solinas, J., et al. Renal response to pyrogen in normotensive and hypertensive man. *Circulation* 36:555, 1967.

23. Greene, L. J., Shapanka, R., Glenn, R. M., et al. Isolation of myocardial depressant factor (MDF) from plasma of dogs in hemorrhagic shock. *Biochem. Biophys. Acta* 491:275, 1977.

24. Gump, F. E., Price, J. B., Jr, and Kinney, J. M. Whole body and splanchnic blood flow and oxygen consumption measurements in patients with intraperitoneal infection. *Ann. Surg.* 171:321, 1970.

25. Haupt, M. T., Gilbert, E. M., and Carlson, R. W. Fluid loading increases oxygen consumption in septic patients with lactic acidosis. *Am. Rev. Respir. Dis.* 131:912, 1985.

26. Hesse, D. G., Tracey, K. J., Fong, Y., et al. Cytokine appearance in human endotoxemia and primate bacteremia. *Surg. Gynecol. Obstet.* 166:147, 1988.

27. Holiday, J. W., and Faden, A. I. Naloxone reversal of endotoxin hypotension suggests role of endorphins in shock. *Nature* 275:450, 1978.

28. Lang, C. H., Bagby, G. J., Ferguson, J. L., et al. Cardiac output and redistribution of organ blood flow in hypermetabolic sepsis. *Am. J. Physiol.* 246:R331, 1984.

29. Lee, K., van der Zee, H., Dziuban, S. W., Jr., et al. Left ventricular function during chronic endotoxemia in swine. *Am. J. Physiol.* 254:H324, 1988.

30. Lucas, C. E., Rector, F. E., Werner, M., et al. Altered renal homeostasis with acute sepsis: Clinical significance. *Arch. Surg.* 106:444, 1973.

31. Maack, T. Renal clearance and isolated kidney perfusion techniques. *Kidney Int.* 30:142, 1986.

32. Maksad, A. K., Chung-Ja, C., Stuart, R. C., et al. Myocardial depression in septic shock: Physiologic and metabolic effects on a plasma factor on an isolate heart. *Circ. Shock. Suppl.* 1:35, 1979.
33. Michie, H. R., Manogue, K. R., Spriggs, D. R., et al. Detection of circulating tumor necrosis factor after endotoxin administration. *N. Engl. J. Med.* 318:1481, 1988.
34. Montgomery, A. B., Stager, M. A., Carrico, C. J., et al. Causes of mortality in patients with adult respiratory distress syndrome. *Am. Rev. Respir. Dis.* 132:485, 1985.
35. Napolitano, L., and Chernow, B. Endorphins in circulatory shock. *Crit. Care Med.* 16:566, 1988.
36. Natanson, C., Fink, M. P., Ballantyne, H. K., et al. Gram-negative bacteremia produces both severe systolic and diastolic cardiac dysfunction in a canine model that simulates human septic shock. *J. Clin. Invest.* 78:259, 1986.
37. Natanson, C., Danner, R. L., Fink, M. P., et al. Cardiovascular performance with *E. coli* challenges in a canine model of human sepsis. *Am. J. Physiol.* 254:H558, 1988.
38. Okusawa, S., Gelfand, J., Ikejima, T., et al. Interleukin 1 induces a shock-like state in rabbits: Synergism with tumor necrosis factor and the effect of cyclooxygenase inhibition. *J. Clin. Invest.* 81:1162, 1988.
39. Parker, M. M., Shelhamer, J. H., Bacharach, S. L., et al. Profound but reversible myocardial depression in patients with septic shock. *Ann. Intern. Med.* 100:483, 1984.
40. Parrillo, J. E., Burch, C., Shelhamer, J. H., et al. A circulating myocardial depressant substance in humans with septic shock. Septic shock patients with a reduced ejection fraction have a circulating factor that depresses in vitro myocardial cell performance. *J. Clin. Invest.* 76:1539, 1985.
41. Pepe, P. E., Potkin, R. T., Reus, D. H., et al. Clinical predictors of the adult respiratory distress syndrome. *Am. J. Surg.* 144:124, 1982.
42. Peters, W. P., Johnson, M. W., Friedman, P. A., et al. Pressor effect of naloxone in septic shock. *Lancet* 1:529, 1981.
43. Reynolds, D. G., Gurll, N. J., Vargish, T., et al. Blockade of opiate receptors with naloxone improves survival and cardiac performance in canine endotoxic shock. *Circ. Shock* 7:39, 1980.
44. Rock, P., Silverman, H., Plump, D., et al. Efficacy and safety of naloxone in septic shock. *Crit. Care Med.* 13:28, 1985.
45. Schaer, G. L., Fink, M. P., and Parrillo, J. E. Norepinephrine alone versus norepinephrine plus low dose dopamine: Improved renal hemodynamics with combination pressor therapy. *Crit. Care Med.* 13:492, 1985.
46. Shine, K. I., Kuhn, M., Young, L. S., et al. Aspects of the management of shock. *Ann. Intern. Med.* 93:723, 1980.
47. Schumer, W. L. Steroids in the treatment of clinical septic shock. *Ann. Surg.* 184:333, 1976.
48. Sprung, C. L., Caralis, P. V., Marcial, E. H., et al. The effects of high-dose corticosteroids in patients with septic shock. *N. Engl. J. Med.* 311:1137, 1984.
49. Sugawa, K. The ventricular pressure volume loop revisited. *Circ. Res.* 43:677, 1978.
50. Tracey, K. J., Beutler, B., Lowry, S. F., et al. Shock and tissue injury induced by recombinant human cachectin. *Science* 234:470, 1986.
51. Tracey, K. J., Fong, Y., Hesse, D. G., et al. Anti-cachectin/TNF monoclonal antibodies prevent septic shock during lethal bacteremia. *Nature* 330:662, 1987.
52. Veterans' Administration Systemic Sepsis Cooperative Study Group. Effect of

high-dose glucocorticoid therapy on mortality in patients with clinical signs of systemic sepsis. *N. Engl. J. Med.* 317:659, 1987.

53. Wangensteen, S. L., Geissinger, W. T., Lovett, W. L., et al. Relationship between splanchnic blood flow and a myocardial depressant factor in endotoxin shock. *Surgery* 69:410, 1971.

54. Wilmore, D. W., Goodwin, C. W., Aulick, L. H., et al. Effect of injury and infection on visceral metabolism and circulation. *Ann. Surg.* 192:491, 1980.

55. Wyler, F., Forsyth, R. P., Nies, A. S., et al. Endotoxin-induced regional circulatory changes in the unanesthetized monkey. *Circ. Res.* 24:777, 1969.

56. Ziegler, E. J., Douglas, H., Sherman, J. E., et al. Treatment of *E. coli* and *Klebsiella* bacteremia in agranulocytotic animals with antiserum to a UDP-Gal epimerase-deficient mutant. *J. Immunol.* 111:433, 1973.

57. Ziegler, E. J., McCutchan, J. A., Douglas, H., et al. Prevention of lethal *Pseudomonas* bacteremia with epismerase-deficient *E. coli* antiserum. *Trans. Assoc. Am. Physicians* 88:101, 1975.

58. Ziegler, E. J., McCutchan, J. A., Fierer, J., et al. Treatment of gram-negative bacteremia and shock with human antiserum to a mutant *Escherichia coli*. *N. Engl. J. Med.* 307:1225, 1982.

Antimicrobial Agents and Infection

Robert A. Salata

During the past 25 years, specialized units for the care of critically ill and unstable patients have come into being [4,39]. The advantages of centralizing care of these severely ill patients in intensive care units (ICUs) are undeniable. Critical care medicine has come to be viewed as synonymous with cutting-edge, high-technology medicine. It is a paradox, however, that lifesaving ICU technology has become a double-edged sword as these invasive devices and techniques predispose to colonization and infection with numerous microbial pathogens [53,88,101]. In addition, many patients admitted to ICUs have sustained injuries or have undergone surgical procedures that significantly impair normal body defenses and further predispose to nosocomial and opportunistic infections. All in all, infection remains the leading cause of death in ICU patients [27,69].

Therapy of infections in ICU patients is complicated by the plethora of potential pathogens, the frequent inability to make a specific etiologic diagnosis, and the increased potential for adverse effects of antimicrobial agents in these patients. Treatment optimally should be directed at specific infectious organisms, with an attempt to balance the efficacy of the antimicrobial agents against the risks of superinfection, drug toxicity, and potential interactions with the many other drugs being employed concurrently in this setting.

This chapter will first detail the epidemiology and spectrum of infections in ICUs. The selected infectious syndromes of pneumonia, urinary tract infection, wound infection, intraabdominal infection, and device-related infectious complications, including candidemia, will be reviewed next. Finally, a practical approach to microbiologic diagnosis and antimicrobial therapy of infectious agents commonly encountered in the ICU setting will be provided. This last section will also provide an update on some of the newer antimicrobials that have become part of our armamentarium.

Table 27-1. Risk factors for developing nosocomial infections in the ICU

---

1. Low birth weight
2. Patent ductus arteriosus
3. Duration of hospitalization
4. Invasive devices and procedures
5. Recent surgery or trauma
6. Extremes of age
7. Broad-spectrum antibiotics
8. Severity of underlying diseases
9. Contaminated life-support systems
10. Overcrowding and transmission by hospital personnel
11. High prevalence of multiply resistant organisms
12. Surgical or burn ICU
13. Steroids or chemotherapy

EPIDEMIOLOGY AND SPECTRUM OF INFECTIONS IN ICUS

Infections in the ICU, for the most part, are acquired nosocomially. In the United States, 5 to 6 percent of all patients admitted to a hospital will acquire an infection [12]. The nosocomial infection rate in intensive care units is two to four times higher and has been estimated to be 15 to 27 percent [19,102]. Surveillance data indicate that 25 percent of all nosocomial infections occur in ICU patients [102]. Several risk factors for developing hospital-acquired infections in ICUs have been identified (Table 27-1). Low birth weight, prematurity, and presence of patent ductus arteriosus have been shown to predispose neonates to nosocomial infections. Severity of underlying disease, duration of hospitalization, invasive procedures and devices (especially endotracheal tubes, urethral and intravascular catheters, intraventricular catheters, and surgical wound drains), contaminated life-support and respiratory therapy equipment, overcrowding, injudicious use of broad-spectrum antimicrobials, and high prevalence of resistant organisms are some of the critical factors in the high rate of infections in ICUs [15,53,102].

Patients in ICUs are particularly prone to develop primary bacteremias (most of which are due to intravascular devices), pneumonias (related to intubation and ventilatory support), and intra-abdominal infections (following trauma or surgery) [53]. In surgical ICUs, 10 percent of patients hospitalized for more than 72 hours will develop hospital-acquired bacteremia [10,17,19,102]. Infection is the most common cause of death in patients who survive major trauma or full-thickness burns and is the most frequent cause of multiple-organ failure in these critically ill patients [27,57,69].

Intensive care units have become the primary hospital areas for epidemics of nosocomial infections, especially those due to antibiotic-resistant pathogens [54,102]. Broad-spectrum antibiotics, liberally used in ICUs, markedly change the normal microflora of patients and predispose to colonization and infection of the skin and the respiratory and gastrointestinal

Table 27-2. Nosocomial infections in adult intensive care units

Type of ICU	Percent of patients infected	Infection rate*	Most frequent sites of infection
Burn	30–50	50–65	Wound, respiratory
Surgical	23–35	40–60	Respiratory, GU, intra-abdominal
Medical	10–24	25–35	Respiratory, GU
Coronary	5–10	1–5	GU

GU = genitourinary.
*Defined as number of infections divided by number of admissions.

tracts. In this setting, methicillin-resistant staphylococci, enterococci, multiply resistant Enterobacteriaceae, *Pseudomonas* species, and *Candida* emerge [25,50,72,99]. Resistant hospital-acquired pathogens from colonized and infected patients are transmitted to other patients in the unit, most frequently on the hands of medical personnel [40,44] and are often perpetuated in urine collection receptacles [80,83], respiratory therapy equipment [31], chamber domes of transducers used in hemodynamic monitoring [20,100], dialysis machines [7,24], fiberoptic endoscopes [84], or bronchoscopes [98].

Nosocomial infection rates vary between hospitals and according to the type of adult ICU population studied (Table 27-2) [8,11,13,15,17,19, 62,66,75,92,102]. Studies have reported rates and types of infections seen in various critical care units. In general, infection rates are highest in burn and surgical ICUs, followed by medical units [8,13]. The lowest rates occur in coronary care units. The greater exposure of surgical patients to invasive procedures and devices of all types likely accounts for the high rates seen in surgical ICUs. Surgical patients have a higher rate of infection caused by enterococci, antibiotic-resistant Enterobacteriaceae (*Klebsiella, Enterobacter,* and *Serratia,* rather then *Escherichia coli*), *Pseudomonas aeruginosa,* and *Candida* [8,13]. These pathogens are selected out by aggressive broad-spectrum antibiotic use and occur frequently as superinfections [8,13,15,53]. It has been observed that surgical patients, as a group, often receive more antimicrobials than do medical ICU patients [15]. Knowing the types of microorganisms likely to be seen in certain ICU patients may help in formulating initial empiric antibiotic therapy when the infecting organisms are unknown (see below).

Mortality rates are higher for medical ICU patients than for patients in surgical units [15]. This increased rate is likely related to the older age of and the variety and complexity of underlying diseases seen in these individuals. Among all ICU patients, the relative risk of mortality is increased three-fold in individuals who acquire a hospital infection.

SELECTED INFECTIOUS SYNDROMES IN ICU PATIENTS
This section is not meant to be an exhaustive review of all infections occurring in ICUs. Rather, some of the most common infections encountered in this setting will be discussed, offering a working approach to selection

of proper treatment for such illnesses. Specific antibiotic choices will be influenced by the sensitivity patterns in one's own ICU.

Pneumonia

Over 1 million cases of pneumonia occur annually in the United States [22]. Despite the advent of antibiotics, pneumonia still is the leading infectious cause of death in this country. Two-thirds of all pneumonia deaths are associated with infections acquired in the hospital setting; mortality rates of 20 to 80 percent continue to be reported [14,32,38, 43,46,56,68,74,82,94,96]. Pneumonia acquired in the hospital may occur in up to 7 to 20 percent of all patients admitted to ICUs [12].

Etiologically, gram-negative bacilli are the pathogens most frequently associated with nosocomial pneumonia [12]. In nationwide surveys, six of the seven most frequently isolated etiologic agents are gram-negative bacilli, with *P. aeruginosa* now being most common [12]. *Staphylococcus aureus* is also a common etiologic agent, especially on medical services. In cases with associated bacteremia, *P. aeruginosa* and *Serratia* are more frequently reported. Mixed infections are being more commonly recognized. The mortality rate seen in gram-negative bacillary pneumonia is greater than that due to infection caused by gram-positives or viruses [14,32,38,43,46,56,68,74,82,94,96].

Several predisposing factors in the development of nosocomial pneumonia have been identified: (1) intubation, particularly with increasing duration of intubation; (2) the ICU environment; (3) prior antibiotic therapy; (4) recent thoracic or abdominal surgery; (5) chronic illness (chronic obstructive pulmonary disease, neoplasia, neutropenia, diabetes mellitus, alcoholism, and neurologic, renal, and hepatic disease); (6) the use of respiratory therapy equipment; (7) extremes of age; and (8) the use of antacids or H_2-blockers [16,21,29,36,82,89,97].

In the patient at risk, normal oropharyngeal defense mechanisms (salivary flow and proteases, fibronectin levels on epithelial cells, and normal oral flora) are overwhelmed, resulting in the development of colonization of the tracheobronchial tree with gram-negative bacilli [82]. Pulmonary defense mechanisms (the mucociliary system, cough reflex, immunoglobulin A levels, PMN, alveoloar macrophages, and lymphocytes) are also compromised. Pneumonia results with the inability to clear an aspirated or aerosolized challenge [82]. Other important elements in the pathogenesis of nosocomial pneumonia include the virulence of the infecting organism and the size of the inoculum [82]. In the hospital setting, pneumonia infrequently results as a consequence of metastatic spread from a bloodstream infection.

Patients who have acquired pneumonia in the hospital, especially in ICUs, may not demonstrate the typical clinical manifestations. The elderly, neutropenic, or bacteremic patient with gram-negative bacillary lower respiratory infection less frequently has cough, dyspnea, fever, and signs of consolidation on presentation [38]. In ICU patients, there may be several alternative causes of fever, leukocytosis, and pulmonary infiltrates, making the clinical diagnosis of pneumonia extremely difficult [3,82,89].

The microbiologic diagnosis of hospital-acquired pneumonia is problematic. Many studies have found that etiology correlates poorly with positive blood or pleural fluid cultures and results of Gram's stain or culture of expectorated sputum [63]. Recent studies have substantiated that Gram's stain analysis and culture of specimens truly representing lower respiratory secretions better reflect etiologic pathogens. In studies done at our institution, serial follow-up of semiquantitatively graded tracheal tube aspirate Gram's stain for neutrophils, bacteria, and intracellular organisms predicted pneumonia in ICU patients with rigidly defined infection [82]. In addition, the presence of elastin fibers in aspirates was associated with nosocomial pneumonia. To obtain specimens for diagnostic evaluation, others have advocated transtracheal aspiration or thin-needle lung biopsy. These procedures are wrought with potential morbidity in these seriously ill ICU patients and are not widely practiced. Other methods, including bronchoalveolar lavage or collection of specimens via bronchoscopy with protected brush, are being evaluated as means of obtaining more-reliable specimens for diagnostic purposes and appear to be very promising [26,37,45,93,104,105].

The choice of antibiotics for hospital-acquired pneumonia must take into account many factors, including results of recent cultures, prior antibiotic therapy (resistant organisms), geographic location in the hospital, sensitivity of nosocomial pathogens in that hospital, ability to make a specific etiologic diagnosis, and status of renal and hepatic function. Often, initial broad empiric therapy directed against gram-negative bacilli (including *P. aeruginosa*) and in some situations against gram-positives is warranted in these critically ill patients [82]. Current controversies in antibiotic therapy of nosocomial pneumonia involve the role of aminoglycosides and the question of whether monotherapy with new broad-spectrum β-lactam antibiotics is sufficient. There have never been prospective, controlled, comparative trials to help answer these questions. It is apparent that the administration of optimal antibiotics in this situation may not significantly impact on the enormous morbidity and mortality associated with nosocomial pneumonia. Attention to handwashing, suctioning techniques, and decontamination of respiratory equipment is still important in the ICU setting [82]. Aggressive use of antacid and H_2-blocker therapy must be questioned. With current advances in biotechnology and in the understanding of the pathogenesis of nosocomial pneumonia, future efforts may provide better means of preventing colonization of the tracheobronchial tree, or of enhancing immune responsiveness against these gram-negative bacilli with vaccination or with antibodies directed against the core glycolipid [5,107].

Urinary Tract Infection

Nosocomially acquired urinary tract infections (UTIs) represent the most common hospital-acquired infection, accounting for over 1 million cases every year [12]. Significant complications include the development of bacteremia, postoperative wound infections, chronic bacteriuria, and antimicrobial toxicity [9,58]. Catherized ICU patients are more susceptible to bacteriuria and serious sequelae such as gram-negative bacteremia and sepsis, chronic and acute renal disease, and increased mortality [9,41,58,67,71].

Although epidemiologic studies have demonstrated that nosocomial UTIs represent a significant problem, the occurrence of the urinary tract as a source of bacteremia and sepsis has recently declined [67]. Closed drainage systems, strict catheter care, and liberal antibiotic use may explain, in part, this decrease of the urinary tract as a frequent source of bacteremia [67]. The best means of preventing UTIs in these patients is to avoid the use of catheters when unnecessary and promptly remove urinary catheters when they are no longer needed [67]. This is particularly important in patients who require long-term care. All studies have shown that systemic antimicrobial therapy is incapable of eradicating catheter-associated infections, other than temporarily. Rather, excessive use of antibiotics has led to the emergence of resistant strains that may be spread rapidly to other patients [42].

A prospective microbiologic evaluation in catherized surgical ICU patients has demonstrated that routine or surveillance cultures of urine is unnecessary [58]. In general, the most frequent pathogens in ICU patients include *E. coli, P. aeruginosa, Enterococcus faecalis, Klebsiella pneumoniae,* and *Proteus mirabilis* [9,41,58,67,71]. Other multiply resistant gram-negative bacilli, such as *Serratia* species or *Enterobacter* species, have also been reported in certain units. *Candida* species in some series has accounted for an increasing proportion of hospital-acquired UTIs in ICU patients [67]. Mixed UTIs have also been seen frequently in catherized ICU patients [67]. Anaerobic bacteria, primarily clostridia, have been reported in critically ill patients. Anaerobes should be suspected if gram-positive or gram-negative rods are seen on Gram's stain but routine urine cultures remain negative. The diagnosis of anaerobic UTI can be confirmed by obtaining anaerobic cultures of a suprapubic aspirate.

Wound Infection

Surgical infection historically has been the greatest threat to patients undergoing surgery and remains a formidable problem in critically ill ICU patients [48]. With effective approaches to infection control, the risk of surgical infection is being reduced. Such a program involves attention to asepsis (keeping microorganisms below the "critical inoculum"), antisepsis (disciplined use of antimicrobials), and host defense mechanisms (altering the factors that reduce immunity).

The general determinants of surgical wound infections are related to the degree of injury, the extent of external contamination, the invasiveness of the specific organism, and host resistance [48]. The diagnosis of wound infections depends on a thorough knowledge of the patient's history, physical examination, and bacteriologic information based on Gram's stain and cultures [42,48,67,85]. Postsurgical and traumatic wounds should be considered as potential sources of bacteremia and sepsis following clean-contaminated or contaminated operations. Early physical examination is vital to exclude developing infection—particularly the rare, rapidly progressive, catastrophic types of infections.

Microbiologically, the spectrum of microorganisms that may be associated with surgical or traumatic wounds is vast. The incubation period for staphylococcal wound infections is usually 4 to 6 days [85]. These infections are often well localized, painful, erythematous, and purulent. Local drainage and antibiotic therapy suffice, in most cases, to eradicate these infections. Gram-negative wound infections usually occur as a result of contamination with enteric bacilli as well as anaerobic streptococci or *Bacteroides fragilis.* The incubation period for most of these infections is 7 to 14 days [85]. These gram-negative wound infections present with fewer local inflammatory signs but often with systemic features, including fever, tachycardia, and sepsis. Drainage of these wounds with attention to potential gastrointestinal (GI) sources, along with antibiotics effective against gram-negative aerobic and anaerobic bacilli, are the mainstays of therapy.

Fever, severe toxicity, and pain in a surgical or traumatic wound within the first 48 hours postoperatively must be highly suspicious of infection due to group-A streptococci or clostridia [67]. Early diagnosis, initiation of appropriate antibiotics, and radical surgical debridement are necessary to prevent mortality, which may occur within 18 to 24 hours without therapy. Wound infections caused by β-hemolytic streptococci and synergistic bacterial infections caused by gram-positive cocci in combination with gram-negative bacilli can cause rapidly progressive infections of the subcutaneous tissue called *necrotizing fasciitis* [52,90]. These infections, which frequently are seen in diabetics, may present with soft-tissue crepitance. The diagnosis depends on demonstrating fascial necrosis and widespread undermining of the skin. In uncertain cases, diagnostic biopsy or surgical exploration may be necessary [52]. Necrotizing fasciitis is a life-threatening infection in which extensive surgical excision combined with appropriate antibiotics is crucial to the survival of the patient [2].

Clostridial myonecrosis is an extremely rapid and progressive infection [85]. This infection, also known as gas gangrene, is fortunately rare and usually follows crushing of muscle in injury contaminated by animal or human feces. Injuries or operations involving the gall bladder or large bowel can, rarely, precede clostridial infections [34,90]. Myonecrosis begins within hours and is accompanied by severe pain. Examination of the wound may reveal only mild local edema and blanching at the wound margins, thickening of the skin, and a cool skin temperature [90]. Gaseous crepitance may be absent early, but a distinctive putrid odor is almost always present [2]. Infection can spread within hours and lead to overwhelming sepsis. A Gram's stain of the wound will show gram-positive rods and few neutrophils [90]. Appropriate antibiotics and radical surgical debridement must be undertaken urgently and must be initiated based on the clinical diagnosis alone.

Significant tissue destruction of extremities and large open abdominal wounds may be the source of bacteremia and sepsis. Sepsis resulting from soft-tissue wounds is seen more frequently in elderly patients, diabetics, and immunocompromised hosts [67].

Intra-abdominal Infection
Intra-abdominal infection may be of several types. The infection may be within the peritoneal cavity (diffuse or localized) or the retroperitoneal

space. Intraperitoneal abscess may form in dependent recesses, such as the pelvic space or Morison's pouch, in the perihepatic spaces, within the lesser sac, or in the major routes of communication between intraperitoneal spaces. In addition, abscesses can be located in intra-abdominal viscera, as with hepatic, pancreatic, tuboovarian, or renal abscesses. Abscesses can also form about involved viscera, as with pericholecystic, periappendiceal, pericolic, or intraloop abscesses.

The diagnosis of intra-abdominal infection, particularly following surgery in critically ill patients, can be extremely difficult. Early diagnosis and drainage are essential for improved survival [18,70]. Because of the limitations of conventional radiographic techniques, computed tomography (CT) has become the preferred method for diagnosing intra-abdominal abscesses [61]. However, given that the postoperative abdomen may contain air, blood, seromas, and areas of tissue necrosis, CT may demonstrate images that are mistaken for purulent areas of abscess [28]. Numerous studies have shown that CT is quite sensitive in depicting well-defined abscesses [81]. Many of these studies, however, do not specifically address the diagnostic accuracy of CT in critically ill patients.

Critically ill patients who develop intra-abdominal infection generally fall into two groups. The first group consists of patients whose host defense reserves are strong enough, so that the offending organisms can be controlled and an intra-abdominal abscess can develop [28]. Generally, these patients do not progress to multiple organ failure. The second group consists of patients whose defense mechanisms are so poor or overwhelmed that they are unable to prevent the onset of sepsis and multiple organ failure, despite aggressive ICU support, antibiotics, and nutritional therapy [67]. These patients are frequently unable to form definite intra-abdominal abscesses [81]. Abdominal exploration may be the only definitive diagnostic test in some instances, especially in patients with unexplained single organ system failure. It is not clear whether reoperation significantly affects outcome in large populations of critically ill patients with multiple organ failure.

The microbiology of intra-abdominal infection in critically ill surgical ICU patients is extensive and generally mixed. The bacterial flora is predominantly anaerobic, including *B. fragilis, Peptostreptococcus,* and *Peptococcus* (anaerobic staphylococci). *E. coli* is the most common aerobic organism. Other gram-negative bacilli, such as *Klebsiella* and *Proteus,* account for only a small part of the total flora, and *Pseudomonas* generally is uncommon. It is important to remember that a patient in whom peritonitis or abscess develops in the hospital or while on antibiotics may have a different aerobic flora; *Klebsiella, Proteus,* or *Pseudomonas* will be present in larger numbers and usually will be resistant to many antibiotics.

Line-related Bacteremia and Candidemia

The relentless progress of medical science and technology has been accompanied by the development of numerous devices, each with its own set of complications. Among the devices, used extensively in the ICU, that can be associated with bacteremia are peripheral and central intravenous catheters, total parenteral nutrition catheters, flow-directed balloon-tipped pulmonary artery catheters, arterial lines, and chronic central venous access catheters such as Hickman or Broviac catheters.

Nosocomial bloodstream infections occur at a rate of 2 to 4 episodes per 1000 general hospital admissions [12,33] and of up to 15 per 100 in teaching institutions [12]. They make up 5 to 15 percent of all nosocomial infections in the United States, affecting 120,000 patients each year [12,33]. The overall mortality rate for these infections ranges from 25 to 50 percent; the direct (attributable) mortality rate has been estimated to be 21 to 31 percent [51,87]. Excess hospital stay has been shown to be at least 14 days for hospital-acquired infections [33,87].

Risk factors associated with device-related infection and bloodstream infections include extremes of ages (≤ 1 year, ≥ 60 years), neutropenia, immunosuppressive chemotherapy, loss of skin integrity (e.g. burns), severity of underlying disease, presence of distant infection, alteration in cutaneous microflora, failure of hospital personnel to perform appropriate handwashing, application of contaminated ointment or cream, contaminated infusate or flush solution, contamination of fluid used in monitoring equipment, frequent manipulations of the system, and formation of a fibrin sheath around the device in the blood vessel [35]. Hospital-related factors that contribute to catheter-associated bloodstream infections include (1) type of catheter (plastic more than steel), (2) location of catheter (central more than peripheral; femoral more than jugular or subclavian), (3) type of placement (cutdown more than percutaneous), (4) duration of placement (72 + hours more than under 72 hours), (5) placement (emergent more than elective), and (6) skill of venipuncturist (others more than IV team) [35]. Microorganisms may gain access to intravascular devices at several points. Although each of the access sites has been responsible for sporadic cases and epidemics of nosocomial bacteremia, the most common point at which microorganisms gain entry is the site at which the device penetrates the skin [54].

Microbiologically, the staphylococci continue to be the most frequently encountered pathogens in device-related infections [35] (Table 27-3). Both *S. aureus* and coagulase-negative staphylococci are frequently seen and together account for one-half to two-thirds of the bacteremias seen with these devices. Studies have suggested that *S. epidermidis* may be able to adhere to plastic catheters better than other organisms. The occurrence of more-unusual isolates (*Enterobacter* species, *Pseudomonas cepacia*, *Citrobacter freundii*) should at least suggest the possibility of a contaminated infusion product or of an aqueous environmental reservoir for these pathogens [54].

Candidemia orginating from intravascular devices has become an increasing problem, especially in ICU patients [35–103]. The incidence of nosocomial candidemia increased three- to tenfold between 1978 and 1984 [12,60]. Between 1962 and 1986, the 12 reported series of nosocomial candidemia reported crude mortality rates ranging from 13 to 90 percent [103]. Candidemia occurs in severely ill patients who have a high probability of dying [23,73,86,91,103]. It is more prevalent among males than females,

Table 27-3. Microbiology of catheter-associated infections

Staphylococcus aureus
Coagulase-negative staphylococci
Klebsiella species[a]
Enterobacter species[a]
Serratia marcescens[a]
Candida albicans[b]
Candida species[b]
Pseudomonas aeruginosa[c]
Pseudomonas cepacia
Citrobacter freundii[a]
Corynebacterium JK[d]

[a]Can be associated with contaminated infusates.
[b]Often associated with total parenteral nutrition.
[c]May arise from a water source.
[d]*Corynebacterium* JK occurs commonly in immunocompromised patients.

and the most common underlying conditions are tumors and hematologic diseases [59]. Other risk factors include prolonged broad-spectrum antibiotics, hyperalimentation, recent GI surgery, central venous lines, corticosteroid use, and evidence of colonization with *Candida* (skin, stool, urine, or sputum) [23,59,73,86,91,103].

Clinical detection of catheter-related sepsis is sometimes very difficult. Signs of local inflammation are present in only 50 percent of cases [54]. Salient distinguishing features of device-associated sepsis include (Table 27-4) (1) local phlebitis or inflammation at the catheter site, (2) lack of other sources of bacteremia/candidemia, (3) embolic disease distal to the cannulated vessel, (4) hematogenous *Candida* endophthalmitis in a patient receiving total parenteral nutrition (TPN), (5) presence of 15 or more colonies of the microorganism on semiquantitative culture of a catheter tip, (6) sepsis refractory to "appropriate" antimicrobial therapy, (7) typical (staphylococci) or unusual (*P. cepacia, Enterobacter agglomerans, Enterobacter cloacae*) microbiology, or (8) clustered infections caused by infusion-associated pathogens. Although none of these features specifically identifies the catheter as the source of the bloodstream infection, the presence of these findings should raise the possibility of device-associated sepsis and lead to line removal.

The semiquantitative culture of the intracutaneous segment of the catheter as described by Maki et al. [55] defines a positive culture if 15 or more colonies grow. This cultural definition, employed in combination with relatively strict clinical criteria for catheter-associated sepsis, has been 76 to 96 percent specific, with a positive predictive value ranging between 16 and 31 percent [80]. The cutoff point of 15 colonies is arbitrary, as most infected catheters yield confluent growth when the semiquantitative technique is used [54].

It is extremely difficult to draw definite conclusions about the relative merits of various blood-culturing techniques in the diagnosis of catheter-

Table 27-4. Features suggesting catheter-associated infections

1. Local inflammation or phlebitis at catheter site
2. No other obvious sources for bloodstream infection
3. Distal embolic (bland or septic) phenomena
4. Candidal retinitis in patient receiving total parenteral nutrition
5. Sepsis refractory to appropriate antibiotics
6. 15 or more colonies on semiquantitative culture of intracutaneous portion of catheter
7. Typical or contaminated infusate microbiology
8. Defervescence after catheter removal

associated infection. Although studies have shown a correlation between blood drawn back through catheters and cultures obtained peripherally [95,106], a 5 percent false-positive and 2 percent false-negative rate for cultures drawn back through catheters has been reported [95].

Another important issue relates to removal of long-term indwelling central venous catheters with proven line-related infection. If tunnel infection is absent by exam and there is no evidence of septic thrombophlebitis or distal embolic phenomena, then infections due to gram-positive organisms, particularly *S. aureus* and coagulase-negative staphylococci, can often be eradicated without catheter discontinuance [35]. Infections caused by *Candida* or aerobic gram-negative bacilli have been more refractory to therapy and most often necessitate catheter removal [35].

ANTIMICROBIAL THERAPY IN ICU PATIENTS

Infecting Organism

In many situations, it is necessary to initiate treatment before the results of cultures are available. Thus, it is important to know what agents are probable in different infections. Such knowledge must be based on consideration of the past hospital history of the patient, since in many instances the ICU patient will be admitted to the unit following a prolonged stay in either another hospital or a different area of the same hospital. Organisms prevalent in one area of the hospital may not be those characteristically seen in another.

Knowledge of the replacement of one type of organism by another is important. For example, the patient with extensive burns is infected with *S. aureus* or *Streptococcus pyogenes* (group-A streptococcus) in the first 3 or 4 days; *P. aeruginosa* or *Proteus* infections occur later [49]. Treatment of such patients with either topical or systemic antimicrobial agents prevents these bacterial infections, but viral infections, such as herpes simplex, or fungal infections with *Candida, Torulopsis,* or *Phycomycetales* may develop [76].

A positive culture does not necessarily mean that the patient is infected with that particular microorganism. All patients become colonized with microorganisms within a few days of entry into the ICU [36]. It is imperative that the physician differentiate between colonization and invasion.

This is a simple matter when considering positive blood cultures, but it becomes complex with culture reports of gram-negative bacilli from tracheal suction.

Specimen Collection

Collection of adequate, appropriate, and representative samples is crucial to successful laboratory evaluation—particularly in ICUs, where basic aseptic precautions may sometimes be omitted in the flurry of activity surrounding a critically ill patient, and where diagnostic material may be unavailable or obtained only after initiation of antimicrobial therapy. Ideal specimens are those collected from normally sterile body sites and not contaminated by organisms of the skin or mucous membranes. Specimens should be adequate, and whenever possible, tissue instead of swabs should be submitted. Specimens should be rapidly transported to protect fastidious organisms and prevent overgrowth of contaminants. If an anaerobic culture is desired, anaerobic transport media should be employed. If possible, specimens should be collected before antimicrobial therapy, and use of topical anesthetics or preservative-containing solutions should be avoided.

Examination of Specimens

Direct microscopic examination of specimens, either as wet mounts (saline, potassium hydroxide, India ink) or stained smears, is extremely important in the diagnosis of multiple infections. Stained smears are commonly performed on a wide variety of specimens and often provide diagnostic information in infectious conditions. Gram's smears of body fluids and exudates can show inflammatory cells as well as bacteria. Clumps of gram-positive cocci suggest staphylococci or peptococci; chains of gram-positive cocci suggest streptococci or peptostreptococci; large gram-positive bacilli suggest clostridia; large gram-negative bacilli suggest Enterobacteriaceae; and small gram-negative bacilli suggest *Pseudomonas, Haemophilus,* or *Bacteroides* species. However, bacterial morphology can be highly variable, particularly in material from abscesses or from patients on antimicrobial therapy, and overinterpretation of smears must be avoided.

Gram's stains of sputum are helpful when inflammatory cells suggest pneumonia; however, if there are oral squamous epithelial cells and a wide variety of organisms, the specimen includes saliva and should be discarded. Pneumonia caused by pneumonococci, *Haemophilus influenzae,* *S. aureus,* and Enterobacteriaceae can often be diagnosed with a high degree of accuracy from a sputum Gram's stain.

Gram's stains of urine are highly suggestive of significant bacteriuria if two or more bacteria are seen per oil-immersion field of well-mixed uncentrifuged urine. Gram-negative bacilli suggest Enterobacteriaceae, and gram-positive cocci suggest enterococci or staphylococci.

A Gram's stain can be easily and rapidly performed by the physician attending the patient. Good results, however, require considerable experience and expertise, because decolorization time depends on the nature of the material being stained. Again, overinterpretation of smears should be avoided. Since many organisms have similar appearances, organisms in gram-stained smears should be described by their morphology as well as their degree of staining.

Mycobacteria do not stain with the Gram method, but they resist acid decolorization and can therefore be identified by various acid-fast stains of sputum and other specimens. Both Ziehl-Neelsen stain using hot carbolfuchsin and Kinyoun stain using cold concentrated carbolfuchsin will stain mycobacteria red. Auramine will stain mycobacteria to a bright yellow under suitable fluorescent illumination.

Fluoroscein-tagged fluorescent antibody stains, available in most microbiology laboratories, are useful in demonstrating various pathogens, such as *Legionella pneumophila.* Other staining methods include silver stains of biopsies for fungi or of biopsies or sputum for *Pneumocystis carinii.*

Culture Methods

The wide variety of bacteria, fungi, viruses, and protozoa that can cause infections require different isolation techniques. Most laboratories choose techniques based on ease of use, local prevalence of various infectious diseases, clinical usefulness, and availability of equipment and facilities. Physicians should be aware of which procedures are routine and which are available on request, either on site or at a referral laboratory. Specimens are usually processed for groups of organisms, such as rapidly growing bacteria (aerobic and anaerobic), mycobacteria, fungi, *Chlamydia,* and viruses.

Antimicrobial Susceptibility Tests

Determining the susceptibility of isolated pathogens to appropriate antimicrobial agents is an important function of clinical microbiology laboratories. This is particularly important in ICUs, where the development and spread of resistant bacteria, such as nosocomial pathogens, as well as the increasing numbers of immunocompromised patients and new antimicrobial agents, magnify the importance of rapid and accurate susceptibility testing of isolates from critically ill patients.

In vivo susceptibility is influenced by several factors: host defense mechanisms; the concentrations of antimicrobial agents at the site of infections; the natural course, nature, and severity of the infection; any delay in starting therapy; and effects of other therapeutic measures, such as surgery. In vitro susceptibility depends on organism, growth medium, atmosphere, inoculum size, and length and temperature of incubation. Since these factors have been standardized for common rapidly growing bacteria, the outcome of infection is mainly affected by in vivo factors.

Organisms are susceptible to an antimicrobial agent if they are inhibited in vitro by a concentration of the agent that is lower than serum concentrations achievable with the usual drug dosage. Resistant organisms are not inhibited or are inhibited only at concentrations above those attainable. Susceptibility and resistance are expressed as the minimal inhibitory concentration (MIC) of an antimicrobial agent required to inhibit growth of a defined population of organisms, or as categories based on antimicrobial levels in various body sites. All susceptibility tests are based on antimicrobial levels in various body sites, are based directly or indirectly on MIC determination, and require strict standardization and quality control. Table 27-5 lists the antibiotic susceptibilities of bacteria commonly encountered in ICUs.

Antimicrobial Agents

General Considerations
Antimicrobial agents may be divided into groups on the basis of their mechanism of action on the microorganism. Agents can interfere with (1) cell-wall biosynthesis, (2) cytoplasmic membrane function, (3) protein synthesis (either transcription or translation), (4) nucleic acid metabolism, and (5) intermediary metabolism within the microorganism. Agents may be bactericidal, killing the microorganism, or bacteriostatic, preventing continued proliferation of the microorganism only while present within the microorganism. In many situations, a bacterostatic agent is as successful as a bactericidal agent would have been. On the other hand, the patient in the ICU, because of the nature of the particular illness or the length of the illness, may be at a special disadvantage. Phagocytic function in critically ill patients is often less effective than it is in healthy persons. Antibody function may be decreased secondary to the administration of other agents. The presence of foreign bodies makes eradication of infecting organisms more difficult with a bacteriostatic agent than with a bactericidal agent. The mechanisms of action of currently available antimicrobial agents against bacteria, fungi, and viruses are given in Table 27-6.

Empiric antibiotic therapy must often be initiated in desperately ill ICU patients. Antibiotics must be given on a timely basis and be appropriate for the causative organisms if significant morbidity and mortality is to be avoided. The choice of antibiotic therapy must take into account several factors: (1) the possible site of infection; (2) community or hospital acquisition; (3) the possibility of a mixed infection, particularly with anaerobes; (4) knowledge of the local hospital or unit pathogens, (5) the type of host; (6) the level of renal and/or hepatic function; (7) allergy history; (8) toxicity of antimicrobials; and (9) combination/synergistic antibiotics in bacteremic neutropenic patients.

For most noninfectious-disease physicians, it is best to learn well a selected number of antibiotics from each class. In special circumstances or when multiply resistant pathogens are involved, consultation with the infectious diseases service should assure that optimal antibiotic regimens for these critically ill individuals are chosen.

Antimicrobial Agents of Choice
The drug of choice for treatment of infections in ICU patients should be the most active drug against the pathogenic organism or the least toxic alternative among several effective agents. Sometimes the choice of drug is modified by the site of an infection, as one drug may penetrate better than another into cerebrospinal fluid, bile, or urine. Characteristics of the

patient that may be extremely important include age, allergy to penicillin, immunocompromised state, and pregnancy. When everything else is equal, the relative cost may be a consideration. Table 27-7 lists first-choice antimicrobials and alternative drugs for infection caused by most of the commonly encountered pathogens in ICUs. In most cases, these recommendations are based on results of microbiologic and clinical trials. For the serious nature of the infections encountered in most ICU patients, parenteral antimicrobial therapy is usually necessary. Table 27-8 lists dosages of frequently utilized antibiotics in the treatment of life-threatening infections in critically ill patients.

Newer Antibiotics Available for Use in ICU Patients
The motivation for development of many new antimicrobials has been the perpetual emergence of resistance among bacteria, particularly hospital-associated strains. This section briefly reviews some of the new antibiotics available to treat serious infections in ICU patients.

β-LACTAMASE INHIBITORS. Currently, the major mechanism of β-lactam resistance seen in both gram-positive and gram-negative organisms is the production of β-lactamases [91]. β-lactamase inhibitors have been developed [47,64]. The two currently available β-lactamase inhibitors, clavulanic acid and sulbactam [47,64], have similar activity, although clavulanic acid primarily inhibits plasmid-mediated (TEM-1) β-lactamases. Both protect β-lactam antibiotics from hydrolysis by β-lactamases. The three β-lactamase inhibitor–β-lactam antibiotic combinations currently available are amoxicillin–clavulanic acid, ampicillin-sulbactam, and ticarcillin–clavulanic acid; the latter two combinations are administered parenterally. Ampicillin-sulbactam and amoxicillin–clavulanic acid have essentially the same antibiotic spectrum. To the usual spectrum of ampicillin-amoxicillin, these β-lactamase inhibitors add activity against β-lactamase–producing strains of *S. aureus, H. influenzae, Branhamella catarrhalis,* and *B. fragilis* [47,64]. The combinations are also active against many β-lactamase–producing gram-negative bacilli, the notable exceptions being *P. aeruginosa* and *Enterobacter* species. However, in many nosocomially acquired infections in which multiply resistant gram-negative bacilli may be involved, ampicillin-sulbactam would be inadequate.

Ticarcillin–clavulanic acid has a somewhat similar spectrum of activity, except that ticarcillin confers activity against many strains of *P. aeruginosa* [78]. This combination has less activity against gram-positive organisms; in particular, activity against enterococci is poor.

NEWER β-LACTAM ANTIBIOTICS. A number of new β-lactams with increased activity against resistant facultative gram-negative bacilli have been developed. Of these, third-generation cephalosporins, imipenem (Primaxin), and aztreonam will be discussed.

The "third-generation" cephalosporins have increased activity against a broad range of gram-negative bacteria. In general, they are less active against gram-positive organisms that are "first-generation" cephalosporins

Table 27-5. Antimicrobial susceptibilities of commonly encountered bacteria in ICUs*

Percent susceptible

Antibiotic	S. pyogenes	Enterococci	Pneumococci	Peptostreptococcus	S. aureus	Methicillin-resistant Sh. aureus	Coagulase-negative Staphylococci	Peptococcus	Clostridium	E. coli	Klebsiella	Enterobacter	Serratia	P. mirabilis	Indole-positive Proteus	P. aeruginosa	Other Pseudomonas Species	Salmonella	Shigella	Acinetobacter	Haemophilus	Neisseria	Bacteroides
Penicillin G	100	20	100	100	25		15	60	100	50	1	2	1	1	1	0	0	85	50	5		90	9
Ampicillin	100	98	100	100	25		55	60	100	50	1	2	1	90	1	0	0	85	50		70	100	
Methicillin and nafcillin	100	5	100		95	0	75													5			6
Ticarcillin,	100	20	100	100	25	0	25	50	100	75	3	72	80	98	50	80	11	88	70	83	85	100	7
mezlocillin, and piperacillin	100	98	100	100	25	0	25	50	100	80	80	80	83	99	97	80	5	89	70	50	85	100	7
Cefazolin	100	0	100	95	90	0	55	89		90	94	0	0	95	1	0	0	95	95	2	80		3
Cefuroxime	100	0	100	100	95	0	95	95		95	95	75	7	95	6	0	0			25	95	100	5
Cefoxitin	100	0	100	100	95	0	95	95	90	98	95	10	11	95	85	0	5			5	95	100	9

Antimicrobial																					
Cefotaxime and ceftriaxone	100	0	100	90	95	0	90	90	95	100	100	85	90	100	20	0	100	100	50	100	100	4
Ceftazidime	100	0	100	90	60	0	70	95	90	100	100	85	90	80	95	49	100	100	98	100	100	9
Imipenem	100	98	100	100	100	50	60	100	98	98	90	80	75	95	30	100	100	98	100	100		9
Aztreonam	10	0	0	0	0	0	95	70	80	100	75	100	90	10	100	100						2
Erythromycin	98	75	100	85	94	0	85	80	95													
Clindamycin	98	100	90	96	0	93	90	95													85	9
Metronidazole																						9
Chloramphenicol	98	75	100	85	88	70	75	80	90	90	85	90	50	3	65	95	10	100	100			9
Gentamicin			90		90		95	95	90	70	98	90	80	5	99	80						
Tobramycin			90		90		98	96	73	98	99	87	7	99	90							
Amikacin			90		98		98	98	98	98	95	98	7	100	90							
Ciprofloxacin	90	85	100	98	98	90	90	99	98	95	85	100	95	85	100	100	90	100	100			

*Values represent the percent susceptible isolates at or below the MIC breakpoint.

Table 27-6. Mechanisms of action of commonly employed antimicrobial agents in the ICU

Antimicrobial agent	Site of action	Mode of action
ANTIBIOTICS		
Penicillins	Cell wall	Bactericidal
Cephalosporins	Cell wall	Bactericidal
Carbapenems	Cell wall	Bactericidal
Monobactams	Cell wall	Bactericidal
Vancomycin	Cell wall	Bactericidal
Aminoglycosides (gentamicin, tobramycin, netilmicin, amikacin)	Protein synthesis, ribosomes	Bactericidal
Carboxyquinolones	DNA gyrase	Bactericidal
Tetracyclines	Protein synthesis, ribosomes	Bacteriostatic
Chloramphenicol	Protein synthesis, ribosomes	Bacteriostatic
Erythromycin	Protein synthesis	Bacteriostatic
Metronidazole	Reductive activity, free radical damage of DNA	Bactericidal
Rifampin	Protein synthesis, RNA polymerase	Either bactericidal or bacteriostatic
Sulfonamides	Competition with PABA	Bacteriostatic
Trimethoprim	Dihydrofolate reductases	Bacteriostatic
ANTIFUNGAL AGENTS		
Nystatin	Cytoplasmic membrane	Either fungicidal or fungostatic
Flucytosine	DNA synthesis	Fungicidal
Amphotericin	Cytoplasmic membrane	Fungicidal
Imidazoles (ketoconazole, miconazole, itraconazole, fluconazole)	Cytoplasmic membrane	Fungicidal
ANTIVIRAL AGENTS		
Acyclovir	DNA synthesis	Viricidal
Amantadine	Interferes with fusion of cell membrane and virus	Viricidal
Ganciclovir	DNA synthesis	Viricidal
Ribaviron	RNA synthesis	Viricidal
Zidovudine (AZT)	DNA chain terminator	Viricidal

Table 27-7. Antimicrobials of choice for commonly encountered microorganisms in the ICU

Organism	Drugs of first choice	Alternative drugs
GRAM-POSITIVE COCCI		
Staphylococcus aureus or coagulase-negative staphylococci		
Non–penicillinase-producing	Penicillin G	A cephalosporin (1st generation), vancomycin, imipenem, clindamycin
Penicillinase-producing	A penicillinase-resistant penicillin (e.g., nafcillin)	A cephalosporin (1st generation), vancomycin, ampicillin-sulbactam, clindamycin, imipenem, ciprofloxacin
Methicillin-resistant	Vancomycin	Ciprofloxacin, trimethoprim-sulfamethoxazole
β-hemolytic streptococci (groups A, B, C, G)	Penicillin G or ampicillin	A cephalosporin (1st generation), vancomycin, erythromycin
Streptococcus, *Enterococcus* endocarditis or severe infection	Penicillin G or ampicillin *plus* gentamicin	Vancomycin *plus* gentamicin
Peptostreptococcus	Penicillin G	Clindamycin, a cephalosporin (1st generation), vancomycin
Streptococcus pneumoniae	Penicillin G	Erythromycin, a cephalosporin (1st generation), vancomycin
GRAM-POSITIVE BACILLI		
Clostridium perfringens	Penicillin G	Chloramphenicol, metronidazole clindamycin
Clostridium tetani	Penicillin G	Tetracycline
Clostridium difficile	Vancomycin (oral)	Metronidazole (oral)
Corynebacterium JK	Vancomycin	
Listeria monocytogenes	Ampicillin with or without gentamicin	Trimethoprim-sulfamethoxazole

Table 27-7 (continued)

Organism	Drugs of first choice	Alternative drugs
GRAM-NEGATIVE COCCI		
Branhamella catarrhalis	Cefuroxime	Trimethoprim-sulfamethoxazole, erythromycin, cefotaxime, ampicillin-sulbactam
Neisseria meningitidis	Penicillin G	Cefuroxime, cefotaxime, chloramphenicol
Haemophilus influenzae meningitis, epiglottis, arthritis, other severe infections	Cefotaxime or ceftriaxone	Cefuroxime, ampicillin *plus* chloramphenicol
GRAM-NEGATIVE BACILLI		
Acinetobacter	Imipenem	An aminoglycoside, ticarcillin, piperacillin, mezlocillin or azlocillin, trimethoprim-sulfamethoxazole
Aeromonas hydrophilia	Trimethoprim-sulfamethoxazole	Gentamicin, tobramycin, imipenem
Bacteroids		
Oropharyngeal strains	Penicillin G	Clindamycin, metronidazole, cefoxitin, chloramphenicol, cefotetan
Gastrointestinal strains	Metronidazole	Clindamycin, cefoxitin, chloramphenicol, imipenem, ampicillin-sulbactam, cefotetan
Campylobacter jejuni	Erythromycin, ciprofloxacin	Gentamicin
Eikenella corrodens	Ampicillin or penicillin G	Erythromycin, ampicillin-sulbactam
Enterobacter	Cefotaxime or ceftriaxone	An aminoglycoside, imipenem, ticarcillin, mezlocillin, piperacillin, azlocillin, trimethoprim-sulfamethoxazole, aztreonam, ciprofloxacin, chloramphenicol
Escherichia coli	Ampicillin	A cephalosporin (1st or 3rd generation), ticarcillin, mezlocillin, an aminoglycoside, azlocillin, aztreonam, trimethoprim-sulfamethoxazole, chloramphenicol

Organism	First choice	Alternative(s)
Klebsiella pneumoniae	Cephalosporin	An aminoglycoside, trimethoprim-sulfamethoxazole, mezlocillin, piperacillin, aztreonam, imipenem, ampicillin-sulbactam
Legionella pneumophilia	Erythromycin	Trimethoprim-sulfamethoxazole with or without rifampin
Pasteurella multocida	Penicillin G	Ampicillin-sulbactam, cefuroxime, a cephalosporin (1st generation)
Proteus mirabilis	Ampicillin	A cephalosporin, ticarcillin, mezlocillin, piperacillin, azlocillin, an aminoglycoside, trimethoprim-sulfamethoxazole, aztreonam, imipenem, ciprofloxacin, chloramphenicol
Proteus, indole-positive	Cefotaxime or ceftriaxone	An aminoglycoside, ticarcillin, mezlocillin, piperacillin, ampicillin-sulbactam, imipenem, aztreonam, trimethoprim-sulfamethoxazole, ciprofloxacin, chloramphenicol
Providencia stuartii	Cefotaxime or ceftriaxone	Imipenem, an aminoglycoside, ticarcillin, mezlocillin, piperacillin, azlocillin, aztreonam, ceftazidime, trimethoprim-sulfamethoxazole, ciprofloxacin, chloramphenicol
Pseudomonas aeruginosa	Ticarcillin, mezlocillin, piperacillin, or azlocillin *plus* tobramycin or amikacin	Tobramycin or amikacin *plus* ceftazidime, imipenem, or aztreonam; ciprofloxacin
Pseudomonas maltrophilia	Trimethoprim-sulfamethoxazole	Ceftazidime, ciprofloxacin
Pseudomonas cepacia	Trimethoprim-sulfamethoxazole	Chloramphenicol, ceftazidime
Salmonella typhi	Trimethoprim-sulfamethoxazole	Chloramphenicol, ciprofloxacin, ampicillin, cefotaxime, or ceftriaxone
Serratia	Cefotaxime or ceftriaxone	Gentamicin or amikacin, imipenem, aztreonam, ceftazidime, trimethoprim-sulfamethoxazole, tricarcillin, mezlocillin, piperacillin, azlocillin, ciprofloxacin

Table 27-7 (continued)

Organism	Drugs of first choice	Alternative drugs
Shigella	Trimethoprim-sulfamethoxazole	Ciprofloxacin, ampicillin
Yersinia enterocolitica	Trimethoprim-sulfamethoxazole	Ciprofloxacin, an aminoglycoside, cefotaxime, or ceftriaxone
Viruses		
Cytomegalovirus	Ganciclovir	
Herpes simplex	Acyclovir	Vidarabine
Influenza A	Amantadine	
Respiratory syncytial virus	Ribavirin	
Varicella-zoster	Acyclovir	Vidarabine
FUNGI		
Aspergillus	Amphotericin B	
Candida	Amphotericin B	Ketoconazole
Coccidioides immitis	Amphotericin B	Ketoconazole, miconazole
Cryptococcus neoformans	Amphotericin B with or without flucytosine	?Fluconazole
Histoplasma capsulatum	Amphotericin B or ketoconazole	
Mucor and other agents of mucormycosis	Amphotericin B	
Pseudallescheria boydii	Ketoconazole or miconazole	

[65]. Activity against *B. fragilis* is poor. Enterococci, listeria, and methicillin-resistant staphylococci are resistant to these agents. Among individual agents, ceftazidime has the greatest activity against *P. aeruginosa*. Cefotaxime and ceftriaxone retain better activity against gram-positives but lack activity against pseudomonads. Rational uses of third-generation cephalosporins include therapy for gram-negative bacillary meningitis or empiric therapy for bacterial meningitis [65]. These agents can be useful in gram-negative bacillary infections acquired in the hospital; an aminoglycoside should be added in neutropenic patients [65]. A case can be made that third-generation cephalosporins should replace aminoglycosides in certain infections, such as initial treatment of pyelonephritis.

Aztreonam is a monobactam with a unique bacterial spectrum [1]. It is active against aerobic and facultative gram-negative bacteria but lacks activity against gram-positive or anaerobic bacteria [1]. Notably, aztreonam appears to have little or no immunologic cross-reactivity with other β-lactams [1]. It thus is useful in treating serious gram-negative infections in patients with major penicillin or cephalosporin allergy.

Imipenem (Primaxin) is a carbapenem with the broadest antibacterial spectrum of any available antibiotic [30,77]. It is active against most clinically important bacteria except *Enterococcus faecium, Pseudomonas maltophilia,* and many strains of *P. cepacia* and methicillin-resistant staphylococci [30,77]. It is a valuable agent for treating infections with multiply drug-resistant bacteria and for treating mixed infections in critically ill patients. It should be used with restraint, however, as resistant bacteria already are beginning to emerge [30,77].

CARBOXYQUINOLONES. The new quinolones are structurally unrelated to other classes of antimicrobial agents and have a unique mechanism of action. They act, at least in part, by inhibition of bacterial DNA gyrase [79]. Many aerobic and facultative gram-negative rods, including *P. aeruginosa* and all of the important enteric pathogens, are susceptible to these agents [79]. Quinolones are active against staphylococci, including methicillin-resistant strains, and have moderate activity against enterococci [79]. The drugs have marginal activity against pneumococci and poor activity against anaerobes [1].

Ciprofloxacin and norfloxacin are the currently available quinolones. Only oral preparations have been released, but an intravenous form of ciprofloxacin is under investigation. Ciprofloxacin achieves good systemic levels, whereas norfloxacin achieves good levels only in the GI and genitourinary tracts. Potential uses of the new quinolones include therapy for complicated urinary tract infections, bacterial enterocolitis, gonorrhea, and bacterial prostatitis, as well as infection prevention in neutropenic patients [79]. Ciprofloxacin, because of its higher systemic and antibacterial activity, also is useful in other selected infections—e.g., osteomyelitis [1].

Drug Interactions
As most ICU patients will be receiving multiple drugs, the potential for adverse drug interactions is substantial and should be carefully considered

Table 27-8. Dosage of antibiotics to be used in the treatment of severe, life-threatening infection[a]

Antibiotic	Total daily dose (gm)	Interval between doses (hr)	Peak serum concentrations (μg/ml)[b]	Average concentration (μg/ml) needed to inhibit susceptible organism	
				Gram-positive	Gram-negative
Penicillin G	$10–12 \times 10^6$ MU	2–4	4–10	0.05–0.5	—
Ampicillin	12	4	10–40	0.05–0.5	1–10
Methicillin	12–16	4	6–10	0.3	—
Oxacillin, nafcillin	8–12	4–6	5–20	0.1–0.3	—
Ticarcillin	18–24	4	50–250	0.1–1	1–64
Mezlocillin	18–24	4	50–250	0.1–1	1–64
Piperacillin	18–24	4	50–250	0.1–1	1–64
Cephalothin	8–12	4	10–30	0.05–1.0	1–16
Cefazolin	4–8	6	20–80	0.05–1.0	1–12
Cefuroxime	4–12	6	20–70	0.1–1	1–12

Cefoxitin	4–12	6	20–70	0.5–4	1–25
Cefotaxime	2–9	6	20–70	0.1–4	0.01–6
Ceftazidime	3–6	8	50–100	0.5–8	0.5–8
Aztreonam	0.5–2	6–12	50–200	—	0.5–25
Imipenem	1–2	6	20–70	0.1–1	0.5–8
Erythromycin	2–4	6	5–15	0.05–1.0	—
Clindamycin	2–5	6	2–20	0.02–1.5	—
Chloramphenicol	50 mg/kg	6	10–20	0.5–2.0	1–10
Gentamicin	3–6 mg/kg	8	4–12	—	0.5–6
Tobramycin	3–6 mg/kg	8	6–10	—	0.5–6
Amikacin	15–20 mg/kg	8	15–25	0.05–0.5	1–10
Ciprofloxacin	1–1.5	12	2–5	0.5–1	0.05–2
Vancomycin	2	6	6–20	0.5–6.0	—

[a]Based on normal renal function.
[b]Based on intermittent therapy program.

whenever new agents, particularly antibiotics, are initiated. Table 27-9 lists some of the important drug interactions involving antimicrobials that may be encountered in critically ill ICU patients. When appropriate, consultations with the clinical pharmacology service or pharmacy department should be obtained.

Antimicrobial Prescribing in the Presence of Renal or Hepatic Failure

A rapidly expanding population of ICU patients is being treated for metabolic disorders, particularly renal and hepatic failure. The ICU physician will frequently need to treat intercurrent infections in patients who are predisposed to adverse drug reactions because of loss of renal or hepatic function. This is especially the case with renal insufficiency, as the biochemical derangements seen in this condition may modify a drug's bioavailability, distribution, pharmacologic action, or elimination [6]. Some practical guidelines for prescribing antimicrobials used in ICU patients in the setting of renal or hepatic failure are provided in Table 27-10. More extensive information on drug prescribing in renal failure can be found elsewhere [6].

SUMMARY

Infection remains one of the most significant problems for the intensivist. Sophisticated medical care in ICUs has prolonged survival of patients but has created hosts and an environment that facilitate nosocomial infection. In order to adequately care for these patients, health care providers in the ICU must become familiar with the epidemiology, clinical nuances, diagnosis, and treatment of infectious complications. Antimicrobial therapy must be chosen wisely and an attempt made to balance the efficacy of the treatment against the risks of superinfection, toxicity, and potential interactions with the many other drugs utilized in this setting. This chapter has provided some insights into the scope and spectrum of infections in ICUs, as well as practical approaches to the identification and management of microorganisms and selected infectious syndromes in these critically ill patients.

Table 27-9. Drug interactions of potential importance in ICUs

Type of interaction and antibiotics	Affected or displaced by	Effect
SERUM CARRIER DISPLACEMENT		
Sulfonamides	Tolbutamide	Hypoglycemia
	Bishydroxycoumarin	Bleeding
	Warfarin	Bleeding
	Bilirubin	Kernicterus
INTERACTION AT TISSUE SITE		
Polymyxins	Curare	Apnea
Aminoglycosides (kanamycin, neomycin, gentamicin)	Succinylcholine	
Aminoglycosides	Polymyxins	Nephrotoxicity
Cephaloridine	Ethacrynic acid, furosemide	Ototoxicity
	Furosemide	Nephrotoxicity
COMPETITION FOR BINDING SITES		
Sulfonamides, chloramphenicol	Tolbutamide, chlorpropamide	Hypoglycemia
Sulfonamides, chloramphenicol	Bishydroxycoumarin	Increased anticoagulation
Chloramphenicol	Bilirubin	Jaundice of the newborn
Isoniazid	Rifampin	Liver toxicity
Isoniazid	Phenytoin	Neurotoxicity

Table 27-10. Use of antimicrobials in renal and hepatic disease

Antibiotic	Removed from body by	Serum half-life (hr) Normal	oliguria	Toxicity in uremia	Intervals between doses with various creatinine clearances — Renal failure Normal (100 ml)	Moderate (24–40 ml)	Severe (<10 ml)	Dose altered by dialysis Hemo-dialysis	Peritoneal	Added to dialysate	Dose in hepatic failure
Penicillin	K-T	0.5	2–4	CNS	4 hr	NC	1 × 10⁶ MU/6 hr	1 × 10⁶ MU/6 hr	No		NC
Ampicillin	K-T	0.5	8	CNS	4 hr	NC	1 gm/8hr	0.5 gm/6 hr	No		NC
Methicillin	K-T	0.5	4	None	4 hr	NC	1 gm/8 hr	No	No		NC
Carbenicillin	K-T, L	1.0	15	CNS, bleeding	4 hr	NC	2 gm/8 hr	1 gm/4 hr	Yes	100 µg/ml	Decreased if renal failure also present
Cephalothin	K-T	0.5	15	None	4 hr	NC	1 gm/8 hr	1 gm/6 hr	Yes	20 µg/ml	NC
Cefotaxime	K	1	2	None	6–8 hr	NC	1 gm/12 hr	Yes	No		Decrease dose
Cefazolin	K-T	1.9	30	None	6–8 hr	NC	24 hr	Yes	Unknown		NC
Cefuroxime	K-T	1.2	15	None	8 hr	8–12 hr	24 hr	Yes	Yes		NC
Ceftazidime	K	1.8	16–25	None	8–12 hr	1 gm/12–24 hr	0.5 gm/24–48 hr	Yes	Yes		NC
Imipenem	K	1	4	CNS	6–8 hr	6–12 hr	12–24 hr	Yes	Yes		NC
Aztreonam	K	1.7–2	6–8.7	None	6–12 hr	12–24 hr	24–36 hr	Yes	Yes		NC
Erythromycin	L	1.5	4–6	None	6 hr	NC	NC	Slight	No		Do not use
Tetracycline-HCl	K-G, L	8.5	100	Renal, hepatic	6 hr	Do not use	Do not use	No	Slight		Do not use

Drug				Toxicity						5–10 µg/ml
Doxycycline	L	17	17	None	12 hr	NC	NC	No	Yes	Do not use
Chloramphenicol	L	1.0–2.5	3–5	None	6 hr	NC	NC	Yes	No	Decrease dose
Clindamycin	L	2.5	10	None	6–8 hr	NC	10 hr	No	No	Decrease dose
Polymyxin B	K-G	4–7	72	Renal, CNS	6–8 hr	24–36 hr	4 days	No	No	NC
Gentamicin	K-G	2–3	70	Ear, renal, CNS	8 hr	Use nomogram or serum levels	Use nomogram or serum levels	Yes	Yes	NC
Tobramycin	K-G	2	70	Ear, renal	8 hr	Use nomogram or serum levels	Use nomogram or serum levels	Yes	Yes	NC
Amikacin	K	2	50	Renal, ear	2 hr	Use nomogram		Check serum level		NC
Ciprofloxacin	K	2.7	8.4	None	12 hr	0.25–0.5/12/hr	0.25–0.5/18–24 hr	No	Yes	NC
Vancomycin	K-G	5	240	Ear, renal	6–12 hr	24 hr	4–6 days	No	No	NC
Isoniazid	K-L	1–4	8	None	24 hr	NC	Decrease dose	Yes	Yes	Decrease dose
Ethambutol	K	4–6	30	Visual	24 hr	Decrease dose	Do not use	Yes	Yes	NC
Rifampin	L-K	1.5–5.0	3–5	None	24 hr	NC	NC	No		Decrease dose
Sulfisoxazole	K	6	12	Renal	12 hr	24 hr	Do not use	Yes	Yes	NC
Trimethoprim	K	10	15–40	Marrow	12 hr	24 hr	48 hr			NC
Amphotericin B	K	24	48–72	Renal	24 hr	3 days	5 days	No	No	NC
5-Fluorocytosine	K	3–8	20	Marrow	6 hr	12–24 days	2 days	25 mg/kg		NC

NC = no change; K = kidney; G = glomerular; T = tubular; L = liver.

REFERENCES

1. Acar, J. F., and Neu, H. C. (eds.). Gram-negative aerobic bacterial infections: A focus on directed therapy, with special reference to aztreonam. *Rev. Infect. Dis.* 7(Suppl. 4):S537, 1985.
2. Ajeski, J. A., and Alexander, J. W. Early diagnosis, nutritional support and immediate extensive debridement improve survival in necrotizing fascitis. *Am. J. Surg.* 145:784, 1983.
3. Andrews C. P., Coalson, J. J., Smith, J. D., et al. Diagnosis of nosocomial pneumonia in acute, diffuse lung injury. *Chest* 80:254, 1981.
4. Bachman, L., Downess, J. J., Richards, C. C., et al. Organization and function of an intensive care unit in a children's hospital. *Anesth. Analg.* 46:570, 1967.
5. Baumgartner, J. D., Glauser, M. P., McCutchan, J. A., et al. Prevention of gram-negative shock and death in surgical patients by antibody to endotoxin core glycolipid. *Lancet* 2:59, 1985.
6. Bennett, W. M., Aronoff, G. R., Morrison, G., et al. Drug prescribing in renal failure: Dosing guidelines for adults. *Am J. Kid. Dis.* 3:155, 1983.
7. Berkelman, R. L., Godley, S., Weber, J. A., et al. *Pseudomonas cepacia* peritonitis associated with contamination of automatic peritoneal dialysis machines. *Ann. Intern. Med.* 96:245, 1982.
8. Brown, R. B., Hosmer, D., Chen, H. C., et al. A comparison of infections in different ICUs within the same hospital. *Crit. Care Med.* 13:472, 1985.
9. Bryan, C. S., and Reynolds, K. L. Hospital-acquired bacteremic urinary tract infection. Epidemiology and outcome. *J. Urol.* 131:494, 1984.
10. Caplan, E. S., and Hoyt, N. Infection surveillance and control in the severely traumatized patient. *Am. J. Med.* 70:638, 1981.
11. Caplan, E. S., Hoyt, N., and Cowley, R. A. Changing patterns of nosocomial infections in severely traumatized patients. *Am. Surg.* 45:204, 1979.
12. Centers for Disease Control. National nosocomial infection surveillance, 1984. *M. M. W. R.* 35:17SS, 1986.
13. Chandrasekar, P. H., Kruse, J. A., and Matthews, M. F. Nosocomial infection among patients in different types of intensive care units at a city hospital. *Crit. Care Med.* 14:508, 1986.
14. Crane, L. R., and Lerner, A. M. Gram-negative pneumonia in hospitalized patients. *Postgrad. Med.* 58:85, 1985.
15. Craven, D. E., Kunches, L. M., Lichtenberg, D. A., et al. Nosocomial infection and fatality in medical and surgical intensive care unit patients. *Arch. Intern. Med.* 148:1161, 1988.
16. Craven, D. E., Kunches, L. M., Klinsky, V., et al. Risk factors for pneumonia in patients receiving continuous mechanical ventilation. *Am. Rev. Respir. Dis.* 133:792, 1986.
17. Daschmer, F. D., Frey, P., Wolff, G., et al. Nosocomial infections in intensive care unit wards: A multicenter prospective study. *Intensive Care Med.* 8:5, 1982.
18. Doberneck, R. C., and Mittleman, J. Reappraisal of the problems of intraabdominal surgery. *Surg. Gynecol. Obstet.* 154:875, 1982.
19. Donowitz, L. G., Wenzel, R. P., and Hoyt, J. W. High risk of hospital-acquired infection in the ICU patient. *Crit. Care Med.* 10:355, 1982.
20. Donowitz, L. G., Marsik, F. J., Hoyt, J. W., et al. *Serratia marcescens* bacteremia from contaminated pressure transducers. *J.A.M.A.* 242:1749, 1979.
21. Driks, M. R., Craven, D. E., Celli, B. R., et al. Nosocomial pneumonia in intubated patients given sucralfate as compared with antacids or histamine type 2 blockers. *N. Engl. J. Med.* 317:1376, 1987.

22. Eichoff, T. C. Respiratory tract infections. Goals for 1995. *Am. J. Med.* 78 (Suppl. 6B):58, 1985.
23. Ellis, C. A., and Spivack, M. The significance of candidemia. *Ann. Intern. Med.* 67:511, 196.
24. Favero, M. S., Peteson, N. J., Boyer, K. M., et al. Microbial contamination of renal dialysis systems and associated health risks. *Trans. R. Soc. Artif. Intern. Organs* 20:175, 1974.
25. Finland, M. Changing ecology of bacterial infections as related to antibacterial therapy. *J. Infect. Dis.* 122:419, 1970.
26. Fletcher, E. C., Mohr, J. A., Leven, D. C., et al. Bacteriologic diagnosis of pneumonia with protected specimen brush and fiberoptic bronchoscopy. *Am. Rev. Respir. Dis.* 121:A134, 1980.
27. Fry, D. E., Pearlstein, L., Fulton, R. L. Multiple system organ failure. The role of uncontrolled infection. *Arch. Surg.* 115:136, 1980.
28. Fry, D. E. The diagnosis of intraabdominal infection in the postoperative patient. *Prob. Gen. Surg.* 1:558, 1984.
29. Garb, J. L., Brown, R. B., Garb, J. R., et al. Differences in etiology of pneumonias in nursing home and community patients. *J.A.M.A.* 240:2169, 1978.
30. Geddes, A. M., and Stille, W. (eds.). Imipenem: The first thienamycin antibiotic. *Rev. Infect. Dis.* 7(Suppl. 3):S353, 1985.
31. Gervich, D. H., and Grout, C. S. An outbreak of nosocomial *Acinetobacter* from humidifiers. *Am. J. Infect. Control* 13:210, 1985.
32. Graybill, J. R., Marshall, L. W., Charache, P., et al. Nosocomial pneumonia. A continuing major problem. *Am. Rev. Respir. Dis.* 108:1130, 1973.
33. Haley, R. W., Culver, D. H., White, J. W., et al. *The nationwide nosocomial infection rate: A new need for vital statistics. Am. J. Epidemiol.* 121:159, 1985.
34. Hart, G. B., Lam, R. C., and Strauss, M. B. Gas gangrene. *J. Trauma* 23:991, 1983.
35. Henderson, D. K. Bacteremia Due to Percutaneous Devices. In G. L. Mandell, R. G. Douglas, and J. E. Bennett (eds.), *Principles and Practices of Infectious Diseases* (2nd ed.). New York: Wiley, 1985. P. 1612.
36. Johanson, W. G., Pierce, A. K., and Sanford, J. P. Changing pharyngeal flora of hospitalized patients. Emergence of gram-negative bacilli. *N. Engl. J. Med.* 281:1138, 1969.
37. Kahn, F. W., and Jones, J. M. Diagnosing bacterial respiratory infection by bronchoalveolar lavage. *J. Infect. Dis.* 155:862, 1987.
38. Karnad, A., Alvarez, S., and Berk, S. L. Pneumonia caused by gram-negative bacilli. *Am. J. Med.* 79(Suppl. 1A):61, 1985.
39. Knaus, W. A., and Thiebault, G. E. Intensive Care Units Today. In B. J. McNeil and E. G. Cravalho (eds.), *Critical Issues in Medical Technology.* Boston: Auburn House Publishing, 1982. P. 193.
40. Knittle, M. A., Eitzman, D. V., and Baer, H. Role of hand contamination of personnel in the epidemiology of gram-negative nosocomial infections. *J. Pediatr.* 86:433, 1983.
41. Krieger, J. N. Kaiser, D. L., and Wenzel, R. P. Nosocomial urinary tract infections: Secular trends, treatment and economics in a University Hospital. *J. Urol.* 130:102, 1983.
42. Kunin, C. M. Genitourinary infection in the patient at risk: Extrinsic risk factors. *Am. J. Med.* 76:131, 1984.
43. Laforce, F. M. Hospital acquired gram-negative rod pneumonias: An overview. *Am. J. Med.* 70:664, 1981.
44. Larson, E. A causal link between hand washing and risk of infection? Examination of the evidence. *Infect. Control Hosp. Epidemiol.* 9:28, 1988.

45. LeGrand, P., Bordelon, J. Y., Gewin, W. C., et al. The telescoping plugged catheter in suspected anaerobic infections: A controlled series. *Am. Rev. Respir. Dis.* 121:A157, 1980.

46. Lerner, A. M., and Federman, J. M. Gram-negative bacillary pneumonia. *J. Inf. Dis.* 124:425, 1971.

47. Lode, H., and Kass, E. H. (eds.). Enzyme-mediated resistance to beta-lactam antibiotics: A symposium on sulbactam/ampicillin. *Rev. Infect. Dis.* 8(Suppl. 5):S465, 1986.

48. Luke, W. P. Surgical infections—The general surgeon's perspective. *Postgrad. Med.* 80:74, 1986.

49. Luterman, A., Dacso, C. C., and Curreri, P. W. Infections in burn patients. *Am. J. Med.* 81(Suppl. 1A):45, 1986.

50. McGowan, J. E. Antimicrobial resistance in hospital organisms and its relation to antibiotic use. *Rev. Infect. Dis.* 5:1033, 1983.

51. McGowan, J. E., Barnes, M. W., and Finland, M. Bacteremia at Boston City Hospital: Occurrence and mortality during 12 selected years (1935–1971), with special reference to hospital-acquired cases. *J. Infect. Dis.* 132:316, 1975.

52. Majeski, J. A. Necrotizing fascitis of the extremities. *Prob. Gen. Surg.* 1:500, 1984.

53. Maki, D. G. Risk factors for nosocomial infection in intensive care. *Arch. Intern. Med.* 149:30, 1989.

54. Maki, D. G. Epidemic nosocomial bacteremias. In R. P. Wenzel (ed.), *Handbook of Hospital Infection.* West Palm Beach, FL: CRC Press, 1981. P. 371.

55. Maki, D. G., Weis, C. E., and Sarafin, H. W. A semiquantitative culture method of identifying intravenous catheter-related infection. *N. Engl. J. Med.* 296:1305, 1977.

56. Malow, J. B. Hospital-acquired bacterial pneumonias. *Compr. Ther.* 8:29, 1984.

57. Marshall, W. G., and Dimick, A. R. The natural history of major burns with multiple subsystem failure. *J. Trauma* 23:102, 1983.

58. Martinez, O. V., Civetta, J. M., Anderson, K., et al. Bacteriuria in the catheterized surgical intensive care patient. *Crit. Care Med.* 14:188, 1986.

59. Meunier-Carpenter, F., Kiehn, T. E., and Armstrong, D. Fungemia in the immunocompromised host. *Am. J. Med.* 71:363, 1981.

60. Morrison, A. J., Frer, C. V., Searcy, M. A. et al. Nosocomial bloodstream infections: Secular trends in a statewide surveillance program in Virginia. *Infect. Control* 7:550, 1986.

61. Mueller, P. R., and Simeone, J. F. Intraabdominal abscesses: Diagnosis by sonography and computed tomography. *Radiol. Clin. North Am.* 21:445, 1983.

62. Munzinger, J., Buhler, M., Geroulanos, S., et al. Nosokomiale infektionen in einem Universitatsspital. *Schweiz. Med. Wochensher.* 113:1787, 1983.

63. Murray, P. R., and Washington, J. A. Microscopic and bacteriologic analysis of expectorated sputum. *Mayo Clin. Proc.* 50:339, 1975.

64. Neu, H. C. (ed.). Beta-lactamase inhibition: Therapeutic advances. *Am. J. Med.* 79(Suppl. 5B):1, 1985.

65. Neu, H. C., and Moellering, R. C. (eds.). Advances in cephalosporin therapy: Beyond the third generation. *Am. J. Med.* 79 (Suppl. 2A):1, 1985.

66. Northy, D., Adess, M. L., Hartsuck, J. M., et al. Microbial surveillance in a surgical intensive care unit. *Surg. Gynecol. Obstet.* 139:321, 1974.

67. Norwood, S. H., and Civetta, J. M. Evaluating sepsis in critically ill patients. *Chest* 92:137, 1987.

68. Pierce, A. K., and Sanford, J. P. Aerobic gram-negative bacillary pneumonia. *Am. Rev. Respir. Dis.* 110:647, 1974.

69. Pink, W., Wertz, M. J., Lennard, E. S., et al. Determinants of organ malfunction or death in patients with intra-abdominal sepsis. A discriminant analysis. *Arch. Surg.* 118:242, 1983.

70. Pitcher, W. D., and Musler, D. M. Critical importance of early diagnosis and treatment of intraabdominal infections. *Arch. Surg.* 117:328, 1982.

71. Platt, R., Polk, F., Murdock, B., et al. Mortality associated with nosocomial urinary-tract infection. *N. Engl. J. Med.* 307:637, 1982.

72. Pollack, M., Charache, P., Niemar, R. E., et al. Factors influencing colonization and antibiotic-resistance patterns of gram-negative bacteria in hospitalized patients. *Lancet* 2:668, 1972.

73. Prasad, J. K., Feller, I., and Thompson, P. D. A ten-year review of *Candida* sepsis and mortality in burn patients. *Surgery* 101:213, 1987.

74. Preheim, L. C., and Sanders, W. E. Nosocomial pneumonia. *Compr. Ther.* 70:20, 1981.

75. Preston, G. A., Larson, E. L., Stamm, W. E. Effect of private isolation rooms on patient care practices: Colonization and infection in an intensive care unit. *Am. J. Med.* 70:641, 1981.

76. Pruitt, B. A., and McManus, A. T. Opportunistic infections in severely burned patients. *Am. J. Med.* 76:146, 1984.

77. Remington, J. S. (ed.). Carbapenems: A new class of antibiotics. *Am. J. Med.* 78(Suppl. 6A):1, 1985.

78. Roselle, G. A., Bode, R., Hamilton, B., et al. Clinical trial of the efficacy and safety of ticarcillin and clavulanic acid. *Antimicrob. Agents Chemother.* 27:291, 1985.

79. Rubinstein, E., Adam, D., Moellering, R., and Waldvogel, F. (eds.) International symposium on new quinolones. *Rev. Infect. Dis.* 10(Suppl. 1):S1, 1988.

80. Rutala, W. A., Kennedy, V. A., Loflin, H. B., et al. *Serratia marcescens* nosocomial infections of the urinary tract associated with urine-measuring containers and urinometers. *Am. J. Med.* 70:659, 1970.

81. Saini, S., Kellum, J. M., O'Leary, M. P., et al. Improved localization and survival in patients with intraabdominal abscesses. *Am. J. Surg.* 145:136, 1983.

82. Salata, R. A., Lederman, M. M., Shlaes, D. M., et al. Diagnosis of nosocomial pneumonia in intubated, intensive care unit patients. *Am. Rev. Respir. Dis.* 135:425, 1987.

83. Schaberg, D. R. Epidemics of nosocomial urinary tract infection caused by multiply resistant gram-negative bacilli: Epidemiology and control. *J. Infect. Dis.* 133:363, 1976.

84. Schliessler, K. H., Rozendaal, B., Taal, C., et al. Outbreak of *Salmonella agona* infection after upper intestinal fiberoptic endoscopy. *Lancet* 2:1246, 1980.

85. Simmons, R. L. Wound infection: A review of diagnosis and treatment. *Infect. Control* 3:44, 1982.

86. Souther, D. I., and Todd, T. R. J. Systemic candidiasis in a surgical intensive care unit. *Can. J. Surg.* 29:197, 1986.

87. Spengler, R. F., and Greenough, W. E. Hospital costs and mortality attributed to nosocomial bacteremias. *J.A.M.A.* 240:2455, 1978.

88. Stamm, W. E. Infections related to medical devices. *Ann. Intern. Med.* 89:764, 1978.

89. Stevens, R. M., Teres, D., Skillman, J. J., et al. Pneumonia in an intensive care unit. A 30-month experience. *Arch. Intern. Med.* 134:106, 1974.

90. Stone, H. H., and Martin, J. D. Synergistic necrotizing cellulitis. *Ann. Surg.* 175:702, 1972.

91. Stone, H. H., Kolb, L. D., Currie, C. A. et al. *Candida* sepsis: Pathogenesis and principles of treatment. *Ann. Surg.* 179:697, 1974.

92. Thorp, J. M., Richards, W. C., and Teffer, A. B. M. A survey of infection in an intensive care unit. *Anesthesia* 34:643, 1979.

93. Thorpe, J. E., Baughman, R. D., Frame, P. T., et al. Bronchoalveolar lavage for diagnosing acute bacterial pneumonia. *J. Infect. Dis.* 155:855, 1987.

94. Tillotson, J. R., and Lerner, A. M. Pneumonias caused by gram-negative bacilli. *Medicine* 45:65, 1966.

95. Tonnesen, A., Peuler, M., Lockwood, W. R. Cultures of blood drawn by catheters vs. venipuncture. *J.A.M.A.* 235:1877, 1976.

96. Valdivieso, M., Gil-Extremera, B., Zornoza, J., et al. Gram-negative bacillary pneumonia in the compromised host. *Medicine* 56:241, 1974.

97. Valenti, W. M., Trudell, R. G., and Bentley, D. W. Factors predisposing to oropharyngeal colonization with gram-negative bacilli in the aged. *N. Engl. J. Med.* 298:1108, 1978.

98. Webb, S. F., and Vail-Spinosa, A. Outbreak of *Serratia marcescens* associated with the flexible bronchoscope. *Chest* 68:703, 1975.

99. Weinstein, R. A. Endemic emergence of cephalosporin-resistant enterobacter: Relation to prior therapy. *Infect. Control* 7(Suppl.):120, 1986.

100. Weinstein, R. A., Stamm, W. E., Kramer, L., et al. Pressure monitoring devices: Overlooked source of nosocomial infection. *J.A.M.A.* 236:936, 1976.

101. Wenzel R. P., Osterman, C. A., Donowitz, L. G., et al. Identification of procedure-related nosocomial infections in high-risk patients. *Rev. Infect. Dis.* 3:701, 1981.

102. Wenzel, R. P., Thompson, R. L., Landry, S. M., et al. Hospital-acquired infections in intensive care unit patients: An overview with emphasis on epidemics. *Infect. Control* 4:371, 1983.

103. Wey, S. B., Mori, M., Pfaller, M. A., et al. Hospital-acquired candidemia. The attributable mortality and excess length of stay. *Arch. Intern. Med.* 148:2642, 1988.

104. Wimberly, N. Y., Bass, J. B., Boyd, B. W. et al. Usage of a bronchoscopic protected catheter brush for the diagnosis of pulmonary infections. *Chest* 81:556, 1982.

105. Wimberly, N. W., Faling, L. J., and Barlett, J. G. A fiberoptic bronchoscopy technique to obtain uncontaminated lower airway secretions for bacterial culture. *Am. Rev. Respir. Dis.* 119:337, 1979.

106. Wing, E. J., Norden, C. W., and Shadduck, R. K., et al. Use of quantitative bacteriologic techniques to diagnose catheter-related sepsis. *Arch. Intern. Med.* 139:482, 1979.

107. Ziegler, E. J., McCutchan, J. A., Fierar, J., et al. Treatment of gram-negative bacteremia and shock with human antiserum to a mutant *Escherichia coli*. *N. Engl. J. Med.* 307:1226, 1982.

Diagnosis and Management of Nonmechanical Bleeding

Michael Metzler
Donald Silver

Prolonged or excessive bleeding may become life-threatening and therefore must be controlled. Fortunately, most bleeding is controlled by natural defenses or by mechanical means (e.g., ligature, cautery, suture, or tamponade.) In order to deal with nonmechanical bleeding disorders, a surgeon must understand normal coagulation, physical and biochemical abnormalities that affect the coagulation system, laboratory tests used to discover specific areas of malfunction, and therapies available for treatment. Consultation with a hematologist or pathologist interested in coagulation disorders is often helpful in the clinical management of nonmechanical bleeding.

COAGULATION SYSTEM OVERVIEW

Disruption of vascular integrity initiates a well-coordinated series of physical and biochemical events that plug the initial vessel breech, produce a fibrin clot, strengthen and contract the clot, lyse excess fibrin, and provide the base for endothelial repair. Usually these events are swift and well-controlled, resulting in a clot limited to the area of injury. A brief overview of the coagulation process and of the cellular and soluble elements that participate in it follows (Fig. 28-1).

Platelets

Platelets are produced in the bone marrow by megakaryocytes and released into the circulation under the regulation of thrombopoietin. Platelet production can increase from 6 to 8 times in response to chronic platelet loss. The normal platelet count is $250,000/\mu l \pm 40,000$. Platelets have an average life span of 9.5 days. Under normal circumstances, two-thirds of the total platelet population is in general circulation, and one-third is in the spleen. The platelets in the spleen exchange freely with those in the general circulation. Up to 90 percent of a patient's platelets may be sequestered in the spleen during times of hypersplenism and thrombocytopenia. Normal platelet turnover rates are $35,000/\mu l \pm 4300/day$.

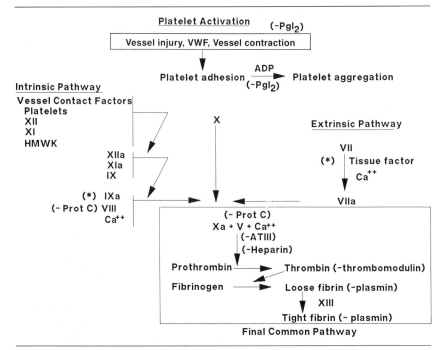

Fig. 28-1. Overview of the coagulation system. "(-substance)" indicates areas of inhibition of coagulation or of clot lysis; see text for explanation of abbreviations. Note that cross-activation of the intrinsic by the extrinsic pathways (and vice versa) may occur at these points (*) if one system is activated.

Platelets contribute to maintenance of hemostasis in three ways: (1) by helping to maintain vascular integrity, (2) by forming the initial hemostatic plug in response to interruption of vascular continuity, (3) by accelerating the coagulation cascade through provision of a reactive surface and the phospholipid requirements for activation of several coagulation factors.

The mechanism(s) by which platelets help maintain normal vascular integrity remain unknown. The reduction to 10 percent or less of circulating platelets contributes to the migration of red cells through the vascular wall and the formation of petechiae and purpura.

When platelets are exposed to vascular basement membrane and collagen in areas of intimal disruption, platelet adhesion with subsequent aggregation is induced. Von Willebrand's factor (VWF), produced by endothelial cells, is necessary to allow adhesion of platelets to the subendothelial surface. Thromboxane A_2 (TxA$_2$), produced by the platelets, causes enhanced platelet aggregation and local vasoconstriction. Platelets release their granule contents during the later stages of aggregation. One of the platelet-release products, adenosine diphosphate (ADP), stimulates other platelets to adhere to the growing mass of platelets and to form the initial hemostatic plug. Irreversible fusion of the platelet mass follows thrombin-induced release of additional platelet constituents.

Platelets have important roles in initiation and acceleration of the two coagulation cascades. The platelet membrane absorbs and transports plasma coagulation factors and provides a surface for their activation. The phospholipid cofactors for several of the reactions of the clotting mechanism are provided by components of the platelet membrane. The fibrin network formed by activation of the coagulation system serves to stabilize the initial platelet hemostatic plug. Contraction of platelet microfilaments in conjunction with the activated factor XIII leads to clot retraction. Platelet factor IV, released during aggregation, has heparin-neutralizing activity.

Soluble Clotting Factors

Twelve clotting factors have been identified, numbered I through XIII. (The original factor VI is an intermediate product and not a true coagulation factor.) Seven factors are proteolytic enzymes; four are cofactors responsible for facilitation, acceleration, and regulation of the reactions catalyzed by the enzymatic factors; and one, fibrinogen, is converted to fibrin to form the hemostatic clot. Table 28-1 lists the plasma half-lives, necessary hemostatic levels, and principal therapeutic sources for replacement therapy.

The initiation of the coagulation process can occur by activation of either the intrinsic or the extrinsic pathway of coagulation. Both pathways produce a common activated clotting factor and share an identical terminal pathway for the production of fibrin from fibrinogen. The activated intrinsic or extrinsic system may activate the other system. The prothrombin time (PT) and activated partial thromboplastin time (APTT) are used to assay the integrity of the extrinsic and intrinsic pathways, respectively.

The intrinsic pathway sequence (Fig. 28-1) usually begins when factor XII is activated by exposure to a foreign substance or negatively charged surface, such as collagen or vascular basement membrane. These "surface factors," plus high-molecular-weight kininogen (HMWK) and kallikrein, activate factor XII to factor XII$_a$, which converts factor XI to its active form (XI$_a$). Factor XI$_a$ then cleaves a single polypeptide bond of factor IX to form factor IX$_a$. Activated factor IX complexes with factor VIII to bring about activation of factor X. Thrombin, the product of the reaction catalyzed by factor X$_a$, modifies factor VIII to increase its specific activity and rate of reaction, producing activated factor X. The phospholipid required for conversion of factor X to factor X$_a$ is supplied by platelets as platelet factor III. Factor X$_a$ subsequently complexes with factor V, calcium, and phospholipid to bring about the conversion of prothrombin to thrombin. Factor V greatly enhances the rate of conversion of prothrombin. Thrombin catalyzes the hydrolysis of four specific arginyl-glycine bonds of fibrinogen with liberation of fibrinopeptides A and B. Following this hydrolytic conversion, the fibrin monomers undergo spontaneous polymerization into a loose gel-like network (loose fibrin). Thrombin also activates factor XIII, the fibrin-stabilizing factor, which catalyzes the formation of peptide bonds between the adjacent fibrin monomers and stabilizes the fibrin network (tight fibrin).

Table 28-1. Factor half-lives, hemostatic levels, and therapeutic sources

Factor	Plasma 1/2 life hours	Level required for hemostasis*	Vitamin K–dependent	Blood component therapeutic source(s)
I (fibrinogen)	90	100 mg/dl	No	Cyro
II (prothrombin)	65	40%	Yes	FFP
V (proaccelerin)	15	10–15%	No	FFP
VII (proconvertin)	5	5–10%	Yes	FFP
VIII (antihemophilic factor A)	10	10–40%	No	Cryo; VIII concentrates
IX (antihemophilic factor B)	20	10–40%	Yes	FFP; IX concentrates
X (Stuart-Prower factor)	40	10–15%	Yes	FFP
XI (plasma thromboplastin antecedent)	45	30%	No	FFP
XII (Hageman factor)	50		No	
XIII (fibrin-stabilizing factor)	120	1–5%	No	FFP

Cryo = cryoprecipitated plasma; FFP = fresh frozen plasma. Factor XII deficiency is not usually treated.
*From C. R. Rizza. Management of Patients with Inherited Blood Coagulation Defects. In A. L. Bloom and D. P. Thomas (eds.), *Haemostasis and Thrombosis.* London: Churchill Livingstone, 1981. Pp. 371–388.

When the extrinsic pathway is initiated (Fig. 28-1), factor X is converted to its activated form by a complex of tissue-derived factor, calcium, and factor VII. Tissue factor is composed of protein and phospholipid subunits and serves as the reactive surface for the activation of factor VII and subsequent enzymatic conversion of factor X to factor X_a. After activated factor X is formed, the coagulation pathway proceeds as described above for the intrinsic system.

Inhibitors

Control of the coagulation process is critical in preventing widespread intravascular coagulation from developing in response to local activation of the clotting process. Vasoconstriction and slowing of blood flow in an injured vessel favors concentration of the biochemical products and cellular elements necessary for clotting. Normal blood flow dilutes the excess activated clotting factors and transports these factors to the liver, where they are cleared.

In addition, several specific controls are operative within the coagulation cascade. Prostaglandin I_2 (prostacyclin, or PGI_2) is synthesized by the endothelium in response to injury and activation of clotting. PGI_2 inhibits platelet aggregation and also causes vasodilatation. Protein C (Prot C) and its cofactor, protein S (Prot S), are produced in response to thrombin binding to an endothelial surface protein, thrombomodulin. Not only does thrombomodulin prevent the thrombin from continuing its action on fibrinogen to produce fibrin, but the resultant Prot C complex inactivates V_a and VIII_a. Antithrombin III (ATIII) is a cofactor of heparin that inhibits factor X_a and thrombin. ATIII is also activated by heparan (an endothelial cell surface protein). The antithrombotic activity of heparin is largely dependent on the presence of ATIII. Plasminogen activators transform plasminogen to plasmin, which is responsible for fibrinolysis.

CLOTTING FACTOR DEFICIENCIES

Congenital Deficiencies

Congenital deficiencies have been described for all clotting factors (Table 28-2). Deficiency states may be characterized by either a low level of the factors or the production of antigenically similar but functionally incompetent factors. Most heterozygous patients with deficiencies do not manifest bleeding symptoms unless challenged by surgery or trauma. Small amounts of factors (5–10% of normal) maintain hemostasis during the normal activities of daily living. Larger amounts (usually >50%) are necessary to maintain hemostasis following trauma or during surgery. Some homozygous patients with low factor levels bleed only when their coagulation systems are sufficiently challenged. Some deficiency states may not cause bleeding because cross-activation of the coagulation pathways may circumvent the area of deficiency.

A brief discussion of the more common congenital bleeding disorders, von Willebrand's disease and hemophilias A and B, follows. Table 28-3 outlines the diagnostic laboratory studies and suggested therapy for congenital factor deficiencies.

Table 28-2. Characteristics of the congenital coagulation deficiencies

Deficiency	Manifestations	Inheritance	Incidence
Factor I	Serious neonatal or infant bleeding episodes.	Autosomal recessive affecting both sexes.	<0.5 per million live births.
Factor II	Serious neonatal or infant bleeding episodes.	Autosomal recessive affecting both sexes.	<0.5 per million live births.
Factor V	Mild excessive bleeding early in life—i.e., epistaxis, menorrhagia, prolonged postoperative bleeding.	Highly penetrant autosomal recessive affecting both sexes.	1 per million live births.
Factor VII	Mild-to-moderate bleeding or purpura.	Autosomal recessive affecting both sexes.	Homozygous form: 1 per 400,000 live births. Heterozygous form more common but may not cause bleeding.
Factor VIII	Neonatal bleeding is unusual. Bleeding becomes manifest at 6–12 mo. Excessive bleeding following dental procedures, hemarthroses, and intraabdominal hemorrhage are common.	Sex-linked recessive with males as bleeders, females as carriers.	Common congenital coagulation factor deficiency; 1 per 25,000 live births.

Factor IX	Excessive bleeding following trauma or surgery in the male. May cause spontaneous CNS hemorrhage. Hemarthroses are uncommon except in severe cases.	Sex-linked recessive with males as bleeders, females as carriers.	1 per 100,000 births.
Factor X	Mild bleeding beginning later in life. Hemarthroses can occur but are rare.	Autosomal recessive with equal frequency in males and females.	Homozygous form: 1 per 400,000 live births; heterozygous form: 1 per 500 live births.
Factor XI	Excessive bleeding following trauma or elective surgery, often as a delayed episode.	Autosomal recessive with equal frequency in males and females.	Approximately 1 per million live births in general population. More common in patients of Jewish ancestry.
Factor XII	Seldom with clinically significant bleeding. Severe deficiency states may be associated with thrombotic episodes.	Autosomal recessive affecting both sexes.	Approximately 1 per million live births.
Factor XIII	Neonatal bleeding is common with cord hemorrhage, ecchymoses, and hematomas.	Autosomal recessive with equal frequency in both sexes.	<0.5 per million live births.
Von Willebrand's disease	Spontaneous epistaxis and easy bruisability in childhood. Gastrointestinal hemorrhage common.	Autosomal dominant with variable expression. Equal frequency in both sexes.	Probably the most common congenital coagulation disorder. Gene frequency up to 10 per 100,000 population.

CNS = central nervous system.

Table 28-3. Diagnosis and therapy of congenital and acquired coagulation deficiencies

Deficiency	Diagnostic tests/results*	Therapy
Factor I	Plasma fibrinogen concentrations decreased, often undetectable. TT, PT, and APTT markedly prolonged.	Cryoprecipitate to rise level to 100 mg/dl.
Factor II	PT and APTT prolonged in the presence of normal concentrations of Factors V, VII, X, and XII.	2 bags cryoprecipitate/10 kg body weight twice daily.
Factor V	PT and APTT prolonged. APTT is corrected by the addition of normal plasma.	20 ml FFP/kg body weight every 12 hr recommended if normal renal and cardiac function are present. 20–25% of normal concentrations are adequate for hemostasis.
Factor VII	PT prolonged. Clotting time, prothrombin consumption time, and APTT normal.	FFP transfusion preferred. 2 units of factor concentrate/kg body weight will increase factor VII concentrations by 3–4%. 20% of normal levels needed for hemostasis. Treat for 8 days following surgery.
Factor VIII	PT normal; APTT prolonged. Clotting times may be normal.	dDAVP for mild bleeding. Cryoprecipitate, glycine-precipitated factor VIII concentrate (AHF, Human). 1 unit of factor VIII/kg body weight will increase plasma levels by 2%. CNS bleeding: 50 units/kg body weight stat., then 40 units/kg/24 hr for 14–21 days. Retropharyngeal and retroperitoneal bleeding: 50 units/kg stat., then 40 units/kg every 12 hr for 3 doses. Surgery: 50 units/kg 1 hr prior to operation; maintain plasma

		level greater than 60% for 4 days; then 40% for 4 days or until all drains and sutures are out. Maintain 15–20% of normal levels for 2 wk following orthopedic procedures. Use of EACA not indicated except in dental procedures. See text for treatment of patients with factor VIII alloantibodies.
Factor IX	PT normal; APTT prolonged.	Fresh frozen plasma or factor IX concentrates. 1 unit of factor IX/kg body weight will increase plasma levels by 1.5%. Treatment regimens are the same as those outlined for factor VIII deficiency.
Factor X	PT and APTT prolonged.	15% level needed for surgical hemostasis. FFP 4–5 units followed by 3 units per day for 7 days.
Factor XI	PT normal; APTT prolonged.	FFP 10–15 ml/kg every 3 days for 1 week.
Factor XII	PT normal; APTT prolonged.	None required.
Factor XIII	PT and APTT normal. Clot is soluble in 5M urea, whereas normal clots are not.	FFP 2 units per week. Frequent transfusions are not necessary due to the 5- to 7-day half-life of factor XIII.
von Willebrand's disease	Bleeding time prolonged and VWF usually decreased, as is VIII:C. Abnormal platelet aggregation studies. APTT may be prolonged due to decreased concentrations of factor VIII activity.	dDAVP 0.3 mg/kg daily for 10 days in cases of mild bleeding in responsive types. Cryoprecipitate is given to maintain the APTT less 100 sec for 7–10 days following surgery. Factor VIII concentrates are not recommended. Platelet transfusions are not indicated.

TT = thrombin time; PT = prothrombin time; APTT = activated partial thromboplastin time; FFP = fresh frozen plasma; CNS = central nervous system; VWF = von Willebrand's factor.
*Specific factor assays are available to determine residual activity levels and define the severity of the deficiency state.

Von Willebrand's Disease (VWD)

Von Willebrand's disease, the most common congenital deficiency syndrome, is characterized by a factor deficiency and related platelet dysfunction. Von Willebrand's factor (VWF) is necessary for normal initial platelet binding to the subendothelium of injured vessels. VWF also facilitates thrombin production by complexing with factor VIII to form factor VIII:C. VWF is a large molecule composed of multimers of smaller subunits. The size and configuration of these multimers have great bearing on the molecular function. VWD follows an autosomal inheritance pattern; therefore, both men and women can be equally affected. The bleeding history in patients with VWD is quite variable but is frequently characterized by episodes of mucosal bleeding. Spontaneous hemarthroses, which frequently occur in patients with classic hemophilia A, are quite rare in patients with VWD.

VWD is further categorized into types I, II, and III; there are also subtypes (e.g., type IIA). A platelet type and an acquired form are also described, as well as miscellaneous subtypes. Classification is based on sophisticated immunoelectrophoretic and platelet aggregation tests that assess the size and function of the VWF molecules, as well as the interaction of platelets with these molecules [6]. The subclassification is important in planning appropriate therapy for these patients.

VWF is found in the cryoprecipitate fraction of plasma and, to a lesser degree, in fresh frozen plasma. Highly purified factor VIII concentrates lack the large VWF multimers and are not good sources for VWF replacement therapy. Recently, 1-deamino-8-D-arginine-vasopressin (dDAVP) has been used to stimulate release of VWF from endothelial cells [20]. The exact mechanism of the action of dDAVP is unknown. Similar release of VWF has been shown following catecholamine infusion [15]. Mild or moderate types I and IIA VWD have the best response to dDAVP treatment. Types IIB, IIC, and III have a poor response. It is important not to use dDAVP therapy in type IIB or platelet type VWD, as an abnormal platelet response causes agglutination and a risk of thrombosis and thrombocytopenia [13]. In patients with acquired VWD associated with myeloproliferative disorders, treatment of the underlying disorder usually improves the VWD. dDAVP is also useful in these patients.

Response to treatment of VWD is characterized as variable, even in the same patient at different times. Factor VIII:C levels of 50 to 80 percent of normal are desirable for a week following severe hemorrhage or major surgery. Cryoprecipitate is the preferred source of VWF when dDAVP treatment is not successful or is contraindicated. Usually, VIII:C levels remain higher for longer periods of time following replacement than they do in hemophilia A patients. Quantitative laboratory tests of factor replacement do not always correlate with clinical hemostasis. Treatment with dDAVP does not always give a uniform response, and patients given repeated doses on a daily basis may show tachyphylaxis. dDAVP also stimulates release of tissue plasminogen. When dDAVP is used for dental extractions or urologic procedures, the concomitant use of epsilon-aminocaproic acid (EACA) is suggested. Burns [4] recommends that 4 gm of

EACA be administered prior to surgery then at 4- to 6-hour intervals for the next 4 days. dDAVP therapy obviates the risk of exposure to blood-borne viral disease. The recommended intravenous dosage of dDAVP, 0.3 μg/kg or 10 μg/m^2 body surface area (24 μg maximum), may cause head-ache, facial flushing, and nausea [18]. These side effects can be minimized by infusion of the dose over 20 minutes in a volume of 50 ml normal saline [16].

Hemophilia A (Factor VIII Deficiency)

Factor VIII deficiency is an X-linked recessive trait; therefore, males usu-ally display the disease and females are carriers. The diagnosis is often made in childhood. Patients with factor VIII levels of less than 1 percent frequently have spontaneous hemorrhages (especially hemarthroses).

A patient with factor VIII deficiency who is bleeding must have factor VIII returned to a level, which will result in hemostasis. The degree of trauma (or severity of planned surgery) and the part of the body affected by the hemorrhage dictate the method and extent of factor replacement. dDAVP may be successful in increasing VIII:C sufficiently to arrest a mus-cle hematoma or mild epistaxis. At the other end of the spectrum, 50 IU/kg of factor VIII may be necessary as initial treatment for major surgery or major trauma with risk of central nervous system injury [8]. Once initial hemostasis is obtained, adequate levels ($\geqslant$60%) must be maintained by reinfusion of factor VIII at half-life (10- to 12-hr) intervals. Adequate levels usually must be maintained for 1 or more weeks following major hemor-rhage or surgery.

Up to 10 percent of hemophiliacs will develop immunoglobulin G (IgG) antibodies to VIII [14]. The presence of antibodies usually makes replace-ment by factor VIII infusion impossible. The customary strategy for pa-tients with antibodies is to bypass factor VIII activation by giving factor IX—in either nonactivated or activated form. Plasmapheresis followed by factor VIII infusion and attempts to overwhelm low levels of antibodies with high doses of factor VIII infusion have been reported [30,31]. Hemo-philiacs often know their usual factor levels and antibody status.

Hemophilia B (Christmas Disease, Factor IX Deficiency)

The hereditary pattern and clinical presentation of factor IX deficiency are the same as those of hemophilia A. Replacement of factor IX from concen-trated forms is the usual treatment for severe bleeding and surgical pro-phylaxis. Antibodies to factor IX occur less frequently than do antibodies to factor VIII but can present problems. Activated prothrombin complex preparations are effective but incur the risk of producing venous throm-bosis. Success has also been reported with attempts to overwhelm inhibi-tors [25].

Elective surgery can be performed safely in patients with hemophilia and hemophilia-like bleeding disorders if the following precautions are observed: (1) the exact nature of the coagulation defect is accurately de-fined, (2) the half-life of the infused factor replacements is determined for the patient, (3) the patient is screened for clotting inhibitors, and (4) the anticipated factor replacement needs are available. The surgeon should also be prepared to continue factor replacement for a week or more postoperatively. The presence of significant clotting inhibitors usually is a contraindication to elective surgery in these patients [12,26].

Acquired Deficiencies

Acquired factor deficiency states may be due to deficient production, dilution, or excessive consumption of one or more of the clotting factors.

Vitamin K Deficiency

Vitamin K intake in the range of 0.3 to 1.5 μg/kg/day [9] is necessary for production of adequate levels of competent vitamin K–dependent factors (Table 28-1). Decreased dietary intake, malabsorption, and antibiotic therapy can decrease vitamin K intake and alter the normal gastrointestinal tract flora—a secondary source of vitamin K. Decreased levels of factors II, VII, IX, and X are manifested by a prolonged PT. Clinical bleeding can occur in patients deficient in vitamin K–dependent factors, especially in the postoperative patient. Ten mg of vitamin K_1, administered parenterally once or twice weekly, will prevent this problem. Vitamin K supplementation should be routine practice in hospitalized patients who are not eating a regular diet, particularly in those receiving antibiotic therapy [22]. Vitamin K–deficient patients should show improvement in their PT within 6 to 8 hours of administration of 2.5 to 25 mg of vitamin K_1 given intramuscularly or subcutaneously. Intravenous administration of vitamin K_1 should not exceed a rate of 1 mg/min.

Liver Disease

All clotting factors except VIII and VWF are produced by the liver. Prolonged PT and APTT and thrombin time (TT) associated with the stigmata of cirrhosis, a history of alcohol abuse, and ascites or jaundice is quite suggestive of a factor deficiency due to decreased production. Administration of vitamin K can be used to distinguish between poor hepatocellular reserve and vitamin K deficiency. The PT corrects with vitamin K administration in the case of deficiency. Occasionally, the signs of liver disease are not obvious. A normal factor VIII level and uniform depression of other clotting factors is diagnostic of decreased hepatocellular synthesis. If platelet and factor VIII levels are also depressed and fibrin degradation products (FDP) are elevated, disseminated intravascular coagulation (DIC) should be suspected. Treatment of factor deficiencies secondary to liver disease consists of factor replacement with fresh frozen plasma and cryoprecipitate.

Massive Transfusion

Massive blood transfusions (greater than 1 blood volume in 4 hours) may produce sufficient dilution of soluble clotting factors and platelets to produce nonmechanical bleeding. The often-attendant problems of hypothermia, acidosis, and poor hepatic perfusion (shock) contribute to the coagulopathy. There are no reliable formulas for replacement of coagulation proteins [21, 29]. The surgeon who cares for multitrauma, emergency vascular, and gastrointestinal hemorrhage patients often encounters a bleeding patient who is in shock and has received 8 to 10 units of packed red cells. The patient will require additional blood transfusions and an operation, but it is uncertain when the shock will be corrected, the operation concluded, and transfusion requirements abated. Our approach to this dilemma is to immediately assess the PT, APTT, fibrinogen level, FDP, and platelet count. Fresh whole blood, if available, is the blood product of choice for immediate transfusion. If component therapy is used, 1 to 2 units of fresh frozen plasma is transfused for each 4 to 6 units of packed red cells until specific guidance can be gained from the above-noted coagulation studies. Platelet transfusions are added if the platelet count is less than 50,000/μl. Monitoring of coagulation studies is continued intraoperatively and postoperatively, on an hourly basis, until these studies begin to normalize and there is no evidence of nonmechanical bleeding. Replacement of factors is governed by results of coagulation studies. In addition, attention is directed toward prevention and treatment of hypothermia (core temperature less than 35°C) and to the restoration of adequate organ perfusion (especially the liver). This approach requires continuing communication among surgeon, anesthesiologist, and blood bank physician.

Disseminated Intravascular Coagulation (DIC)

DIC is not a disease entity; rather, it is a manifestation of several disease processes characterized by excessive activation of the coagulation system [24]. PT, APTT, and TT are prolonged, and the platelet count is usually less than 100,000/μl, indicating consumption of soluble coagulation factors and platelets by the process. FDPs are greater than 100 μg/ml in 80 percent of the cases [11]. Trauma, sepsis, obstetric complications, and malignancy are common causes of DIC.

The most effective treatment is removal of the inciting event. If the DIC process does not then readily abate, anticoagulation with heparin (to inhibit further factor consumption) is a logical next step. It is suggested that the whole blood clotting time (not the APTT) be used to monitor heparin therapy, as the effects of DIC on the APTT are difficult to separate from those of heparin. Although it seems paradoxical to give heparin to patients who are bleeding from DIC, heparin is useful if the cause of the DIC cannot readily be found and eliminated. Heparin is used to halt the coagulation process and may be given as a single bolus dose (15,000–20,000 units IV). As activation of the coagulation system is controlled, clotting factor replacement can exceed consumption, so that when the heparin anticoagulation wanes (usually after several hours), bleeding will be controlled. Others give smaller amounts of heparin (400–500 units/hr by constant IV infusion) to slow factor consumption and allow bleeding to be controlled over a period of 8 to 12 hours. Following anticoagulation by heparin therapy, replacement of factor deficiencies is indicated. Fibrinogen should be replaced to a level of greater than or equal to 150 mg/dl. Cryoprecipitate is used for this purpose. Platelet replacement should be aimed at keeping the platelet count greater than 50,000/μl. Inhibition of fibrinolysis with EACA should be done cautiously, because one may induce thrombosis

[10]. Removal of the inciting event, support of the circulation, red cell transfusion, anticoagulation, and factor replacement should interdict the DIC process.

HYPERFIBRINOLYSIS

The fibrinolytic system is one of the body's basic defense systems, capable of restoring and maintaining the patency of blood vessels and other tubular structures at risk of being occluded by fibrin. Plasminogen, the inactive precursor of plasmin, is tightly bound to fibrinogen and when clotting occurs, is incorporated into the fibrin clot. Intravascular fibrin deposition causes elaboration of plasminogen activator(s) that convert plasminogen to plasmin, an endopeptidase, which digests fibrin, fibrinogen, and other plasma proteases. Plasmin activity may also be increased through the administration of plasminogen activators such as urokinase or streptokinase. Fibrin is the preferred substrate of plasmin; however, plasmin will nonspecifically digest other components of the coagulation system when released in large quantities.

Fibrinolysis occurs whenever plasmin is present in amounts greater than can be inhibited by the naturally occurring antiplasmins. Also, α-2-macroglobulin and α-1-globulin inhibitor (α-1-antitrypsin) inactivate plasmin, but at a much slower rate than do the specific antiplasmins. Hyperfibrinolysis may be primary (related solely to excess plasmin release) or secondary (occurring in response to DIC). Both primary and secondary hyperfibrinolysis may cause bleeding into body cavities, into the retroperitoneum, or around intravascular catheters, as well as delayed surgical or traumatic bleeding.

Primary Hyperfibrinolysis

Primary hyperfibrinolysis is a rare cause of nonmechanical bleeding and may be confused with DIC. It is usually associated with conditions causing sudden death (e.g., major trauma, electrical shock, massive myocardial infarction, and acute hypoxemia) that result in release of massive quantities of fibrinolytic activators. Rapid clot lysis and/or the absence of clot formation may be manifestations of increased fibrinolytic activity. Plasma fibrinogen levels are decreased and the PT and APTT are prolonged. Nonspecific proteolysis of clotting factors (principally factors V, VIII, IX, and XI) occurs as a result of the excess plasmin. The platelet count is usually normal in this disorder—a finding that distinguishes it from DIC. Laboratory studies will demonstrate shortening of the whole blood lysis time (normal range, 90–120 min) and euglobulin lysis time (normal range, 6–24 hr), as well as increased lytic activity of plasma incubated on fibrin plates. Management is directed toward adequate resuscitation from the catastrophic event that precipitated the excess release of plasmin. In most instances, hyperfibrinolysis resolves as normal conditions are restored. If primary hyperfibrinolysis persists, EACA can be given intravenously to directly inhibit the plasminogen activators. The usual dosage is 5 gm initially and 1 gm/hour for 6 to 8 hours. Rapid intravenous administration of EACA should be avoided, as this has been associated with hypotension, bradycardia, and arrhythmias. It is difficult to prevent primary hyperfibrinolysis, since the inciting event is usually unexpected and frequently not preventable.

Secondary Hyperfibrinolysis

Secondary hyperfibrinolysis is much more common than primary hyperfibrinolysis but is a less frequent cause of bleeding than is the DIC, which frequently causes it. The diagnosis is similar to that of primary hyperfibrinolysis, but evidence of DIC (consumption of coagulation factors *and* platelets) will also be present. Treatment should be directed toward eliminating the cause of the DIC. If excessive fibrinolytic activity persists after coagulation has stopped and coagulation factors have been restored, EACA may be utilized in the same manner and with the same precautions as in the management of primary hyperfibrinolysis.

CONGENITAL PLATELET DISORDERS

Essential Thrombocythemia

Essential thrombocythemia is characterized by spontaneous bleeding and thrombosis. It is often associated with splenomegaly and usually occurs in patients over 30 years of age. Gastrointestinal bleeding is common, and there is an increased incidence of both arterial and venous thromboses. Purpuras are usually not present. Essential thrombocythemia is a rare disorder that affects both sexes. The platelet count is greater than 1 million, and the platelets have bizarre shapes and possess functional abnormalities, as evidenced by abnormal aggregation studies. An associated leukocytosis and iron deficiency anemia may be present. The bleeding and the thromboses produced are often improved by reduction of the platelet count, usually with the use of alkylating agents such as melphalan. The use of aspirin (300 mg 4 times a day) and dipyridamole (50 mg 4 times a day) may also help to impair platelet aggregation while their numbers are decreasing. Splenectomy is contraindicated in this disorder, since it may be associated with an exacerbation of thrombocythemia, thrombosis, hemorrhage, and death [33].

Hereditary Thrombocytopenia

Five hereditary thrombocytopenic states—all uncommon—have been described:

1. *Bernard-Soulier syndrome.* In this syndrome, the platelets are larger than normal and are often decreased in number. The bleeding tendency is not directly related to thrombocytopenia.
2. *Wiskott-Aldrich syndrome.* This is characterized by thrombocytopenia and reduced levels of immunoglobulin M, which is responsible for the recurrent pyogenic infections and eczema. The platelets are small and have a decreased life span.
3. *Thrombocytopenia with absent radius.* In this condition, the platelets are decreased in number, and megakaryocytes are abnormal. Other skeletal abnormalities are frequently present in addition to the absent radius.

4. *May-Hegglin anomaly.* In this syndrome, giant platelets are present with Dohle bodies (areas of basophilic cytoplasm) in the leukocytes. Most patients are asymptomatic, but bleeding can occur.
5. *Hereditary thrombocytopenia resembling idiopathic thrombocytopenia purpura.* These patients, whose symptoms begin early in life, have a positive familial history of purpura. The in vitro assay for antiplatelet antibodies is negative, whereas in idiopathic thrombocytopenic purpura it is often positive.

Abnormal Platelet Function

Thrombasthenia (Glanzmann's Disease)

The signs of thrombasthenia are petechiae, ecchymoses, mucous membrane hemorrhages, and severe anemia. Thrombasthenia occurs early in life; the frequency of bleeding episodes tends to decrease with age. It is rare and is inherited as an autosomal recessive trait. Characteristically, defective clot retraction is associated with an abnormal platelet count, PT, and APTT. Abnormal platelet morphology is present. The bleeding time may or may not be prolonged. ADP does not induce platelet aggregation, and platelet adhesiveness is reduced. Platelet transfusions are recommended for treatment of hemorrhage, but their effectiveness varies.

ACQUIRED THROMBOCYTOPENIA

Idiopathic Thrombocytopenic Purpura (ITP)

Idiopathic thrombocytopenic purpura is an immune disorder that results in accelerated platelet destruction by the spleen secondary to recognition of antibodies and antibody complexes bound to the platelet membrane. ITP is divided into chronic, acute, and neonatal forms. Chronic ITP is usually seen in adults; the exact cause is unknown. Acute ITP is seen in children, usually following a viral illness; the majority of patients show spontaneous remission within a few months of onset. Neonatal ITP is seen in newborns of mothers with ITP secondary to immune complexes that cross the placenta and bind to platelets of the fetus.

ITP is characterized by a decreased platelet count and a prolonged bleeding time with normal PT and APTT. Purpuras and gingival bleeding are common. Initial treatment is usually steroid therapy, aimed at decreasing phagocytosis of platelets by the reticuloendothelial system. If the disease does not abate and requires high-dose steroid therapy that cannot be tapered, splenectomy will produce improvement in up to 90 percent of patients (50% complete remission) [2, 19]. Platelet transfusions are indicated only for acute bleeding secondary to thrombocytopenia. Treatment of neonatal ITP involves peripartum steroid treatment of the mother. Vaginal delivery, as opposed to cesarean section, is associated with a higher incidence of intracranial hemorrhage in thrombocytopenic infants [35].

Thrombotic Thrombocytopenic Purpura (TTP)

Thrombotic thrombocytopenic purpura is a rare platelet disorder characterized by microangiopathic anemia, thrombocytopenia, fever, and neurologic and renal manifestations. The characteristic clinical findings are secondary to occlusions of the microcirculation with a hyalinelike material. Over 400 cases have been reported, and multiple etiologies for the disorder have been proposed. It affects females slightly more than males and has a peak incidence in the third decade of life. If untreated, it rapidly progresses and is often fatal [36]. Laboratory findings include schistocytes and other evidence of microangiopathic anemia, marked thrombocytopenia, and renal dysfunction with proteinuria, hematuria, and rising blood urea nitrogen (BUN) and creatinine. The diagnosis may be conclusively established with a gingival biopsy that demonstrates occlusion of the microcirculation with hyalinelike material and intimal proliferation, but no evidence of vasculitis. No therapy is uniformly successful [27]. High-dose corticosteroids combined with antiplatelet drugs such as aspirin and dipyridamole have met with some success. Splenectomy is offered to patients who fail to respond to steroids and antiplatelet agents.

Secondary Thrombocytopenia

Thrombocytopenia may be secondary to numerous agents and conditions that can cause either decreased platelet production or increased destruction. Factors that affect decreased production include malignancy, drug toxicity, radiation, and aplastic anemia. Increased destruction can also be caused by drugs and by autoimmune phenomenon, infection, DIC, hypersplenism, and alloantibodies secondary to multiple transfusions. Thrombocytopenia is likely to be responsible for bleeding only if the platelet count is less than 30,000/µl. Clinical manifestations of secondary thrombocytopenia may vary, but petechiae and mucosal purpura, as well as occult gastrointestinal bleeding, are frequent. The underlying cause of secondary thrombocytopenia should be eliminated if possible. If platelets are needed to control hemorrhage, transfusion with ABO type-specific is desirable. HLA-A–cross-matched platelets will minimize development of alloantibodies [7], which can significantly shorten the life span of subsequently infused platelets.

ABNORMAL PLATELET FUNCTION

Aspirin, other nonsteroidal antiinflammatory drugs (NSAID), dipyridamole, certain antibiotics, and other drugs affect platelet function to varying degrees. Aspirin irreversibly acetylates platelet aggregation systems. As the platelet is a cell without a nucleus and is incapable of renewing its enzyme systems, the aspirin affect is operative for the life of the circulating platelet. The constant turnover of platelets and the pulsed dosing of aspirin prevents a totally inhibited circulating platelet pool. Other drugs, such as ibuprofen, exert reversible affects on platelet aggregation. Although the affects of these drugs may be readily apparent in vitro with platelet aggregation studies, clinical hemorrhage is rarely the sole result of decreased platelet aggregation. Nevertheless, platelet dysfunction, in addition to such primary processes as peptic ulcer, trauma, surgery, and renal failure, may contribute to overt hemorrhage. The primary underlying cause of hemorrhage should be treated directly; however, platelet transfusion may be necessary to permit surgical therapy. dDAVP treatment of bleeding associated with uremia is often successful [18].

EXCESSIVE ANTICOAGULATION

Heparin

Heparin, the most widely used and reliable anticoagulant available today, is a mucopolysaccharide of varying molecular weight with a strong negative charge that permits it to bind with specific lysine residues of ATIII. Heparin alone has essentially no anticoagulant activity. When combined with ATIII, heparin mediates a conformational change in the ATIII molecule, making the arginine reactive center of the ATIII more accessible to binding with the active serine center of thrombin and other serine proteases of the coagulation cascade. ATIII alone can slowly inactivate the active forms of serine protease clotting factors; however, in the presence of heparin, this reaction is almost instantaneous. The heparin-ATIII complex has been shown to inhibit the actions of activated factors IX, X, XI, and XII and to inactivate thrombin and plasmin [32].

Different concentrations of heparin affect the coagulation cascade at different sites. The minidose heparin regimen appears to be effective primarily through inactivation of factor X_a, whereas larger doses of heparin administered in the therapy of thromboembolic disease interfere with function of all activated serine protease clotting factors. The most common complication of heparin therapy is hemorrhage. However, allergic reactions, alopecia, and hyperaldosteronism have been reported. A more recently recognized complication of heparin therapy, heparin-induced thrombocytopenia (HIT) with associated thromboembolic complications rather than hemorrhage, is now being reported with increasing frequency [17].

Diagnosis of Bleeding from Heparin

The patient's history usually suggests that heparin may be the cause of bleeding. A significant prolongation of the clotting time (>30–40 min), APTT greater than 100 seconds, or activated clotting time (ACT) greater than 200 seconds is usually present. To rule out associated coagulation factor deficiencies or fibrinolysis, TT and protamine-corrected thrombin times (PCTT) should be done. If the ACT is abnormal and the TT is normal, coagulation factor deficiencies exist. If both the ACT and the TT are abnormal and the PCTT is normal, incomplete heparin neutralization is present. Abnormal PCTT, ACT, and TT indicates that fibrinogen deficiency exists, and a workup for DIC should be performed.

Management

Bleeding secondary to overanticoagulation with heparin is best managed by immediate discontinuation of the heparin. Its short half-life (1–2 hr) makes the need for heparin neutralization rare. Should heparin reversal be indicated, protamine can be used. When clotting time or APTT is utilized for heparin monitoring, protamine sulfate should be given slowly until the clotting time or APTT returns toward normal. The amount of protamine required depends on the amount of heparin given, the interval between the administration of heparin and the protamine, and the status of the patient's renal and hepatic functions. It is best to give protamine in repeated small amounts until the coagulation studies return toward normal. The rule of 1 to 2 mg of protamine to neutralize 100 units of heparin is a useful approximation of the required dose. However, it is best to administer smaller amounts of protamine than thought to be necessary and to give additional protamine as indicated by coagulation testing. Rapid injection of protamine sulfate may produce hypotension. If the ACT method of anticoagulation monitoring is utilized, it may be possible to calculate the amount of protamine needed from a heparin dose-response curve. This curve is derived by plotting the ACT versus the heparin dose administered for both control and 5-minute postheparin administration samples and joining these two points with a straight line. A protamine dose equal to 1.3 times the calculated residual heparin usually provides adequate heparin neutralization [23,38].

Vitamin K Antagonists
Dicumarol, warfarin, and other vitamin K antagonists interfere with the action of vitamin K in the synthesis of factors II, VII, IX, and X. A vitamin K–dependent carboxylase has been identified that is responsible for conversion of glutamyl residues on the clotting factor precursors to γ-carboxyglutamyl residues. This conversion is necessary for the binding of calcium, a cofactor in the reactions catalyzed by the affected clotting factors. Patients receiving vitamin K antagonists produce clotting-factor precursors that are antigenically similar to normal factors but are without procoagulant activity, due to their abnormal calcium-binding characteristics. The reduction of clotting factors that retain normal activity slows clotting by reducing the amount and rate at which thrombin is produced.

Diagnosis of Bleeding Secondary to Administration of Vitamin K Antagonists
The PT is frequently used to monitor the effects of vitamin K antagonists. Bleeding often occurs when the PT exceeds twice the control value. Prolongation of the PT may occur from an overdose of the prescribed drug or from synergistic effects between the vitamin K antagonists and other drugs. The list of drugs that interact either directly or indirectly with warfarin is quite long. The effects of these drugs may enhance or counteract the warfarin effect.

Management
If bleeding is not life-threatening, clotting abnormalities are best treated by discontinuing the vitamin K antagonist and allowing the coagulation factors to return toward normal. Complete reversal of the vitamin K antagonists' effect can be obtained within hours by giving 5 to 25 mg of vitamin K_1 parenterally (see section on vitamin K deficiency). It must be recognized that rapid and total correction of anticoagulation induced by vitamin K may contribute to thrombotic events for which the original anticoagulation therapy was instituted (clotting on heart valves or deep venous thromboses). Alternative methods of anticoagulation should be considered once hemorrhage is controlled. If instantaneous correction of vitamin K–depen-

dent factor deficiency is needed, transfusion with fresh frozen plasma immediately provides levels of active factors II, VII, IX, and X. Vitamin K should also be considered for those patients treated by FFP infusions, as the factor levels from FFP will wane according to their half-lives (Table 28-1).

DIAGNOSIS OF BLEEDING DISORDERS

History

The type of bleeding experienced by the patient, its course, and its frequency may help determine the etiology of the bleeding. Prolonged or excessive bleeding with circumcision, tooth extractions, menstruation, trauma, or operative procedures, or a history of spontaneous bleeding, chronic iron deficiency anemia, and repeated blood transfusions may indicate congenital defects in the hemostatic mechanism. If a family history of bleeding is present, the clinician should try to establish its cause and pattern of inheritance. A history of drug therapy with direct or indirect anticoagulants, platelet depressants, broad-spectrum antibiotics, or chemotherapy may suggest the etiology of the excessive bleeding. Local or systemic diseases such as leukemia, uremia, collagen-vascular disorders, and liver disease may aggravate or even cause a hemorrhagic diathesis.

Physical Examination

One should look for the presence and distribution of petechiae, purpuras, ecchymoses, jaundice, and hemangiomas. Raised petechiae are more commonly associated with vasculitis, whereas flat petechiae, principally in areas of increased hydrostatic pressure, are usually indicative of thrombocytopenia. Widespread ecchymoses in combination with hematuria and gastrointestinal hemorrhage are common in acquired coagulation defects. Hemarthroses, residual joint deformities, and hematomas are common sequelae of congenital coagulation factor deficiencies. Splenomegaly may be associated with thrombocytopenia. Lymphadenopathy or hepatosplenomegaly may indicate the presence of an infiltrative malignancy affecting organs responsible for clotting factor synthesis or platelet production. The stigmata of chronic liver disease, such as ascites and portosystemic collateral channels, should alert one to the possibility of deficiencies in clotting factors synthesized by the liver.

Laboratory Testing

The etiology of nonmechanical bleeding can usually be determined by performing a battery of screening tests and, when needed, specific quantitative tests of coagulation and lysis. The screening battery should include the following: complete blood count and platelet count, PT, APTT, fibrinogen level, and TT. If the TT is prolonged, a protamine titration test should be performed. If hyperfibrinolysis is suspected, whole-blood lysis times or euglobulin clot lysis time and fibrin split product concentrations should be measured. Template bleeding time is useful in determining platelet dysfunction when platelet counts are greater than $100,000/\mu l$. More-sophisticated platelet aggregation studies are performed when indicated. If an inhibitor is thought to be present, a 50 : 50 mixture of patient and normal plasma can be used for repeating the abnormal coagulation test. Correction of the test by addition of normal plasma indicates a factor deficiency in the patient tested; noncorrection indicates the presence of an inhibitor.

The results of a screening battery (Table 28-4) should permit further characterization of the bleeding. Specific testing and history will distinguish between the various acquired and congenital coagulation deficiencies. The whole-blood lysis time and euglobulin lysis time are shortened in both primary and secondary hyperfibrinolysis. If primary lysis is excessive, coagulation proteins may also be lysed and the tests of coagulation prolonged. The main differentiating feature between primary and secondary hyperfibrinolysis is the normal platelet count found with primary hyperfibrinolysis.

Low platelet counts may be detected during episodes of thrombocytopenia and DIC. Coagulation factors are markedly decreased during DIC, but they are normal in thrombocytopenia. Significant bleeding is much more common in DIC than in thrombocytopenia. Normal coagulation factors, normal platelet counts, normal lysis times, and a prolonged thrombin time that is corrected with protamine suggests the presence of heparin contamination. Normal platelets, TT, and lysis times with prolonged PT and APTT suggest depletion of vitamin K–dependent coagulation factors. Normal PT and prolonged APTT suggest either hemophilia or one of the parahemophilias.

BLOOD AND BLOOD COMPONENT THERAPY

Blood transfusions have traditionally been used to restore blood volume, increase the oxygen-carrying capacity of the blood, and provide coagulation proteins and platelets. Rather than storing large quantities of whole blood, freshly donated blood is separated into components: (1) cellular (red cells, platelets, and white cells); (2) cryoprecipitate; (3) cryoprecipitate-poor plasma, which frequently is further divided into other components. These components, with appropriate processing, can be stored for long periods of time and thus are available for the needs of a large number of patients. The component system has permitted storage of reliable quantities of coagulation products and red cells that would not be available if the blood-banking system were limited simply to storage of whole blood. A thorough knowledge of blood and blood component therapy is essential for safe and effective hemotherapy. Table 28-5 outlines the compositions, unit volumes, and indications for use of the commonly available blood components.

Transfusion Reactions

Transfusion reactions vary from mild febrile responses to severe hemolytic reactions with anemia, DIC, and renal impairment or failure. Allergic reactions are encountered in up to 5 percent of patients receiving blood transfusions—usually characterized by development of hives, pruritus, or diffuse rash. True anaphylactic reactions are rare. Hemolytic transfusion reactions occur at the rate of 1 in every 15,000 to 20,000 transfusions. The

Table 28-4. Results of screening battery in various nonmechanical bleeding disorders

Type of bleeding disorder	Fibrinogen level	Prothrombin time (PT)	Activated partial thromboplastin time (APTT)	Thrombin time (TT)	Lysis time	Platelet count	Fibrin/fibrinogen degradation products (FDP)
Congenital coagulation deficiencies	N-A	N-A[a]	N-A[a]	N-A	N	N	N
Disseminated intravascular coagulation	A	A	A	N-A	A	A	A
Decreased platelet number	N	N	N	N	N	A	N
Decreased platelet function[b]	N	N	N	N	N	N	N
Hyperfibrinolysis	N-A	N-A	N-A	N-A	A	N	N-A
Heparin	N	A[c]	A[c]	A[c]	N	N	N
Vitamin K antagonists	N	A	A	N	N	N	N

A = abnormal; N = normal.

[a] A normal PT and APTT excludes hemophilia and the parahemophilias (except von Willebrand's disease) as a cause of bleeding and indicates that the vitamin K factors are present in adequate amounts. If either the PT or APTT is abnormal, variations of the APTT can be used to determine the specific coagulation defect and the factor level.

[b] Specific tests of adhesion or aggregation are necessary to define abnormalities of platelet function.

[c] Heparin interferes with most tests of coagulation. If the heparin is "neutralized" with protamine, the PT, APTT, and thrombin time will become normal if the coagulation factors are normal.

hemolytic reactions are caused by preformed antibodies in the recipient or the donor producing marked hemolysis. Hemolytic transfusion reactions are important in a discussion of nonmechanical bleeding, as they may be attended by DIC and profound hypotension. Hemolytic transfusion reaction should be suspected when fever, chills, flushing, headache, flank pain, and hypotension develop within the first 20 to 30 minutes of transfusion therapy. Management of transfusion reactions consists of immediately discontinuing the blood transfusion and treating hypotension and hypovolemia with intravenous fluids. Forced diuresis with the aid of mannitol or a loop diuretic and alkalinization of the urine is also recommended. Once the transfusion is stopped and adequate volume restored, DIC, if evident, should abate. If DIC persists, it should be treated as described above.

The transfusion of red cells, liquid plasma, FFP, cryoprecipitate, and/or platelets should respect ABO compatibility.

Posttransfusion Purpura (PTP)

Posttransfusion purpura is a rare, life-threatening thrombocytopenia that occurs approximately 1 week following transfusion. It is believed to be due to production of an antibody against a common platelet antigen (PL^{A1}). This antibody develops when PL^{A1}-negative recipients are transfused with platelets containing the PL^{A1} antigen. The resulting antibody is then adsorbed to the surface of the patient's own platelets, resulting in their destruction. The disease is often self-limiting. Specific treatments involving steroids, plasmapheresis, and saturation of antibody-binding sites with large doses of IgG have been reported [39]. No one therapy is uniformly effective.

Disease Transmission by Blood Transfusions and Blood Component Therapy

The safety of biologic transfusion products in regard to disease transmission depends on a number of factors: (1) the original donor source, (2) the ability to test either donor or product for disease, and (3) the preparation and storage process involved in making the transfusion product. Hepatitis A, B, and non-A/non-B (NANB), cytomegalovirus (CMV), human immunodeficiency virus (HIV), and bacterial diseases have been transmitted by blood product transfusion. Generally speaking, the following statements regarding disease transmission by transfusion are true.

Volunteer blood sources are safer than commercial ones.
Fresh transfusion products favor disease transmission over heated and/or lyophilized products with extended storage times.
Products made of pooled plasma from multiple donors convey a higher risk than do single-donor or pooled single-donor products.
Infusion of blood products at suggested rates following refrigerated storage minimizes secondary bacterial contamination.
The only way to ensure complete absence of viral contamination of biologic products is to manufacture them with the techniques of genetic engineering in a virus-free environment.

Table 28-5. Blood components: composition, volume, indications for use

Component/product	Composition	Approximate volume	Indications
Whole blood	RBC; plasma; WBC; platelets.	500 ml	Increase both red cell mass and plasma volume (WBC and platelets not functional; plasma deficient in labile clotting factors V, VIII)
Red blood cells	RBC; reduced plasma, WBC, and platelets; avg. HCT = 70%	250 ml	Increase red cell mass in symptomatic anemia (WBC and platelets not functional)
Red blood cells, adenine-saline added	RBC; reduced plasma, WBC and platelets; 100 ml of additive solution	330 ml	Increase red cell mass in symptomatic anemia (WBC and platelets not functional)
Leukocyte-poor RBC (prepared by filtration, centrifugation or saline washed)	RBC; few WBC and platelets; minimal plasma	200 ml	Increase red cell mass; minimize febrile or allergic (if washed) reactions due to leukocyte antibodies or plasma proteins
Frozen-thawed-deglycerolized RBC	RBC; minimal WBC and platelets; no plasma	180 ml	Increase red cell mass; minimize febrile or allergic transfusion reactions; used for rare blood storage
Granulocyte-platelet concentrate (centrifugation leukapheresis)	Granulocytes; lymphocytes; platelets ($>1.0 \times 10^{10}$ PMN/unit; $>2.0 \times 10^{11}$ platelets/unit); some RBC	220 ml	Provide granulocytes for septic leukopenic patients; platelets present will treat thrombocytopenia (24-hr shelf life)
Platelet concentrate (random donor)	Platelets; some WBC; plasma ($>5.5 \times 10^{10}$ platelets/unit); some RBC	50 ml	Bleeding due to thrombocytopenia or thrombocytopathy (5-day shelf life) expect 5000–7000 increase in platelet count/μl for each unit transfused

Component	Contents	Volume	Indications
Platelet concentrate (single donor plateletpheresis)	Platelets; some WBC; plasma; ($>3 \times 10^{11}$ platelets/unit); some RBC	300 ml	Bleeding due to thrombocytopenia in patients with HLA antiplatelet antibodies; product often HLA-matched (24-hr or 5-day shelf life; varies with storage bag)
Fresh frozen plasma	Plasma; all coagulation factors; complement, (no platelets)	220 ml	Treatment of some coagulation disorders
Liquid plasma	Plasma; stable clotting factors; no platelets	220 ml	Treatment of stable clotting-factor deficiencies (II, VIII, IX, X, XI)
Cryoprecipitate-depleted plasma (modified plasma)	Plasma; stable clotting factors; no platelets	200 ml	Treatment of stable clotting-factor deficiencies (II, VII, IX, X, XI)
Cryoprecipitated AHF, also called cryoprecipitate	Fibrinogen; factors VIII and XIII, von Willebrand factor; fibronectin	15 ml	Deficiency of factor VIII (hemophilia A), factor XIII, fibrinogen; treatment of von Willebrand's disease
Lyophilized VIII	Factor VIII	25 ml	Hemophilia A (VIII deficiency)
Lyophilized II, VII, IX, X	Factors II, VII, IX, X	25 ml	Hereditary II, VII, IX, or X deficiency
Albumin/plasma protein fraction	Albumin, some α, β globulins	(5%); (25%)	Volume expansion; increase oncotic pressure
Immune serum globulin	IgG antibodies	Varies	Treatment of hypo- or agammaglobulinemia; disease prophylaxis

Adapted from Snyder, E. L. (ed.) *Blood Transfusions Therapy, A Physician's Handbook* (2nd ed.). American Association Blood Banks, 1987.

The widespread availability of gene-manufactured coagulation products is not presently a reality. Disease is transmitted by blood and blood product transfusion despite efforts that curb, but do not eliminate, the problem. It is important that potential benefit of transfusion be weighed against potential risk. In cases in which a medication (e.g., dDAVP) will provide necessary factor levels, the medication should be used in preference to the blood product.

Hepatitis following transfusion remains a problem. Serologic tests for hepatitis B (HepB) are available. Immunization against HepB is recommended as protection for patients, such as hemophiliacs, who are exposed to repeated transfusions. Serologic testing for NANB virus is under development. Screening of donors for elevated liver enzymes is common practice. Nevertheless, NANB presently accounts for 75 to 90 percent of hepatitis transmitted by transfusion [5].

CMV is a problem for neonates and adult patients who are immunosuppressed as the result of malignancy or therapy following organ transplantation. Screening of transfused blood products may have a positive impact [27].

HIV has introduced the specter of a uniformly fatal disease capable of being transmitted by biologic products. Although serologic tests are available for donor screening and have been in routine use since 1985, problems remain. The period between HIV exposure and seroconversion may be weeks to months [28]. During this time of viremia, the donor may not test positive. The risk of HIV exposure by single-donor transfusion is estimated to be 1 in 250,000 units [1]. Heat treatment and lyophilization of factor concentrates from pooled plasma substantially decrease the HIV transmission risk. The Centers for Disease Control in January 1988 reviewed reports of 18 cases from worldwide populations that met reasonable guidelines for possible HIV seroconversion following exposure to heat-treated factor concentrates. Twelve cases had documented exposure to nonheated factor concentrates. The remaining six cases could have been caused by transfusion of heat-treated factor concentrates. Nevertheless, data were cited from the surveillance of 1489 seronegative patients who had collectively received a total of 75,000,000 units of heat-treated, donor-screened, pooled coagulation factor concentrates over the last 2 years—none of this group had seroconverted. Inactivation of HepB and NANB by the same factor treatment processes has been less successful than with HIV [34].

REFERENCES

1. Bove, J. R. Transfusion-associated hepatitis and AIDS. *N. Engl. J. Med.* 317:242, 1987.
2. Brennan, M. F., Rappaport, J. M., Maloney, W. C., and Wilson, RE. Correlation between response to corticosteroids and splenectomy for adult idiopathic thrombocytopenic purpura. *Am. J. Surg.* 129:490–2, 1975.
3. Bukowski, R. M., Hewlett, J. S., Harris, J. W., et al. Exchange transfusions in the treatment of thrombotic thrombocytopenic purpura. *Semin. Hematol.* 13:219, 1976.

4. Burns, E. R. *Clinical Management of Bleeding and Thrombosis.* Boston: Blackwell, 1987. P. 135.
5. Coffin, C. M. Current issues in transfusion therapy: Risks of infection. *Postgrad. Med.* 80:219, 1986.
6. Coller, B. S. Von Willebrand Disease. In R. W. Colman, J. Hirsch, V. J. Marder, and E. W. Saltzman (eds.), *Hemostasis and Thrombosis: Basic Principles and Clinical Practice* (2nd ed.). Philadelphia: Lippincott, 1987. P. 77.
7. Curtoni, E. S., and Gabrielli, A. Platelet transfusion. *Hematologica* 61:498, 1976.
8. Eyster, M. E., Gill, F. M., Blatt, P. M., et al. Central nervous system bleeding in hemophiliacs. *Blood* 52:1179, 1978.
9. Frick, P. G., Reidler, G., and Brogli, H. Dose response and minimum daily requirements for vitamin K in man. *J. Appl. Physiol.* 23:387, 1967.
10. Granlnick, H. R., and Griepp, P. Thrombosis with epsilon-aminocaproic acid therapy. *Am. J. Clin. Pathol.* 56:151–4, 1971.
11. Hamilton, P. J., Stalker, A. L., and Douglas, A. S. Disseminated intravascular coagulation: A review. *J. Clin. Pathol.* 31:609–18, 1978.
12. Hilgartner, M. The Management of Hemophilia. In F. S. Morrison (ed.), *Hemophilia.* Washington, D.C.: American Association of Blood Banks, 1978.
13. Holmberg, L. Nilsson, I. M., Borge, L., et al. Platelet aggregation induced by 1-deamino-6-D-arginine vasopressin (DDAVP) in type IIB von Willebrand's disease. *N. Engl. J. Med.* 309:816, 1983.
14. Jones, P. Developments and problems in the management of hemophilia. *Semin. Hematol.* 14:375, 1977.
15. Koch, B., Luban, N. L., Galioto, F. M., et al. Changes in coagulation parameters with exercise in patients with classic hemophilia. *Am. J. Hematol.* 16:227, 1984.
16. Kolbrinsky, N. L., Gerarrard, J. M., Watson, C. M., et al. Shortening of bleeding time by 1-deamino-8-D-arginine vasopressin in various bleeding disorders. *Lancet* 1:1145, 1984.
17. Laster, J., Cikrit, D., Walker, N., and Silver, D. The heparin-induced thrombocytopenia syndrome: An update. *Surgery* 102:763, 1987.
18. McEvoy, G. K. (ed.). *Drug Information 88.* Bethesda, MD: American Society of Hospital Pharmacists, 1988. P. 1816.
19. MacPherson, A. I. S., and Richmond, J. Planned splenectomy and treatment of idiopathic thrombocytopenic purpura. *Br. Med. J.* 1:64–6, 1975.
20. Mannucci, P. M. Desmopressin (dDAVP) for treatment of disorders of hemostasis. *Prog. Hemost. Thromb.* 8:19, 1986.
21. Martin, D. J., Lucas, C. E., Ledgerwood, A. M., et al. Fresh frozen supplement to massive red cell transfusion. *Ann. Surg.* 202:505, 1985.
22. Metzler, M. H. Antibiotic-related coagulopathies. In D. Silver (ed.), *Seminars in Vascular Surgery,* 1:233, 1988.
23. Mollitt, D. L., Gartner, D. J., and Madura, J. A. Bedside monitoring of heparin therapy. *Am. J. Surg.* 135:801, 1978.
24. Nichols, W. K. Disseminated Intravascular Coagulation. In D. Silver (ed.), *Seminars in Vascular Surgery,* 1:190, 1988.
25. Nilsson, I. M., Hedner, U., and Bjorlin, G. Suppression of factor IX antibody in hemophilia by factor IX and cyclophosphamide. *Ann. Intern. Med.* 78:91, 1973.
26. Nilsson, I. M., Hedner, U. Ahlberg, A. S., et al. Surgery of hemophiliacs—20-year experience. *World J. Surg.* 1:55, 1977.
27. Onaroto, I.M., Morens, D. M., Martone, W. J., et al. Epidemiology of cyto-

megaloviral infections: Recommendations for prevention and control. *Rev. Infect. Dis.* 7:479, 1985.

28. Ranki, A., Valle, S. L., Krohn, M., et al. Long latency precedes overt seroconversion in sexually transmitted human-immunodeficiency-virus infection. *Lancet* 2:589–93, 1987.

29. Reed, L. R., Ciavarella, D., Heimbach, D. M., et al. Prophylactic platelet administration during massive transfusion. *Ann. Surg.* 203:40, 1986.

30. Rizza, C. R. Management of Patients with Inherited Blood Coagulation Defects. In A. L. Bloom and D. P. Thomas (eds.), *Haemostasis and Thrombosis.* London: Churchill Livingstone, 1981. Pp. 371–388.

31. Rizza, C. R., and Matthews, J. M. Effective frequent replacement on a level of factor VIII antibodies in hemophilia. *Br. J. Haematol.* 52:13, 1982.

32. Rosenberg, R. D. Biological actions of heparin. *Semin. Hematol.* 14:427, 1977.

33. Rubinowitz, M. J. Thrombocytosis: Practical approach to diagnosis and treatment. *Rocky Mt. Med.* 75:261, 1978.

34. Safety of therapeutic products used for hemophilia patients. *J.A.M.A.* (Leads from the MMWR) 260:901, 1988.

35. Scott, J. R., Cruikshank, D. P., Kochenour, N. K., et al. Fetal platelet counts in obstetrical management of immunologic thrombocytopenic purpura. *Am. J. Obstet. Gynecol.* 136:495,1980.

36. Scott, J. R., Cruikshank, D. P., Kochenour, N. K., et al. Fetal platelet counts in obstetrical management of immunologic thrombocytopenic purpura. *Am. J. Obstet. Gynecol.* 136:161, 1980.

37. Slocumbe, G. W., Newland, A. C., Colvin, M. P., and Colvin, B. T. The role of intensive plasma exchange in the prevention and management of hemorrhage in patients with inhibitors to factor VIII. *Br. J. Haematol.* 47:577, 1981.

38. Vitez, T. S. Intraoperative anticoagulant management. *Contemp. Surg.* 13:29, 1978.

39. Vogelsang, G., Kickler, T. S., and Bell, W. R. Post-transfusion purpura: A report of five patients and a review of the pathogenesis and management. *Am. J. Hematol.* 21:259, 1986.

SELECTED READINGS

Burns, E. R. *Clinical Management of Bleeding and Thrombosis.* Boston: Blackwell, 1987. A very readable and concise text dealing with treatment of bleeding disorders.

Colman, R. W., Hirsh, J., Marder, V. J., and Salzman, E. W. *Hemostasis and Thrombosis: Basic Principles and Clinical Practice* (2nd ed.). Philadelphia: Lippincott, 1987. This authoritative reference provides substantial background into the biochemical details of coagulation.

Snyder, E. L. (ed.). *Blood Transfusion Therapy: A Physician's Handbook* (2nd ed.). Arlington, VA: American Association of Blood Banks, 1987. Details standard transfusion practices of the AABB.

Blood Substitutes

Konrad Messmer

Substitutes replacing all the complex functions of whole blood (e.g., carrier function, clotting function, and immunologic defense function) are not yet on the horizon, despite extensive work in this direction. Homologous blood, even when stored only for a short period of time, does not meet all these functions. Clearly, the substitute of choice is fresh autologous blood. Fortunately, the use of autologous blood has increased during recent years; the new interest in autologous blood and autotransfusion procedures was fostered mainly by the appearance of the acquired immunodeficiency syndrome (AIDS), although the risk of transfusion-transmitted human immunodeficiency virus (HIV) infection is very low when compared with the risk of transmission of non-A/non-B hepatitis. Furthermore, it is reported with increasing frequency that transfusions of homologous blood can induce immunosuppression and thereby affect the patient's resistance to infections, recurrences of tumors, and metastasis formation [44]. All these risks can safely be excluded by autotransfusion, because the patient's own blood is the safest blood [20,45]. Autotransfusion is currently used in three different forms:

1. Blood donation before surgery and storage (predonation or predeposit programs) [35,48,50]
2. Acute preoperative hemodilution [30,31]
3. Intraoperative blood salvage and retransfusion by cell savers [50].

All three procedures alone, but particularly when combined, have been shown to reduce the need for homologous blood. However, even when autotransfusion techniques are practiced under optimal conditions, the transfusion requirements of patients suffering major blood loss from trauma and surgery cannot always be met.

In order to avoid side effects from blood components that for a given patient are either inactive or unnecessary, the concept of blood component therapy should be used more vigorously. This concept includes the identification of the individual component deficit (oxygen carrier, clotting factors, colloids, immunoglobulins) and selective substitution for the deficiency.

There is general agreement that restoration of the circulating volume is the most important single step in blood replacement therapy; this goal can be achieved simply by the infusion of plasma substitutes. However, because they dilute key components of the patient's remaining blood, plasma substitutes have their limits in restoration of blood volume. Clinical studies with pre- and intraoperative normovolemic hemodilution have clearly revealed that surgical patients will tolerate hemoglobin levels of 8 to 10 dl/100 ml without the risk of reduced oxygen delivery and ensuing tissue hypoxia, provided circulating blood volume and cardiac output are adequately maintained by the plasma substitutes. Increased oxygen demands in the postoperative period (e.g., fever) or in coronary disease with the inability to raise stroke volume with increasing preload call for a higher number of red blood cells: i.e., higher hemoglobin concentration [30,31].

The following sections discuss the plasma substitutes available for clinical use, with special regard paid to their capacity to restore the circulating volume and to promote nutritional blood flow.

PHYSICOCHEMICAL CHARACTERISTICS OF PLASMA SUBSTITUTES

Plasma substitutes, by definition, aim to replace the lost fluid, which is a colloidal solution containing various proteins. Of these proteins, albumin has the highest concentration and colloid-osmotic water-binding capacity.

Infusion solutions free of colloid molecules cannot be considered plasma substitutes, because the characteristic features of plasma—namely, the colloid content and, hence, the colloid-osmotic power—are lacking. Nevertheless, the circulating volume can be rapidly restored by either crystalloid or colloid solutions. Although maintenance of the normal colloid-osmotic pressure (COP) of plasma is not an absolute prerequisite for hemodilution, it is difficult to establish and maintain normovolemia with crystalloids alone. In addition, significant fluid shifts occur into other fluid compartments (third space) as COP is reduced. To establish and maintain normovolemia exclusively with crystalloids requires volumes 2.5 to 4 times the volume lost; close monitoring of the patient is needed to adjust the infusion volume and infusion speed to the actual hemodynamic status, in order to avoid hypovolemia on the one hand and circulatory overloading with pulmonary edema on the other.

Therefore, for the sake of practicality and safety, we strongly advocate initial replacement of plasma deficits with colloid solutions, which provide predictable, long-lasting volume effects. These depend upon the physicochemical properties of the colloid molecules. Colloidal molecules of a weight below 50,000 pass the glomerular membrane and are rapidly excreted by the kidney [15]. In contrast, albumin, by virtue of its molecular weight of 69,000, is retained in the circulatory system. It should be noted that none of the artificial colloids has the monodisperse form of albumin; the artificial colloidal solutions are polydisperse in nature and thus provide a mixture of different species of molecules, the weights of which are distributed in a Gaussian curve.

Hence, the intravascular persistence of artificial colloids depends, first, on the molecular weight of the majority of molecules and, second, on the width of distribution of molecular weights. The ratio of average molecular weight (MW) to average molecular number (MN) indicates the degree of polydispersity (see Table 29-1). Unity of the ratio MW/MN describes a monodisperse colloid, such as albumin.

The water-retaining capacity or the colloid-osmotic imbibing power of colloid solutions depends on the MW/MN ratio and the colloid content of the solutions. Solutions with higher tonicities than plasma will attract water mainly from the interstitial space; as a consequence, these solutions will lead to an expansion of the plasma volume—at the expense of the interstitial and or intracellular fluid volume. The effectiveness of colloids in restoring plasma deficits can be predicted from their physicochemical properties; these predictions have been verified in numerous experimental and clinical studies [15,18,29]. A plasma substitute should not impair the rheologic properties of the blood: i.e., the fluidity of the blood and its cellular elements. Protracted volume loss and shock are characteristically associated with a disturbance of microcirculatory flow and with a decrease in blood fluidity. Both microcirculatory flow and blood fluidity can be more efficiently improved by colloids than by crystalloids, provided the viscosity of the colloid solution itself does not exceed the viscosity of whole blood [18]. In addition, colloids may provide specific properties, such as the antithrombotic effect of dextran.

NATURAL COLLOIDS

Among the natural colloids, 4% pasteurized protein solution (Plasmanate) and 5% human serum albumin (HSA) are highly suitable for plasma volume replacement; both solutions yield a volume effect in vivo that roughly equals the amount of volume infused [15]. These protein preparations are free from the risk of transmitting infectious diseases, but not free from the risk of anaphylactoid reactions (immediate and delayed) with severe hypotension [2,42,43]. The occasional occurrence of adverse reactions is not, however, a contraindication to routine use. (This statement is valid for all colloids in clinical use today.)

Because of these shortcomings, and for economic reasons (1 gm HSA costs about 15 times as much as 1 gm dextran), these natural colloids should never be used for routine plasma volume replacement; they should be reserved for those hypovolemic patients with significant hypoproteinemia. Also, for the same reasons, routine intraoperative volume replacement with protein solutions cannot be justified. Several authors have investigated whether posttraumatic respiratory insufficiency or acute respiratory distress can be prevented by early administration of HSA; as yet, there is no conclusive evidence that HSA is superior to artificial colloids in patients without significant hypoproteinemia.

Homologous fresh frozen plasma (FFP) carries the same risk of transmitting hepatitis, HIV, etc. and should therefore not be used for volume

Table 29-1. Artificial colloids for plasma volume substitution[a]

Colloid	Generic name	Colloid content	Mean MW	Mean MW : Mean MN	Intravascular persistence (hr)	Remarks
Dextran (Dx)	Dx 60[b]	6 gm/dl	60,000	2.0	6	Antithrombotic effect
	Dx 70	6 gm/dl	70,000	1.85	6	Antithrombotic effect
	Dx 40	10 gm/dl	40,000	1.4	2–3	Antithrombotic effect
Starch (HES)	HES 450/0.7	6 gm/dl	450,000	6.3	6	
	HES 200/0.5	10 gm/dl	200,000		6	
	HES 200/0.62	6 gm/dl	200,000		6	
	HES 40/0.5	6 gm/dl	40,000	2.0	2–3	Diuretic effect
Gelatin	Urea-linked gelatin	3.5 gm/dl	35,000	2.3	2–3	Diuretic effect
	Modified fluid gelatin (MFG)	4 gm/dl	35,000	2.2	2–3	Diuretic effect
	Oxypolygelatin	5.5 gm/dl	30,000	1.5	2–3	Diuretic effect

[a]According to data from literature and manufacturers.
[b]Dx 60: mean MW 60,000, available in Germany and Austria; properties nearly identical to those of Dx 70.

replacement; its indications are limited and have been specified by an NIH Consensus Conference in 1985 [39].

ARTIFICIAL COLLOIDS
The literature on artificial colloids contains a number of controversies concerning the advantages versus the disadvantages of various artificial colloids. The physicochemical properties of the colloids in question constitute the only criteria for any comparative judgment. Table 29-1 lists the most important data for the most frequently used artificial colloids. Since the sources, data for MW and MN, colloid content, and noncolloidal solutes vary widely among different countries and are sometimes changed, our discussion will be restricted to representative colloid substitutes (for detailed information, see Gruber [15] and Lutz [29]).

Dextrans
Dextrans are high- or macromolecular-weight polysaccharides consisting of glucose molecules connected mainly by 1.6 glucosidic linkages. The clinically used dextrans are obtained by hydrolytic fractionation. Dextran 60/70 (Macrodex) and dextran 40 (Rheomacrodex) are the most important dextran preparations. The 6% solution of dextran 60/70 exerts a colloid-osmotic effect, expressed as water-retaining capacity per gram of the nondiffusing polymer, of 20 to 25 ml—higher than that of albumin or plasma proteins. Therefore, dextran 60/70 seems particularly suitable for primary volume replacement and maintenance of adequate intravascular volume over a longer period of time [15,18,32].

Dextran 40, with an average molecular weight of 40,000, is available as a 10% solution, which, compared with plasma, is strongly hyperoncotic. For this reason, the initial volume effect of dextran 40 is about twice the volume infused. Owing to the lower MW, dextran 40 is more rapidly excreted; 3 to 4 hours after infusion the intravascular volume gain approximately equals the volume infused. The initial volume gain is due to transcapillary fluid shift at the expense of the interstitial fluid. As a rule, equal volumes of isotonic electrolytes are given intravenously with or after 10% dextran 40 solution in order to avoid interstitial dehydration. Along the colloid-osmotic gradient, interstitial fluid is drawn into the intravascular space, particularly on the venous side of the microcirculation; for this reason, microcirculatory flow is rapidly restored by dextran 40 infusions, because additional hemodilution takes place in the most vulnerable part of the microcirculation, the postcapillary venules. This effect depends on the colloid-osmotic pressure gradient across the microvascular membrane and is thus not specific for dextran 40. Dextran 40 is indicated particularly in patients with protracted shock and with microcirculatory disorders [18,32].

Dextrans are completely excreted or metabolized after short-term storage in the reticuloendothelial system (RES) and tubular cells of the kidney. Both dextrans possess antithrombotic properties, which differ from dextran's influence on the clotting mechanism; the latter is observed only when the dose limit of 1.5 mg/kg of body weight per day is exceeded. The antithrombotic properties of dextran are due to a decrease of platelet adhesiveness, depression of factor VIII activity, increased susceptibility of thrombi to fibrinolysis, and blood flow improvement [1,16]. The literature—mostly European—documents that in addition to their volume effect, both dextran preparations safely prevent postoperative deep venous thrombosis and fatal pulmonary embolism [16,17]. Besides their effect on blood clotting when the dose limit is exceeded, dextrans, like all other colloids, carry the rare risk of severe anaphylactoid/anaphylactic reactions, which are now preventable by hapten inhibition (see below).

Gelatin

Gelatin is the oldest clinically used colloidal plasma substitute. Three types, differing in source of raw material (collagen) and method of production, are in clinical use (Table 29-1).

The major difference between gelatins and other clinical colloids (dextran 70 and hydroxyethylstarch solutions with high or medium molecular weight—see below) is that gelatins have a lower average molecular weight. For this reason, the intravascular persistence of gelatin is shorter and the initial volume effect is less pronounced when compared with identical volumes of dextran 70. Nevertheless, animal studies and clinical experience indicate that normovolemia can be achieved by infusion of initially higher amounts and can be maintained by more frequent reinfusions. Since no dose limit—apart from the dilutional fall in red cell mass—exists for gelatin, considerable plasma volume replacement can be performed [28]. Lundsgaard-Hansen et al. [28] stress in particular the absence of a specific gelatin effect on the blood-clotting mechanism; conversely, however, gelatin has no antithrombotic properties (for side effects, see below), and recent reports suggest that it may interfere with the immunodefensive (opsonizing) and wound-healing functions of fibronectin [6,19,37].

Hydroxyethylstarch (HES)

HES is manufactured from amylopectin and consists of hydroxyethylated glucose molecules linked by α-1.4 bindings. In Europe at present, three main preparations are commercially available from different manufacturers.

High-molecular-weight Hydroxyethylstarch (HES 450/0.7)

The average molecular weight of this 6% solution is 450,000 in vitro, and the degree of substitution is 0.7, which indicates that 7 out of 10 glucose molecules are substituted by hydroxyethyl groups. The initially very large molecules are degraded in vivo by serum α-amylase rather rapidly to molecules in the range of about 70,000 MW; thus, the intravascular volume effect of HES 450/0.7 is comparable with that of dextran 70. Expansion of plasma volume in excess of the infused volume was not observed [22]. Jesch et al. [22] were the first to report on the increase of serum α-amylase as a result of infusion of HES. Although apparently of no pathogenic importance, this effect must be taken into account in patients with increased serum amylase levels, so as to avoid the false diagnosis of pancreatitis. The formation of an HES-amylase complex (macroamylase) has been demonstrated to cause this phenomenon [24] (for side effects, see below). The elimination of HES 450/0.7 follows a different pattern from that of dextran 70/60, because it is stored in the cells of the RES for a prolonged time [5,32]. To circumvent this problem, starch preparations with lower MW and faster elimination patterns have been introduced in Europe. In addition to its dilutional effect, HES 450/0.7 influences the clotting system by decreasing factor VIII activity [46]. Recent reports on fatalities suggest that large and repeated doses should be used with caution, to avoid bleeding complications [8,47]. Despite this problem, there is no clinical evidence that HES prevents thromboembolism.

Medium-molecular-weight Hydroxyethylstarch (HES 200/0.5, HES 200/0.62)

Medium molecular weight molecules, with an MW of 200,000 and a substitution degree of 0.5 to 0.62 (HES 200/0.5 and 200/0.62), have been employed for clinical use in form of hyperoncotic (10%) and isooncotic (6%) solutions. The volume-expanding effect appears comparable to 10% dextran 40 and 6% dextran 60/70, respectively. When used as a volume substitute, HES has no specific demonstrated advantages over dextran; whether the lower solution viscosity of these HES solutions is of any clinical significance remains to be demonstrated.

Low-molecular-weight Hydroxyethylstarch (HES 40/0.5)

HES 40/0.5 provides a volume effect comparable with the effect of gelatin preparations. During progressive hemodilution with HES 40/0.5, the colloid osmotic pressure of the plasma is not maintained; hence, HES 40/0.5 cannot be considered a satisfactory colloidal plasma substitute. Serum α-amylase increases in response to infusion of HES 40/0.5, as observed with the other HES preparations.

SIDE EFFECTS OF COLLOIDAL PLASMA SUBSTITUTES

Neither human serum albumin nor plasma protein solutions are free from the risk of anaphylactoid reactions. The majority of these reactions are mild and affect mainly the skin (flush, erythema, etc.); however, severe reactions, even fatal outcome from cardiac arrest, have been reported over the years. The incidence of adverse reactions is not high when compared with that of other drugs, but the risk of fatal outcome calls for special awareness. The incidence of adverse reactions to the various colloids varies considerably in the literature, most probably due to conceptual differences of the underlying studies; in general, retrospective studies have yielded lower figures than have prospective, randomized trials [42]. The situation can be summarized as follows.

1. Severe adverse reactions with severe hypotension and cardiac arrest have been observed after infusion of HSA and plasma protein solutions, with an overall incidence of less than 0.1 percent. A clinically applicable prophylaxis is not known.

2. The incidence of dextran-induced anaphylactoid/anaphylactic reactions (DIAR) is 0.07 to 1.1 percent [42, 43]. Cardiac arrest was observed in a higher frequency with DIAR than with plasma proteins, HES, or gelatin. This problem, however, has been solved by the introduction of an efficient prophylaxis by means of preinjection of monovalent hapten-dextran. Based on the finding that patients experiencing DIARs upon infusion of dextran solution do have high titers of preformed dextran-reactive antibodies of the immunoglobulin G (IgG) class that form noxious complexes with dextran molecules and thereby elicit anaphylactic reactions, the concept of hapten-inhibition of DIAR was developed [25,41]. By preinjection of 20 ml of monovalent hapten-dextran (MW 1000), the binding sites of the dextran reactive antibodies can be blocked and the formation of complexes prevented; consequently, the clinical reactions (DIAR) will not occur. This concept has been proven to work efficiently in the majority of all patients at risk [25,26,34].

3. The incidence of adverse reactions to gelatin depends on the type of gelatin preparation. The figures vary from 0.05 to about 10 percent [28,42,43]. Life-threatening and fatal reactions have been reported. Prophylaxis by histamine receptor (H_1 and H_2)–antagonists has been successfully introduced into the clinical routine by Lorenz et al. [27].

4. HES has not yet been used to the same extent as dextran and gelatin. The incidence of adverse reactions to HES appears to be around 0.1 percent. Life-threatening reactions also occur, although less often than with dextran 70 before hapten inhibition was introduced in 1981 [3]. The pathomechanism of these reactions remains unknown; since prophylactic measures against HES-induced side effects are not available, constant awareness for the risk of side-effects is required.

The clinician using colloids should be conscious of the possibility of untoward reactions and the principles behind their treatment. However, the low risk of these reactions and availability of prophylactic and therapeutic measures justify the use of either of these colloids.

OXYGEN-CARRYING SUBSTITUTES
Stromafree hemoglobin solution (SFH) and perfluorochemicals (PFC) appear to be the most promising candidates for blood substitutes in the future, provided the term *blood substitute* is restricted to oxygen-carrying capacity and volume properties. Preparations of both hemoglobin solution and PFCs have been administered to a few volunteers and to desperately ill patients. However, neither substance has been perfected for clinical use at this time.

Stromafree Hemoglobin Solution
Hemoglobin solution has been studied intensively as a potential blood substitute since Rabiner et al. [40] described a method for preparing hemoglobin solutions without stromal lipid contaminants (SFH). It was noted, however, that SFH, which should neither induce coagulation disturbances nor impair kidney function, presents two major disadvantages [23,33]. First, SFH leaves the intravascular space rapidly (with a half-life of 100–140 min) and is thus unable to maintain blood volume over an extended period of time. Second, due to the lack of the red cell membrane and the

subsequent bereavement of its intraerythrocytic milieu, the free hemoglobin exhibits a higher affinity for oxygen as compared with the intraerythrocytic hemoglobin [9,23, 33]. Therefore, SFH cannot serve as a blood substitute, even though it has a high oxygen-carrying capacity when compared with small amounts of oxygen physically dissolved in artificial colloids.

Various research groups in Europe and in the United States have put greater efforts into attempts to prolong the intravascular persistence and to reduce the oxygen affinity of SFH [4,7,9,14]. SFH was modified with the aims of stabilizing the tetrameric hemoglobin molecule by intramolecular bridging to prevent dissociation into dimers that are readily excreted or of creating hemoglobin polymers by intermolecular bridging. A promising approach to decreasing the high oxygen affinity of SFH is the introduction of a pyridoxal phosphate group; this concept was first tested in vivo by Jesch et al. [21,33] and subsequently by other authors [9,36,49]. Although both approaches have yielded hemoglobin solutions with prolonged intravascular persistence and acceptable oxygen affinity, a hemoglobin compound that could be applied in patients has not yet emerged. Further work is needed in order to determine whether the potential benefits (availability, long-term storage, absence of risk of transmitting diseases, etc.) will finally outweigh the imminent risks (immunogenicity, general and organ toxicity) of chemically modified SFH [11].

Perfluorochemicals
PFCs are solutions of dispersed perfluorocompounds, which became attractive candidates as substitutes for blood by virtue of their ability to dissolve oxygen in quantities comparable with the amount of oxygen bound chemically by hemoglobin. Owing to the linear relation between oxygen content and partial pressure (PO_2) with PFCs a high oxygen content is achieved only at an inspired oxygen fraction (FiO_2) of 0.7 to 1.0. Definite proof of the ability of PFCs to carry and to unload oxygen at the tissue level was demonstrated in experiments with total blood exchange for PFC or perfusion of isolated organs with PFC as sole oxygen carrier [12,38]. To use PFC as a blood substitute, it is mandatory to demonstrate that in dilutional anemia, in which some red cells are still circulating, oxygen is unloaded at the tissue level not only from the red cells, but, to a significant degree, also from PFC. The results from experiments with measurements of oxygen extraction from the red cell hemoglobin and the circulating PFC have so far not been convincing. With regard to in vivo storage and complete elimination from the body, the recently developed compounds (Fluosol-43, Fluosol-DA*) are definitely superior to the earlier fluorocarbons [38]. However, the elimination by excretion through the lungs of the material stored is protracted; the long-term sequelae of incorporated PFC have not been identified.

Since a high oxygen content of the PFC blood can be obtained in vivo only by means of ventilation with a high FiO_2, the detrimental effects of

*Green Cross Corp., Osaka, Japan.

high FiO$_2$ will necessarily limit the use of PFC in patients [13]. Although at present there is no PFC solution available for blood replacement in the clinical setting, the present and forthcoming perfluorocompounds can be useful for organ preservation [10].

SUMMARY

Plasma volume replacement is achieved most efficiently and safely with colloidal solutions, which provide a long-lasting volume effect and oncotic power without impairing the fluidity of the blood. The natural colloids (human serum albumin, pasteurized plasma protein solution), dextran 60/ 70, and some new hydroxyethylstarch (HES) solutions fulfill these criteria and are thus suitable for plasma volume replacement and treatment of hypovolemic shock. The specific physiochemical properties of gelatins limit the values of these solutions for long-term volume support. Low-molecular-weight starch (HES 40/0.5) cannot be considered a colloidal plasma substitute.

All colloids carry the risk of occasional anaphylactoid reactions; however, this is not a contraindication to their clinical use.

Neither human protein solutions nor human serum albumin should be used for volume replacement but should be preserved exclusively for patients with significant hypovolemia and hypoproteinemia.

Hemodilution induced by replacement of blood losses by plasma substitutes will not jeopardize the patient's oxygen delivery as long as the hemoglobin concentration does not fall below 8 dl/100 ml. Respiratory and coronary disease as well as increased oxygen demands might, however, motivate higher hemoglobin levels.

With respect to their volume effect, their specific antithrombotic effect, and the possibility of preventing anaphylactoid/anaphylactic reactions to dextran by preinjection of monovalent hapten-dextran, dextran solutions offer definite advantages.

New concepts and new efforts are needed before oxygen-carrying substitutes, such as stromafree hemoglobin and perfluorochemicals, can become clinically applicable as substitutes of blood.

REFERENCES

1. Åberg, M., Hedner, U., and Bergentz, S. E. Effect of dextran on factor VIII (antihemophilic factor) and platelet function. *Ann. Surg.* 189:243, 1978.
2. Alving, B. M., Hojima, J., Pisano, J. J., Mason, B. L., Buckingham, R. E., Mozen, M. M., and Finlayson, J. S. Hypotension associated with prekallikrein activator (Hageman Factor Fragments) in plasma protein fraction. *N. Engl. J. Med.* 299:66, 1978.
3. Beez, M., and Dietl, H. Retrospektive Betrachtung der Häufigkeit anaphylaktoider Reaktionen nach Plasmasteril® und Longasteril®. *Infusionstherapie* 6:23, 1979.
4. Bellelli, A., Brunori, M., Condo, S. G., and Giardina, B. Human hemoglobin cross-linked through the polyphosphate-binding site. *J. Biol. Chem.* 262: 2624, 1987.
5. Boon, J. C., Jesch, F., Ring, J., and Messmer, K. Intravascular persistence of hydroxyethyl starch in man. *Eur. Surg. Res.* 8:497, 1976.

6. Broden, B., Hesselvik, F., and von Schenck, H. Decrease of plasma fibronectin concentration following infusion of a gelatin-based plasma substitute in man. Scand. J. Clin. Lab. Invest. 44:529, 1984.
7. Chang, T. M. S., and Varma, R. Pyridoxalated heterogenous and homologous polyhemoglobin and hemoglobin: Systemic effects of replacement transfusion in rats previously received immunizing doses. Biomat. Art. Cells Art. Org. 15:443, 1987.
8. Damon, L., Adams, M., Stricker, R. B., and Ries, C. Intracranial bleeding during treatment with hydroxyethyl starch. N. Engl. J. Med. 317:964, 1987.
9. DeVenuto, F., and Zegna, A. I. Distinctive characteristics of pyridoxylated-polymerized hemoglobin. Progr. Clin. Biol. Res. 122:29, 1983.
10. Faithfull, N. S. Fluorocarbons. Current status and future applications. Anaesthesia 42:234, 1987.
11. Feola, M., Simoni, J., Canizaro, P. C., Tran, R., Raschbaum, G., and Behal, F. J. Toxicity of polymerized hemoglobin solutions. Surg. Gynecol. Obstet. 166:211, 1988.
12. Geyer, R. P. "Bloodless" rats through the use of artificial blood substitutes. Fed. Proc. 34:1499, 1975.
13. Gould, S. A., Rosen, A. L., Seghal, L. R., Seghal, H. L., Langdale, L. A., Krause, L. M., Rice, C. L., Chamberlin, W. H., and Moss, G. S. Fluosol-DA as a red-cell substitute in acute anemia. N. Engl. J. Med. 314:1653, 1986.
14. Gould, S. A., Rosen, A. L., Seghal, L. R., Seghal, H. L., and Moss, G. S. Efficacy of polymerized pyridoxylated hemoglobin solution as an O_2 carrier. Biomat. Art. Cells Art. Org. 15:359, 1987.
15. Gruber, U. F. Blood Replacement. New York: Springer, 1969.
16. Gruber, U. F. Dextran and the prevention of postoperative thromboembolic complications. Surg. Clin. North Am. 55:679, 1975.
17. Gruber, U. F., Saldeen, T., et al. Comparison of the incidence of fatal pulmonary embolism with dextran 70 and low dose heparin prophylaxis. An international multicenter trial. Br. Med. J. 280:69, 1980.
18. Gruber, U. F., Sturm, V., and Messmer, K. Fluid replacement in shock. In I. Ledingham (ed.), Shock, Clinical and Experimental Aspects. Amsterdam: Excerpta Medica, 1976. P. 231.
19. Imavari, M., Hughes, R., Gove, C., and Williams, R. Fibronectin and Kupffer cell function in fulminant hepatic failure. Digest. Dis. Sci. 30, 11:1028, 1985.
20. Isbister, J. P., and Davis, R. Should autologous blood transfusion be rediscovered? Anaesth. Intens. Care 8:168, 1980.
21. Jesch, F., Hobbhahn, J., Endrich, B., Peters, W., and Messmer, K. Improved in vivo oxygen delivery from stromafree hemoglobin by pyridoxilation. Pflüg. Arch. Europ. Physiol. 362:R16, 1976.
22. Jesch, F., Kloevekorn, W. P., Sunder-Plassmann, L., Seifert, J., and Messmer, K. Hydroxyäthylstärke als Plasmaersatzmittel. Untersuchungen mit isovolämischer Hämodilution. Anästhesist 24:202, 1975.
23. Jesch, F. H., Peters, W., Hobbhahn, J., Schoenberg, M., and Messmer, K. Oxygen-transporting fluids and oxygen delivery with hemodilution. Crit. Care Med. 10:270, 1982.
24. Köhler, H., Kirch, W., Weihrauch, T. R., Prellwitz, W., and Horstmann, H. J. Macroamylasemia after treatment with hydroxylethyl starch. Eur. J. Clin. Invest. 7:205, 1977.
25. Laubenthal, H., Peter, K., and Messmer, K. Prevention of dextran anaphylaxis. Münch. Med. Wochenschr. 124:951, 1982.
26. Ljungström, K.-G., Renck, H., Hedin, H., Richter, W., and Wiholm, B.-E. Hapten inhibition and dextran anaphylaxis. Anaesthesia 43:729, 1988.

27. Lorenz, W., Doenicke, A., Dittmann, I., Hug, P., and Schwarz, B. Anaphylactoid reactions following administration of plasma substitutes in man. Prevention of side-effects of Haemaccel by premedication with H_1- and H_2-receptor antagonists. *Anaesthesist* 26:644, 1977.
28. Lundsgaard-Hansen, P., and Tschirren, B. Modified fluid gelatin as a plasma substitute. *Prog. Clin. Biol. Res.* 19:227, 1978.
29. Lutz, H. *Plasmaersatzmittel* (4th ed.). Stuttgart: Thieme, 1986.
30. Messmer, K. Hemodilution. *Surg. Clin. North Am.* 55:659, 1975.
31. Messmer, K. F. W. Acceptable hematocrit levels in surgical patients. *World J. Surg.* 11:41, 1987.
32. Messmer, K. F. W. The use of plasma substitutes with special attention to their side effects. *World J. Surg.* 11:69, 1987.
33. Messmer, K., Jesch, F., Schaff, J., Schönberg, M., Pielsticker, K., and Bonhard, K. Oxygen supply by stroma-free hemoglobin. *Prog. Clin. Biol. Res.* 19:175, 1978.
34. Messmer, K., Ljungström, K., and Gruber, U. F. Prevention of dextran-induced anaphylactoid reactions by hapten-inhibition. *Lancet* 1:975, 1980.
35. Milles, G., Langston, H. T., and Dalessandro, W. *Autologous Transfusions.* Springfield, IL: Thomas, 1971.
36. Moos, G. S., Gould, S. A., Sehgal, H. L., and Rosen, A. L. Hemoglobin solution: From tetramer to polymer. *Surgery* 95:249, 1984.
37. Nagelschmidt, M., Becker, D., Bönninghoff, N., and Engelhardt, G. Effect of fibronectin therapy on fibronectin deficiency on wound healing. *J. Trauma* 27, 11:1267, 1987.
38. Naito, R., and Yokoyama, K. *Perfluorochemical Blood Substitutes "Fluosol-43", Fluosol DA 20% and 35%.* Technical Information Ser. No. 5. Osaka, Japan: Green Cross, 1978.
39. NIH Consensus Conference. Fresh-frozen plasma. *J.A.M.A.* 253:551, 1985.
40. Rabiner, S. F., Helbert, J. R., Lopas, H., and Friedman, L. H. Evaluation of stroma-free hemoglobin solution for use of a plasma expander. *J. Exp. Med.* 126:1127, 1967.
41. Richter, W., and Hedin, H. J. Dextran hypersensitivity. *Immunol. Today* 3:132, 1982.
42. Ring, J. Anaphylactoid Reactions. In *Anaesthesiology and Intensive Care Medicine* (Vol. 111). New York: Springer, 1978.
43. Ring, J., and Messmer, K. Incidence and severity of anaphylactoid reactions to colloid volume substitutes. *Lancet* 1:466, 1977.
44. Schriemer, P. A., Longnecker, D. E., and Mintz, P. D. The possible immunosuppressive effects of perioperative blood transfusion in cancer patients. *Anesthesiology* 68:422, 1988.
45. Surgenor, D. M. The patient's blood is the safest blood. *N. Engl. J. Med.* 316:542, 1987.
46. Stump, D. C., Strauss, R. G., Henriksen, R. A., and Saunders, R. Effect of hydroxyethyl starch on blood coagulation, particularly factor VIII. *Transfusion* 25:349, 1985.
47. Symington, B. E. Hetastarch and bleeding complications. *Ann. Intern. Med.* 105:627, 1986.
48. Toy, P. T. C. Y., Strauss, R. G., Stehling, L. C., Sears, R., Price, T H. et al. Predeposited autologous blood for elective surgery. A national multicenter study. *N. Engl. J. Med.* 316:517, 1987.
49. Tye, R. W., Medina, F., Bolin, R. B., Knopp, G. L., Irion, G. S., and McLaughlin, S. K. Modification of hemoglobin-tetrameric stabilisation. *Progr. Clin. Biol. Res.* 122:41, 1983.

50. Wasman, J., and Goodnough, L. T. Autologous blood donation for elective surgery. *J.A.M.A.* 258:3135, 1987.

SELECTED READINGS

Bergentz, S.E. (ed.). Program symposium—Hemotherapy. World J. Surg. 11:1, 1987.

Tuma, R.F., White, J. V., Messmer, K. The role of hemodilution in optimal patient care. *Zuckschwerdt München* pp. 1–146.

Management of the Critically Ill Immunodeficient Patient

Richard E. Wilson

It is crucial that physicians and surgeons caring for patients in an acute care situation be aware of the fact that the immunodeficient individual is at much higher risk for complications and death than is the patient with normal immune status. A patient whose immune functions are depressed requires special consideration in almost every aspect of care. These individuals require strong and constant psychologic support, as well as physical efforts, in order to do well. The major problem is that immunodeficient patients are usually chronically as well as acutely ill. Therefore, one often cannot separate the acute illness that rendered critical care necessary from the chronic disease that either was responsible for the acute episode or may complicate it. These patients require fluid and electrolyte homeostasis, hormone balance, sepsis management—both therapeutic and prophylactic—and, frequently, some sort of surgical procedure. Surgeons may often enter the scene late in the course of the illness, and it is essential that in such circumstances the surgeon be familiar with the major aspects of the underlying problems, with what type of surgery has been performed in the past, and with what sort of response has been achieved from surgery. The surgeon must also have a full knowledge of what medications are being administered, the reason for their use, and their potential risks. Only by careful attention to all aspects of the usually complex past and present status of these patients will one avoid serious acts of commission or omission in their management.

This chapter is divided into four sections, so as to best define the problems. The first section describes immune mechanisms in health, so that the reader can understand how the body usually responds to an immunologic challenge. New data are constantly being derived as we learn more about the various components of the immune system, but this broad overview will provide an update on the current status. The second section identifies alterations in the normal immune response system that can result in the immunodepressed state for patients. Specific deficits, when known, will be presented for the various components of the host response. The third section describes the types of patients seen in clinical practice who have deficits in their immune responses and points out the options available to the physician that might stabilize or improve responsiveness—or certainly, avoid a worsening of the defect. The fourth section discusses approaches to the clinical management of immunodeficient individuals and particularly concentrates on the responsibilities of and concepts for the surgeon faced with this patient population. Frequently, an event in the life of a patient with chronic immune deficiency makes a surgical procedure necessary, placing that patient in a situation requiring critical care.

IMMUNE MECHANISMS IN HEALTH

The human immune response system is very complex, but its primary function is to protect us from foreign antigens, particularly invasive organisms such as bacteria, viruses, and fungi. It has vast capabilities for identifying and responding to dangerous substances that have entered the body through the usual protective barriers, although many questions remain unanswered as to the ways in which one can control and orchestrate this system in any therapeutic manner. Homeostasis of all body mechanisms is the key, and it must be pointed out that acute disease states themselves can alter the homeostatic system and enhance any underlying deficiency state. It is necessary to study the component parts of the system and to define how the component parts interact to achieve the desired result.

Components of the Immune System

The two major components responsible for normal immune response are serum factors and cellular factors. Most of the serum factors are proteins, and many are produced either in the liver or in lymphoid tissues. Of the several immunoglobulins (Ig), IgG, IgA, and IgM are the three most involved with clinical immune responses. These have different functions, can be varied in their activities to match the stimulating antigen protein, and can work with or without another protein factor called *complement*. The production and activity of complement in itself is the subject of extensive investigations. There are yet other proteins present in the serum, whose exact functions, as well as how they integrate with antibody and cellular activities, have yet to be identified.

Antibodies themselves are secretions of B lymphocytes, usually manufactured in lymph nodes and the spleen. Complement, properidan, and clotting factors are primarily produced in the liver. Macrophages are responsible for interleukin 1 (IL1) whereas activated T lymphocytes are the natural sources of IL2, IL4, and IL6.

The level of IgG in the serum is 800 to 1500 mg/100 ml; of IgM, 40 to 120 mg/100 ml; and of IgA, 50 to 200 mg/100 ml. Further, four additional subclasses of IgG help to define differences in interaction with cells and complement. The immunoglobulin structure consists of a long Fc fragment (heavy chain) that reacts with complement and two Fab fragments (made up partly of the heavy chain and partly of light chains) that recognize and attach to antigens, giving the molecule unique specificity. Variable regions of the heavy chains give further specificity of response. The entire field of monoclonal antibody biochemistry is based on these unique capabilities of response of the IG molecule.

White cell populations circulating in the blood, and present within organs, are produced by the lymphoid tissue and bone marrow. They play an equally critical role in the immune response system. Leukocytes from the bone marrow are most responsible for attacking and engulfing acute bacterial infections, whereas lymphocytes—comprising many classes—are more involved with recognizing and responding to foreign tissues, viruses, fungi, and other microorganisms. The cellular and serum factors work in concert, stimulating each other, secreting additional factors, binding certain substances, and dealing with specific problems as they arise in the total immune effort. Macrophages play a tremendous role in the way the host recognizes foreign antigens. They provide information to the lymphocytes that permits appropriate responses and then serve to "mop up" the operation later. Macrophages are probably produced in the bone marrow, in lymph nodes, and in the liver and spleen and are part of the reticuloendothelial system of the body. We now know that there are many classes of lymphocytes, and with monoclonal antibodies to define the surface characteristics, their exact in vivo functions are constantly becoming better understood. Some lymphocytes can kill other foreign cells or microorganisms directly, some require coupling with additional lymphocytes, and some require interaction with complement. Growth factors secreted by macrophages and activated lymphocytes—such as the interleukins—are exceedingly important in the processes by which the body responds properly to disease-producing organisms. Without the appropriate "helper T" lymphocyte, immunoglobulin is not produced by plasma cells. Without the appropriate interleukin, lymphocytes cannot become activated and respond. These are only some of the incredibly broad aspects of the components we now understand are responsible for orchestrating the immune response system.

As stated, cellular responses are achieved by white cells and macrophages, without the requirement for antibody or complement. This type of cell-to-cell contact and destruction of foreign cells requires specific "activation," usually of T lymphocytes, which produce a large array of mediators that are critical for normal immune responses (Fig. 30-1). It is certainly not yet known how all these factors work and how many more will be defined, but their identification has entirely changed the concepts of the immune response system. Just to demonstrate how incredibly complex this system is, contact between a T lymphocyte and a specific antigen leads to the production of a host of mediators that probably serve to carry out the immune function of the activated T lymphocyte. These mediators include migration inhibition factor (MIF); macrophage-activating factor (MAF); skin reactive factor; transfer factor; cytotoxic factor, or lymphotoxin; interferon; macrophage-specific chemotactic factors; lymphocyte permeability factor; osteoclast-activating factor; aggregation factor; soluble suppressor factors; and growth-stimulating factors, including macrophage growth factor, IL1, T-cell growth factors, IL2, and others.

The various lymphocyte populations have been defined by their surface membrane characteristics as identified by specific monoclonal antibodies

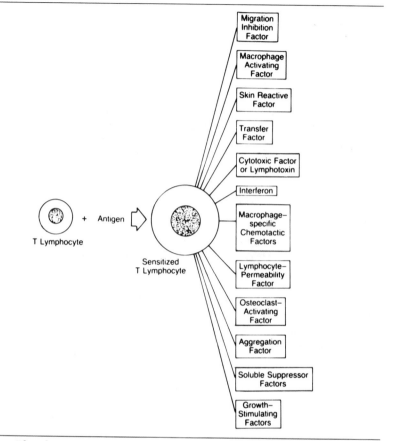

Fig. 30-1. This diagram emphasizes the large number of factors that may be released from a sensitized T lymphocyte. Not all of the biologic functions of these lymphokines are known. Many of them can now be produced by genetic engineering techniques in large quantities and used for clinical therapy. This is particularly true of such specific products as interferon and the interleukins, which are growth-stimulating factors. (From R. E. Wilson, *Surgical Problems in Immuno-Depressed Patients.* Philadelphia: Saunders, 1984. P. 5.)

to their surface structures. Types of lymphocytes that have been classified are cytotoxic T lymphocytes, suppressor T lymphocytes, helper T lymphocytes, null lymphocytes (no surface markers), and natural killer lymphocytes, as well as B lymphocytes—precursors of plasma cells that secrete antibody. The large variety of cells and mediators is probably produced to allow careful modulation and exquisite control of the entire immune system in the normal state.

Measurement of Immune Responses

Efforts to measure immune responses have been much more crude than have those that have been directed toward identifying its components.

Many factors are known to be present, but their functions are only partially understood. Likewise, the ability to measure the quantity of a given cell does not necessarily tell us that the cell is doing anything. Nonetheless, we must make the attempt to define with some degree of accuracy what an individual's immune response is. We can carry out skin testing for foreign antigens to tell us whether responses are either delayed or immediate. Delayed responses are generally cell-mediated in nature, whereas immediate responses are usually antibody-mediated. Antibodies are measured either in the test tube (if there is an antigen that it can respond to appropriately) or by surface testing, either in the eye or on the skin. When a known antigen is placed intradermally, antibody response can occur with immediate redness or a wheal; cellular responses are represented by reaction with the antigen at a later time—usually 24 to 72 hours. The delayed reaction is an intradermal reddened and locally tender nodule that eventually subsides. The response can be quantitated by the size of the nodule in 48 hours, and various standard substances can be used to test the host reactivity. Responses to a new antigen (dinitrochlordenzene) can be used as a standard quantitative mechanism and has been applied to study patients with cancers and trauma. Investigators now can identify types of lymphocytes in the circulating blood that change in response to acute and chronic disease, in hopes that this type of quantitation will be more valuable. It is by this technique, for instance, that patients with acquired immune deficiency syndrome (AIDS) have been defined. They have a specific defects in the distribution of their T-cell subpopulations.

The most important facts for the clinician to be aware of are that: (1) immune responses are multifactoral in nature, (2) they are generally working to strengthen the host immune response in the most efficient manner, and (3) there are many pathways through which interactions of the various components can achieve a satisfactory result. However, the complexity of immune responses also makes it possible for alteration, dysfunction, and, sometimes, total failure. This is what leads to immunodeficient patients.

CIRCUMSTANCES THAT RESULT IN IMMUNE DEPRESSION
Simply put, three general categories of abnormalities are responsible for immune alterations: (1) congenital deficiencies of components of the immune system, (2) drugs and other therapeutic agents that induce alteration of immune responses, and (3) disease states that are either autoimmune or result from invading microorganisms, particularly viruses, that alter the responses of the host. This last-named category also includes acute trauma; operative procedures, including splenectomy; and anesthetic effects.

Congenital Deficiencies
These abnormalities are generally grouped together under the term *immunodeficiency diseases*. The most profound of the primary immunodeficiency diseases are types of "severe combined immunodeficiency" (SCID), which involves both T and B cells. It should be recognized that essentially all of these syndromes occur in children, and most of them are associated with shortened life spans and a high incidence of tumor induction. There are four subtypes of SCID, depending on the type of stem cell

that is deficient. It is possible for children to have preservation of B-cell function with primarily a T-cell abnormality, whereas other patients may have an abnormality in B-cell function resulting in hypogammaglobulinemia, with T cells being relatively normal. Many of these individuals have other types of congenital dysfunction as well. Finally, some groups have defects in effective function but have cell populations apparently present and available. In the most common of these disorders, Wiskott-Aldrich syndrome, there appears to be an abnormality in the way the cells interact in the afferent loop of the immune response.

Drug-Induced Immune Suppression

A very common group of patients whose immune functions are less than normal comprises those receiving one or another type of drug therapy. Probably the most common drugs in clinical use that affect immune responses are the adrenal corticosteroids. Unfortunately, these are used widely for a tremendous number of illnesses. Because they are often very effective, it is common for patients on steroid therapy to take these drugs chronically—sometimes intermittently, sometimes constantly. Steroids are used following organ transplants; as part of chemotherapy courses for malignancy, especially in patients with leukemia, lymphomas, brain tumors, or breast cancer; and frequently, as part of the treatment for chronic asthma, inflammatory bowel diseases, and autoimmune syndromes. They are often administered rather indiscriminately for arthritis and many other common inflammatory diseases without concern for their consequences.

Corticosteroids have many effects on both macrophage and lymphocyte function—which, of course, is why they are such effective antiinflammatory agents (Fig. 30-2). Macrophages are the major site of production of IL1, and this action is reduced by corticosteroids. In addition, there is decreased DNA synthesis, decreased membrane stabilization, and reduced RNA synthesis within the lymphocytes. Liposomal membranes in the lymphocyte lose their stability and rupture more easily. Finally, the general lympholytic action reduces the actual number of lymphocytes available. Alterations in acute responses to infection, antibody release, and wound healing are all part of the price one has to pay for treating patients with corticosteroids. In the acute care situation, one must be particularly alert to the "muting" effect of the normal inflammatory response in both acute disease and trauma, as well as the requirement for exogenous corticosteroid support to keep up with increased demands of both physical and mental stress. Corticosteroid administration depresses adrenocorticotrophic hormone (ACTH) production by the pituitary, thus preventing the normal response by the adrenal gland to stressful circumstances.

Immunosuppressive therapy for transplant recipients almost always includes corticosteroids. Several other agents usually added to steroids all have specific actions against portions of the immune system. Azathioprine (Imuran) alters purine metabolism and has a marked effect on cell replication and DNA synthesis. Since all cellular components of the immune system require a recruitment of cells, there is a purposeful reduction in T-cell replication which affects both antibody and cellular responses.

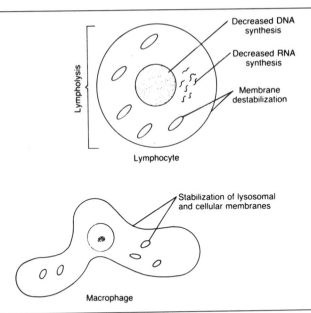

Fig. 30-2. This figure demonstrates the dramatic cellular effects on lymphocytes and macrophages of corticosteroid therapy. In the lymphocyte, there is decreased DNA and RNA synthesis and destabilization of cell surface and intracellular membranes. There is a general reduction in the numbers of lymphocytes, as well. Macrophages demonstrate stabilization of intracellular lysosomal membranes, reducing effective phagocytosis and chemotaxis. (From R. E. Wilson, *Surgical Problems in Immuno-Depressed Patients.* Philadelphia: Saunders, 1984. P. 52.)

Antilymphocyte sera directly attack lymphocytes; depending on the markers against which the sera have been raised, one or another population of circulating T cells is more susceptible. The same is true of antithymocyte serum, which directs its attack against the cytotoxic T lymphocyte. Cyclosporine A, which is of much more recent vintage, apparently directs its action toward preventing graft rejection and establishing immunologic unresponsiveness to a graft by preventing precursor cytotoxic T lymphocytes (CTL) from ever becoming responsive to IL2. Without IL2, these cell populations will not grow and proliferate in a manner necessary for any immune response. B cells and macrophages do not seem to be affected by the cyclosporine A. At one time it was thought that cyclosporine also stimulated the production of suppressor T cells and reduced the number of CTLs in vivo. As new information about the intercellular metabolism of immune responding cells becomes available, reevaluation of the roles of substances that affect immune responses must be carried out, as has been done with cyclosporine A. Other drugs used in cancer chemotherapy have an immunosuppressive effect, including methrotrexate, which is a purine metabolism inhibitor; and 5-fluorouracil, which competes with the production of pyrimidines. Many drugs widely used in cancer therapy have not been specifically tested for immune alteration, but since all of them affect cell growth, it would be no surprise if all had some immuno-suppressive effect.

Disease States Responsible for Altered Immune Function

Most of the disease states that result in abnormalities of immune function are related to viral infections. Cytomegalovirus (CMV), Epstein-Barr virus (EBV)—responsible for infectious mononucleosis—and various hepatitis viruses are all believed to be, to varying degrees, sources of immune-suppressed states. Currently, the most catastrophic of viral agents responsible for alteration in immune function is the human immunodeficiency virus (HIV), which is responsible for AIDS. Viruses have unique ways of getting into cells once they have attached to the cell membrane, and they can even be carried for generations. During an individual's life span or in the life of his or her offspring, virus particles may become activated to produce abnormal disease states. One of the ways that oncogenes may be activated is through the presence of a viral infection that changes the membrane characteristics of a specific cell. Many mutations thought to be spontaneous in the body may actually be induced by this mechanism. The net result, however, is that viral infections can reduce immune activity and, sometimes, totally eradicate component parts of the immune arc in a random manner.

This seems to be the mechanism by which HIV produces its destructive effect. It appears to induce a progressive, time-dependent destruction of T4 helper lymphocytes, possibly by blocking T4 receptor sites. The absence or marked reduction of the T4 helper-inducer cells and a marked disproportion in their relationship to the T8 suppressor cells are incompatible with normal immune function. This reversal of the T4 : T8 ratio, which normally is approximately 2:1 in favor of T4, was one of the initial methods of diagnosing AIDS. Now, HIV itself can often be recognized by antibody titer levels. Apparently, the ubiquitous and unstable protein coat of the virus is what makes vaccine production unsuccessful. The best test on the horizon for identifying HIV infection is definition of HIV antigenemia.

Other patients have diseases secondary to immune disorders. These diseases, almost all of which are associated with some sort of vasculitis, include polyarteritis, systemic lupus erythematosus, Sjögren's syndrome, polymyositis, adult and juvenile rheumatoid arthritis, and scleroderma. These patients all can be demonstrated to have abnormal immune complexes. Autoimmune reactions against the patient's own tissues produce a great variety of lesions that are usually associated with some sort of alteration of the immune system. In many of these patients, antinuclear antibodies (ANA) also provide part of the evidence of the disease.

Finally, traumatic injuries or surgery, such as splenectomy, can increase the risk for some degree of immune suppression. Increased suppressor cells are seen in patients with splenectomy, along with inadequate production of IgM antibodies—the first response to acute infection. However, most adult splenectomy patients without underlying hematologic disorders do not suffer from these immune suppressive effects.

TYPES OF PATIENTS IN CLINICAL SETTINGS WITH IMMUNE DEFICIENCY

Organ Transplant Recipients

Most numerous in this group are patients who receive kidney transplants; less common are recipients of liver, heart, pancreas, and even lung transplants. Most kidney transplant recipients resume relatively normal lifestyles, so they are subject to the same diseases and injuries as the normal population. Thus, such a patient might easily appear in a critical care situation in a hospital following trauma. In order for their transplants to survive and function, these patients must suffer from general lymphocyte depletion. They demonstrate relative increases in suppressor T lymphocytes—which make cytotoxic T cell activity much more limited—and have all of the abnormalities of corticosteroid administration. Cyclosporine-A is also being administered to more and more transplant recipients, at least for the short term, and its effect on IL2 is dramatic.

The main problem in all transplant recipients is sepsis. The physician should be alert to this possibility and consider both administering prophylactic antibiotics in the apparently healthy patient put under a critical care situation and proceeding with aggressive and early antibiotic therapy for anybody who demonstrates a febrile process. Transplant recipients may be faced with a host of ancillary problems, so whenever such a patient is under critical care for one disease, the physician must be alert to the possibility that many of the patient's organ systems may also become less efficient. Many patients—particularly renal transplant recipients—have undergone splenectomy, one should be aware of whatever long-term effect this may have on the management of acute infection. Finally, corticosteroid administration can produce a significant incidence of steroid-induced diabetes in transplant recipients, and this must be carefully monitored in transplant patients who are acutely ill.

AIDS Patients

Patients with AIDS are no longer a rarity, particularly in large urban centers. Their immune depression is dramatic. HIV initiates a progressive killing off and disappearance of T4 lymphocytes from the circulation, and thus the immune system deteriorates. The most severe problem in the AIDS patient is that posed by infectious complications (see below). Patients with pre-AIDS may already have a degree of immune suppression that makes them more susceptible to the complications of AIDS without inducing full-blown T4 lymphocyte elimination. Unusual septic complications combined with the spontaneous initiation of malignancies—particularly Kaposi's sarcoma—constitute the most lethal aspects of the HIV infection.

Corticosteroid Therapy

All patients treated with corticosteroids have decreased cellular immune responses. The most disturbing aspect of corticosteroid therapy is the dampening of inflammatory responses, which makes it more difficult to diagnose acute illness. Unfortunately, many individuals receive corticosteroids, especially prednisone, and a large number do not even know they are taking one of these drugs. Corticosteroids are often given for rashes, all sorts of inflammatory states, and joint and muscle discomfort, as well as in situations in which documentation of disease has not even been made. In a critical care situation, therefore, one must be certain to quiz patients and their families to learn whether they have been on corticosteroids within the past year. It should be remembered that steroids are sold under many names! Even though the patient may appear to be perfectly normal, the adrenal and pituitary do not function adequately for at least a year after the last steroid treatment. Replacement therapy is absolutely essential, and failure to implement it may result in hypotension, shock, and, eventually, death.

Malignant Disease as a Cause of Immune Suppression

Certain specific diseases, particularly Hodgkin's lymphoma, are associated with a relative degree of cellular immune alteration. Skin grafts will survive longer in Hodgkin's patients, and they are considered to be poorly responsive to skin testing. These immune changes seemingly have nothing to do with the prognosis of Hodgkin's lymphoma and do not affect all patients with this disease. Advanced-stage malignancy is also associated with a reduction in immune response, although for different reasons. Protein synthesis is remarkably abnormal, and cachexia from continued growth of the tumor is apparent. There is very little evidence that patients with early malignancy have any immune alteration. Certainly, no specific factors have been successfully identified, and until recently there has been very little evidence that any form of immune therapy has altered the survival rate of patients with advanced cancer. New studies with substances such as lymphocyte-activated killer cells (LAK) with IL2, interferons, tumor-infiltrating lymphocytes (TIL), and tumor necrosis factor (TNF) may change this outlook. Untoward effects with these agents must always be looked for, particularly pulmonary congestion and water retention.

Chemotherapy

Chemotherapeutic agents generally have a major effect on immune responses, as has already been mentioned. The type of agent(s) and the dosage(s) used are best correlated with the immune effects. Alkylating agents, such as cyclophosphamide, and the nitrogen mustards affect cell replication on the part of the host and greatly alter bone marrow function. Antimetabolites, which interfere with purine and pyrimidine metabolism, do not allow adequate immune cell reproduction in the face of specific requirements. Other chemotherapeutic agents, such as intercalators and alkaloids, apparently are less immunosuppressive. Nonetheless, anyone on chemotherapy—either as adjuvant therapy or for advanced disease—should be more carefully monitored and specifically supported as necessary.

Splenectomized Patients

Whether the operation was done therapeutically or for trauma, splenectomized patients have altered responses in their immune functions. For most, the alteration becomes less significant with time. IgM production, in response to bacterial antigen, is markedly slowed in this circumstance, and there is also some T-cell alteration initially after splenectomy. Children—especially those with hematologic disorders—have a significantly greater immune deficiency and should always receive prophylactic antibiotics. At the present time, all patients with splenectomy or a history of splenectomy are given pneumococcal vaccine (Pneumovax) to protect against infection with pneumococci and other encapsulated organisms.

Immune Suppression Associated with Acute and Chronic Diseases

It is well known that all major surgical procedures, as well as just general anesthetic, are associated with some increase in suppressor cells, reduction in T4 lymphocytes, and significant alterations in lymphokine production. These changes are usually short-lived and are directly related to the size and extent of the operative procedure and the length of administration of the anesthetic. If normal recovery is complicated, however, the postoperative changes can be much more protracted and important.

Patients being treated with chronic hemodialysis have significant alterations in T-cell function, but these are not sufficient to allow skin grafts to survive permanently. Patients with chronic burns and acute septic processes, such as thermal burn, pneumonia, and undrained abscesses, all demonstrate reduced capability of the host to respond to an immunologic challenge. Chronic infections that alter immune function are mostly viral. However, patients with inflammatory bowel diseases, hepatitis, and chronic draining infectious sinuses will often have severe nutritional deficiencies. When placed in a critical care situation, such patients are far more susceptible to the consequences of immune dysfunction.

GENERAL AND SPECIFIC APPROACHES TO THE MANAGEMENT OF IMMUNE-SUPPRESSED PATIENTS

It is critical that patients with acute medical and surgical problems be screened for alterations in immune function. Recognition of immune defects is the key first step in trying to counter them. (This is not nearly so true in the chronic situation, in which added stress and additional problems are not impacting on the patient's immune capabilities.) Upon recognition, one must look for associated problems that can be corrected.

Should a deficit in immune responsiveness be identified, or even suspected, then it is important to define the defect. In some circumstances, specific therapy can be instituted; on other occasions, techniques of immune augmentation might be available. Finally, it is crucial to either treat the defect or take it into account when managing a patient with any type of critical injury. In many patients in critical care situations, the physician has so many simultaneous problems to consider that the potential for immune abnormality is forgotten. Other diseases and injuries may obscure the presentation, so the physician must be even more alert to this problem when people are ill.

Recognition of Immune Deficit

The history is by far the most important source of information about these patients prior to the manifestation of an immune deficiency. Information from the patient's history, the family, and any available records is crucial. In looking for evidence of immune insufficiency, the physician should pay particular attention to the intraoral and lung areas, the presence of adenopathy, splenic enlargement or its absence, the cardiopulmonary status, and skin lesions. Colorectal abnormalities—particularly diverticulitis and constipation—must also be protected against in this group of patients. For individuals with transplants, knowledge of the drugs used and the function of the transplant is necessary. For patients with malignancies, information as to the stage of the disease and prior treatment is required, and the use of radiation therapy should also be documented. Once again, the potential for occult steroid therapy is very important, as is knowledge of whether or not the patient is taking chemotherapy.

Chronic illnesses, such as ulcerative colitis and inflammatory bowel disease or rheumatoid autoimmune states, should also be sought for and well-documented. One must look for metabolic derangements in these patients, as in any patient, and be certain that electrolytes are in good order. Acute burn injuries are associated with increased suppressor cell activity, decreased macrophage function, and lymphokine abnormalities, and this combination may increase immune deficiency. Prophylactic antibiotic therapy for potential sepsis must always be part of the management of these individuals in an acute care situation.

Associated Problems in Immunosuppressed Patients

In the critical care setting, whatever the instigating factor of the illness, the most frequent association between reduced immune function and critical injury is the development of sepsis. Although standard antibody production is reduced in many of these patients, it is white cell alteration, including leukocytes, lymphocytes, and monocytes, that usually contributes to sepsis as the major cause of death in immunosuppressed patients. There are vague aspects to the problem, such as a decrease in the host resistance, difficult to quantify; reduced repair function for damaged tissue; alteration in psychologic response producing depressive states; and finally, the fact that the diagnosis of the injury or illness for which the patient is in the critical care facility may have only been made with difficulty and after significant delay. It must be reiterated that the entire panoply of interactive immune functions—including the addition of complement, lymphokines, and receptors—must function effectively to combat potentially lethal components of major illness.

It is not redundant to stress that the consideration of sepsis is critical with patients who are known to be immunodepressed and who are in acute care situations. Aggressive workup for sepsis, be it potential or proven, must be done with rapid culture for any potential source—as a patient with a fever of unknown origin would be evaluated. Remember that unusual organisms can be present in unusual locations in these patients. The infections are often opportunistic ones by organisms that usually are not significantly pathogenic in man. One must consider selection of antibiotic therapy before the diagnosis is completely established, in order to provide as early an attack on the sepsis process as possible. Knowledge of the spectrum of organisms in these patients helps to decide which antibiotics one should select.

The patient with AIDS has the most serious risk of sepsis of almost any group of individuals with immunodeficiency. In a recent paper, Glatt et al. [1] identified six basic principles associated with the diagnosis and treatment of HIV-associated infections. These principles may be paraphrased as follows.

1. Fungal, parasitic, and viral infections may be controlled during an acute infectious episode, but they are almost impossible to cure. Long-term suppressive therapy is required to keep these infections under control, and they tend to flare up intermittently as changes in immune response occur.
2. As is the case with other severely immunodepressed individuals, most HIV-associated infections result from endogenous organisms that were acquired in the past and do not represent a threat to the medical staff or the family. Only tuberculosis, herpes zoster, and, possibly, salmonellosis can be transmitted.
3. Infections are usually multiple, with multiple organisms involving many sites. Second infections, rather than drug failure, may be the cause of a poor response.
4. The frequency of specific fungal and parasitic infections observed in HIV-infected patients depends to some degree on the ambient incidence of these infections in the community. This is particularly true for fungal infections. Diagnosis of HIV-associated infections will be helped by knowledge of where the patient came from and what exposure he or she may have had to such opportunistic infections.
5. Certain bacterial infections are now accepted as HIV-associated diseases. The association may specifically be that functional defects in B cells in HIV patients permit these organisms to invade and grow in the host more effectively.
6. Infections associated with HIV disease are usually more severe and more disseminated than they are in other patients. They are frequently characterized by a very high density of organisms, making therapy even more difficult.

This is not a chapter on sepsis, but the AIDS patient is an obvious example of the complex problems involved in the total management of immune-deficient critically ill patients. An acute awareness of the complicating features in patients with HIV infections on the part of the lay public and the medical profession will impact on all other patients with immunodepressed states.

More than 80 percent of patients with AIDS will acquire *Pneumocystis carinii* pneumonia, and in 60 percent it is the initial opportunistic infection. As would be expected, the presenting findings may be either typical or atypical. Other infections in this population include central nervous system toxoplasmosis, cryptococcal meningitis, disseminated avium-intracel-lulare, tuberculosis, disseminated CMV infection, herpes simplex, herpes zoster, salmonellosis, candidiasis, and cryptosporidiosis. Fortunately, tri-methoprim and sulfamethoxazole (Bactrim) and the newer agent zidovu-dine, an antiretroviral drug, have produced a significant number of re-sponders with many of these diseases. Glatt et al. [1] cover the major pathogens in advanced HIV disease and discuss what can be done for them.

AIDS complications represent a tremendous exaggeration of all the other septic problems seen with immune-suppressed patients. The enormity of the distribution of infection, the total loss of the T4 subsets of lymphocytes, and the incurable status of the disease make the maximum complicating circumstance of loss of immune control. Many other patients with de-creased immune responses who are in critical care facilities are not so un-treatable, however. In either case, the lessons are clear: one must find sep-sis and treat it as early as possible, preserving as much immune capacity within the patient's own system as possible. Pulmonary, oral, central ner-vous system (CNS), enteric, urologic, and wounded tissue are the most common sites of sepsis in these patients. Extra care should be taken to evaluate each of these locations, and cultures should be repeated fre-quently. This is the only way that meaningful reduction in septic compli-cations will occur in a patient who is capable of responding. One must be aware of the risks associated with infected indwelling central venous cath-eters in the acute care facility. This may be especially true because these catheters may have been inserted in an emergency situation. One should not hesitate to change central lines over a wire, or to remove the lines com-pletely, to rule out that site as a septic source.

Underlying gastrointestinal problems, such as esophagitis, perforated and bleeding ulcers of the upper gastrointestinal tract, perforated diverti-culitis, and perianal abscesses, can be very insidious in this patient popu-lation and much harder to diagnose than in normal individuals. Acute pan-creatitis and acute cholecystitis occur in people with gallstones who have been unable to eat and then resume eating too quickly. Beware of the ste-roid diabetic, since those patients require additional insulin when they are acutely ill. Finally, one must be concerned about thrombophlebitis and pulmonary embolism in this patient population. To begin with, these pa-tients are often chronically ill, many have some degree of cardiac disease, and most are much less ambulatory than they might have been previously. Significant changes occur continually in the platelet level and other coag-ulopathy factors during any critical illness. Should an operation be re-quired, the development of phlebitis and emoblization is an obvious po-tential complication for which these patients are at greater risk than any other type of nonoperative individual. The use of subcutaneous heparin and protective stockings and boots should always be considered part of the management.

Cardiovascular complications are not rare in immunosuppressed pa-tients, because in many of them cardiovascular abnormalities are part of the disease process responsible for reduced immune competence. Hypertension and coronary artery disease are common in patients who had been in renal failure prior to renal transplant and who received many months or years of hemodialysis. The key is to recognize underlying disease processes while managing the acute problem that brought the patient to a critical care facility.

Surgical Care in the Immunodeficient Critically Ill Patient

Key factors to remember in attempting to achieve a successful outcome for surgical therapy in this patient population include the following.

1. These patients are extremely fragile, and maintenance of homeostatic mechanisms is far more difficult than it is even in other critically ill individuals.
2. Utilize extra efforts in planning and executing surgical procedures.
3. Do not hesitate to obtain expert consultation to help manage complicating aspects of the patient's care.
4. It may be necessary to vary the usual surgical approach for a given problem: operative procedures may require staging, more-straightforward or simplified approaches may be necessary, and special attention should be given to methods of drainage and wound closure.
5. Exaggerated postoperative risks require more-aggressive postoperative approaches. More monitoring, more-thorough and more-frequent evaluations, and earlier reoperation should be considered if surgical-type complications develop.
6. Healing is frequently delayed after any surgical procedure in the majority of these patients, usually because of underlying therapeutic aspects of their care. This holds true for surgery performed in any part of the body. Corticosteroids are the most serious offender in this regard.

The critically ill immune-depressed patient with acute abdominal complaints typifies the clinical problem for the surgeon. The evaluation and care of the "acute abdomen" serves as a prototype for the surgeon's dilemma in all aspects of this field.

Although the patient's history of the present illness remains the most valuable method of identifying acute abdominal disease, the symptoms may often be minimal. Complaints may be delayed or altered, and bizarre settings may exist in presentation. Pain, distention, nausea, vomiting, and a history of fever or jaundice are pressing issues and must be considered promptly. Evaluation of each and every complaint, no matter how small, must be reviewed in the critically ill individual. The surgeon must examine all complaints in the light of the patient's critical episode and with the previous history in mind. Findings on physical examination, even in patients complaining of acute abdominal problems, may be less apparent or outright confusing. For example, pain and tenderness in the scrotum may actually be the result of perforated diverticulitis in a transplant recipient who has total absence of abdominal pain and demonstrates only slight abdominal tenderness.

The examiner must look for subtle deviations from the norm. Always think of those problems that could be lethal to the patient—such as perforation of a viscus (stomach, gallbladder, bowel), an undiagnosed abdominal abscess, mesenteric vascular injury, or undefined bleeding. After the initial evaluation, frequent follow-up examination may be necessary to finally identify a specific acute disease state. These reexaminations may have to be done as often as every 2 or 3 hours. Obviously, in approaching the acute abdomen, the surgeon is always reevaluating the question of whether or not laparotomy should be performed, and when. Peritoneal tap or lavage may frequently help to define problems that require laparotomy. The exploratory laparotomy is still the surgeon's method of identifying intraabdominal disease when all other approaches are inconclusive. Laparotomy should neither be rushed into too early nor delayed until nothing can be accomplished for the patient. If pathologic processes are found, simple procedures should be employed in the critical care situation. "Divert, drain, and decompress" should be the watchwords.

Fortunately, many new diagnostic tests and procedures are now available to help the surgeon avoid unnecessary laparotomy, including endoscopy of both the upper and lower gastrointestinal tracts, endoscopic examination of the biliary tract and pancreatic ducts, real-time ultrasound (with the potential for ultrasound-directed needle biopsy or aspiration), and HIDA and other radionuclide scans to define biliary disease in the acute situation. More complex to obtain but extremely valuable are computed tomography (CT) scanning and magnetic resonance imaging (MRI). Both of the last-named tests require sophisticated equipment that is not available at all hospitals, and both present greater logistic difficulties in terms of performance on a given patient. The CT scan is most useful for studying the spleen (looking for infarct or rupture), the kidney, and the liver and for diagnosing diverticulitis, both ruptured and unruptured. Ultrasound is especially valuable for defining gallbladder disease, searching for abscesses, and studying the female pelvis. Barium studies can be most useful in looking for mucosal disease of the intestinal tract. Plain x-rays of the abdomen, as well as selected barium studies, are best for evaluating obstructive complaints. The experience of the surgeon, in collaboration with the radiologist, should guide selection of the best and most effective examinations to be performed.

In the final analysis, however, the surgeon must decide what steps to take in patients presenting with an acute abdomen. In immunodepressed patients, the diagnosis is more difficult, but the risks of delay can be greater. Immunodepressed individuals who are critically ill with abdominal disease may not survive such an acute episode unless the problem is corrected. The chronic state of debility from which many of these patients suffer limits the "physiologic reserve" to deal with sepsis and trauma. Natural defense mechanisms are often reduced or nonfunctional, and reparative processes are much less efficient. Successful treatment of the critically ill immune-deficient patient requires aggressive and expeditious evaluation of the problem, experienced decision making to correct the acute disease whenever possible, and the extensive use of supportive therapy—such as blood products and antibiotics—in an attempt to improve patient response. It is especially important to avoid splenectomy for splenic injury. Many approaches are available to achieve splenic preservation (Fig. 30-3).

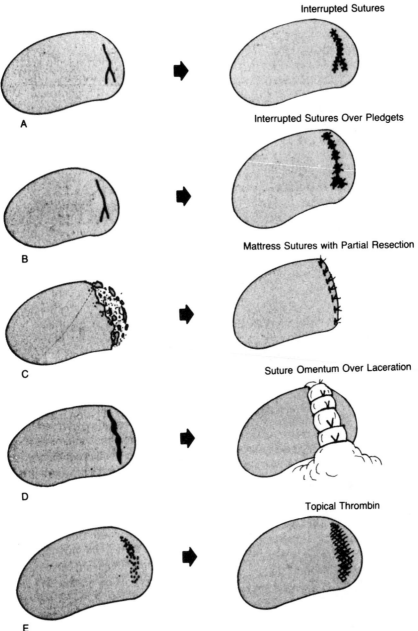

Interrupted Sutures

Interrupted Sutures Over Pledgets

Mattress Sutures with Partial Resection

Suture Omentum Over Laceration

Topical Thrombin

A

B

C

D

E

Fig. 30-3. In this diagram, several techniques of splenorrhaphy are demonstrated. Whenever possible, traumatic injury of the spleen should be treated with splenic preservation. Shallow lesions, as in A and B, can be treated with single interrupted sutures over pledgets. Partial resection and control of hemostasis by through-and-through mattress sutures may be required (C), and deep lacerations may be controlled by plication of omentum into the wound (D). Superficial bleeding may sometimes be controlled by pressure and topical thrombin or other coagulating agents (E). (From R. E. Wilson, *Surgical Problems in Immuno-Depressed Patients.* Philadelphia: Saunders, 1984. P. 85.)

Sometimes it is possible to temporarily reverse the immune abnormality and allow recovery from a life-threatening complication. With better understanding and diagnosis of the specific immune deficit, more-effective therapy can be selected to accomplish this goal. The use of lymphokine infusions, growth factors, cytotoxic lymphocyte and macrophage preparations, and large doses of monospecific antibodies are techniques that are on the horizon. Thus, it is imperative that the expertise of many scientific disciplines be called into play to help manage this very special, and ever-enlarging, group of complicated patients.

REFERENCES

1. Glatt, A. E., Chirgwin, K., and Landesman, S. H. Treatment of infections associated with human immunodeficiency virus. *N. Engl. J. Med.* 318:1439, 1988.

31

Critical Care of the Transplant Patient

Lucile E. Wrenshall *David E.R. Sutherland*
Arthur J. Matas *R. Morton Bolman*
William D. Payne *Frank B. Cerra*

GENERAL PRINCIPLES OF PRE- AND POSTOPERATIVE CARE

Organ transplantation has become an accepted form of therapy for end-stage disease in many organ systems. Improvements in graft and patient survival have increased the numbers of centers offering this form of therapy to the patient populations they service. Concomitantly, indications for transplantation have broadened, and age limitations have expanded to include both younger and older patients. The list of contraindications has decreased as well, so that increased numbers of less-healthy patients are being considered as possible candidates for transplantation. Consequently, the need for intensive care unit (ICU) monitoring/therapy in the pre- and postoperative care of these patients continues to grow, making the ICU team an integral part of any transplant program. Finally, without ICU support of the potential donor, the majority of this work would, of course, be impossible.

In general, the need for ICU therapy in the transplant recipient is determined by the type of transplant planned, as well as the medical status of the patient. This may be determined by a thorough preoperative evaluation. Routinely, this assessment begins with a complete history and physical examination, a chest x-ray, an electrocardiogram (ECG), and several laboratory studies (see Table 31-1), including blood and tissue typing.

Patients with evidence of coronary artery disease should undergo cardiac sonogram and further evaluation by a cardiologist. Coronary angiography should be performed, if warranted, so that clinical lesions may be corrected prior to transplantation.

Similarly, patients with a history of or symptoms consistent with peptic ulcer disease should undergo endoscopy and if ulcer disease or gastritis is found, appropriate medical therapy. Transplantation should be deferred until the ulcer is no longer present. In some instances, definitive surgical therapy may be necessary prior to transplantation. Routine gallbladder ultrasound is also performed on all patients, with pretransplant cholecystectomy considered if cholelithiasis is found (except for liver transplant recip-

729

Table 31-1. Laboratory and radiologic evaluation of the transplant patient

Laboratory	Radiologic
Hepatitis B profile	Chest x-ray
Viral titers	Gall bladder ultrasound
Urine, throat culture	Upper GI series*
CBC, electrolytes, liver function tests	Lower GI series*
VDRL	Cardiac catheterization*
HTLV III	

*When indicated by patient history.

ients). This eliminates the risk of sepsis secondary to cholecystitis after transplantation.

Assessment of compliance is another important part of the pretransplant evaluation. At the University of Minnesota, potential renal transplant recipients who have demonstrated noncompliance on dialysis are given a trial period of 6 months. If during this time they show a willingness to comply with prescribed medications, diet, etc., they are then considered for transplantation.

Finally, other general preoperative considerations include weight loss for the overweight/obese patient, cessation of smoking, and treatment of any acute/chronic infections.

The pretransplant evaluation allows for definition of the individual risks of each potential recipient. General contraindications to transplantation include disseminated malignancy and active sepsis. Relative contraindications include acquired immunodeficiency syndrome (AIDS), a history of substance abuse, noncompliance, hepatitis, and advanced disease in an organ system outside that being considered for transplantation.

Once the patient is accepted as a transplant candidate, the decision as to whether he or she will need postoperative ICU monitoring can usually be made prior to transplantation. This decision is, of course, always subject to change, depending on the patient's intraoperative and immediate postoperative course. Some patients, and especially heart transplant recipients, will need preoperative ICU management as well. Liver and cardiac transplant recipients routinely require ICU care postoperatively. Kidney and pancreas transplant recipients may need ICU monitoring, depending on the age of the patient, extent of debilitation due to primary disease, or other risk factors such as significant coronary artery disease. Patients with ischemic or valvular heart disease may additionally benefit from preoperative pulmonary artery catheterization with optimization of end diastolic volume and systemic vascular resistance.

Postoperative management of a transplant recipient follows the general principles of postoperative care, with special attention to parameters that indicate proper functioning of the allograft received. Liver and cardiac transplant recipients routinely require mechanical ventilation for at least 24 hours posttransplantation. Nasogastric suctioning is utilized for recipients with intraabdominally placed grafts until gastrointestinal function returns. Patients requiring mechanical ventilation are maintained on nasogastric suction as well. Once the nasogastric tube is discontinued, oral alimentation may usually be initiated as tolerated. Pneumatic stockings are routinely worn intraoperatively and postoperatively until the patient is able to ambulate frequently, in order to prevent thromboembolism. Early ambulation is both encouraged and enforced by the nursing staff.

Laboratory data—such as hemoglobin, electrolytes, arterial blood gases, and liver function tests—are monitored closely in the early postoperative period. The emphasis on which tests are obtained most frequently varies with the type of transplant performed. Serial chest x-rays are often obtained, both for assessment of the lung fields and for confirmation of correct placement of all lines and tubes.

Common prophylactic medications are administered irrespective of the type of transplant received. Antacids are given for protection against stress ulceration and the ulcerogenic side effects of steroids. Parenteral antibiotics are utilized for perioperative antibacterial coverage. Nonabsorbable antifungal agents are administered for oral *Candida* prophylaxis, and trimethoprim/sulfamethoxazole is utilized for prophylaxis against *Pneumocystis carinii*. Finally, at the University of Minnesota, oral Acyclovir is given to most solid-organ transplant recipients for the first 3 months posttransplantation, in an attempt to prevent lethal cytomegalovirus infection.

A three-drug immunosuppression regimen consisting of azathioprine, cyclosporine A (CSA), and prednisone is utilized at the University of Minnesota for recipients of all types of solid-organ transplants. Antilymphocyte globulin is included in some protocols as well. The drug dosages differ for each type of transplant, however, as illustrated in Table 31-2. Adjustments in drug dosages may be necessitated by the toxic side effects of these immunosuppressive agents. Specifically, azathioprine dosage may be decreased or withheld for patients whose white blood cell count falls below 4000 cells/μl. Similarly, with patients receiving cyclosporine A, renal function must be followed closely, because of the well-documented nephrotoxicity of this drug. An increase in serum creatinine may necessitate a decrease in or temporary withdrawal of CSA therapy.

The general principles of pre- and postoperative care of the transplant patient are similar, irrespective of the organ received. Dissimilarities exist, however, in certain aspects of patient selection, in the timing of the transplantation, and in the extent of ICU therapy needed in the perioperative period. Parameters for monitoring graft function and specific complications vary as well. These differences are outlined for each type of transplant in the following sections.

RENAL TRANSPLANTS

Renal transplantation has become the treatment of choice for most patients with end-stage renal disease. Improved quality of life and decreased cost are two major advantages of this form of treatment over dialysis. The fact that postoperative ICU monitoring/therapy is not necessary for most renal transplant patients aids in increasing the cost-effectiveness of this procedure. Patients requiring ventilation or invasive pulmonary artery catheter

Table 31-2. Immunosuppression protocols for solid organ transplants at the University of Minnesota for the first postoperative month

	Immunosuppressive drug dosage (mg/kg/day)							
Type of allograft	CSA	POD#	AZA	POD#	P	POD#	ALG	POD#
Kidney—LRD	10 (bid)* 8 Dosage adjusted to maintain CSA levels 100–200 ng/ml.	−2, −1 1–30	5 (qd) 4 3 2.5	0–2 3–5 6–11 12–30	1 (qid) 0.75 (bid) 0.5 0.45 0.4	0–5 6–8 9–17 18–20 21–30	None	
Kidney—cadaver	8 (bid) Dosage adjusted to maintain CSA levels 100–200 ng/ml.	6–30	5 (qd) 2.5	0 1–30	1 (qid) 0.75 (bid) 0.5 0.45 0.4	0–2 3–8 9–17 18–20 21–30	20 (IV)	0–7
Liver	0.75 (IV continuous infusion) gradually increased to 3 → adjusted to maintain trough level 250–350 ng/ml. 10 (po) replaces IV CSA when oral intake initiated		2.5	1–30	1 (IV) 2	0 1 → taper to 0.1 by 3 months	None	

Pancreas—cadaver	14	0.125 (mg/kg/h continuous IV infusion) → adjusted to maintain trough level 300 ng/ml. 8 (po) replaces IV CSA when oral intake initiated → CSA level maintained at 200 ng/ml.	0	5 2.5	0–6 7–30	2 1	0 1 → taper to 0.5 by day 30	Randomized to ALG 20 (IV) or OKT$_3$ 5 (IV) for 1st postoperative week
Heart	8–10 (bid) Adjust to keep CSA levels approximately 200 ng/ml.	1–30		2.5	1–30	1	1 → taper to 30 mg/day by end of first end of first month	None

qd = single daily dose; bid = two divided doses; qid = four divided doses; IV = intravenous administration.

monitoring and those with hemodynamic instability may require the ICU for short periods of time, however. Identification of the high-risk patient who may need ICU monitoring is facilitated by the preoperative evaluation.

Several risk factors in renal transplantation must be considered in the initial assessment of each patient. Relative contraindications to transplantation include a history of hepatitis B, chronic cardiac failure, aortoiliac disease, chronic pulmonary disease, and noncompliance. In patients having renal diseases with a high recurrence rate, the benefits of transplantation must be weighed against the probability of recurring disease in the transplanted organ. Diseases such as oxalosis, scleroderma, focal segmental glomerulonephritis, mesangiocapillary, glomerulonephritis types 1 and 2, and Henoch-Schonlein purpura are included in the latter category. Patients with renal failure secondary to systemic disease (diabetes mellitus, amyloidosis, systemic lupus erythematosus, etc.) need a thorough assessment of the degree to which other organs have been affected by the disease process. Diabetics, for example, with a high documented incidence of coronary artery disease and decreased symptomatology, should routinely undergo a complete cardiac evaluation prior to transplantation. Finally, patients with a recent history of malignancy also need special consideration. Those with localized disease that is judged to be eradicated are observed for 1 year following treatment. If there is no evidence of recurrence during this time, the patient is then considered as a possible transplant candidate.

For the patient with a history of genitourinary problems, special attention is directed toward assessment of the urinary tract. This is best accomplished by the use of a voiding cystourethrogram. Vesicoureteral reflux, outflow obstruction, bladder dysfunction, and significant postvoid residual volume must be ruled out. Due to the risk of infection in the native kidneys, most patients with significant (grade III or IV) vesicoureteral reflux should undergo bilateral nephrectomy with excision of both ureters at the ureterovesical junction. Other indications for pretransplant nephrectomy include (1) renin-dependent hypertension that cannot be controlled medically, (2) renal failure resulting from pyelonephritis with persistent bacilluria, (3) polycystic kidney disease complicated by infection or hemorrhage, (4) proteinuria producing uncontrollable nephrotic syndrome, and (5) kidneys diverted into GI conduits or skin ureterostomies [7].

Pretransplant blood transfusions are a part of the preoperative regimen in many transplant centers. Prior to the use of CSA, recipient transfusions from random third-party donors were found to have a beneficial effect on both living related and cadaveric graft survival. With the advent of CSA, the continued practice of random pretransplant blood transfusion has been controversial. In one study, the use of pretransplant transfusions with CSA was found to be beneficial; in another, equally successful results were obtained in untransfused cadaver recipients immunosuppressed with CSA [9, 15].

For recipients of living related donor (LRD) kidneys, many centers have incorporated donor-specific transfusion (DST) into their pretransplantation protocols. The DST procedure involves the administration of 200 ml of fresh whole blood (or packed cell equivalent) on three separate occasions at 2-week intervals. Azathioprine is administered concomitantly to decrease donor-specific sensitization. DST has been shown to increase long-term graft survival in one-haplotype-matched donor recipient pairs. Limited experience with short-term follow-up of zero-haplotype-matched pairs has also shown an increase in graft survival [26]. The DST effect in light of cyclosporine A usage is currently under study.

At the University of Minnesota, random donor transfusions are utilized for cadaver, living related, and living unrelated donor recipients. DST is no longer used, because of the risk of sensitization (despite the use of azathioprine) of the recipient.

At the time of operation, immediate pretransplant preparations involve optimizing the patient's metabolic and volume status. Acidosis, hyperkalemia, and volume overload may be corrected by dialysis. Patients utilizing continuous ambulatory peritoneal dialysis may actually be volume-depleted and require restoration of plasma volume preoperatively. Unless indicated by evidence of tissue ischemia, as on ECG, transfusing patients up to a hemoglobin of 10 to 12 gm/dl is not routinely practiced. In settings of advanced ischemic or valvular heart disease with previous or current medical/surgical therapy, preoperative pulmonary artery catheterization with optimizing of end-diastolic volume and systemic resistance may be a beneficial therapeutic tool on a case-by-case application. As noted in Table 31-2, immunosuppression is instituted in the immediate pretransplant period as well. As a final preparative step, a Foley catheter is inserted in all recipients, and the bladder is irrigated with an antibiotic solution prior to initiation of the operation.

Postoperative management consists of the previously outlined postsurgical care, with special attention paid to fluid and electrolyte balance. The patient should not be allowed to become hypovolemic. Assessment of volume status can be facilitated by the use of central venous pressure (CVP) monitoring. The CVP is used in conjunction with physical parameters such as heart rate, blood pressure, and urine output to maintain a euvolemic state. In high-risk settings or whenever the clinical setting warrants, a pulmonary artery catheter with measurements of cardiac output, systemic vascular resistance, and capillary wedge pressure can be very helpful. If the graft is immediately functional, urine output is replaced cc/cc for the first 24 hours, after which time a decreasing percentage of the urine output is replaced. The patient is tapered to a maintenance fluid replacement, which is discontinued when the patient has an adequate oral intake. The Foley catheter is kept in place for 3 to 5 days. In the immediate postoperative period, patients (especially LRD recipients) may have a urine output exceeding 500 cc/hour. For these patients, as well as diabetics, an intravenous solution of $D_1 0.45NS$ is utilized. Nondiabetics with urine outputs less than 500 cc/hour receive $D_5 0.45NS$. Potassium chloride may be added to the intravenous solution at a concentration of 10 to 20 mEq/liter or greater, depending on the serum and urine potassium. Serum potassium is monitored every 4 hours for the first 24 hours posttransplantation. Other electrolytes, as well as blood urea nitrogen (BUN) and serum creatinine, are obtained in the recovery room and then repeated on a daily basis. Serial hemoglobins (every 4 to 6 hr) are also obtained for the first 24 hours.

The above intravenous fluid regimen is appropriate for the polyuric patient. Some (primarily cadaveric) grafts, however, do not function immediately. Multiple donor, preservation, and recipient factors have been implicated in the pathogenesis of delayed graft function (DGF). Once the diagnosis of DGF is made, the fluid intake of the patient is minimized. Dialysis also may be needed until renal function is initiated. Correct diagnosis of the etiology of oliguria/anuria is extremely important, as management of the possible diagnoses differs widely. A schema for the logical evaluation of oliguria/anuria is depicted in Figure 31-1.

Rejection, as noted in Figure 31-1, is another important cause of oliguria/anuria in the early posttransplant period. Types of rejection occurring at this time point include hyperacute, accelerated acute, and acute. Hyperacute rejection is mediated by preformed antibodies in the recipient and is usually evident at the time of operation. The kidney will be soft and dusky in color despite patent anastomoses. Immediate nephrectomy is the only treatment. Accelerated acute rejection occurs in the first few days posttransplantation and is probably due to undetectable presensitization to donor human leukocyte antigens (HLA) or vascular endothelial cell (VEC) antigens. Acute cellular (T cell) rejection does not usually occur before the first 1 to 2 weeks posttransplantation. It is manifested clinically by low-grade fever, mild hypertension, weight gain, and graft tenderness. Urinary output and creatinine clearance are decreased, accompanied by an increase in serum creatinine. Other possible causes of decreased urinary output must be ruled out, as previously discussed. Diagnosis of acute rejection is suggested by decreased uptake and excretion of 131I-Hippuran, as well as edematous renal papillae demonstrable by ultrasound. Definitive diagnosis requires biopsy of the graft. Most of the many existing protocols for treatment of rejection include an initial increase in steroid dosage (intravenously or orally) and the subsequent addition of ALG or OKT3 if no improvement is seen. At the University of Minnesota, acute rejection episodes are initially treated by an increase in prednisone dosage to 2 mg/kg/day. This dose is subsequently tapered at the rate of 0.25 mg/kg every three days. The decision to administer OKT3 or ALG is based on (1) histologic diagnosis, (2) initial clinical response to prednisone, and (3) number and proximity of prior rejection episodes.

The immunosuppression protocol used at the University of Minnesota is designed to minimize both the number of rejection episodes and the risk of CSA nephrotoxicity in the early posttransplant period [27]. Cadaver recipients, who are particularly at risk for delayed graft function, receive ALG for the first postoperative week. CSA, which has been shown to prolong delayed graft function, is withheld until the fifth postoperative day. This regimen has been known to lower the number of early rejection episodes and to shorten hospital stay in cadaver recipients with documented delayed graft function [18]. LRD recipients, with a significantly lower risk of delayed graft function, do not receive ALG. They are begun on CSA

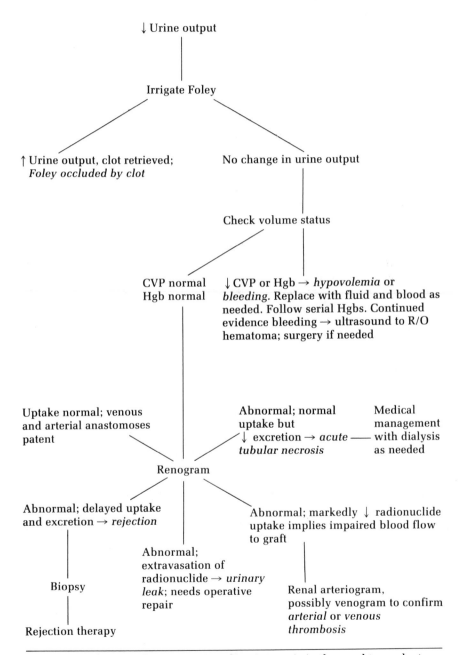

Fig. 31-1. Evaluation of postoperative oliguria/anuria in the renal transplant recipient.

preoperatively, which is continued immediately following transplantation. Specific dosages and routes of administration are outlined in Table 31-2. Routine prophylactic medications are administered as previously discussed.

Several complications of renal transplantation may occur in the early posttransplant period. These include primarily vascular, urologic, and, less commonly, infectious sources. Vascular complications, previously reported to be as high as 30 percent, have decreased to 0.1 to 0.3 percent [32]. The primary manifestations of vascular complications in the early postoperative period are hemorrhage and occlusion. Anastomotic leaks and unligated bleeding vessels may present within the first few hours of operation. Rupture of the allograft is an unusual cause of massive hemorrhage [11]. Delayed hemorrhage is commonly due to infection and may result in anastomotic disruption or formation of a false aneurysm.

Arterial occlusion within the first few hours postoperatively is usually due to mechanical trauma, technical error, or hyperacute rejection. Allograft loss is almost inevitable. Arterial thrombosis occurring later than the initial postoperative period is usually a result of immunologic sequelae.

Venous occlusion, which occurs less commonly than arterial occlusion, is manifested by swelling of the graft and proteinuria. Iliac vein thrombosis is often revealed by swelling of the ipsilateral lower extremity. Common causes of venous thrombosis include external compression, technical error, and extension of deep venous thrombosis. Successful venous thrombectomy has been reported, but nephrectomy is usually required [32]. Noninvasive Doppler ultrasound is useful in the evaluation of iliofemoral venous blood flow.

Urologic complications occur in approximately 1 to 15 percent of renal transplants. Up to 60 percent of these complications are ureteral leaks, which may be due to a damaged blood supply with subsequent necrosis, technical complications, or poor healing secondary to infection or immunosuppression [4]. Urinary extravasation is manifested by a decrease in urine output, flank pain and fullness, or leakage of fluid through the wound. The diagnosis is established by ultrasound or hippuran scan, as well as by comparison of serum, urine, and fluid creatinine. Surgical repair is indicated; results of repair vary widely.

Infection, although a significant cause of morbidity and mortality in the transplant patient, is less commonly problematic in the immediate postoperative period. Causes of infection in this time period include pretransplant infection of the recipient, infection of the allograft, and infection related to the surgical procedure itself. Examples of pretransplant recipient infection include hepatitis and "cold abscesses" secondary to *Staphylococcus aureus* or *Mycobacterium tuberculosis* [34]. These abscesses may become activated in the posttransplant period, resulting in disseminated disease. The primary concern in acquisition of infection from the allograft is the possible transmission of hepatitis B or human T-cell leukemia virus type III (HTLV-III). Therefore, *all* donors should be tested for these diseases. Any donor in the high-risk group for AIDS should be disqualified, regardless of serology. Infections related to the surgical procedure itself include wound infection, urinary tract infection, and pneumonia. These can be prevented or significantly decreased by rigorous attention to detail during the surgical procedure (preventing hematomas, urinary leaks, etc.), perioperative antibiotics, sterile technique while placing all lines and catheters, and subsequent removal of these objects as soon as possible.

LIVER TRANSPLANTS
Within the last two decades, liver transplantation has changed from an experimental procedure to an accepted form of therapy for end-stage liver disease and some metabolic disorders. From 1978 to the present, 1-year survival rates have increased from 30 to 70 percent and 5-year survival rates have risen from 18 to 60 percent [12]. Better patient selection, improvements in perioperative care, and cyclosporine have contributed to these increased survival rates. Concomitantly, the number of centers performing liver transplantation has increased as well, although such centers generally are confined to those with 24-hour in-house physician coverage. Knowledge of potential problems in the perioperative care of the liver transplant patient should therefore be included in the data base of the surgical resident.

Criteria for selection of potential transplant candidates include the presence of progressive, irreversible liver disease; medical/surgical intractability; and absence of absolute contraindications. Despite the aforementioned improvements in survival, these requirements have remained fairly constant. There has been an increasing trend, however, toward moving back the time in the progression of the patient's disease when transplant is considered to a point at which the mortality risk in the next year exceeds 50 percent. This practice has resulted in greater numbers of recipients of improved risk for major operative intervention.

Contraindications to liver transplantation include active extrahepatic sepsis, extrahepatic malignancy, advanced cardiac disease, and AIDS. Relative contraindications—such as advanced chronic renal disease, advanced age, portal vein thrombosis, hepatitis B surface antigen and E antigen positivity, extensive right upper quadrant surgery, and alcoholic liver disease—are also carefully considered when determining appropriate candidates for liver transplantation. The most common liver diseases for which patients receive liver transplants are chronic active hepatitis, primary biliary cirrhosis, and sclerosing cholangitis.

The timing of the transplant is important. Although the most critically ill patients are given the highest priority on waiting lists, it is mandatory to attempt transplantation while the patient is still able to withstand the surgical stress. This is not a minor consideration, in that the surgery may exceed 12 hours in duration and is frequently accompanied by significant transfusion requirements. Complications of liver disease that indicate the necessity for transplantation include refractory ascites, recurrent variceal bleeding, recurrent spontaneous bacterial peritonitis, recurrent cholangitis, severe hepatic osteodystrophy, and intractable pruritus. Patients with recurrent spontaneous bacterial peritonitis or cholangitis should be treated for a minimum of 4 to 5 days preoperatively with systemic antibiotics, to prevent infection following transplantation. Complications that postpone liver transplantation usually involve organ systems outside the liver and include infection, ischemic heart disease, cardiomyopathy, and acute pulmonary disease [10].

The recipient of a liver transplant enters the ICU in the immediate postoperative period. Almost all patients have an increased extravascular fluid volume with a reduced intravascular volume. Frequently, left ventricular compliance is reduced, and mild acute lung injury with increased lung water is present. Several days of mechanical ventilation are often required. There is usually a coagulopathy as well, both from the significant intraoperative blood loss and from hepatic malfunction due to temporary ischemic damage in the revascularized grafted liver. A fresh frozen plasma infusion of 50 to 100 ml/hour is usually necessary for control of this problem, along with platelet transfusions to keep the platelet count at 75,000 to 100,000 cells/μl. The citrate load frequently contributes to a metabolic alkalosis. This metabolic alkalosis frequently is only responsive to hydrochloric acid infusion, 0.1 or 0.2 N, by central vein.

Early postoperative care at the University of Minnesota consists of continuous monitoring of blood pressure via arterial line, assessment of filling pressures and cardiac function via Swan-Ganz catheter, and close attention to urine output. Resuscitation is pursued until a state of flow-independent oxygen consumption is achieved. This approach ensures adequate perfusion of the graft and vital organs. Laboratory assessment consists of every-6-hour coagulation parameters (prothrombin time, partial thromboplastin time, thrombin time), hemoglobin, electrolytes, and arterial blood gases. Clotting factors V and VIII, as well as fibrinogen, are obtained twice daily. Liver function tests are obtained daily. Graft function is monitored primarily through production of clotting factors and the clearance of bilirubin, lactate, and amino acids. Mental status, urine output, and biliary tube (if present) output are important clinical indicators of early graft function [12]. Biliary drainage output tends to decrease over the first 36 to 72 hours and then to increase again in the well-functioning liver. Biliary tube drainage may not reflect this pattern.

Radiologic studies are obtained as indicated. A hepatobiliary nuclear scan is obtained on postoperative day 1 and as needed thereafter. Liver excretory function, patency of the biliary tract, and possible biliary leakage can be assessed with this study. A duplex ultrasound is also obtained on the first postoperative day, to confirm patency of the vascular anastomoses. Finally, if a biliary tube is present, a cholangiogram is obtained on the fifth postoperative day to evaluate the biliary tract.

Multiple medications are routinely necessary in the early postoperative period, for support of cardiac and renal function, fluid management, immunosuppression, and infectious disease prophylaxis. Loop diuretics are often required to remove excess fluid volume acquired intraoperatively. Spironolactone may be helpful as well, both for diuresis and for conservation of serum potassium. In most cases, a period of myocardial dysfunction occurs that may require the use of inotropic agents, such as dopamine/dobutamine, or preload/afterload-reducing agents, such as nitroprusside/

nitroglycerin, to maintain an adequate cardiac output and prevent or treat pulmonary edema. This myocardial dysfunction is usually a combination of both reduced compliance and reduced contractility, with the former usually dominating. The Swan-Ganz catheter is extremely helpful in determining the need for and efficacy of the above agents. In most patients, postoperative hypertension will occur. It is usually catecholamine-mediated and responds well to calcium-channel blockers.

Routine prophylactic agents are administered as previously noted. Immunosuppression for liver transplant recipients is given as outlined in Table 31-2. CSA, which requires bile salts for absorption, must be administered intravenously in the initial postoperative period to maintain adequate whole-blood trough levels. The intravenous CSA is discontinued when oral alimentation is initiated. The initial oral dose (10 mg/kg/24 hr) is adjusted to maintain therapeutic levels and to avoid nephrotoxicity. Continuous attention to the patient's renal function is essential. In the immediate postoperative period, intravenous CSA is frequently associated with acute oliguria and sodium retention in the presence of adequate perfusion. High doses of loop diuretics, along with maintenance of adequate blood volume, may overcome the problem. If a rapid response does not occur, CSA may have to be temporarily reduced or discontinued, until adequate urine flow is restored (1.0–1.5 ml/kg/hr).

Nutritional support is usually begun on the second postoperative day by the enteral and/or parenteral route. Enteral nutrition is administered by nasoduodenal or nasojejunal tube. Calories are supplied as glucose, 5 gm/kg/day, with the use of long-chain fatty acids restricted for the first 5 to 7 days. These are subsequently begun at a dose of 0.5 to 1.0 gm/kg/day. Protein supplementation is initiated at 1.5 to 2.0 gm/kg/day, usually as high branched-chain amino acid. The dose is adjusted to achieve nitrogen equilibrium with a BUN less than 110 mg/dl and a respiratory quotient (RQ) below 0.9.

Hepatically metabolized drugs, such as narcotic analgesics and tranquilizers and sedatives, should be used in low doses and as infrequently as possible. Their metabolism appears to be unpredictable in the first 5 to 7 days posttransplantation.

Surgical complications following liver transplantation most commonly involve bleeding and patency of the vascular and biliary tract anastomoses. Bleeding is often a problem due to the large raw surface area created in a patient with a decreased clotting capacity. The risk of bleeding is greatest within the first 48 hours following transplantation. The status of clotting-factor production is not necessarily a reliable indicator of hepatic function. Reasonable levels can be maintained in the presence of a poorly functioning graft. Late postoperative bleeding may occur as well, often as a result of percutaneous diagnostic procedures.

Vascular complications may involve the portal vein, hepatic artery, or inferior vena cava. Thrombosis is most often seen in the hepatic artery [16]. Clinical manifestations of hepatic artery thrombosis vary in severity from asymptomatic to septic shock secondary to hepatic necrosis. Fever with gram-negative septicemia is seen in most cases of hepatic artery thrombosis. Other common clinical patterns include delayed biliary fistula and relapsing bacteremia, persistent hypermetabolism with multiple organ failure syndrome, and hepatic abscesses with absence of liver tissue in some areas. Laboratory examination reveals elevated transaminase levels. Serum bilirubin eventually rises as cholestasis ensues. Blood cultures often grow gram-negative organisms. Doppler ultrasound can be utilized to assess patency of the hepatic artery anastomosis and to detect any biliary leaks. Arteriography is recommended for confirmation of the vascular diagnosis. Treatment of clinically significant hepatic artery thrombosis almost invariably requires retransplantation.

Inferior vena caval stenosis or thrombosis is an occasional occurrence that presents as a Budd-Chiari syndrome, with hepatic vein dilatation, hepatic congestion, and progressive ascites refractory to medical therapy. In addition, lower-extremity venous hypertension with or without thrombosis may occur. Stenosis may be managed by balloon dilation; thrombosis is treated symptomatically and may require retransplantation.

Portal vein thrombosis also occurs occasionally. It may be asymptomatic or may present as bowel edema and pseudoobstruction, pancreatitis, or ascites. Treatment is symptomatic; retransplantation may be necessary.

The incidence of biliary complications in liver transplant patients is approximately 13 percent [16]. The majority occur within weeks of transplantation, although complications such as stricture can occur late. The most common early postoperative complication related to the biliary tract is leakage. Bile leaks most frequently occur at the biliary tube choledochotomy but can occur at the anastomotic site as well. Leakage from the donor biliary tree at sites other than the anastomosis is especially serious and most likely represents bile duct necrosis secondary to hepatic artery occlusion. Clinically, bile leakage is manifested by abdominal pain, fever, leukocytosis, anomalous bile drainage, increased serum bilirubin, alkaline phosphatase, and gamma GTP. Precise location of the leak is best determined by cholangiography. Small leaks at the biliary tube exit site in an asymptomatic patient may be treated conservatively. All other larger, clinically significant leaks are repaired surgically.

The second major biliary tract complication, obstruction, usually becomes apparent later in the postoperative course. Causes of this complication include ischemic stricture (anastomotic and nonanastomotic), retained biliary stent, T-tube dysfunction, allograft cystic duct remnant mucocele, and common duct redundancy. Clinical presentation can follow one of several patterns: cholangitis with fever, chills, abdominal pain, and gram-negative bacteremia; recurrent low-grade fevers with fluctuating liver enzymes; and gradual rise in liver function tests without associated symptoms. The manifestations of gradual obstruction, although less severe, may be mistaken for rejection. Ultrasound may be used as an initial screening test, but the false-negative rate is high. Definitive diagnosis is made by cholangiography. Localized obstructions warrant a trial of percutaneous balloon dilatation. Treatment failures or generalized dilatations require surgical treatment.

Other surgically related complications include intestinal obstruction, perforation, abdominal sepsis, and wound infection or hematoma.

Medical problems following transplantation include infection, hepatic dysfunction, and renal insufficiency. The side effects of immunosuppression contribute to some of these problems. Major bacterial infections occur in 40 percent of patients in the early posttransplant period. Common types of bacterial infection in these patients are pneumonia and abdominal abscess. Fungal infections can also occur in the early posttransplant period, with *Candida* and *Aspergillus* serving as the major pathogens. Preoperative steroid and antibiotic administration, operating time greater than 6 hours, and increased use of postoperative antibiotics and immunosuppressants all increase the risk of fungal infection. Viral hepatitis is the most common infectious cause of hepatic dysfunction in the postoperative period. Cytomegalovirus infection primarily manifests betweeen 3 and 6 weeks following transplantation. Therefore, it is especially important to avoid the false diagnosis of allograft rejection during this time period. This can be done by obtaining a liver biopsy if rejection is suspected. Recurrent hepatitis B, which may also be problematic for the liver transplant patient, rarely occurs prior to the second postoperative month [16].

Hepatic function is monitored by serum levels of bilirubin and liver enzymes. An early elevation in serum transaminase (prior to day 3) may indicate primary graft dysfunction, which usually results from injury at the time of harvest or preservation. Other signs/symptoms of ischemic injury include sluggish bile flow, progressive jaundice, severe coagulopathy, and metabolic acidosis. Diagnosis is made by biopsy, and the outcome is variable. In most cases the lesion is reversible, but retransplantation may be the only treatment choice in severe cases.

Rejection is another significant cause of hepatic dysfunction in the immediate postoperative period and may occur as early as 5 days following transplantation. Clinical signs/symptoms are nonspecific and include fever, malaise, abdominal pain, hepatosplenomegaly, and increasing ascites. A decrease in or change in the character of bile output may occur as well. Laboratory abnormalities consist of increases in alkaline phosphatase, transaminase, and bilirubin levels, although rejection may be present in the face of normal laboratory values as well. Definitive diagnosis is made by biopsy. Treatment in most centers entails use of increased corticosteroids (up to 1 gm intravenously), with a subsequent taper as initial management. ALG or OKT3 is utilized for severe cases or those that are steroid-resistant.

Renal insufficiency is a common complication following liver transplantation. Contributing factors include preexisting renal failure, intraoperative hypotension, allograft failure, and use of nephrotoxic agents (CSA, nephrotoxic antibiotics). Treatment includes maintenance of urine output with adequate volume and diuretics, decrease in dose or temporary withdrawal of nephrotoxic agents, and correction of underlying factors (such as allograft failure).

PANCREAS TRANSPLANTS

The first human pancreas transplant was performed by Kelly and Lillehei at the University of Minnesota in 1966. As of December 1988, 1830 pancreas transplants had been performed worldwide. Significant improvements in immunosuppression and surgical technique have been made since 1966. Nevertheless, this procedure is still considered to be an experimental treatment for diabetes mellitus. From 1984 to March 1989, graft and patient survivals were 52 percent and 92 percent, respectively, for cases performed at the University of Minnesota [28]. The major causes of graft failure are rejection and technical problems.

Due to the potential complications and cost of this procedure (pancreas transplantation is covered by some but not all insurance/government programs), patient selection is especially important. Pancreas transplant recipients at the University of Minnesota generally fall into three categories: (1) nonuremic, nonkidney transplant recipients; (2) prior renal transplant recipients; and (3) those undergoing simultaneous pancreas and renal transplantation [29]. Patients in group 1 are transplanted if their current or potential complications of diabetes are worse than the side effects of chronic immunosuppression. Patients with preproliferative retinopathy or albuminuria (both markers for progressive disease in their respective organs) are good candidates for this group. Simultaneous pancreas and kidney transplantation is somewhat controversial [30]. The benefit of this approach is that the kidney can be monitored more easily for rejection, thus leading to an earlier diagnosis of rejection in the pancreas. Also, it spares the recipient a second operation. The disadvantage of simultaneous kidney-pancreas transplantation is that if complications with the pancreas graft occur, loss of the renal allograft is more likely than if the graft were well-established. Functional survival rates of pancreases transplanted concurrently with or following prior renal transplantation, however, do not differ significantly [13]. Current recommendations from the University of Minnesota are to transplant both organs simultaneously if feasible.

Laboratory review of the potential recipient is designed to evaluate the function of all organs predominantly affected by diabetes mellitus. This evaluation is then continued at yearly or biannual intervals following transplantation. The specific tests performed include glucose tolerance tests, 24-hour metabolic profile, urine and serum C peptide levels, islet hormone secretogogue stimulation, glycosylated hemoglobin, islet cell antibody titer, and insulin withdrawal if no history of ketosis is present. Full neurologic, cardiovascular, renal, ophthalmic, and psychiatric evaluations are performed as well. The cardiovascular evaluation may include cardiac catheterization if a positive stress test occurs or a strong past medical history of coronary artery disease is present. Subsequent angioplasty or coronary artery bypass grafting may then be indicated prior to pancreas transplantation.

In general, the emphasis at the University of Minnesota has shifted from transplantation in the diabetic with advanced, irreversible disease to transplantation in the nonuremic, nonrenal patient with potentially reversible end-organ damage to retina, kidney, and peripheral nerves. The benefit of transplantation in this patient group is currently undergoing evaluation.

The postoperative care of the pancreas transplant recipient somewhat depends on the surgical technique used. Three methods of pancreatic duct management have been utilized: enteric drainage, bladder drainage, and duct injection. As bladder drainage is the most commonly used technique at the University of Minnesota, the care outlined below will refer primarily to this type of patient.

The basic principles of postoperative management are applicable to the general care of these patients (see the section on General Principles). One minor difference of note is that in bladder-drained patients, the Foley catheter is kept in place until the seventh postoperative day. Accidental early removal has not resulted in complications, however. In general, ICU care is not required in the postoperative period, and the patients are usually admitted to the transplant nursing unit, where adequate nursing and physician personnel are present. Occasionally, in the immediate postoperative period, adult respiratory distress syndrome may occur. The origin in most cases is obscure; in some, it seems related to graft thrombosis, OKT3 administration, or perigraft infection. Graft removal is sometimes necessary.

Laboratory evaluation includes frequent monitoring (every 2 hours) of glucose for the first 24 hours postoperatively, and every 4 hours thereafter. Twenty-four-hour urine amylase is monitored daily while the patient is hospitalized. This is the most sensitive indicator of graft function for the pancreas transplant recipient with a bladder-drained graft [22].

Several medications are administered in the immediate postoperative period. An insulin infusion (regular humulin) is utilized as needed to maintain the blood glucose at less than 150 mg/dl. Chronic hyperglycemia has been shown to be detrimental to islet cells and is therefore avoided. Prophylactic agents are administered as previously discussed.

A three-drug regimen is again utilized for immunosuppression, the specifics of which are outlined in Table 31-2. Dosages vary somewhat for living related donor versus cadaver recipients. Cadaver recipients are additionally randomized to receive seven doses of ALG or OKT3 for the first postoperative week. Adjustments are also made for patients with renal allografts already in place.

As previously mentioned, monitoring of graft function in the bladder-drained recipient is best accomplished by following the urine amylase. A decrease in urine amylase has been found to precede a rise in serum glucose during graft rejection. Rejection is suspected with a decrease in urine amylase activity (urine amylase per hour) of 25 percent and virtually certain with a decline of 50 percent. Following the patient's discharge, rejection is monitored both by measurement of urine pH (the pancreas excretes bicarbonate into the urine), as well as urine amylase collections two or three times per week. A decrease in urine pH to less than 7.0 warrants further evaluation. Although urine pH may be used as an initial screening test, urine amylase is still considered to be the more critical test in diagnosing rejection. Plasma glucose is followed in patients with all types of ductal drainage. Levels of less than 200 mg/dl should be maintained if the graft is functional. Serum C peptide levels are helpful in confirming partial graft function during an episode of hyperglycemia. Insulin levels are not measured, as most recipients have circulating antibodies to insulin for at least the first 2 months posttransplant (secondary to an immune response to injection of heterologous insulin). Finally, serum amylase is followed in all pancreas transplant recipients. Levels may sharply drop, or increase and then drop, to herald the onset of rejection. Changes in serum amylase may therefore be difficult to interpret.

Recipients of combined kidney-pancreas transplants are additionally monitored by serum creatinine. An increase in serum creatinine will usually precede a drop in urine amylase as an indicator of pancreatic graft rejection [23]. Occasionally, however, the pancreas may show evidence of rejection prior to the renal allograft.

Several complications of pancreas transplantation may potentially occur in the early postoperative period. The most common immediate problem is that of graft thrombosis, which occurs in approximately 12 percent of pancreas transplants [31]. For this reason, some centers use systemic anticoagulation for several days postoperatively. Graft thrombosis is heralded by hyperglycemia and an increase in insulin requirements within the first few days of transplantation. A technetium flow study should initially be obtained if this diagnosis is suspected. If the pancreas is not visualized, an arteriogram should then be performed for confirmation. Successful thrombectomy has never been accomplished; therefore the treatment of choice is transplant pancreatectomy.

The most common complication leading to graft loss is intraabdominal infection. In a series of 116 pancreas transplants at the University of Minnesota, 22% developed intraabdominal infections. *Escherichia coli,* enterococci, and anaerobes were cultured from patients with enteric ductal drainage, and *Candida* was cultured from all patients regardless of technique. Eighteen patients required graft removal. The mortality rate was 27 percent in the patients with intra-abdominal infections, versus 7 percent in the remaining 90 cases. Of the six patients who died due to other causes, four succumbed to cardiovascular disease [14].

The presence of an intra-abdominal abscess should be suspected in any patient complaining of abdominal pain. Fever is an unreliable diagnostic sign in this immunosuppressed patient population. Diagnostic studies include blood, urine, sputum cultures (for suspected infection of unknown origin), with subsequent ultrasound or computed tomography (CT) scan. A fluid collection, if found, may be treated by aspiration alone if sterile. For true abscesses (pus and/or bacteria), percutaneous drainage alone has rarely been successful. Operative drainage with graft removal and cessation of immunosuppression is usually required.

Overall, the most common cause of graft loss is rejection. This may be indicated (depending on the procedure performed) by hyperglycemia, a decrease in urine amylase, or an increased serum creatinine, as previously outlined. Diagnosis of suspected rejection is essentially made by ruling out other causes of graft dysfunction. Biopsy may be performed in bladder-drained grafts via cystoscopy, but laparotomy may be required if sufficient tissue is not obtainable by this technique. Treatment usually includes an increase in prednisone to 2 mg/kg/day, with the addition of ALG or OKT3. Single-drug treatment may be utilized if the rejection is felt to be mild. Insulin is administered as needed to maintain plasma glucose levels at less than 200 mg/dl.

Pancreas transplantation, when successful, can effectively treat many of the manifestations of type-I diabetes mellitus. Technical complications and the side effects of immunosuppression currently preclude widespread use of pancreas transplantation as a treatment of type-I diabetes mellitus. If and when these problems are overcome, pancreas transplantation may become the treatment of choice for this disease.

HEART TRANSPLANTS
Improvements in cardiac transplantation have resulted in the emergence of this procedure as an accepted form of therapy for end-stage heart disease. The first successful heart transplant was performed by Christian Barnaard in 1967. By 1985, over 75 centers were offering heart transplantation to the patient populations they served. Heart transplant recipients may now expect 80 percent 1-year and 50 percent 5-year survival rates with improved quality of life and increased capacity for physical activity [3].

As with all types of transplants, patient selection contributes significantly to a successful outcome. The primary criteria for selection of heart transplant recipients is the presence of disease that is untreatable by other medical/surgical therapies and from which the patient will succumb in less than 6 to 12 months. All candidates should be in the New York Heart Association class IV, as well. Absolute contraindications to cardiac transplantation include active infection, recent pulmonary infarct, and pulmonary vascular resistance greater than 8 woods units. Relative contraindications—such as diabetes mellitus, renal or hepatic dysfunction not secondary to cardiac disease, peripheral vascular disease, hyperlipidemia, age greater than 60, chronic obstructive pulmonary disease (with FEV_1/ FVC less than 45% of predicted), history of substance abuse, or history of medical noncompliance—may preclude transplantation in individual cases. Some centers have modified their criteria to include some diabetic and older patients. In a recent series from the University of Pittsburgh, diabetic heart transplant patients were not found to have a higher incidence of graft atherosclerosis or acute rejection episodes. A significantly higher lethal infection rate was noted in this patient population, however [17].

The preoperative evaluation, in addition to the routine studies previously outlined, concentrates on the pulmonary and cardiovascular systems. Further pulmonary workup includes arterial blood gases and pulmonary function testing. The cardiac evaluation is completed with Holter monitoring, rest and exercise (if possible), nuclear scan, and cardiac catheterization (with endomyocardial biopsy). Decompensated congestive heart failure may result in a restrictive defect and make interpretation of the pulmonary function tests more difficult. Preexisting pulmonary function tests performed when the patient was not in congestive heart failure, if available, should also be reviewed.

After acceptance as potential recipients, up to 20 percent of patients will die while waiting for an acceptable donor [33]. These patients fall into three general categories that determine the extent of preoperative management needed [20]. Status 3 defines patients who are stable and can be managed at home; status 2 includes patients stable in the hospital on medical therapy who cannot be discharged due to severe congestive heart failure or arrhythmias. Status 1 includes patients who are unstable and require ICU therapy and monitoring, which may include anything from parenteral inotropic support to mechanical circulatory assist devices such as an intra-aortic balloon pump, left ventricular assist device, or an artificial heart. Approximately 60 percent of patients awaiting cardiac transplantation can be managed at home.

One common but difficult to manage problem in these patients is that of arrhythmias. Multifocal premature ventricular complexes (PVCs) and non-sustained ventricular tachycardia are often present in patients with dilated cardiomyopathy. Unfortunately, none of the antiarrhythmic agents to date have been effective in treating these arrhythmias. Most deaths in patients awaiting transplantation are sudden and probably secondary to ventricular arrhythmias. Potential cardiac transplant recipients with symptomatic complex ventricular ectopy are therefore recommended for early transplantation.

The initial postoperative management of the cardiac transplant recipient occurs in the ICU and resembles that of any open heart surgical patient. Fluid status and cardiac function are monitored by Swan-Ganz catheter and arterial pressure monitoring. This instrumentation may also be used to judge the need for and efficacy of inotropic support. In general, oxygenation is maintained by mechanical ventilation for the first 24 to 48 hours. Loop diuretics may be utilized to facilitate diuresis. Salt-poor albumin may also be helpful in mobilizing third-space fluid. Bradycardia is a common dysrhythmia in cardiac transplant recipients; isoproterenol can be helpful in this regard, for both its chronotropic and its inotropic effects. The heart rate can more reliably be maintained, however, by sequential atrioventricular pacing. Selection of the optimal heart rate can be performed by increasing the paced rate and then measuring the cardiac output. The optimal heart rate is the rate that yields the best cardiac output with the least myocardial work.

Multiple medications are required in the postoperative period, both for cardiac support and for immunosuppression. Inotropic drugs are routinely begun intraoperatively and subsequently weaned as tolerated. Most patients require inotropic support for the first 24 to 48 hours following transplantation. Drugs most commonly used in this category are dopamine and isoproterenol. Isoproterenol is especially useful due to its chronotropic effects, as the cardiac output of the transplanted heart is rate-dependent. Positive inotropic support is also needed as therapy for the myocardial depression usually present secondary to temporary ischemic damage in the revascularized cardiac allograft.

Patients with low blood pressure and low cardiac output may be treated with agents that affect both α and β receptors, such as dopamine and epinephrine. Care must be taken not to increase the systemic vascular resistance to the extent that the increased afterload increases myocardial work. Dopamine may also be utilized in low doses (2 to 3 μg/kg/min) if renal perfusion is felt to be impaired.

Hypertension, secondary to stress, pain, and preexisting atherosclerosis, is commonly present in the postoperative period. In many cases, CSA may also induce elevations of blood pressure. Agents such as nitroprusside and nitroglycerin can be utilized for rapid titration of the blood pressure. If hypertension persists, oral vasodilators such as nifedipine or hydralazine may be necessary for chronic maintenance.

Pulmonary hypertension, if present, requires immediate correction, as the donor heart is intolerant to an increased pulmonary vascular resistance and right heart failure can quickly ensue. This condition is treatable by the use of inotropes, diuretics, pulmonary vasodilators and by avoidance of acute hypoxemia and hypercarbia. Agents effective in dilating the pulmonary bed include isoproterenol, prostaglandin E, and nitroprusside. Nitroglycerin may also help, by increasing venous capacitance and therefore decreasing the blood volume in the pulmonary vasculature.

Antiarrhythmics are often necessary in the care of the cardiac transplant recipient. Initial management of arrhythmias should always include a search for and correction of etiologies such as electrolyte abnormalities, hypoxia, acidosis, rejection, or mechanical irritation. Ventricular arrhythmias are usually suppressible by lidocaine with minimal adverse effects. The ventricular response to an atrial arrhythmia may be regulated with digoxin. Conversion of atrial fibrillation to normal sinus rhythm can be attempted with the addition of quinidine to the previously digitalized patient. Emergency and elective countershock may also be utilized for conversion of ventricular and atrial arrhythmias to normal sinus rhythm. Rapid atrial pacing is often effective for conversion of atrial flutter to normal sinus rhythm. This method is not useful for the treatment of atrial fibrillation, however, due to the inability of the external current to successfully capture the atrium [19]. Agents, such as propranolol, that interfere with the catecholamine stimulation of the (denervated) donor heart should be used with caution [5]. Verapamil has a variable effect on atrioventricular conduction and should probably be avoided [6].

Other medications administered postoperatively include potassium, analgesics, antacids, and dipyridamole (Persantine). Routine antifungal, antiviral, and antibacterial prophylaxis is carried out as well (see the section on General Principles). Immunosuppression is again achieved via a three-drug regimen of azathioprine, prednisone, and CSA. Dosages and routes of administration are listed in Table 31-2.

As with any transplant, the physician must be aware of the several complications that may occur in the early posttransplant period. Most cardiac transplant recipients are kept on Coumadin preoperatively, to prevent formation of mural clot with subsequent embolism. These patients are therefore at risk for bleeding in the postoperative period. Parenteral vitamin K administered preoperatively will at least partially reverse the effects of Coumadin. Hemostasis is also important for the prevention of cardiac tamponade and infection.

A second complication that may occur in the early posttransplant period is low cardiac output. This problem is easily detectable with a Swan-Ganz catheter. Common causes include harvest-reperfusion–induced myocardial injury, acute rejection, hypovolemia, tamponade, sepsis, and medications. Hypovolemia may be assessed by the use of the Swan-Ganz catheter (low filling pressures) combined with clinical assessment. Tamponade may be suspected if there is equalization of filling pressures and collapse of the right ventricle in diastole, or if significant clot is seen on echocardiography. A large effusion and indentation of the right atrium may be seen as well [1]. Sepsis is evaluated by culture of all body fluids and replacement of all intravenous/intra-arterial lines. If other causes of low cardiac output have been ruled out, acute rejection and myocardial injury must be differentiated. This is best carried out by transvenous endomyocardial biopsy. If both injuries are present to the extent that circulatory support cannot be maintained, retransplantation with possible intermediary support by mechanical devices must be employed.

Common neurologic complications in the postoperative period include cerebrovascular accident, disorientation/confusion, and seizures. Air embolus and rebound hypertension are the two primary causes of cerebrovascular accident during this time period. Confusion/disorientation may have multiple etiologies, such as hypoxia, sepsis, electrolyte abnormalities, and ICU psychosis. Cyclosporine has been noted to have several neurologic side effects, including ataxia, paraparesis, quadriparesis, mental status changes, seizures, and visual hallucinations [2, 8, 21, 24]. These may occur despite maintenance of therapeutic blood levels.

As with any transplant patient, rejection may be problematic for the new cardiac transplant recipient. Formerly, rejection was indicated by the presence of right heart failure, peripheral edema, jugular venous distention, and decreased voltage by ECG. These findings may not be present in patients on cyclosporine, however. Rejection in the CSA era is diagnosed primarily by biopsy. All patients are therefore monitored for acute rejection by weekly endomyocardial biopsy for the first 1 to 2 months posttransplant [3]. Acute rejection usually does not occur before the first 5 to 7 days following transplantation. Changes in rhythm (especially atrial abnormalities) and low cardiac output may be indicators of acute rejection in the early transplant period [19]. If other etiologic factors are ruled out, these conditions should be evaluated by endomyocardial biopsy. Mild rejection episodes usually require no change in immunosuppression. Moderate-to-severe rejection is treated by an increase in oral or intravenous prednisone dosage. ALG may be utilized for steroid-resistant or recurrent rejection episodes.

Discharge from the hospital is possible when the patient has mastered the immunosuppression regimen and rehabilitation has progressed to the point at which the patient can ambulate short distances and perform the activities of daily living. On average, the cardiac transplant recipient is ready for discharge within 10 to 14 days of transplantation.

SUMMARY

In summary, transplantation offers an increased survival rate and improved quality of life to many patients with end-stage organ failure. Despite the advances in this field, many complications (primarily related to the degree of immunosuppression required to prevent rejection) persist. Some of these complications may be minimized by diligent perioperative care. By this means the ICU team, in conjunction with the transplant surgeon, may significantly contribute to a successful outcome for the transplant recipient. Finally, the role of the ICU team in providing medical support of the potential donor cannot be overemphasized.

REFERENCES

1. Armstrong, W. F., Schilt, B. F., Helper, D. J., et al. Diastolic collapse of the right ventricle with cardiac tamponade: An echocardiographic study. *Circulation* 64:1491, 1982.
2. Atkinson, K., Biggs, J., Darveriza, P., et al. Cyclosporine, associated central nervous system toxicity after allogenic bone marrow transplantation. *Transplantation* 38:34, 1984.
3. Barnhart, G., and Lower, R. Cardiac Transplantation. In J. Cerilli (ed.), *Organ Transplantation and Replacement*. Philadelphia: Lippincott, 1988.
4. Bennett, A. Urologic Complications of Renal Transplantation. In J. Cerilli (ed.). *Organ Transplantation and Replacement*. Philadelphia: Lippincott, 1988.
5. Bexton, R. S., Milne, J. R., Cory-Pearce, R., et al. Effect of beta blockage on exercise response after cardiac transplantation. *Br. Heart J.* 49:584, 1983.
6. Bexton, R. S., Nathan, A. W., Cory-Pearce, R., et al. Electrophysiological effects of nifedipine and verapamil in the transplanted human heart. *Heart Transplant.* 3:97, 1984.
7. Birtch, A. Patient Selection for Renal Transplantation. In J. Cerilli (ed.), *Organ Transplantation and Replacement*. Philadelphia: Lippincott, 1988.
8. Boogaerts, M., Zachee, P., and Verwilghen, R. Cyclosporine, methylprednisolone and convulsions. *Lancet* 2:1216, 1982.
9. Cecka, J., Cicciarelli, J., Mickey, M., and Terasaki, P. Blood transfusions and HLA matching—An either/or situation in cadaveric renal transplantation. *Transplantation* 45:81, 1988.
10. Dindzans, V., Schade, R., and Van Thiel, D. Medical problems before and after transplantation. *Gastroenterol. Clin. North Am.* 17:19, 1988.
11. Goldman, M., DePauw, L., Kinnaert, P., et al. Renal allograft rupture. *Transplantation* 32:153, 1981.
12. Gordon, R., Iwatsuki, S., Esquivel, C., et al. Liver Transplantation. In J. Cerilli ed., *Organ Transplantation and Replacement*. Philadelphia: Lippincott, 1988.
13. Hanto, D., and Sutherland, D. Pancreas transplantation: Clinical considerations. *Radiol. Clin. North Am.* 25:333, 1987.
14. Hesse, U., Sutherland, D., Najarian, J., and Simmons, R. Intraabdominal infections in pancreas transplant recipients. *Ann. Surg.* 203:153, 1986.
15. Kerman, R., Van Buren, C., Lewis, M., and Kahan, B. Successful transplantation of 100 untransfused cyclosporine-treated primary recipients of cadaveric renal allografts. *Transplantation* 45:37, 1988.
16. Koneru, B., Tzakis, A., Bowman, J., et al. Postoperative surgical complications. *Gastroenterol. Clin. North Am.* 17:71, 1988.
17. Ladowski, J., Kormos, R., Hardesty, R., et al. Heart transplantation in diabetic recipients. Abstract. *American Society of Transplant Surgeons,* May 1989:42.
18. Matas, A., Tellis, V., Quinn, T., Glicklich, D., Soberman, R., and Veith, F. Individualization of immediate posttransplant immunosuppression. *Transplantation* 45:406, 1988.
19. Murray, K., and Howanitz, E. Perioperative and Postoperative Management of the Heart Transplant Patient. In P. Myerowitz (ed.), *Heart Transplant.* Mt. Kisco, NY: Futura, 1987.

20. Myerowitz, P. Selection and Management of the Heart Transplant Recipient. In P. Myerowitz (ed.), *Heart Transplantation.* Mt. Kisco, NY: Futura, 1987.
21. Noll, R., and Kulkarni, R. Complex visual hallucinations and cyclosporine. *Arch. Neurol.* 41:329, 1984.
22. Prieto, M., Sutherland, D., Fernandez-Cruz, L., et al. Experimental and clinical experience with urinary amylase monitoring for early diagnosis of rejection in pancreas transplantation. *Transplantation* 43:73, 1987.
23. Prieto, M., Sutherland, D., Fernandez-Cruz, L., et al. Diagnosis of rejection in pancreas transplantation. *Transplantation* 19:2348, 1987.
24. Powell-Jackson, P. R., and Carmichael, F. J. L. Adult respiratory distress syndrome and convulsions associated with administration of cyclosporine in liver transplant recipients. *Transplantation* 38:341, 1984.
25. Reitz, B. Cardiac and cardiopulmonary transplantation. In D. McGoon (ed.), Cardiac surgery. *Cardiovasc. Clin.* 17:347, 1987.
26. Salvatierra, O. The Role of Blood Transfusions in Transplantation. In J. Cerilli (ed.), *Organ Transplantation and Replacement.* Philadelphia: Lippincott, 1988.
27. Simmons, R., Canafax, D., Strand, M., et al. Management and prevention of cyclosporine nephrotoxicity after renal transplantation: Use of low doses of cyclosporine, azathiaprine, and prednisone. *Transplant Proc.* 17:266, 1985.
28. Sutherland, D., Dunn, D., Goetz, F., et al. A ten year experience with 290 pancreas transplants at a single institution. (In press.)
29. Sutherland, D., Goetz, C., and Najarian, J. Pancreas transplantation at the University of Minnesota: Donor and recipient selection, operative and postoperative management, and outcome. *Transplant Proc.* 19:63, 1987.
30. Sutherland, D. Selected issues of importance in clinical pancreas transplantation. *Transplant Proc* 16:661, 1984.
31. Sutherland, D., Moudry, K., and Najarian, J. Pancreas Transplantation. In J. Cerilli (ed.), *Organ Transplantation and Replacement.* Philadelphia: Lippincott, 1988.
32. Tellis, V., Matas, A., and Veith, F. Vascular Complications of Transplantation. In J. Cerilli (ed.), *Organ Transplantation and Replacement.* Philadelphia: Lippincott, 1988.
33. Thompson, M., Kormos, R., Zerbe, A., et al. Patient selection and results of cardiac transplantation in patients with cardiomyopathy. In J. Shaver (ed.), Cardiomyopathies: clinical presentation, diagnosis, and management. *Cardiovasc. Clin.* 19:263, 1988.
34. Tolkoft-Rubin, N., and Rubin, R. Infection in the Organ Transplant Recipient. In J. Cerilli (ed.), *Organ Transplantation and Replacement.* Philadelphia: Lippincott, 1988.

Recent Advances in Computers and Microprocessors in Critical Care Medicine

William H. Chamberlin, Jr.
Charles L. Rice

The effect that computers have had in the medical environment are apparent to most personnel working the intensive care unit (ICU). Whereas the 1979 *Index Medicus* listed three headings with four pages devoted to references on computers in medical care, the 1987 *Index* had seven major headings, 19 cross-references, and 12 pages devoted to articles from the more than 10 journals dealing with computers in the health sciences.

Devices made possible only by microprogramming technology have become necessary to deliver care in the increasingly technical atmosphere of the ICU. Some pundits believe that technology rather than reason and compassion rule the day in ICU care, but that question is not for this chapter to decide. Rather, that technical world and the support available for the ICU physician will be explored.

Electronic circuits are used for two general-device categories: microprocessors and general computers. The microprocessor is generally dedicated to a single task, such as a measurement or a computation, and is not usually flexible enough for programming by the user. Examples are the pulse oximeter, the cardiac output "computer", and the metabolic cart. Electronic circuitry makes and controls complex measurements and derives values based on certain accepted clinical dicta. Computers, on the other hand, are multitask devices that can be programmed by the user for various tasks. Computers often control many microprocessors. They come in three varieties: the mainframe, the minicomputer, and (since 1975) the microcomputer. It is the last of these that has truly revolutionized the information world—providing a cheap source of information processing that has put computers on the desktop. The IBM-PC and Apple Macintosh products are examples of such devices.

MICROPROCESSORS

Microprocessors can perform as sensors and as monitors. For our purposes, a sensor is a device directly responsible for measurement. In the pulse oximeter, for example, microprocessors have permitted the union of two technologies (plethysmography and spectrometry) to create a tool for the noninvasive measurement of hemoglobin saturation. Older oximeters were too bulky or inaccurate to use at bedside. Microprocessors have reduced the device to the size of a small cigar box and improved the accuracy significantly.

Monitors can be considered to be devices for the display of sensed data. They frequently convert analog or continuous waveform data into digital or numbered information. In the ICU, "snapshots" of a patient are taken frequently, and patients are characterized by pulse or blood pressure or urine output at hourly intervals. ICU theory dictates that by watching for change in these variables, dangerous trends can be detected and wrong made right. Our understanding of complex physiologic processes has been limited by our ability to measure various parameters, as well as by the sensory overload that occurs when we try to appreciate changes in more than a few variables. In most ICUs, monitors display constantly measured parameters, and it becomes the responsibility of the personnel to interpolate this information for care. In traditional recordkeeping such information is essentially lost for the more complex relationships. The newest trend in such information management is to send monitored data from the bedside into computerized data bases. This is opening a new era in which complex relationships among physiologic data can be explored for better understanding of life and death processes.

Microchip technology, in the meantime, has created more variables that can be measured in real time. The pulse oximeter measures constant oxyhemoglobin saturation, as do fiberoptic devices that can be placed in the pulmonary artery for continuous display of mixed venous oxygen saturations. Indwelling arterial lines, nasogastric tubes, and urimeters can now measure constant pH of their respective fluids. One monitor reportedly used to estimate colonic ischemia was a pH probe placed in the rectum of a postoperative patient following aortic surgery.

Monitors all have one thing in common. A parameter presumed vital to patient health is measured at frequent intervals (sometimes constantly) and displayed for interpretation. Current methods alert care personnel when simple changes occur in the data. For instance, the heart rate alarm sounds when high or low rate limits are exceeded. The arterial pressure alarms indicate similar changes. In many systems, ventricular tachycardia may go unnoticed if the rate limit is not exceeded. A change in respiratory rate from 20 beats per minute (bpm) to 30 bpm may go unnoticed as the first sign of pulmonary edema. Our use of monitors is limited but is advancing quickly.

Cardiac Monitors

Rhythm Monitors

The simplest device for following cardiac status is the rate and rhythm monitor. Since heart rate frequently has significance as an indicator of ischemia or impending tamponade, it has proved very useful and constitutes the first electronic device brought to the bedside. Although rate and rhythm remain the standbys for any ICU system, more-complex arrhythmias are now analyzed for P-wave morphology and S–T segment changes. The latter, in particular, are likely to revolutionize the approach to ischemic heart disease. Anesthesiologists are using S–T segment monitoring during operations as one of the earliest indicators of active ischemia and are reporting a reduction in cardiac morbidity.

Cardiac Function
Echocardiography is available at the bedside with smaller mobile devices that permit rapid analysis of ventricular function, valvular disease, and pericardial fluid. Echocardiography with an ultrasound probe in the esophagus is currently a research technique that provides sensitive information about the state of the myocardium and currently is used during operations to monitor wall motion for evidence of ischemia.

Another device combines ultrasound with Doppler analysis to permit noninvasive and accurate measurement of cardiac output. We use this particular tool to avoid invasive cardiac devices, such as the thermodilution right heart catheter. The latter device, of course, has the capacity to measure and display cardiac outputs, right-sided vascular pressures, and mixed venous oxygen saturations. Additionally, bedside measurement of function through nuclear medicine studies is available in some medical centers.

Respiratory Monitors

Gas Exchange
Pulse oximetry utilizes two wavelengths of light that are absorbed at different intensities depending on the amount of oxyhemoglobin and deoxyhemoglobin in the blood. A similar principle works with saturations measured with indwelling arterial or venous catheters. Fiberoptic bundles are used to transmit and receive light, and microchips are used to do the complex derivations and associations that permit the display of continuous saturation to the clinician. These devices have found widespread use in the care of patients in ventilatory failure, where changes in mixed venous saturation reflect alterations in pulmonary shunt or cardiac output.

In addition to saturation determination, devices are also available to monitor changes in arterial oxygen, mixed venous oxygen, and exhaled carbon dioxide tensions. Capnography has been used in some centers to monitor the patients' carbon dioxide levels during the weaning process. During neurosurgical procedures in the sitting position, many institutions employ the capnograph to detect air embolism. Transcutaneous oxygen sensors work on the principle that oxygen diffusing to the skin surface from the dermal capillary bed reacts with the metal surface of the electrode to create current. The current is proportional to the oxygen tension. Although used successfully in neonates, these monitors have met with only partial success in adults, since the relationship between transcutaneous oxygen pressure and arterial oxygen pressure depend on factors such as skin thickness, capillary flow, cardiac output, and skin temperature. Some investigators have therefore utilized not the absolute value, but the trend of such information to draw conclusions about the state of the circulation rather than arterial oxygenation. Transconjunctival oxygen sensors overcome some of the technical difficulties, since skin thickness and the need for a heated sensor are no longer relevant, but this technique likewise has met with very limited acceptance.

Ventilatory Monitors
Noninvasive devices such as the Respitrace are gaining widespread acceptance for diagnostic as well as monitoring purposes. Bands placed around the abdomen and thorax have sensors that permit recognition of disordered breathing patterns as well as respiratory rate. Microchips record this information to provide patterns that can be examined at the convenience of the physician, to help determine the course of weaning from mechanical ventilators or to document obstructed breathing patterns in sleep apnea.

Mechanical Ventilators
Ventilators have probably been the most visible devices affected by microchip technology. Ventilators can now monitor a patient's minute ventilation and support with intermittent positive pressure when the determined minimum has not been met. Airway pressure recordings combined with flow meters permit flow-loops to be constructed during routine care. Compliance determinations from static lung pressures and volumes are routinely determined and recorded. Some ventilators have features that permit measurement of exhaled and inhaled gas tensions, to determine metabolic rates. Additionally, microchip memory in many ventilators today permits storage of the parameters for recall, collation, and printing at a time remote from recording.

Neurologic Monitoring
Although clinical examination remains the most important tool for neurologic evaluation, several techniques clearly complement physical assessment. Measurement of intracranial pressure has been a practical clinical reality since the 1950s. Recent innovations include the use of fiberoptic devices that are placed above the dura and reduce the risk of infection from that associated with the use of bolts and intraventricular drains. Modules are available to measure continuous electroencephalograms (EEGs) and monitor therapy for continuous seizures. Electrical impulses from the brain are also available for analysis of brainstem evoked potentials. This technique utilizes microprocessors to detect and amplify the small electrical activities that result from controlled stimulation of specified neural pathways in the brain. In this manner, the brain stem can be analyzed in ways impossible with normal EEGs. Visual evoked potentials and brain stem evoked potentials are variations of the technique. The information obtained permits more-precise localization of deficits, as well as information of prognostic value.

Near-infrared absorbance technology also has been applied to study of the brain. With this technology, brain oxygen tensions can be measured. Positron emission tomography permits characterization of the brain metabolism, and bedside nuclear medicine studies permit characterization of regional cerebral blood flow.

Nutritional Monitoring

Great strides have been made understanding the metabolic derangements that occur with sepsis, trauma, and stress. Individualization of therapy has been less aggressively pursued, however, in part because of difficulties in measuring metabolic requirements. Clinicians generally project basic metabolic need with equations such as the Harrison-Benedict and then multiply by "fudge" factors to account for the stress of the patient's own disease or injury process. Two methods have now been firmly established to measure oxygen metabolism and project more accurately the nutritional needs of the critically ill patient. Volumetric methods have been available for some time but are now being applied to the ventilated patient on enhanced inspired oxygen fraction. A new "open" method of gas analysis provides reproducible results for patients breathing room air. Such methods have demonstrated that use of the Harrison-Benedict–based models overestimate caloric needs by greater than 30 percent. Microcomputers wed to such devices estimate respiratory quotients (RQ) and, by accepted formulas, project, not only caloric requirement, but also protein, fat, and carbohydrate contents.

Renal Function

Monitoring of urine output has, of course, been a standby for years. Devices utilizing ultrasound to detect volume changes now collect urine and display hourly outputs, flow rates, and body temperature on a continuous basis. This information has been fed directly into computerized data bases for general data management, as will be described below.

COMPUTERS IN THE INTENSIVE CARE UNIT

Commercial systems for the collection, collation, and display of bedside information have been in use for well over 10 years. These systems were invariably minicomputers that took information entry from nurses, physicians, and technicians at bedside terminals. These devices rarely interfaced directly with any laboratory or bedside device and represented little more than glorified typewriters for elegantly printed output of clinical information. Clinical personnel had to do without the 24-hour bedside flow sheets that still dominate most ICU environments.

This situation is changing dramatically. The microcomputer's role has long been limited to the performance of individual though related tasks at the bedside or central station. Rarely has it integrated information from diverse sources. One computer measures cardiac outputs. Another brings lab results back to the ICU. Another calculates drug doses. Integration of the information depends upon the "sneaker" network. That is, the information is transported manually from program to program and computer to computer. This no longer need be the case.

The information environment in today's ICU is integrated by microcomputers. Computers are now in the position of aiding and abetting the care givers with what they do best: collect, organize, integrate, analyze, display, and store.

Data Collection

Information no longer need be gathered by hand and placed through a keyboard into the computer. Ventilators, urine collection devices, cardiac output computers, metabolic carts, intravenous pumps, and heart rate/ pressure monitors can all communicate directly with a computer. Increasingly, laboratories communicate across electronic links directly with bedside display devices. On-site ICU laboratory devices communicate directly with ICU computers. In our ICU, blood gas results can be back at the bedside within 1 to 2 minutes of the draw—barely more than the time necessary for analysis.

Accumulation of bedside information has been slowed due to the lack of standardization of medical information. Currently, to link a new device into a system, a separate communications protocol is necessary to establish an interface with the computer for each device. Each intravenous pump, for instance, may require its own hardwired link, as well as software protocol. Manufacturers have made "ports" available on each device that can be hooked into the computer across these links. This setup vastly escalates the cost of each equipment interface and slows the process of integration considerably. The Institute of Electrical and Electronic Engineers is working to publish standards for a medical information bus that should lead to enhanced communication between medical devices. The bus translates hardware and software protocols from one device to another to permit the sharing of information. This should reduce the software and hardware overhead of enhancing the communication of the many devices found at bedside. Additionally, with devices in direct communication with computers, better documentation of the intravenous changes can occur. A twist of the dial on the intravenous pump can be recorded automatically, thus relieving the nurse of recording responsibilities. At least one intravenous solution vendor currently sells such a product.

Data Organization

Tabular and graphic display of information clearly helps the clinician interpret patient-care data. The computer easily collates and organizes information in a way that reduces or eliminates the need for human updating of flow sheets. Our ICU is only one of many across the country that have virtually eliminated the need for hand-written flow sheets. Laboratory results, hemodynamic evaluations, and vital signs are all recorded into the computer, which displays that collated information to the clinician, nurse, and technician. The newest technologies utilize high-resolution video devices that continuously display the flow-sheet information in a format most units traditionally use for data display on written records. This greatly enhances the "user-friendly" nature of the computer and improves acceptance of the computer in the environment.

Data Analysis

Timely analysis of data is one of the most important tools the computer brings to the bedside. Given the availability of information, complex analyses can be made within moments of receipt of the data. This process may be as simple as the integration and analysis of hemodynamic information.

In our ICU, results entered directly from the blood gas device are combined with blood pressure and heart rates from the nurses, vital signs, and cardiac outputs from the technician to present the clinician with information such as oxygen delivery, oxygen extraction ratios, and stroke volume indices.

Another example of collation and calculation in the ICU is the analysis of nutritional information. Tables have been created containing the constituents of hyperalimentation fluid. On demand, a program searches the input/output records for intravenous or oral feedings, analyzes the fluid and volume to determine the amounts of fat, carbohydrate, and protein given the patient, and reports the estimated caloric input on a daily basis. Displayed with that data is the basal energy expenditure calculated from the Harrison-Benedict equation.

To perform these calculations by hand may require considerable time and effort. By using the computer, the health-care provider is free to use the information, not required to generate it.

Display

The revolution in data interpretation has only begun. Currently in medicine, we use fairly primitive graphics to interpret data. Heart rate, blood pressure, and temperature are charted by the nurse, and review of records is enhanced for the physician with the most commonly employed graph for this purpose—a time line. Computer graphics open up possibilities for other characterizations to be accomplished routinely—modeling for antibiotics, Starling curves, effects of therapy, etc. The time saving is substantial, and hardware enhancements permit a real-time display of flow-sheet information. The primary benefit of such display will be a more friendly system that reproduces the traditional environment, ensuring better data entry by reinforcing the display value of the information.

INFORMATION USES

The ability to store data in a central computer storage bank is a valuable tool for physicians. Use of this quantitative data promises real advances in understanding and documentation of care. Information routinely collected at bedside can be used to generate, for example, Therapeutic Intervention and Severity Scores (TISS), Acute Physiology Scores (APS), and Acute Physiology and Chronic Health Evaluation (APACHE II) scores. With computers, the data is captured at the time of entry by the health care professionals. The fact that separate data-entry personnel are unnecessary to the process reduces the cost of quality-assurance studies. More important, the data are now available for quantifying care. Combining bedside information with demographics and diagnostic information permits substantial reductions in the number of personnel needed for audit studies, which are routinely and increasingly required to meet federal requirements. Additionally, severity scores generated with such information may become important for reimbursement from third-party payers if the Health Care Financing Administration has its way. The data will be generated painlessly and accurately.

CONCLUSION

Computers and microchips are revolutionizing data management in the ICU. Sophisticated devices are available whose tasks are made possible by the chips. Calculations and evaluations are made routine by taking advantage of the speed and reproducibility of the computers' work. Most important, perhaps, we have entered a new era of data analysis. Never before have physicians had such a cost-effective tool for the analysis of quantitative information. Following outcomes and using "patient care monitors" routinely should permit improvement of our understanding of the role of ICUs in patient care. Computers have enhanced our capacity to do quality control work in the ICU to take us out of the "dark ages" of information.

SELECTED READINGS

Ellis, J. E., Roizen, M. F., Aronson, S., et al. Frequency with which ST segment trends predict intraoperative myocardial ischemia. *Anesthesiology* 67 (Suppl. 3A):A2, 1987.

A flight simulation for general anesthesia training. *Comput. Biomed. Res.* 20:64, 1987.

Gardner, R. M. Computerized management of ICU patients. *MD Comput.* 3:36, 1986.

Golding, J. Cardiac rhythms and arrhythmias: A teaching program. *Comput. Methods Programs Biomed.* 23:331, 1986.

Hashimoto, F., et al. A computer simulation program to facilitate budgeting and staffing decisions in an ICU. *Crit. Care Med.* 15:156, 1987.

Henderson, J. V. Interactive videodisc to teach combat trauma life support. *J. Med. Syst.* 10:271, 1986.

Kotter, G. S., Kotrly, K. R., Kalbfleisch, H., et al. Myocardial ischemia during cardiovascular surgery as detected by an ST segment trend monitoring system. *J. Cardiothoracic Anesth.* 1:190, 1987.

Overton, D. T. A computer assisted emergency department chart audit. *Ann. Emer. Med.* 16:68, 1987.

Petrini, M. F. Distribution of ventilation and perfusion: A teaching model. *Comput. Biol. Med.* 16:431, 1986.

Physiologic data display during anesthesia. *IMJCM Comp.* 3:123, 1986.

Shabot, M. D., Leyerle, B. J., and LoBue, M. Automatic extraction of intensity-intervention scores from a computerized surgical intensive care unit flow-sheet. *Am. J. Surg.* 154:72, 1987.

Tutor, F. M. A computer aided instruction system for teaching fetal monitor interpretation. *Am. J. Obstet. Gynecol.* 156:1045–8, 1987.

Vozeh, S. Computer assisted individualized lidocaine dosage. *Am. Heart J.* 113:928, 1987.

Appendixes

1. Abbreviations, Definitions, and Normal Values

Abbreviation	Definition	Normal value
BSA	Body surface area	Meters (square)
$\overline{AP}$	Mean systemic arterial pressure	85–95 mm Hg
CVP	Central venous pressure	5–12 cm H_2O
$\overline{PA}$	Mean pulmonary artery pressure	10–17 mm Hg
$\overline{PCWP}$	Mean pulmonary capillary wedge pressure	5–12 mm Hg
CO	Cardiac output	5–6 liters/min
CI	Cardiac index	2.5–3.5 liters/min/M^2
SVR or TPR	Systemic vascular resistance Total peripheral resistance	900–1200 dynes · sec · cm^{-5}
PVR	Pulmonary vascular resistance	150–250 dynes · sec · cm^{-5}
HR	Heart rate	60–90 beats/min
SV	Stroke volume	60–70 ml/beat
SI	Stroke index	35–45 ml/beat/M_2
RVSW	Right venticular stroke work	8–12 gmM/M^2
LVSW	Left ventricular stroke work	51–61 gmM/M^2
CBV	Central blood volume	750–800 ml/M^2
EF	Ejection fraction	0.67
EDV	End-diastolic volume	70 ml/M^2
dp/dt	First time derivative of left ventricular pressure	1500–1800 mm Hg/sec (normal value varies with method and equipment)
MTT	Mean transit time Calculated from indicator dilution curve Time from venous injection to peak concentration in artery	13–14 sec
P_AO_2	Mean partial pressure of oxygen in the alveolus	104 mm Hg

Abbreviation	Definition	Normal value
P_ACO_2	Partial pressure of carbon dioxide in the alveolus	40 mm Hg
PaO_2	Partial pressure of oxygen in arterial blood	Will vary with patient's age and the F_IO_2 on room air: 80–95 mm Hg on 100% O_2: 640 mm Hg
$PaCO_2$	Partial pressure of carbon dioxide in arterial blood	40 mm Hg
$P\bar{v}O_2$	Partial pressure of oxygen in mixed venous blood	Will vary with the F_IO_2, cardiac output, and oxygen consumption from 35–40 mm Hg
$P\bar{v}CO_2$	Partial pressure of carbon dioxide in mixed venous blood	41–51 mm Hg
$P(A–a)O_2$	Alveolar-arterial oxygen gradient	25–65 mm Hg at $F_IO_2 = 1.0$
SaO_2	Percent oxyhemoglobin saturation of arterial blood	97% (air)
$S\bar{v}O_2$	Percent oxyhemoglobin saturation of mixed venous blood	75% (air)
CaO_2	Arterial oxygen content	Will vary with hemoglobin concentration and PaO_2 on air from 19–20 ml/100 ml
$C\bar{v}O_2$	Mixed venous oxygen content	Will vary with CaO_2, cardiac output, and O_2 consumption from 14–15 ml/100 ml
$C(a–v)O_2$	Arteriovenous oxygen content difference	4–6 ml/100 ml
O_2 avail	Oxygen availability	550–650 ml/min/M²
O_2 ext ratio	Oxygen extraction ratio	0.25
P_B	Barometric pressure	
$\dot{V}O_2$	Oxygen consumption (STPD[a])	115–165 ml/min/M²
$\dot{V}CO_2$	Carbon dioxide production (STPD[a])	192 ml/min
R or RQ	Respiratory quotient	0.8
FRC	Functional residual capacity (BTPS[b])	2400 ml
VC	Vital capacity (BTPS[b])	65–75 ml/kg
IF	Inspiratory force	75–100 cm H_2O

Abbreviation	Definition	Normal value
EDC	Effective dynamic compliance	35–45 ml/cm H_2O females 40–50 ml/cm H_2O males
V_D	Dead space (BTPS[b])	150 ml
V_T	Tidal volume (BTPS[b])	500 ml
V_D/V_T	Dead space to tidal volume ratio	0.25–0.40
$\dot{Q}s/\dot{Q}T$	Right-to-left shunt (percent of cardiac output flowing past nonventilated alveoli or the equivalent)	5–8%

[a]Standard temperature pressure, dry.
[b]Body temperature pressure, saturated.
Note: See Chapter 6 for additional values.

2. Table of Formulas

$\overline{AP}$ estimate: diastolic pressure plus ⅓ pulse pressure

$$CI \text{ (liters/min/M}^2) = \frac{\text{cardiac output (liters/min)}}{\text{body surface area (M}^2)}$$

$$SVR \text{ (TPR) (dynes} \cdot \text{sec} \cdot \text{cm}^{-5}) = \frac{(\overline{AP} \text{ [mm Hg]} - CVP \text{ [mm Hg]}) \times 79.9}{\text{(cardiac output [liters/min])}}$$

$$PVR \text{ (dynes} \cdot \text{sec} \cdot \text{cm}^{-5}) = \frac{(\overline{PA} \text{ [mm Hg]} - \overline{PCWP} \text{ [mm Hg]}) \times 79.9}{\text{cardiac output (liters/min)}}$$

$$SV \text{ (ml/beat)} = \frac{\text{cardiac output (ml)}}{\text{heart rate}}$$

$$SI \text{ (ml/min/M}^2) = \frac{\text{stroke volume}}{\text{body surface area}}$$

$$RVSWI \text{ (gmM/M}^2) = \frac{SV \times (\overline{PA} \text{ [mm Hg]} - CVP \text{ [mm Hg]})}{BSA} \times 0.0136$$

$$LVSWI \text{ (gmM/M}^2) = \frac{SV \times (\overline{AP} \text{ [mm Hg]} - \overline{PCWP} \text{ [mm Hg]})}{BSA} \times 0.0136$$

CO_2 (ml O_2/100 ml blood or vol%) = (Hb × 1.39) SaO_2 + (PaO_2 × 0.0031)

$C(a-v)O_2$ (ml/100 ml or vol%) = CaO_2 − $C\overline{v}O_2$

$\dot{V}O_2$ (ml/min/M²) = CI × $C(a-v)O_2$ × 10

$$RQ = \frac{\dot{V}CO_2}{\dot{V}O_2}$$

O_2 avail (ml/min/M²) = CI × CaO_2 × 10

CBV (ml/M²) = MTT × CI × 16.7

$$O_2 \text{ ext ratio} = \frac{C(a-v)O_2}{CaO_2}$$

$$\dot{Q}s/\dot{Q}T(\%) = \frac{CcO_2 - CaO_2}{CcO_2 - CvO_2} \times 100$$

$$\dot{Q}_S/\dot{Q}_T(\%) = \frac{0.0031 \times P(A-a)O_2}{(C[a-v]O_2) + (0.0031 \times P[A-a]O_2)} \times 100$$

Valid only when arterial blood is 100% saturated

$$EDC \ (ml/cm \ H_2O) = \frac{tidal \ volume \ (ml)}{peak \ airway \ pressure \ (cm \ H_2O)}$$

$$V_D/V_T = \frac{PaCO_2 - P\overline{E}CO_2}{PaCO_2}$$

$$P(A-a)O_2 \ (mm \ Hg) = PAO_2 - PaO_2$$

$$Ejection \ fraction = \frac{SV}{EDV}$$

$$MTT = \frac{\int_0^\infty tc(t)dt}{\int_0^\infty c(t)dt}, \ where \ c = dye \ concentration \ and \ t = time$$

3. Nomograms

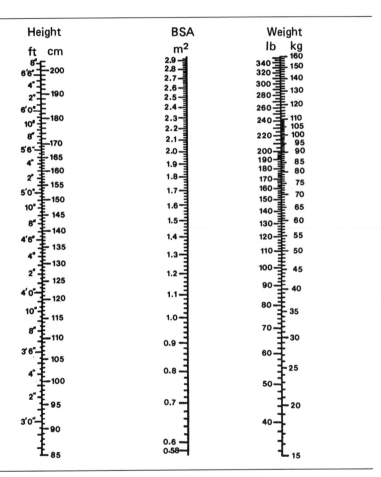

DuBois nomogram for calculating the body surface area of adults. To find body surface of a patient, locate height in inches (or centimeters) on Scale I and weight in pounds (or kilograms) on Scale III and place straight edge (ruler) between these two points. This will intersect Scale II at patient's surface area. (From E. J. DuBois, *Basal Metabolism in Health and Disease.* Philadelphia: Lea & Febiger, 1936. Copyright 1920 by W. M. Boothby and R. B. Sandiford.)

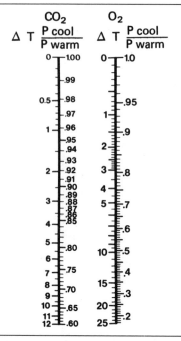

Nomogram for Severinghaus PO_2 and PCO_2 temperature correction factors for blood. These are applicable to either in vitro or in vivo conditions. Factors on right side of the columns are multiplied by the tensions at warmer temperature to correct to cooler temperature. Conversely, factors are divided into tensions at cooler temperature to correct to warmer temperature.

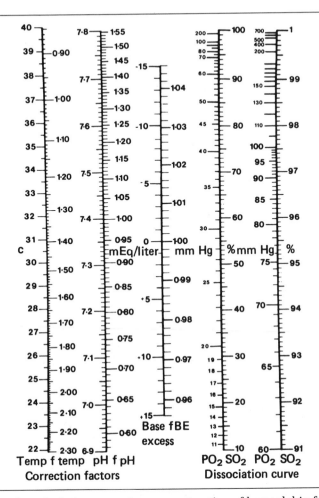

Nomogram for calculating percent oxygen saturation of hemoglobin from measured PO₂. Line charts representing oxyhemoglobin dissociation curve (temperature = 37°C, pH = 7.40, base excess = 0 mEq/liter) are on right. Remaining line charts are factors (left to right: temperature, pH, and base excess) by which measured PO₂ should be multiplied before entering standard dissociation curve. (From G. R. Kelman and J. F. Nunn, Nomograms for correction of blood PO₂, PCO₂, pH, and base excess for time and temperature. *J. Appl. Physiol.* 21:1484, 1966.)

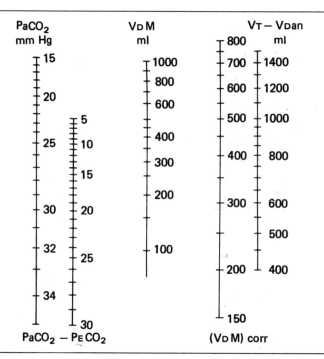

Nomogram for calculating dead-space requirement during prolonged artificial ventilation. Mechanical dead space (VDM) required to raise $PaCO_2$ to approximately 40 mm Hg can be predicted from this nomogram. $PaCO_2$ is the observed arterial carbon dioxide tension before introduction of mechanical dead space; VT is tidal volume, and $V_{D_{an}}$ is anatomic dead space. For patient with normal pulmonary and circulatory status, line in middle gives required value for VDM. In presence of pulmonary disease or circulatory failure, a correction must be made by connecting points on the ($PaCO_2$ − P_ECO_2) line and VDM line, then extending it to right. Read value on (VDM) correction line. $V_{D_{an}}$ is two-thirds of body weight (in pounds), plus dead space of tracheostomy tube and ventilator.

Example: A patient is being ventilated at given respiratory frequency with tidal volume of 1130 ml. $PaCO_2$ is measured and found to be 25 mm Hg. Patient's body weight is 150 lb; dead space of tracheostomy tube and ventilator is 30 ml. $V_{D_{an}}$ = two-thirds of body weight + ventilator and tracheostomy dead space = 130 ml. Since VT = 1130 ml, VT − $V_{D_{an}}$ = 1000 ml. The two points, 1000 for VT − $V_{D_{an}}$ and 25 for $PaCO_2$, are connected, and we read off the center line that VDM should be 430 ml. Assuming reasonably normal lungs, insertion of dead space of 430 ml should raise this patient's $PaCO_2$ to approximately 40 mm Hg. It is emphasized that respiratory frequency and tidal volume must remain unchanged.

If patient's lung function is not normal, P_ECO_2 is determined also and found to be 10 mm Hg; $PaCO_2$ − P_ECO_2 is then 25 mm Hg − 10 mm Hg = 15 mm Hg. Connect this point ($PaCO_2$ − P_ECO_2 = 15 mm Hg) with already obtained VDM of 430 ml; extend connecting line to right and read off corrected VDM (on the line [VDM] corr.). Corrected value is 600 ml. (From K. Suwa et al, A nomogram for dead space requirement during prolonged artificial ventilation. *Anesthesiology* 29:1206, 1968.)

4. Conversion Factors

Temperature

Fahrenheit-Centigrade Conversion Table*

°F	°C
93	33.9
94	34.4
95	35.0
96	35.6
97	36.1
98	36.7
98.6	37.0
99	37.2
100	37.8
101	38.3
102	38.9
103	39.4
104	40.0
105	40.6
106	41.1
107	41.7
108	42.2

*Fahrenheit to Centigrade: $°C = (°F - 32) \times 5/9$.
 Centigrade to Fahrenheit: $°F = °C \times 9/5 + 32$.

Pressure
1 mm Hg = 1.36 cm H_2O
1 cm H_2O = 0.73 mm Hg

Length
1 inch (in.) = 2.54 cm
1 cm = 0.394 in.

Weight
1 pound (lb) = 0.454 kg
1 kilogram (kg) = 2.2 lb
1 grain (g) = 60 mg

Index